AF585153

Australian Nurses' Dictionary
7th edition

Australian Nurses' Dictionary
7th edition

Jennie King
RN, BA (Hons), PhD
Clinical Nurse Consultant (Nursing and Midwifery Research),
Central Coast Local Health District;
Clinical Senior Lecturer, Sydney Nursing School, The University of Sydney;
and Conjoint Senior Lecturer, School of Nursing and Midwifery,
University of Newcastle

Rhonda Hawley
RN, RMN, Cardio-Thoracic Cert, Dip Teach. BA, MEd, PhD
Independent Nurse Consultant;
Formerly Senior Lecturer, School of Nursing, Midwifery and Paramedicine
(NSW and ACT), Australian Catholic University

Adapted from the *Baillière's Dictionary: For Nurses and Health Care Workers*
edited by

Jayne Taylor
RN HV RNT DipN (Lond) Bsc (Hons) MBA PhD
Head of Organisational Development, West Hertfordshire
Hospitals NHS Trust Watford, UK Edinburgh

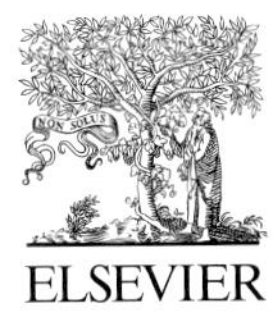

ELSEVIER

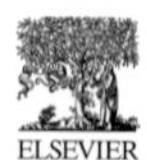

ELSEVIER

Elsevier Australia. ACN 001 002 357
(a division of Reed International Books Australia Pty Ltd)
Tower 1, 475 Victoria Avenue, Chatswood, NSW 2067

ISBN 9780702072796
International ISBN 9780702072789

This adaptation of Baillière's Dictionary: For Nurses and Health Care Workers, 27e, by Jayne Taylor, was undertaken by Elsevier Australia and is published by arrangement with Elsevier Ltd.

Australian Nurses' Dictionary; 7th Edition

ISBN: 978-0-7295-4349-1

National Library of Australia Cataloguing-in-Publication Data

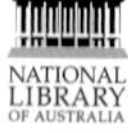

A catalogue record for this book is available from the National Library of Australia

Senior Content Strategist: Melinda McEvoy
Content Project Manager: Kritika Kaushik
Edited by Margaret Trudgeon
Proofread by Tim Learner
Cover Design by Lisa Petroff
Internal design: Avril Makula
Typeset by GW Tech India
Printed in China by RR Donnelly

Last digit is the print number: 9 8 7 6 5

Contents

Preface

This 7th edition of the *Australian Nurses' Dictionary* brings a thoroughly revised and updated text that takes account of recent developments in nursing and midwifery practice. The dictionary, first adapted from the *Baillière's Nurses' Dictionary* in 1991, continues to provide comprehensive coverage of the ever-expanding vocabulary of the nursing and midwifery professions to reflect advances in practice, education, technology, research and innovation. This edition has been expanded to include new, relevant terminologies, several appendices relevant to clinical practice and an extended, abridged version of the atlas of human anatomy. Students, in particular, need extra assistance when learning the numerous structures that make up the body systems. We trust you will agree that the addition of the atlas makes it an ideal visual display and easy reference for learning body systems. The hope is that the dictionary remains relevant to nursing and midwifery needs in a rapidly changing healthcare environment. We continue to present this dictionary in its easy and ready-to-use format to enable you to access up-to-date information wherever and whenever it is required.

The guiding principles in the revision have been to establish direct relevance to Australian conditions, and to provide a quick reference source for students and nurses in the clinical setting. For a more extensive background to specific entries, the reader is referred to encyclopaedic nursing dictionaries, and to pharmacology, anatomy and physiology texts. In a dictionary of this size, it is impossible to include every generic and brand name of drugs in common use; therefore, only the class of drug (e.g. antibiotic, diuretic and steroid) has been included.

This edition has relied on the support of nurses and allied health personnel in many areas. Thank you to the reviewers of the 6th edition, who provided valuable feedback, comments and recommendations for this 7th edition; and to Tony Smith and John Hawley for their continued encouragement and support in meeting deadlines.

Jennie King, Rhonda Hawley

Acknowledgment

The publisher would like to thank the American College of Surgeons for their kind permission to reproduce the figure in the Lund and Browder chart.

The authors would like to thank Sanofi-Aventis Group for permission to reproduce medication labels, a blister pack and tablet for inclusion in Appendix 5. Thank you also to the Australian Commission on Safety and Quality in Health Care for granting permission to use sections of the National Inpatient Medication Chart (NIMC) – Acute (2018) (Appendix 5); and Department of Health for permission to include the National Immunisation Program (NIP) Schedule (Appendix 7); and the World Health Organisation for permission to include the 5 Moments of Hand Hygiene (Appendix 10); and the Australian and New Zealand Committee on Resuscitation (ANZCOR) for permission to include the Basic Life Support Flowchart (Appendix 6).

References

Baillière's Dictionary for Nurses and Health Care Workers. 27th ed. Edinburgh: Churchill Livingstone; 2019.

Dorland's Illustrated Medical Dictionary. 32nd ed. Philadelphia: Saunders; 2019.

Forrester K, Griffiths D. *Essentials of Law for Health Professionals.* 4th ed. Sydney: Mosby; 2014.

Gatford JD, Phillips N. *Nursing Calculations.* 9th ed. Edinburgh: Churchill Livingstone; 2015.

Harris P, Nagy S, Vardaxis N. *Mosby's Dictionary of Medicine, Nursing and Health Professions.* 3rd Australian and New Zealand edition (rev.). Sydney: Elsevier; 2018.

Schneider Z, Whitehead D, LoBiondo-Wood G et al. *Nursing and Midwifery Research: Methods and Appraisal for Evidence-based Practice.* 5th ed. Sydney: Mosby; 2016.

Pronunciation guide

All pronunciations in this dictionary are transcribed using ordinary English-spelling letters, with the exception of the upside-down 'e' or 'schwa' (ə). All pronunciations are given in parentheses immediately following the bold headword and reflect general Australian English in *current, spoken usage*. Where alternative pronunciations for a word are given, or where alternative spellings or synonyms are given, these are separated by commas. For example:

medicine ('medəsən, ˌmedsən)

neurone (neuron) (ˌnyoo·rohn, ˌnyoo·ron)

Alternative pronunciations are often given in truncated form with hyphens. For example:

encephalic ('enkəˌfalik, 'ensə-)

Single letters represent single sounds. Where two or more characters are combined, as in the lists below, these also represent precise sounds.

Vowel sounds			
a	as in **bad** (bad)	o	as in **body** (ˌbodee)
ah	as in **father** ('fahthə)	oh	as in **choke** (chohk)
air	as in **hair** (hair)	oo	as in **boot** (boot)
aw	as in **water** ('wawtə)	oo	as in **cure** (kyooə)
ay	as in **fatal** ('fayt'l)	ow	as in **now** (now)
e	as in **bed** (bed)	ow	as in **hour** (owə)
ee	as in **fetus** ('feetəs)	oy	as in **goitre** ('goytə)
i	as in **film** (film)	oyə	as in **soya** ('soyə)
ie	as in **bite** (biet)	u	as in **tongue** (tung)
i·ə	as in **chloropsia** (klaw'ropsi·ə)	uh	as in **foot** (fuht)
		ə	as in **mother** ('muthə)
iə	as in **fear** (fiə)	ər	as in **bird** (bərd)
ieə	as in **diet** ('dieət)	y	as in **yet** (yet)

Consonant sounds			
b	as in **baby** ('baybee)	nh	as in **en passant** (onh 'pasonh)
ch	as in **chat** (chat)		
d	as in **digit** ('dijət)	ny	as in **nutrition** (nyoo'trishən)
f	as in **fever** ('feevə)	p	as in **pelvis** ('pelvəs)
g	as in **gag** (gag)	r	as in **rod** (rod)
h	as in **heal** (heel)	s	as in **sac** (sak)
j	as in **jump** (jump)	sh	as in **fish** (fish)
k	as in **king** (king)	t	as in **test** (test)
l	as in **light** (liet)	th	as in **thirst** (thərst)
m	as in **man** (man)	v	as in **vein** (vayn)
n	as in **need** (need)	w	as in **weight** (wayt)
ng	as in **sung** (sung)	z	as in **zero** ('ziə·roh)
		zh	as in **pleasure** ('plezhə)

Stress marks

Stress marks are used where the word or term has more than one syllable. The stress mark is placed before the syllable to be stressed. The primary stressed syllable is indicated by a superior stress mark (ˈ) and secondary stress by a subscript stress mark (ˌ). For example:

respiration (ˌrespəˈrayshən)

respirator (ˈrespəˌraytə)

respiratory (rəsˈpirətree)

Apostrophe

Where a consonant is preceded by an apostrophe, this indicates that the consonant should be pronounced as a separate syllable. For example:

hospital (ˈhospət'l)

Centred full stop

Where two letters occur together that may be mistaken for a different sound from that intended, a centred full stop is added to separate the characters. For example:

myopia (miəˈohpi·ə)

Sub-entries

Sub-entries are listed alphabetically under the main entry, with the initial letter(s) of the main entry repeated. For example:

abdomen

Acute a.
Pendulous a.
Scaphoid (navicular) a.

Atlas of human anatomy

SKELETAL SYSTEM

ANTERIOR VIEW OF SKELETON

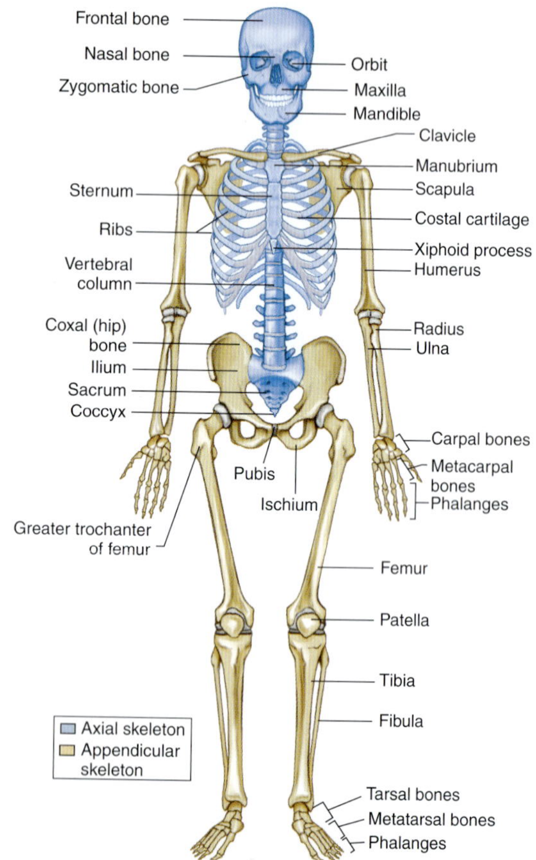

POSTERIOR VIEW OF SKELETON

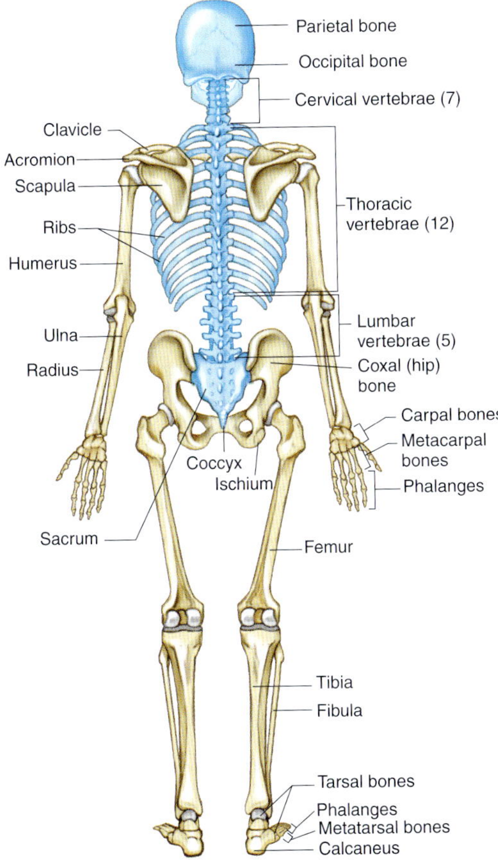

CLASSIFICATION OF BONES BY SHAPE

ANTERIOR VIEW

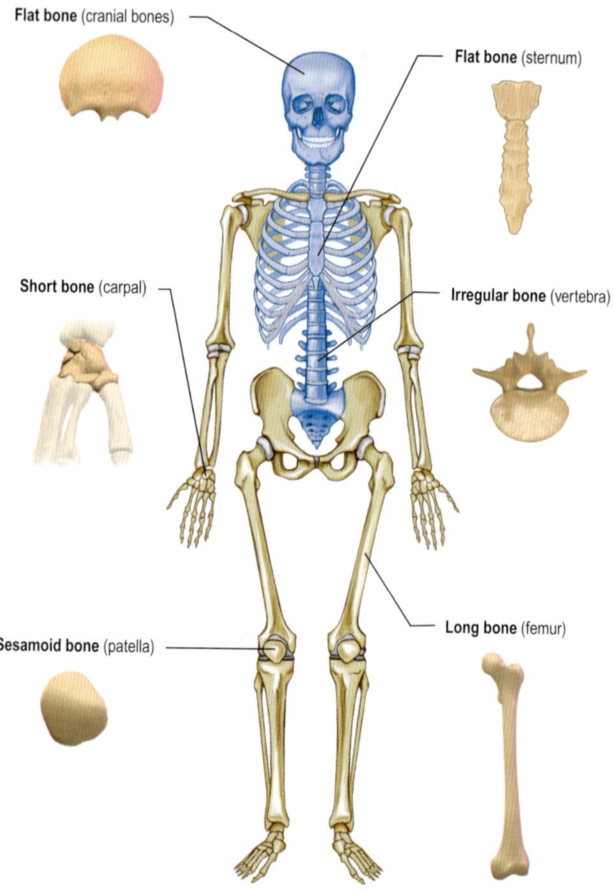

MUSCULAR SYSTEM

ANTERIOR VIEW

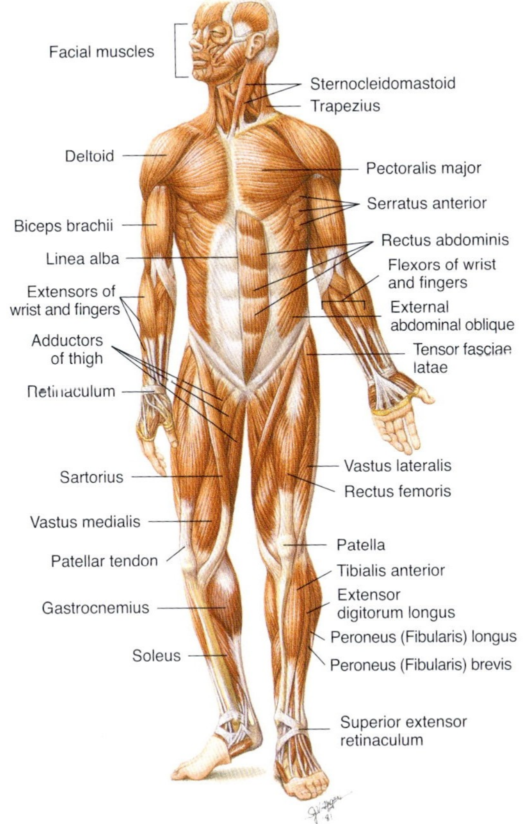

POSTERIOR VIEW

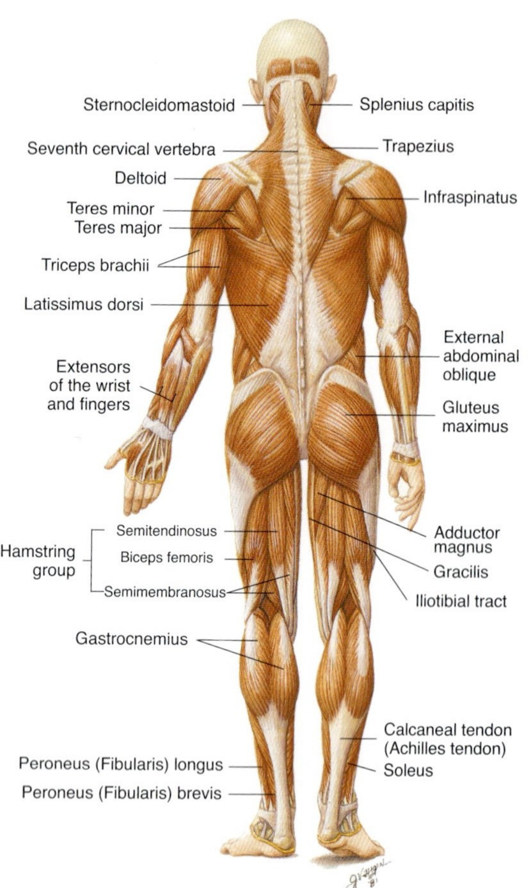

STRUCTURE OF LONG BONE

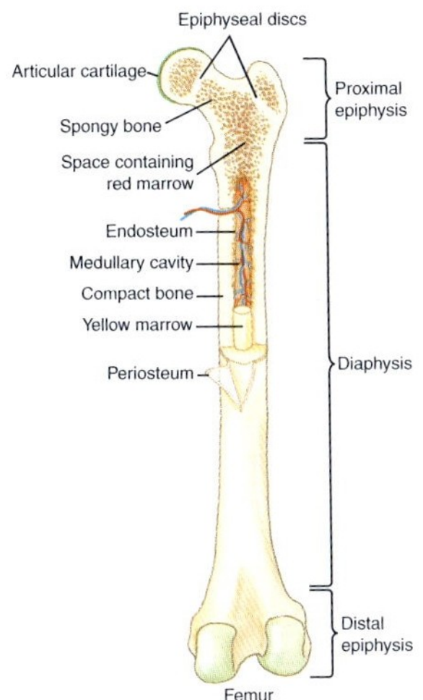

Femur

MICROSCOPIC STRUCTURE OF BONE

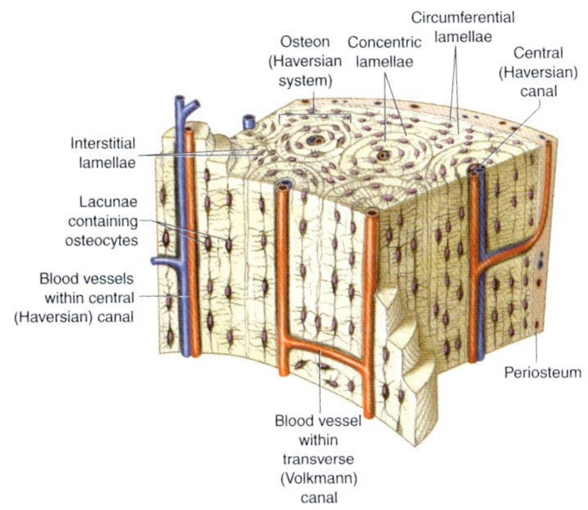

TYPES AND STRUCTURE OF MUSCLE

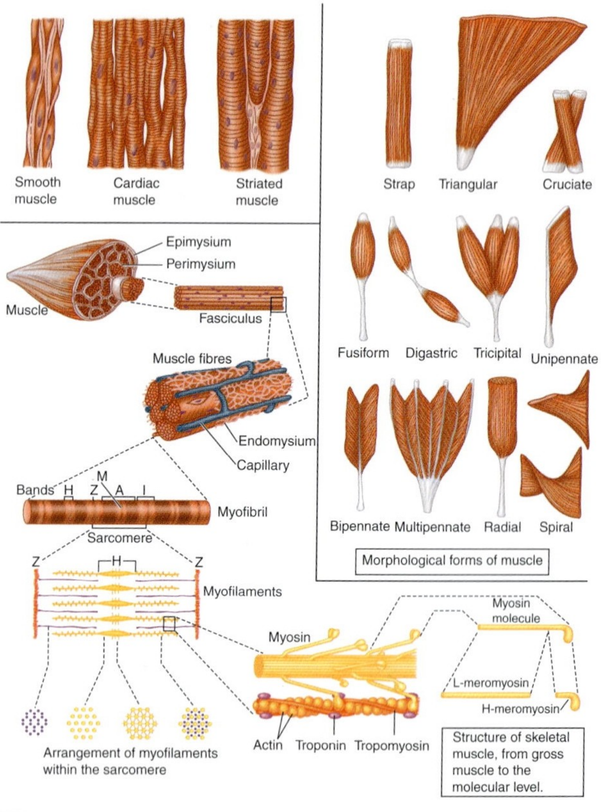

Morphological forms of muscle

Structure of skeletal muscle, from gross muscle to the molecular level.

CIRCULATORY SYSTEM

PRINCIPAL ARTERIES

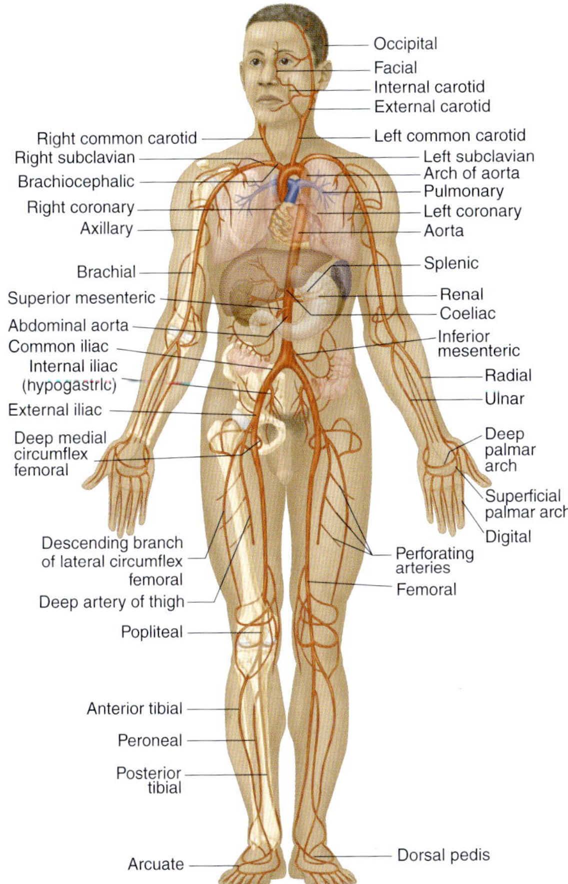

PRINCIPAL VEINS

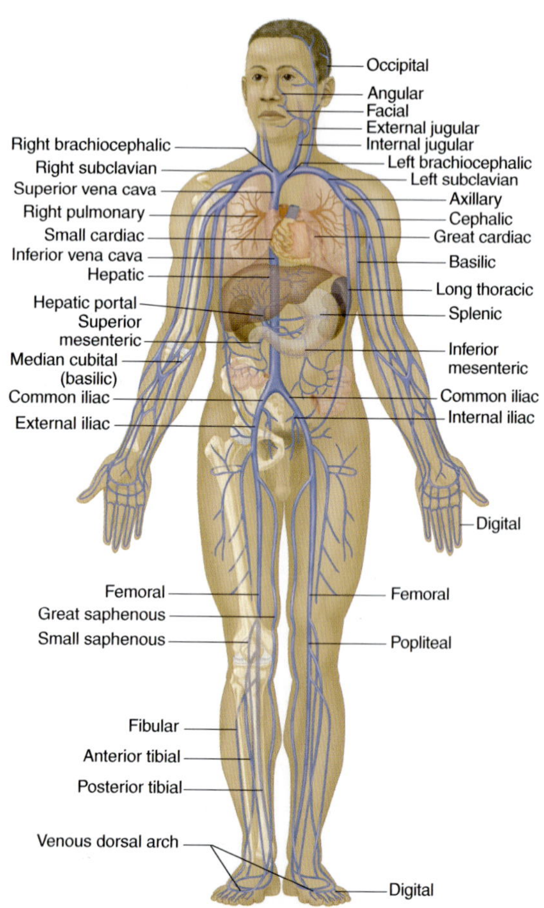

ANTERIOR VIEW OF THE HEART

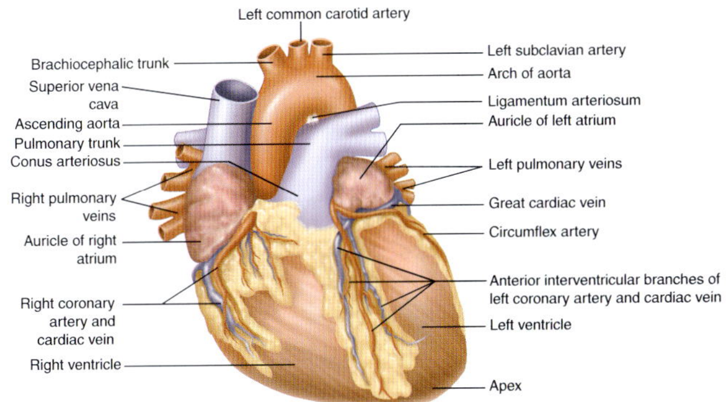

POSTERIOR VIEW OF THE HEART

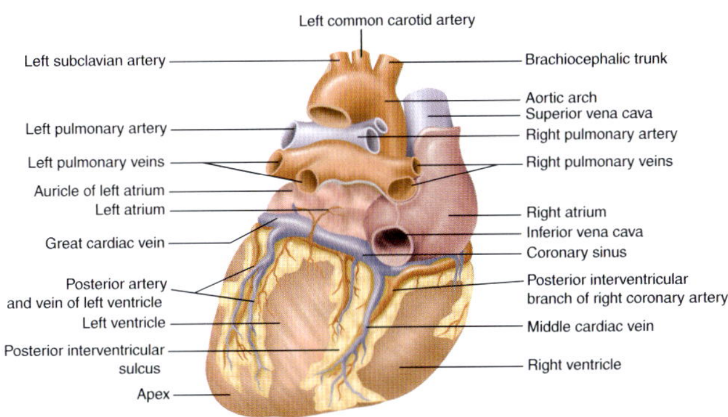

STRUCTURES OF THE HEART

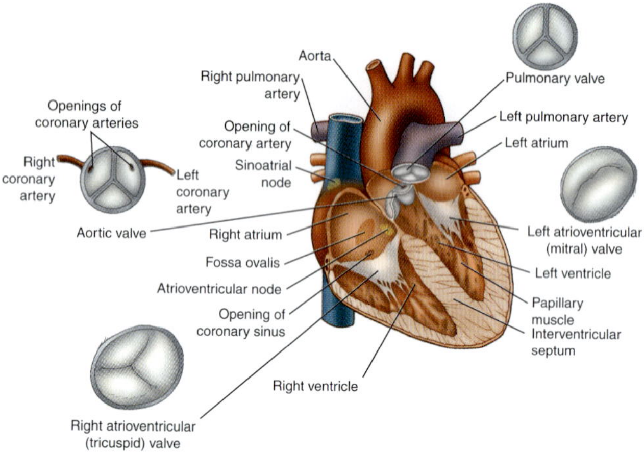

Openings of coronary arteries
Right coronary artery
Left coronary artery
Aortic valve
Aorta
Right pulmonary artery
Opening of coronary artery
Sinoatrial node
Right atrium
Fossa ovalis
Atrioventricular node
Opening of coronary sinus
Right ventricle
Right atrioventricular (tricuspid) valve
Pulmonary valve
Left pulmonary artery
Left atrium
Left atrioventricular (mitral) valve
Left ventricle
Papillary muscle
Interventricular septum

CONDUCTING SYSTEM OF THE HEART

Flow of cardiac impulse
Spread of conduction impulses from SA node to left atrium
SA node
Internodal pathways
LA
RA
LV
RV
Left bundle branch
Posteroinferior fascicle of left bundle branch
AV node
Bundle of His
Right bundle branch
Anterosuperior fascicle of left bundle branch
Purkinje fibres
Septum

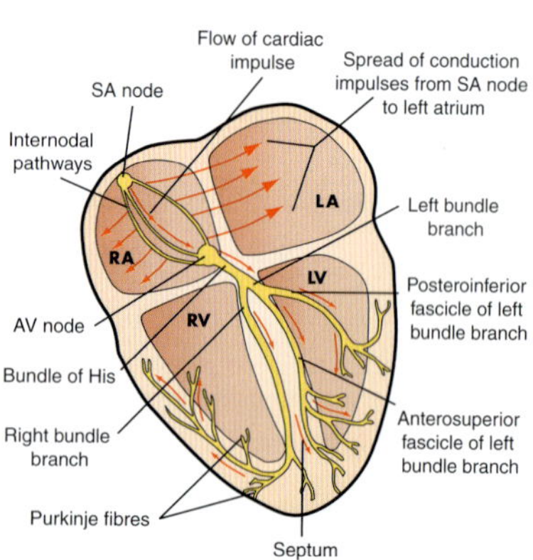

ENDOCRINE SYSTEM

GLANDS OF THE ENDOCRINE SYSTEM

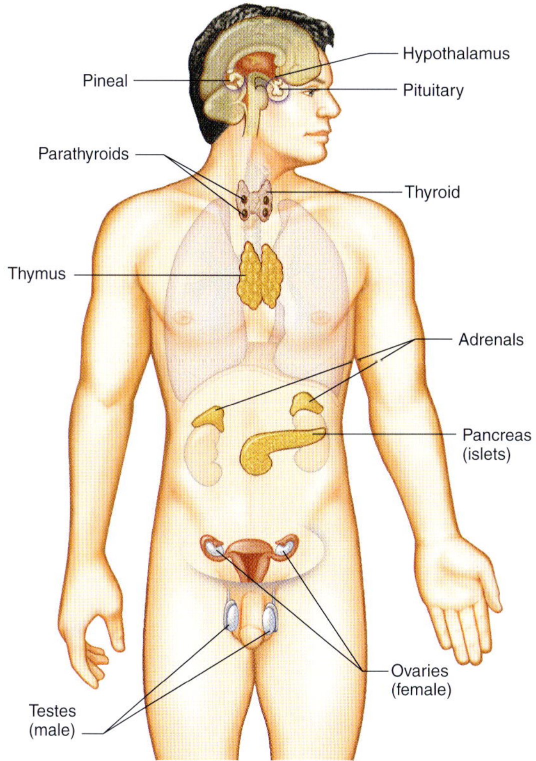

LYMPHATIC SYSTEM

GLANDS OF THE LYMPHATIC SYSTEM

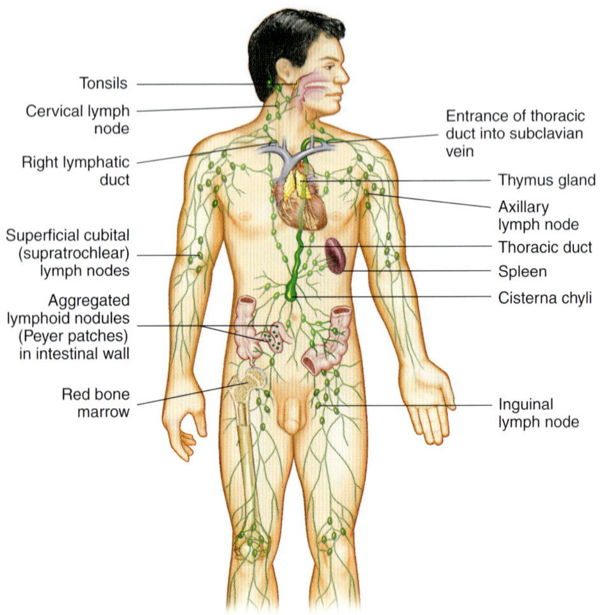

NERVOUS SYSTEM

SIMPLIFIED VIEW OF THE NERVOUS SYSTEM

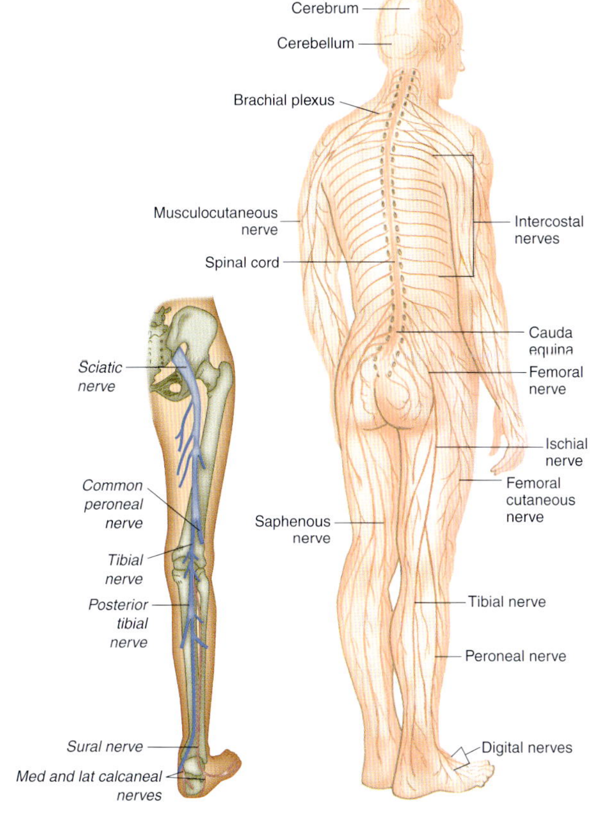

GROSS ANATOMY OF THE SPINAL CORD

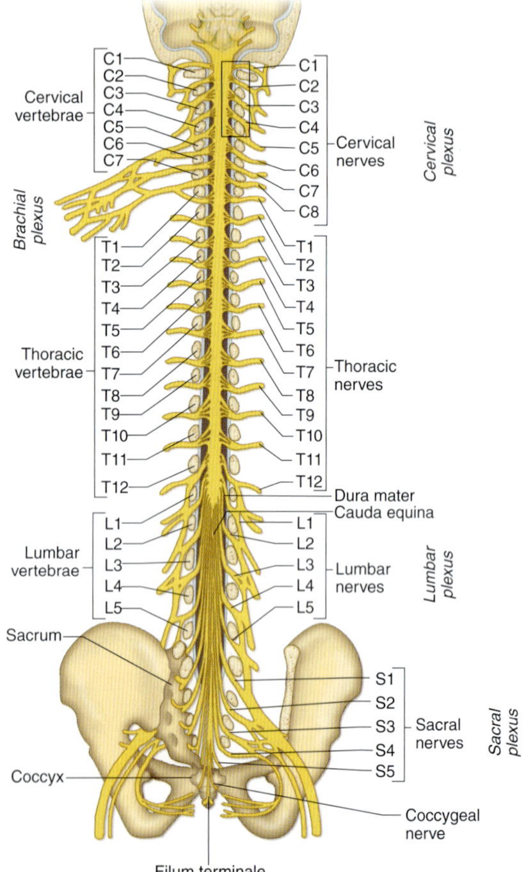

FUNCTIONAL AREAS OF THE CEREBRAL CORTEX

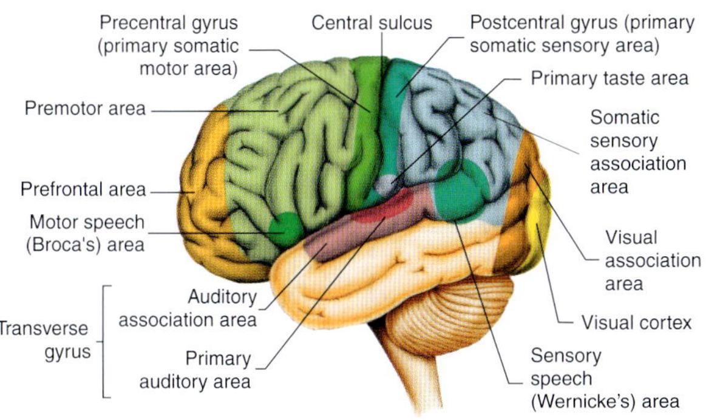

RETICULAR ACTIVATING SYSTEM

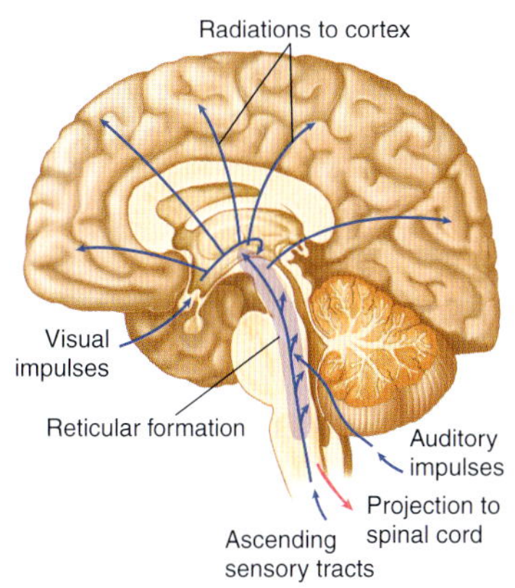

BASE OF THE BRAIN

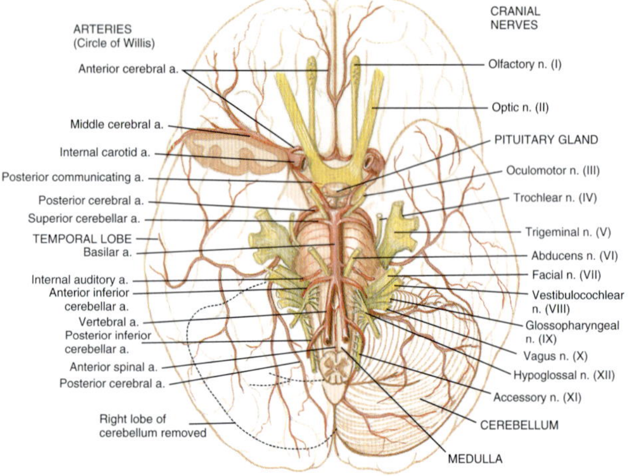

ARTERIES
(Circle of Willis)
Anterior cerebral a.
Middle cerebral a.
Internal carotid a.
Posterior communicating a.
Posterior cerebral a.
Superior cerebellar a.
TEMPORAL LOBE
Basilar a.
Internal auditory a.
Anterior inferior cerebellar a.
Vertebral a.
Posterior inferior cerebellar a.
Anterior spinal a.
Posterior cerebral a.
Right lobe of cerebellum removed
CRANIAL NERVES
Olfactory n. (I)
Optic n. (II)
PITUITARY GLAND
Oculomotor n. (III)
Trochlear n. (IV)
Trigeminal n. (V)
Abducens n. (VI)
Facial n. (VII)
Vestibulocochlear n. (VIII)
Glossopharyngeal n. (IX)
Vagus n. (X)
Hypoglossal n. (XII)
Accessory n. (XI)
CEREBELLUM
MEDULLA

BRAINSTEM AND DIENCEPHALON

Intermediate mass
Thalamus
Optic chiasma
Hypothalamus
Diencephalon
Cerebral peduncle
Midbrain
Pons
Medulla oblongata
Olive
Pyramid
Diencephalon
Brain-stem
Thalamus
Pineal body
Diencephalon
Superior colliculi
Inferior colliculi
Midbrain
Cerebral peduncle
Pons
Middle cerebellar peduncle of pons
Superior cerebellar peduncles
Fourth ventricle
Inferior cerebellar peduncles of pons
Olive
Medulla oblongata

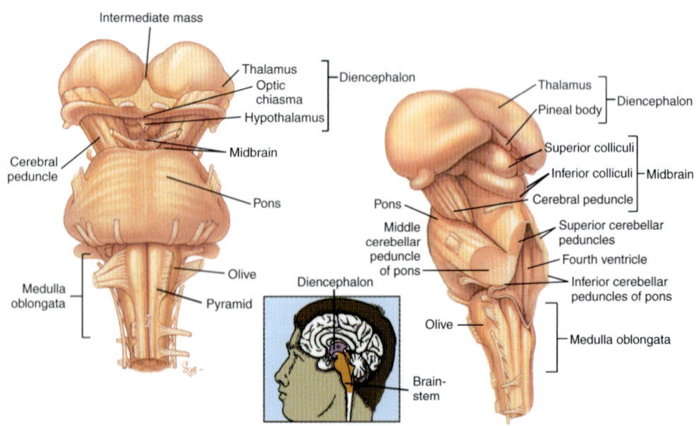

BASIC STRUCTURE OF THE NEURONE

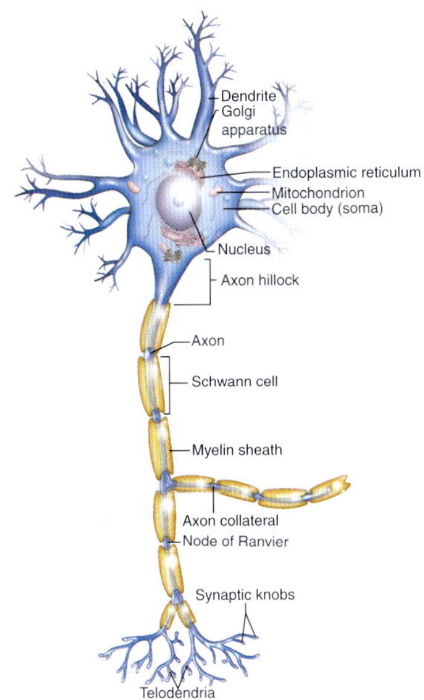

MYELINATED AXON

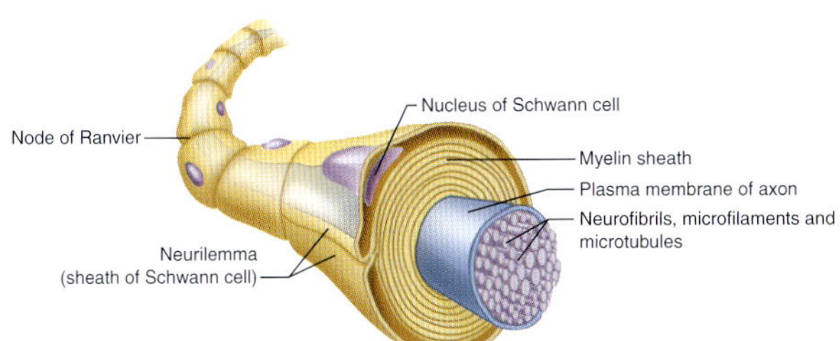

RESPIRATORY SYSTEM

ORGANS OF THE RESPIRATORY SYSTEM

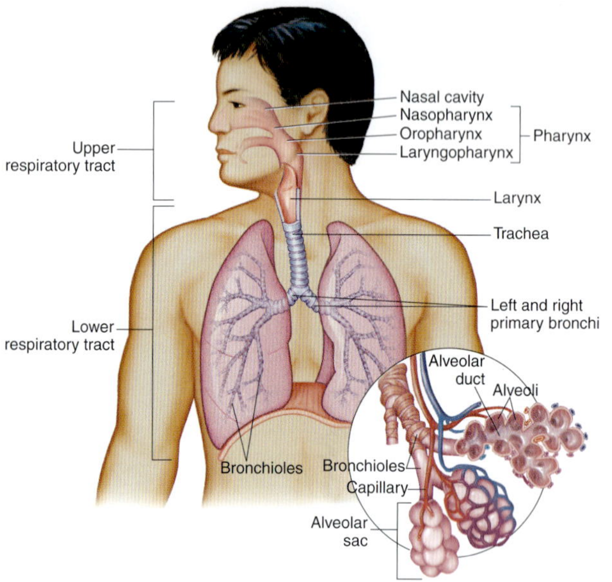

LUNGS

Trachea
First rib
Sternum
(manubrium)
Right
superior lobe
Left
superior lobe
Right primary
bronchus
Left primary
bronchus
Horizontal
fissure
Body
of sternum
Right
middle lobe
Oblique
fissure
Oblique
fissure
Seventh rib
Right
inferior lobe
Left
inferior lobe
Sternum
(xiphoid process)

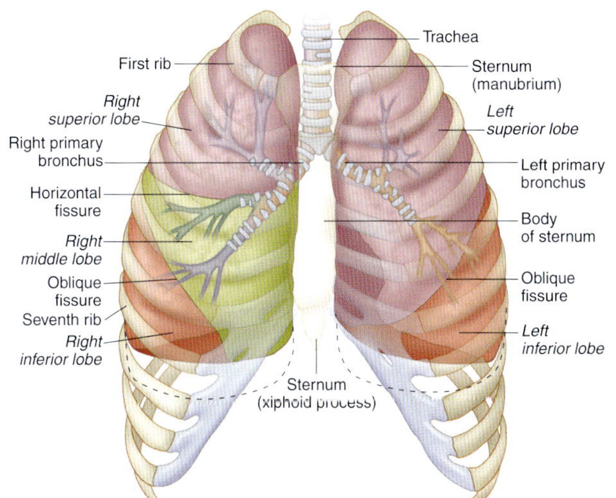

RIGHT LUNG

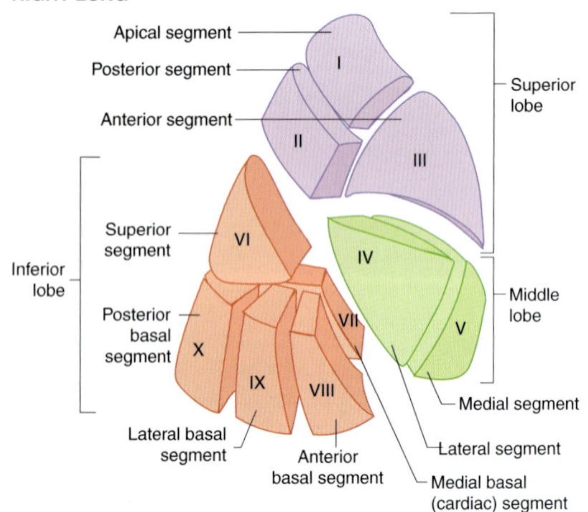

LEFT LUNG

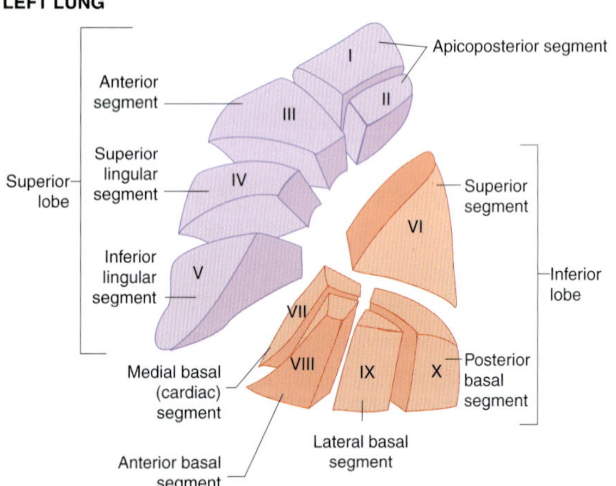

DIGESTIVE SYSTEM

ORGANS OF THE DIGESTIVE SYSTEM AND SOME ASSOCIATED STRUCTURES

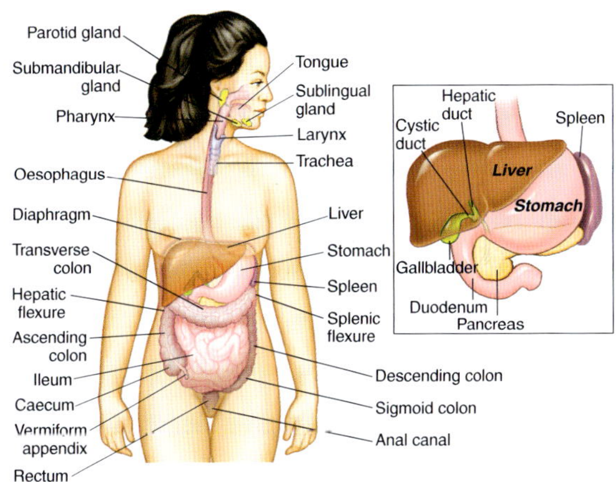

WALL OF THE GASTROINTESTINAL TRACT

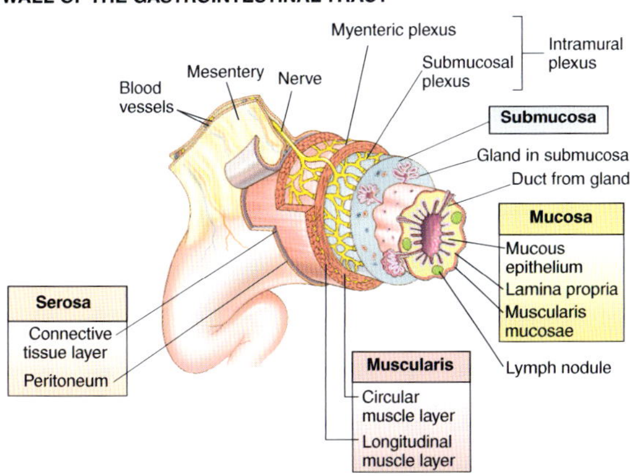

LOCATION OF THE SALIVARY GLANDS

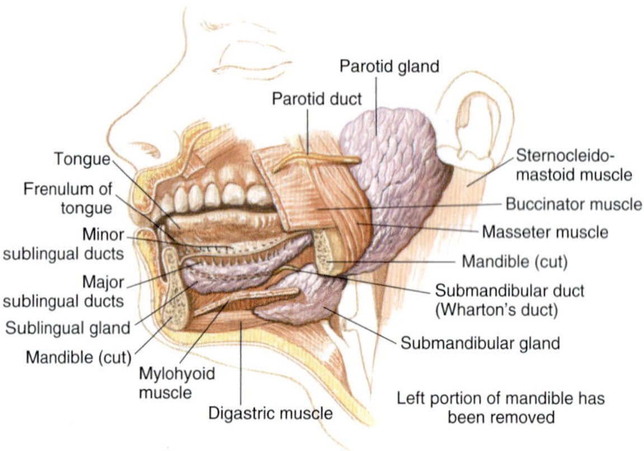

Parotid gland
Parotid duct
Tongue
Frenulum of tongue
Minor sublingual ducts
Major sublingual ducts
Sublingual gland
Mandible (cut)
Mylohyoid muscle
Digastric muscle
Sternocleido-mastoid muscle
Buccinator muscle
Masseter muscle
Mandible (cut)
Submandibular duct (Wharton's duct)
Submandibular gland
Left portion of mandible has been removed

SOURCES OF INTESTINAL SECRETIONS

Bile from the bladder, pancreatic juice from the exocrine pancreas, and mucus secretion from Brunner's glands in the duodenal wall.

Stomach
Cystic duct
Common hepatic duct
Gallbladder neck
Gallbladder
Common bile duct
Villi
Brunner's glands
Ampulla
Duodenum
Pancreatic duct
Pancreas (head)
Pancreas (tail)
Spleen

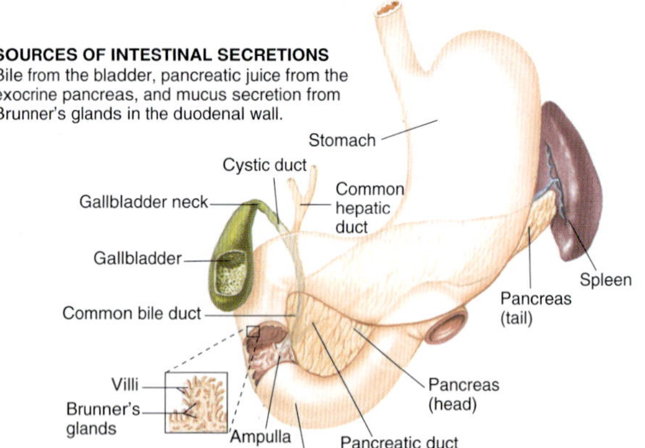

LARGE INTESTINE

Enlarged detail of the large intestine, rectum and anus shows the junction between the large and small intestines and the valve-like entry of the ileum into the caecum.

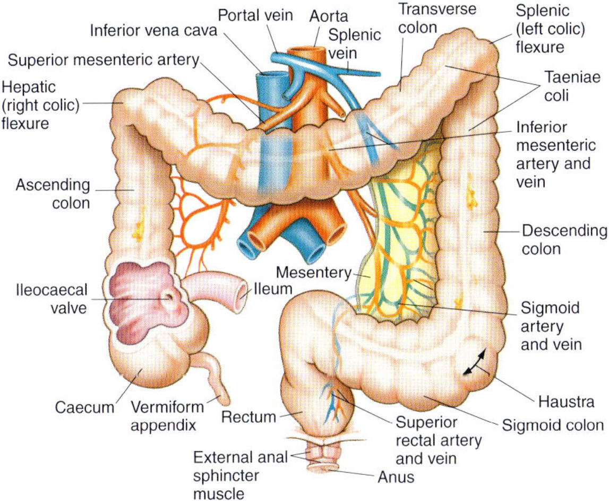

Portal vein
Aorta
Transverse colon
Splenic (left colic) flexure
Inferior vena cava
Splenic vein
Superior mesenteric artery
Taeniae coli
Hepatic (right colic) flexure
Inferior mesenteric artery and vein
Ascending colon
Descending colon
Mesentery
Ileocaecal valve
Ileum
Sigmoid artery and vein
Haustra
Caecum
Vermiform appendix
Rectum
Superior rectal artery and vein
Sigmoid colon
External anal sphincter muscle
Anus

CAECUM AND TERMINAL ILEUM

Ascending colon
Ileum
Ileocaecal fold flaps
Caecum
Appendix

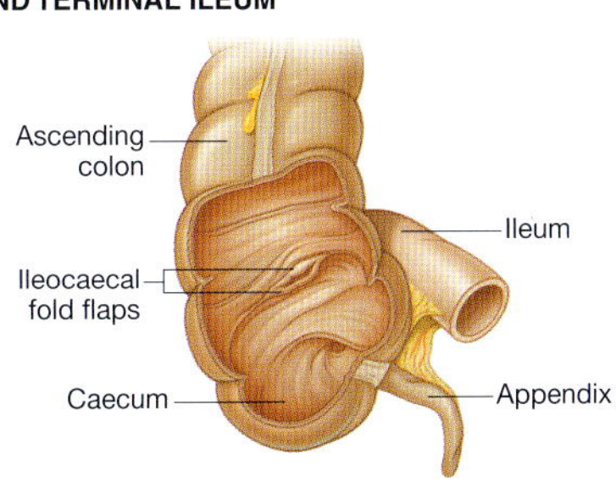

REPRODUCTIVE SYSTEM

LATERAL VIEW OF FEMALE REPRODUCTIVE ORGANS AND ASSOCIATED STRUCTURES

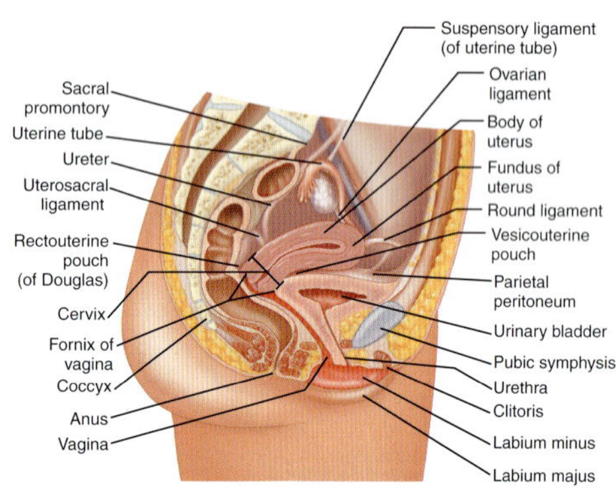

ANTERIOR VIEW OF PELVIC FEMALE ORGANS

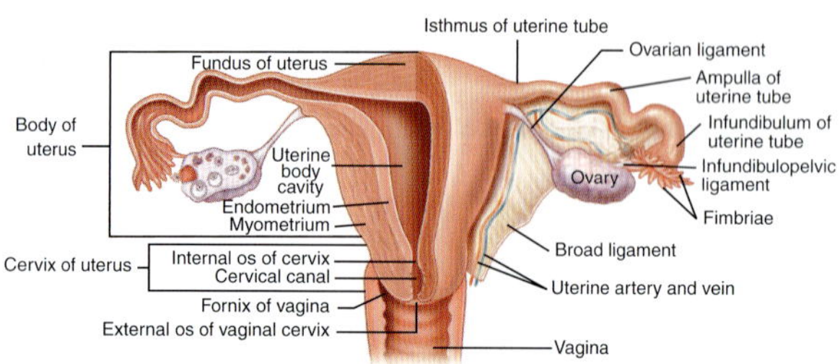

FEMALE BREAST

Clavicle
Intercostal muscle
Fascia of pectoral muscles
Pectoralis major muscle
Alveolus
Ductule
Duct
Lactiferous duct
Lactiferous sinus
Nipple pores
Adipose tissue
Suspensory ligaments
(of Cooper)

Pectoralis
major
muscle
Alveoli
Areola
Nipple

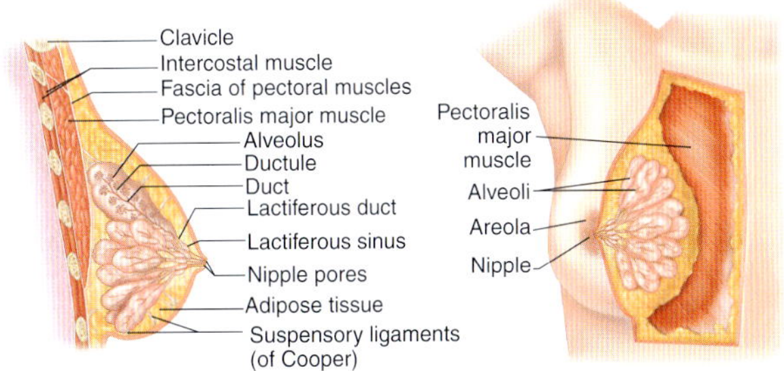

LYMPHATIC SYSTEM AND THE FEMALE BREAST

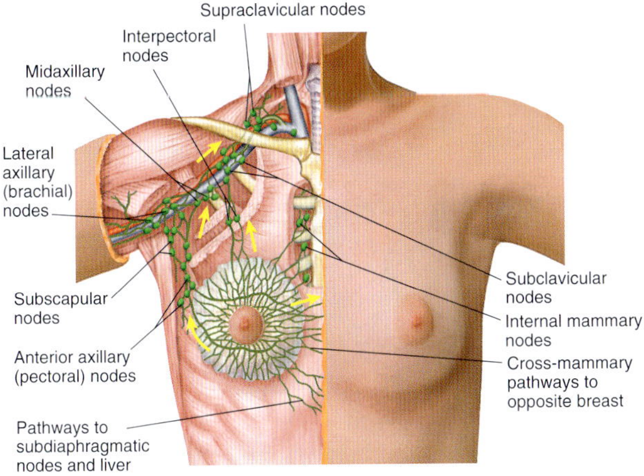

Supraclavicular nodes
Interpectoral
nodes
Midaxillary
nodes
Lateral
axillary
(brachial)
nodes
Subscapular
nodes
Anterior axillary
(pectoral) nodes
Pathways to
subdiaphragmatic
nodes and liver
Subclavicular
nodes
Internal mammary
nodes
Cross-mammary
pathways to
opposite breast

MALE REPRODUCTIVE ORGANS AND ASSOCIATED STRUCTURES

Seminal vesicle
Ejaculatory duct
Prostate gland
Rectum
Bulbourethral (Cowper's) gland
Anus
Ureter
Urinary bladder
Pubic symphysis
Vas (ductus) deferens
Urethra
Penis
Foreskin (prepuce)
Epididymis
Testis
Scrotum

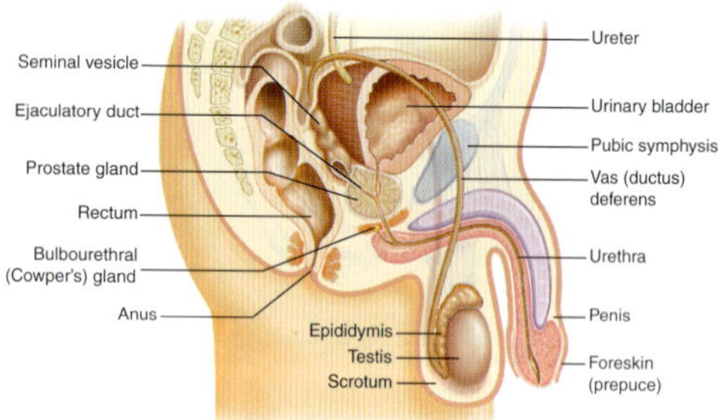

ANTERIOR VIEW OF MALE REPRODUCTIVE STRUCTURES

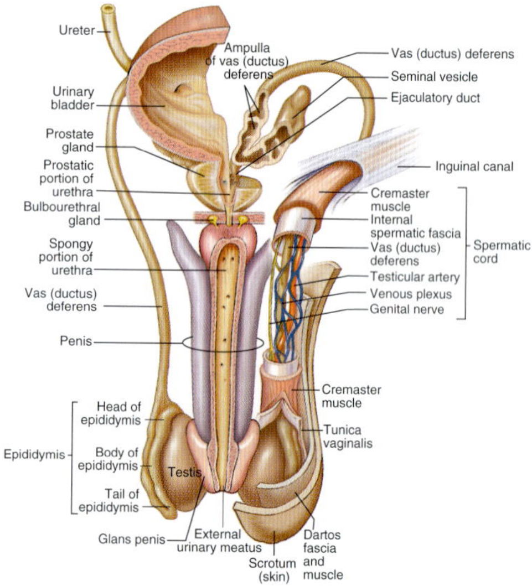

Ureter
Urinary bladder
Prostate gland
Prostatic portion of urethra
Bulbourethral gland
Spongy portion of urethra
Vas (ductus) deferens
Penis
Epididymis
Head of epididymis
Body of epididymis
Tail of epididymis
Testis
Glans penis
External urinary meatus
Scrotum (skin)
Dartos fascia and muscle
Ampulla of vas (ductus) deferens
Vas (ductus) deferens
Seminal vesicle
Ejaculatory duct
Inguinal canal
Cremaster muscle
Internal spermatic fascia
Vas (ductus) deferens
Testicular artery
Venous plexus
Genital nerve
Spermatic cord
Cremaster muscle
Tunica vaginalis

TUBULES OF THE TESTIS AND EPIDIDYMIS

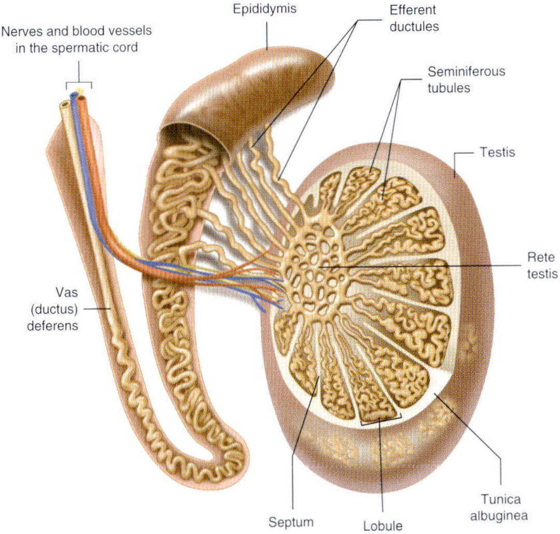

Epididymis
Efferent ductules
Nerves and blood vessels in the spermatic cord
Seminiferous tubules
Testis
Rete testis
Vas (ductus) deferens
Tunica albuginea
Septum
Lobule

SPERMATOZOON

Acrosome
Head
Nucleus
Midpiece
Centrioles
Mitochondria
Tail
Tail

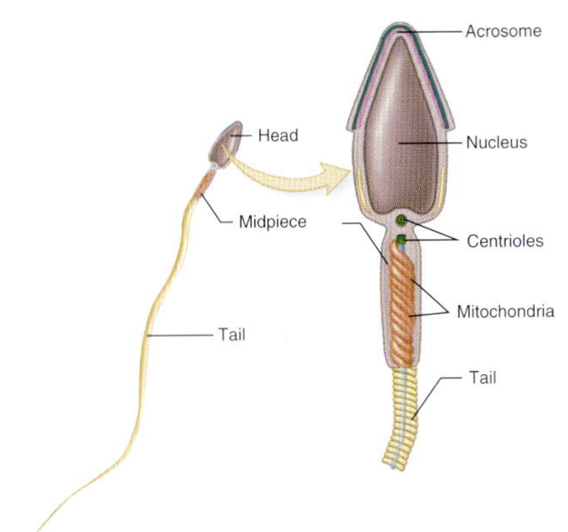

URINARY SYSTEM

URINARY SYSTEM AND SOME ASSOCIATED STRUCTURES

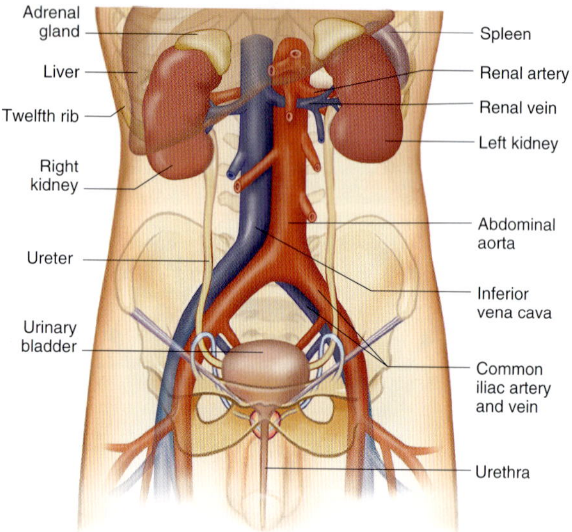

Adrenal gland
Liver
Twelfth rib
Right kidney
Ureter
Urinary bladder
Spleen
Renal artery
Renal vein
Left kidney
Abdominal aorta
Inferior vena cava
Common iliac artery and vein
Urethra

Inferior vena cava
Peritoneum
Renal vein
Abdominal aorta
Peritoneal cavity
Muscle
Renal fat pad
Renal artery
Left kidney
Spinous process of vertebra

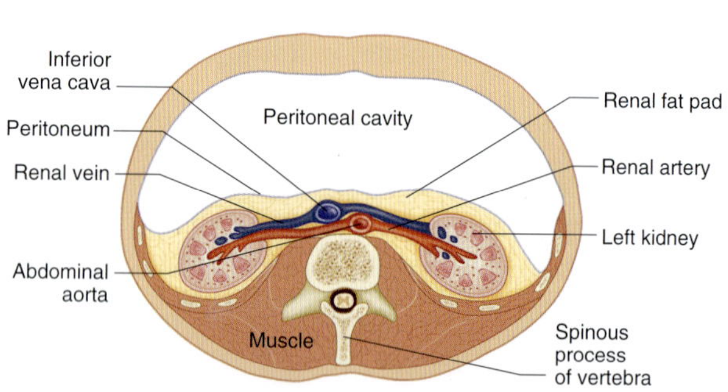

BLADDER

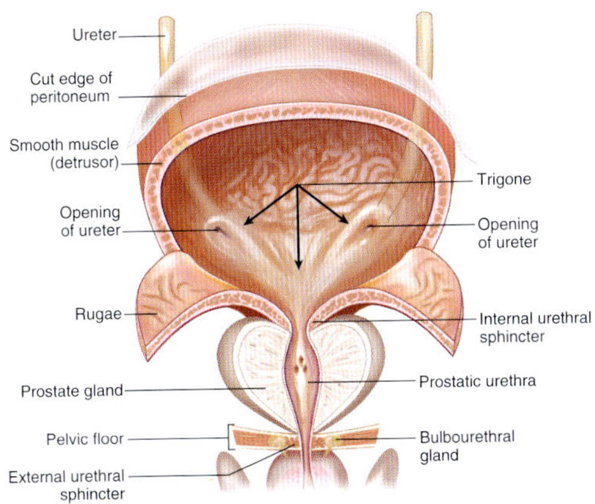

INTERNAL STRUCTURE OF THE KIDNEY

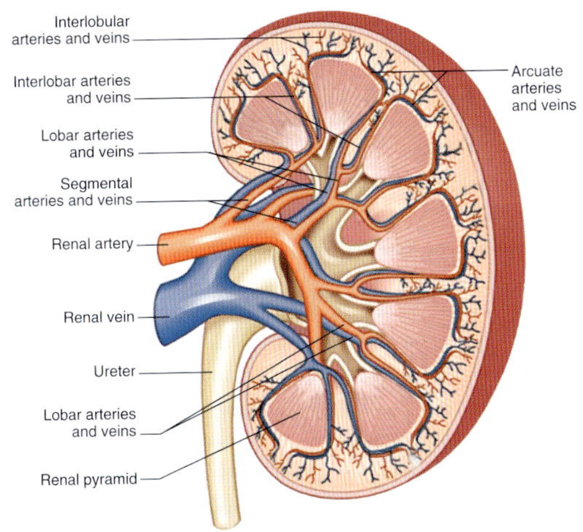

NEPHRON

Bowman's capsule
Glomerulus
Renal corpuscle
Distal convoluted tubule (DCT)
Proximal convoluted tubule (PCT)
Cortex
Medulla
Descending limb of Henle (DLH)
Renal tubule
Collecting duct (CD)
Thick ascending limb of Henle (TAL)
Henle (nephron) loop
Thin ascending limb of Henle (TALH)
Papilla of renal pyramid

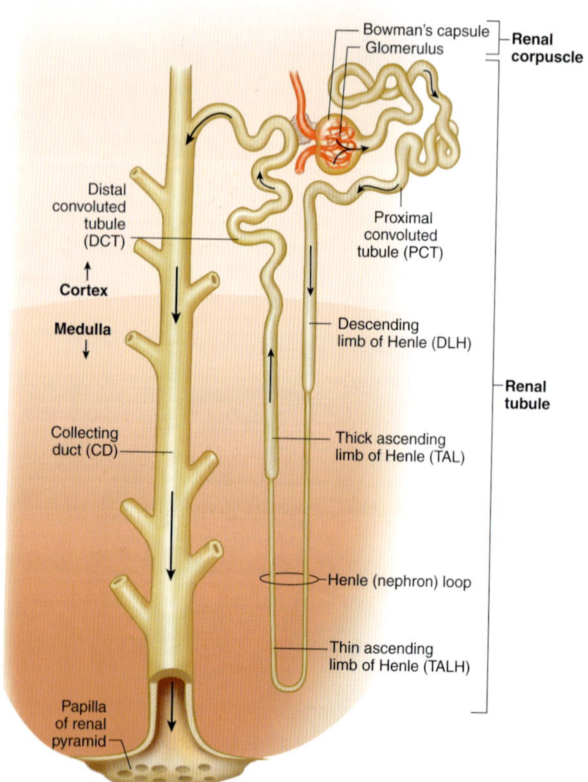

SPECIAL SENSES

GROSS ANATOMY OF THE EAR

External ear (not to scale)
Middle ear
Inner ear
Auricle (pinna)
External acoustic meatus
Temporal bone
Tympanic membrane
Semicircular canals
Oval window
Facial nerve
Vestibular nerve
Cochlear nerve
Vestibulocochlear nerve (CN VIII)
Cochlea
Vestibule
Round window
Auditory (eustachian) tube
Malleus
Incus
Stapes
Auditory ossicles

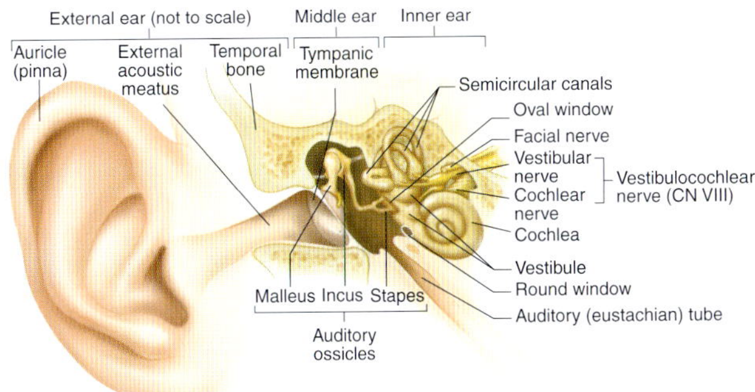

STRUCTURE OF THE SKIN

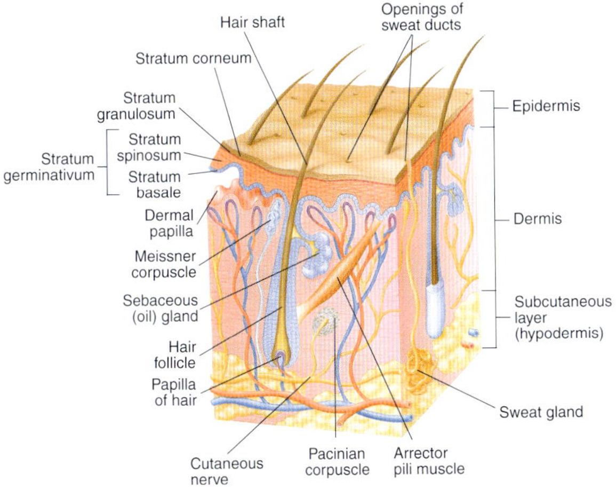

Hair shaft
Openings of sweat ducts
Stratum corneum
Stratum granulosum
Stratum germinativum
Stratum spinosum
Stratum basale
Dermal papilla
Meissner corpuscle
Sebaceous (oil) gland
Hair follicle
Papilla of hair
Cutaneous nerve
Pacinian corpuscle
Arrector pili muscle
Sweat gland
Epidermis
Dermis
Subcutaneous layer (hypodermis)

CROSS-SECTIONAL VIEW OF THE EYE

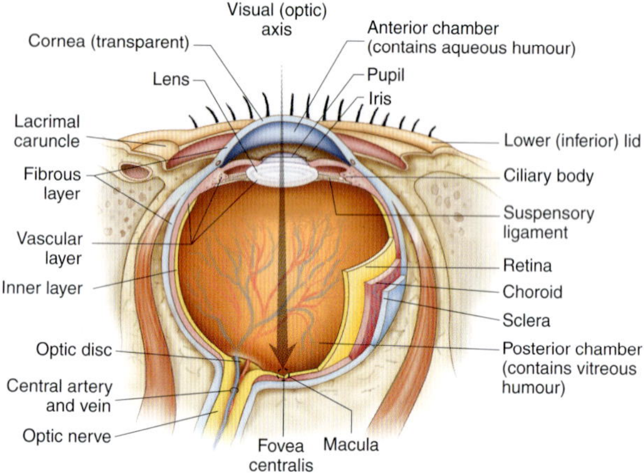

Visual (optic) axis
Cornea (transparent)
Anterior chamber (contains aqueous humour)
Lens
Pupil
Iris
Lacrimal caruncle
Lower (inferior) lid
Fibrous layer
Ciliary body
Suspensory ligament
Vascular layer
Retina
Inner layer
Choroid
Sclera
Optic disc
Posterior chamber (contains vitreous humour)
Central artery and vein
Optic nerve
Fovea centralis
Macula

Sclera
Choroid
Retina
Scleral venous sinus (canal of Schlemm)
Ciliary muscle
Iris
Ciliary ring
Ciliary body
Posterior chamber
Ciliary processes
Anterior chamber
Suspensory ligaments
Cornea
Lens

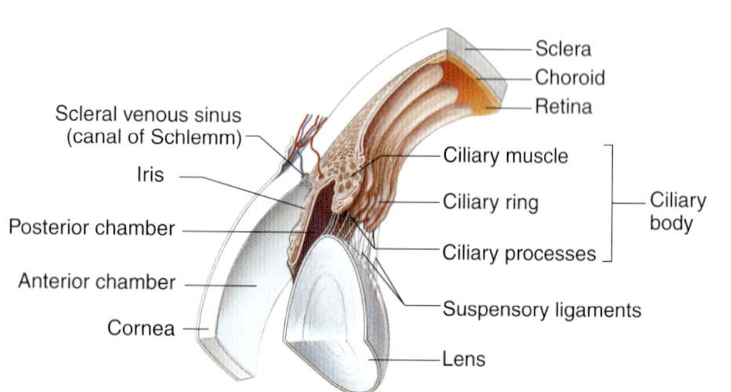

Aa

A abbreviation for *accommodation*; *adenine*; *anode (anodal)*; *anterior*; *axial*; symbol for *ampere* and *mass number*.

AAA *see* ABDOMINAL AORTIC ANEURYSM.

abatement (əˈbaytmənt) a decrease in the severity of a pain or a symptom.

abdomen (ˈabdəmən) the cavity between the diaphragm and the pelvis, lined by a serous membrane, the peritoneum, and containing the stomach, intestines, liver, gallbladder, spleen, pancreas, kidneys, suprarenal glands, ureters and bladder. For descriptive purposes, its area can be divided into nine regions (*see* figure). *Acute a.* any abdominal condition urgently requiring treatment, usually surgical. *Pendulous a.* a condition in which the anterior part of the abdominal wall hangs down over the pubis. *Scaphoid (navicular) a.* a hollowing of the anterior wall, presenting a concave rather than convex contour.

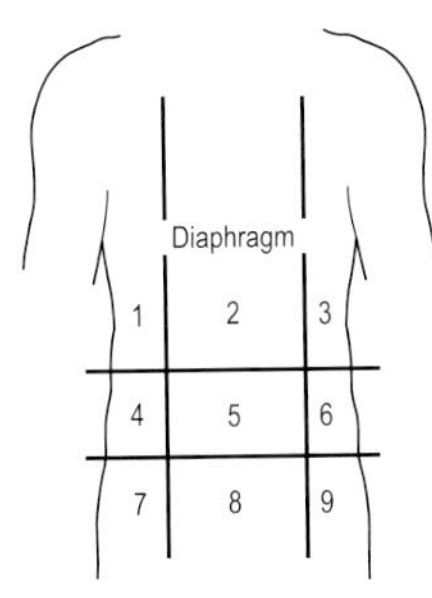

1. Right hypochondriac region
2. Epigastric region
3. Left hypochondriac region
4. Right lumbar region
5. Umbilical region
6. Left lumbar region
7. Right iliac fossa
8. Hypogastric region
9. Left iliac fossa

Regions of the abdomen.

abdominal (abˈdomənəl) pertaining to the abdomen. *A. aorta* that part of the aorta below the diaphragm. *A. aortic aneurysm (AAA)* a dilatation of the abdominal aorta, usually in an area of severe atherosclerosis. This type of aneurysm is four times more common in men than women over the age of 65 years. Rupture of this aneurysm is a surgical emergency and carries a high risk of cardiovascular morbidity and mortality. *A. adhesion see* ADHESION. *A. breathing* a pattern of inhalation and exhalation in which most of the ventilation work is done with the abdominal muscles. *See also* DIAPHRAGMATIC BREATHING. *A. cavity* the space within the abdominal walls between the diaphragm and the pelvic area. Contains a number of crucial organs, including the liver, stomach, intestines, spleen, gallbladder, kidneys and associated tissues, and blood and lymph vessels. *See also* PERITONEAL

CAVITY. *A. examination* a systematic physical assessment of the abdomen by visual inspection and the use of palpation, percussion and auscultation. The purpose is to identify abnormalities, if any, based on any change in size, shape, consistency or sound on percussion of the organs found therein. During pregnancy, the purpose is to determine the equality of uterine size with the calculated period of gestation and later in the pregnancy to determine the position of the fetus. Postnatally, the examination is used to ascertain that the uterus is regaining its former non-pregnant size and position. *A. reflex* reflex contraction of abdominal wall muscles observed when skin is lightly stroked. *A. section* incision through the abdominal wall. *A. thrust formerly called the Heimlich manoeuvre* an emergency procedure for dislodging a bolus of food or a foreign object from the trachea to prevent asphyxiation. Abdominal thrusts may be effective in clearing the airway but have also been associated with complications so are not routinely recommended.

abdominocyesis (ab͵domənoh-ˈsieˈeesəs) an abdominal pregnancy.

abdominopelvic (ab͵domənohˈpel-vik) concerning the abdomen and the pelvic cavity.

abdominoperineal (ab͵domənoh-͵periˈneeəl) pertaining to the abdomen and the perineum. ***A. resection*** a surgical procedure using both anterior abdominal and perineal incisions to treat cancer low in the rectum or in the anus and sigmoid colon.

abdominoplasty (ab͵domənoh-ˈplastee)͵a surgical procedure to remove redundant skin and fat from the abdominal wall. Also called tummy tuck.

abduce (abˈdyoos) to abduct or to draw away.

abducent (abˈdyoosənt) leading away from the midline. *A. muscle* the external rectus muscle of the eye, which rotates it outwards. *A. nerve* the cranial nerve that supplies this muscle.

abductor (abˈduktə) a muscle that draws a limb away from the midline of the body. The opposite of adductor.

aberrant (aˈberənt) 1. pertaining to a wandering from the usual or expected course, such as various ducts, nerves and vessels in the body, or cardiac conduction. 2. (in botany or zoology) pertaining to certain atypical individuals in a species.

aberration (͵abəˈrayshən) deviation from the normal. In optics, failure to focus rays of light. *Mental a.* mental disorder with a deviation from linear or normal thinking.

ability (əˈbilətee) the power to perform an act, either mental or physical, with or without training. *A. test* a test that measures a person's level of performance or estimates future performance. Sometimes also known as an intelligence test, achievement test or aptitude test. *Innate a.* the ability with which a person is born.

ablation (abˈlayshən) the removal or destruction, by surgical or radiological means, of neoplasms or other body tissue.

abnormal (͵abˈnawm'l) varying from what is regular or usual.

ABO system *see* BLOOD GROUPS.

abort (əˈbawt) 1. to terminate a process or disease before it has run its normal course. 2. to remove or expel from the womb an embryo or fetus before it is capable of independent existence.

abortifacient (əˌbawtiˈfayshənt) an agent or drug that may induce abortion.

abortion (əˈbawshən) 1. premature cessation of a normal process. 2. expulsion from the uterus of the products of conception before the fetus is viable. 3. the product of such an abortion. *Complete a.* one in which the contents of the uterus are expelled intact. *Criminal a.* the termination of a pregnancy for reasons other than those permitted by law (i.e. danger to mental or physical health of mother or child or family) and without medical approval. *Incomplete a.* one in which some part of the fetus or placenta is retained in the uterus. *Induced a.* the intentional emptying of the uterus. *Inevitable a.* abortion where bleeding is profuse and accompanied by pains, the cervix is dilated and the contents of the uterus can be felt. *Missed a.* one where all signs of pregnancy disappear and later the uterus discharges a blood clot surrounding a shrivelled fetus, i.e. a carneous mole. *Septic a.* abortion associated with infection. *Therapeutic (legal) a.* one induced on medical advice because the continuance of the pregnancy would involve risk to the life of the pregnant woman, or injury to the physical or mental health of the pregnant woman or any existing children of her family, greater than if the pregnancy were terminated; or because there is a substantial risk that if the child were born it would suffer from such physical or mental abnormalities as to be seriously handicapped. *Threatened a.* the appearance of signs of premature expulsion of the fetus; bleeding is slight, the cervix is closed. *Tubal a.* the termination of a tubal pregnancy caused by rupture of the uterine tube.

abrasion (əˈbrayzhən) a superficial injury where the skin or mucous membrane is rubbed or torn, sometimes called a graze. *Corneal a.* condition in which the surface of the cornea has been removed, e.g. by a scratch or other injury.

abreaction (ˌabriˈakshən) the reliving of a painful experience, with the release of repressed emotion.

abruptio placentae (əˌbrupshioh- pləˈsentie, -tioh) premature detachment of the placenta, causing maternal shock.

abscess (ˈabsəs) a collection of pus in a cavity. Caused by the disintegration and replacement of tissue damaged by mechanical, chemical or bacterial injury. *Alveolar a.* an abscess in a tooth socket. *Brodie's a.* a bone abscess, usually on the head of the tibia. *Cold a.* the result of chronic tubercular infection; and so called because there are few, if any, signs of inflammation. *Psoas a.* a cold abscess that has tracked down the psoas muscle from caries of the lumbar vertebrae. *Subphrenic a.* an abscess situated under the diaphragm.

absorbent (əbˈsawbənt, -ˈzaw-) 1. able to take in, or suck up and incorporate. 2. a tissue structure involved in absorption. 3. a substance that absorbs or promotes absorption.

absorption (əbˈsawpshən, -ˈzaw-) 1. in physiology, the taking up by suction of fluids or other substances by the tissues of the body. 2. in psychology, great mental concentration on a single object or activity. 3. in radiology, uptake of radiation by body tissues.

abstinence (ˈabstənəns) a refraining from the use of (or indulgence in) food, stimulants or coitus. *A. syndrome* the withdrawal symptoms that occur after abstinence from a drug, especially a narcotic, to which a person is addicted.

abstract (ˈabstrakt) a brief, comprehensive summary of a research study or other academic report.

abuse (əˈbyoos) misuse, maltreatment or excessive use; may be physical, sexual, psychological or neglect. Can apply to any group of people, e.g. the vulnerable, children, women, people with learning disabilities or older people. May also apply to the misuse of power, authority, drugs and other substances, e.g. solvents and equipment.

abuse of the older person (əˈbyoos of the oldə ˌpərˈsən) *see* ELDER ABUSE.

abusive head trauma (əˈbyoosˌiv hed ˈtrawmə) a form of non-accidental brain injury and encompasses shaking and impact brain and head injuries of infants and young children. *See* SHAKEN BABY SYNDROME.

Acarus (ˈakə·rəs) a genus of small mites. *A. scabiei* (*Sarcoptes scabiei*) the cause of scabies.

acataphasia (ˌaykatəˈfayzi·ə) loss of the ability to express connected thought, resulting from a cerebral lesion.

acceleration (akˌseləˈrayshən) 1. an increase in the speed or velocity of an object or reaction. 2. an increase in the fetal heartbeat of at least 15 beats per minute over the baseline rate for at least 15 seconds.

access to health records (akˌsesˈ tooˈ helth ˈreˌkordz) the right of patients or clients to inspect, discuss and amend their own health records depending on a particular state or territory law, e.g. Victoria introduced its *Health Records Act (2001)* in 2002 and NSW introduced its *Health Records and Information Privacy Act (2002)* in 2004. There is also a national *My Health Record Act (2012)*.

accessory (akˈsesəree, ˈək-) supplementary. *A. nerve* the 11th cranial nerve. It is made up of two portions: the cranial and the spinal.

accident (ˈakˌseedənt) any unexpected or unplanned event that may result in injury. *A. form* a form, also known as an incident form, which provides a record of any accident to any person occurring in a healthcare facility. Employers require that the form is completed as soon after the accident as possible.

accident and emergency (ˈakˌseedənt and əˈmərjənsee) sometimes referred to as casualty or trauma medicine. A setting for dealing with problems which require immediate attention and where patients may be directed or referred by a general practitioner or the emergency services.

accommodation adjustment (əˌkoməˈdayshən əˈjustmənt). In ophthalmology, the term refers specifically to adjustment of the ciliary muscle, which controls the shape of the lens. *Negative a. a.* the ciliary muscle relaxes and the lens becomes less convex, giving long distance vision. *Positive a. a.* the ciliary muscle contracts and the lens becomes more convex, giving near vision.

accountable (əˈkowntəb'l) liable to be held responsible for a course of action. A qualified nurse has a duty of care according to law; in nursing, being *accountable* refers to the responsibility the qualified nurse takes for prescribing and initiating nursing care. Nurses are *accountable* to their patients, their peers and their employing authority, according to codes of conduct for nurses and midwives. (*See* Appendix 8.)

accreditation (əkˌredəˈtayshən) 1. the action of officially recognising someone as having particular status or being qualified to perform particular activity. 2. an acknowledgement of a person's responsibility or achievement of something. 3. the public recognition by a healthcare accreditation body, such as the Australian Council of Healthcare Standards, of the satisfactory achievement of specified standards by the health care organisation. *A. for Prior Learning (APL)* a system used by academic institutions and other establishments to grant credit for previous academic achievements. Usually used to gain credit transfer between institutions leading to academic qualifications.

accretion (əˈkreeshən) growth. The accumulation of deposits (e.g. of salts) to form a calculus in the bladder. In dentistry, the growth of tartar on the teeth.

acculturation (əkolchəˈrayshən) the process by which a person absorbs the beliefs, values and customs of another culture, usually through direct contact, e.g. migrants resident in another country.

ACE inhibitors (ays inˈhibətəz) a group of drugs used in the treatment of hypertension. The name 'angiotensin-converting enzyme (ACE) inhibitors' explains part of their mode of action, although it is thought that some of their other actions may also be important in reducing blood pressure.

acet- (ˈasət-) combining form denoting acid. From the Latin *acetum*, vinegar.

acetabuloplasty (ˌasəˈtabyəloh-ˌplastee) corrective surgery on the acetabulum to restore its normal shape.

acetabulum (ˌasəˈtabyələm) the cup-like socket in the innominate bone, in which the head of the femur moves.

acetate (ˈasəˌtayt) a salt of acetic acid.

acetic acid (əˈseetik ˈasəd) the acid of vinegar. Used in the manufacture of some pharmaceutical preparations, including antimicrobial solutions for the treatment of superficial infections of the external auditory canal.

acetoacetic acid (ˌasətoh·əˈseetik ˈasəd, əˌsee-) diacetic acid. A product of fat metabolism. It occurs in excessive amounts in diabetes and starvation, giving rise to acetone bodies in the urine.

acetonaemia (ˌasətəˈneemi·ə, əˌsee-) the presence of acetone bodies in the blood.

acetone (ˈasəˌtohn) a colourless flammable liquid with a characteristic odour. Traces are found in the blood and in normal urine. *A. bodies* ketones found in the blood and urine of patients with uncontrolled diabetes and also in those with acute starvation as a result of the incomplete breakdown of fatty and amino acids.

acetonuria (ˌasətəˈnyoo·ri·ə, əˌsee-) the presence of an excess quantity of acetone bodies in the urine, giving it a peculiar sweet smell.

acetylcholine (ˌasətielˈkohleen, ˌasitil-) a chemical transmitter that is released by some nerve endings at the synapse between one neurone and the next or between a nerve ending and the effector organ it supplies. These nerves are said to be cholinergic, e.g. the parasympathetic nerves and the lower motor neurones to skeletal muscles. Acetylcholine is rapidly destroyed in the body by cholinesterase (an enzyme).

acetylcholinesterase (ˌasətiel-ˌkohlənˈestə·rayz) an enzyme that reduces or prevents excessive firing of neurones at neuromuscular junctions.

acetylcoenzyme A (ˌasətielkoh-ˈenziem, ˌasətəl-) the active form of acetic acid, to which carbohydrates, fats and amino acids that are not needed for protein synthesis are converted.

achalasia (akəˈlayzi·ə) failure of the relaxation of a muscle sphincter, causing dilatation of the part above, e.g. of the oesophagus above the cardiac sphincter (*see* figure below).

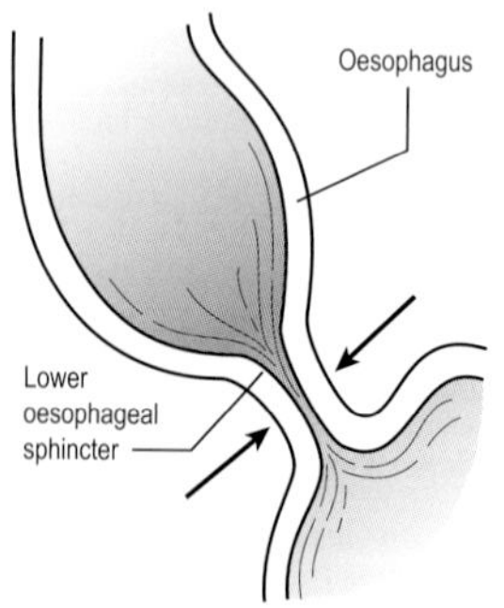

Achalasia.

ache (ayk) a dull, continuous pain.

Achilles (əˈkileez) Greek mythological hero who could be wounded only in the heel. *A. tendon* tendocalcaneus, connecting the soleus and gastrocnemius muscles of the calf to the heel bone (calcaneum or os calcis). Tapping the Achilles tendon normally produces the *Achilles reflex* or ankle jerk.

achlorhydria (ˌayˈklorˈhiedri·ə) the absence of free hydrochloric acid in the stomach. May be found in pernicious anaemia, pellagra and gastric cancer.

acholia (ayˈkohli·ə) a lack of secretion of bile.

acholuria (ˌaykəˈlyoo·ri·ə) a deficiency or lack of bile in the urine.

acholuric (ˌaykəˈlyoo·rik) pertaining to acholuria. *A. jaundice* jaundice without bile in the urine.

achondroplasia (ayˌkondrohˈplay-zi·ə) an inherited condition in which there is early union of the epiphysis and diaphysis of long bones. Growth is arrested, resulting in short stature.

achromasia (ˌaykrohˈmayzi·ə) 1. lack of colour in the skin. 2. absence of normal reaction to staining in a tissue or cell.

achromatopsia (ˌaykrohməˈtopsi·ə) complete colour blindness caused by disease or trauma. It may be congenital.

achylia (ayˈkieli·ə) an absence of hydrochloric acid and enzymes in the gastric secretions. *A. gastrica* a condition in which gastric secretion is reduced or absent.

acid (ˈasəd) 1. sour or sharp in taste. 2. a substance which, when combined with an alkali, will form a salt. Any acid substance will turn blue litmus paper red. Individual acids are given under their specific names *A.–alcohol-fast* descriptive of stained bacteria that are resistant to decolourisation by both acid and alcohol. *A.–base balance* the normal ratio between the acid ions and the basic (or alkaline) ions required to maintain the pH of the blood and body fluids. Most of the body's metabolic processes produce acids as their end-products, but a somewhat alkaline body fluid is required as a medium for vital cellular activities. Therefore, chemical exchanges of hydrogen ions must take place continuously in order to maintain a state of equilibrium. An optimal pH (hydrogen ion concentration) between 7.35 and 7.45 must be maintained; otherwise, the enzyme systems and other biochemical and metabolic activities will not function normally.

acidaemia (ˌasəˈdeemi·ə) abnormal acidity of the blood which contains an excess of hydrogen ions, in which the pH of the blood falls below 7.35.

acidity (əˈsidətee) 1. sourness or sharpness of taste. 2. the state of being acid.

acidosis (ˌasəˈdohsəs) a pathological condition resulting from accumulation of acid or depletion of the alkaline reserve (bicarbonate content) in the blood and body tissues, and characterised by increase in hydrogen ion concentration (decrease in pH to below 7.30). *Metabolic a.* acidosis resulting from accumulation in the blood of ketoacids (derived from fat metabolism) at the expense of bicarbonate, thus diminishing the body's ability to neutralise acids. Occurs in diabetic ketoacidosis, lactic acidosis and failure of renal tubules to reabsorb bicarbonate. *Respiratory a.* acidosis resulting from ventilatory impairment and subsequent retention of carbon dioxide. Carbon dioxide accumulates in the blood and unites with water to form carbonic acid, thus reducing plasma pH. The condition can be acute with a sudden onset, or it can develop gradually as lung function deteriorates. *See also* KETOSIS.

acidotic (ˌasəˈdotik) 1. pertaining to acidosis. 2. a person suffering from acidosis.

acinus (ˈasənəs) *pl.* acini. a minute saccule or alveolus of a compound gland, lined by secreting cells. The secreting portion of the mammary gland consists of acini.

acme (ˈakmee) 1. the peak or highest point, e.g. the peak of intensity of a uterine contraction during labour. 2. the crisis of a fever when the symptoms are fully developed.

acne (ˈaknee) an inflammatory condition of the sebaceous glands in which blackheads (comedones) are usually present together with papules and pustules. *A. keratitis* inflammation of the cornea associated with acne rosacea. *A. rosacea* a redness of the forehead, nose and cheeks due to chronic dilatation of the subcutaneous capillaries, which may become permanent with the formation of pustules in the affected areas. *A. vulgaris* a form of acne that occurs commonly in adolescents and young adults, affecting the face, chest and back.

acneiform (akˈnee·əˌfawm) resembling acne.

acousma (əˈkoosmə) the hearing of imaginary sounds.

acoustic (əˈkoostik) relating to sound or the sense of hearing. *A. neuroma* a benign tumour that develops from the eighth cranial nerve. Depending on the size and location of the tumour hearing and balance may be affected. Also known as vestibular schwannoma.

acquired (ə'kwieəd) pertaining to disease, habits or immunity developed after birth; not inherited.

acquired immunodeficiency syndrome *see* AIDS.

acrocephalia (ˌakrohke'fayli·ə, -se-) malformation of the head, in which the top is pointed.

acrochordon (akro'kaw'dun) benign pedunculated growth commonly found on the eyelids, neck, axilla or groin. Also called skin tag.

acromegaly (ˌakroh'megəlee) a chronic condition producing gradual enlargement of the hands, feet and bones of the head and chest. Associated with overactivity of the anterior lobe of the pituitary gland in adults.

acromioclavicular (əˌkrohmioh-ˌklə'-vikyələ) pertaining to the joint between the acromion process of the scapula and the lateral aspect of the clavicle.

acromion (ə'krohmi·ən) the outward projection of the spine of the scapula, forming the point of the shoulder.

acroosteolysis (ˌakrohˌostee·oh·-'lisəs) an occupational disease that affects people working with polyvinylchloride (PVC) plastics.

acroparaesthesia (ˌakrohˌparəs-'theezi·ə) a condition in which pressure on the nerves of the brachial plexus causes numbness, pain and tingling of the hand and forearm.

acrophobia (ˌakroh'fohbi·ə) extreme or irrational fear of height.

acrosclerosis (ˌakrohsklə'rohsəs) a combination of RAYNAULD'S DISEASE and SCLERODERMA that affects the hands, feet, face or chest.

acrosome ('akrəˌsohm) part of the head of a spermatozoon containing enzymes that break down the cell membrane of the ovum and allow penetration.

ACTH adrenocorticotrophic hormone; corticotrophin.

actigraph ('aktəˌgraf) an instrument that records changes in the activity of an organism and produces a graphic record of the process.

actin ('aktən) the protein of myofibrils responsible for contraction and relaxation of muscles.

actinic keratoses ('aktən'ikˌ kerə'tohsəz) also known as solar keratoses; rough patches of skin caused by sun exposure over a prolonged period of time. Most often affects the face, ears and hands.

actinodermatitis (ˌaktənohˌdərmə-'tietəs) inflammation of the skin due to the action of ultraviolet or X-rays.

Actinomyces (ˌaktənə'mieseez) a genus of branching, spore-forming, vegetable parasites which may give rise to actinomycosis and from which many antibiotic drugs are produced, e.g. streptomycin.

actinomycosis (ˌaktənohmie'kohsəs) a chronic systemic disease, characterised by deep lumpy abscesses, chiefly affecting the lung and jaw, and more rarely in the intestines and pelvis.

actinotherapy (ˌaktənoh'therəpee) the use of ultraviolet, other parts of the spectrum of the sun's rays, or X-rays to treat various disorders, particularly skin diseases.

action ('akshən) the accomplishment of an effect, whether mechanical or chemical, or the effect so produced. *A. potential* the change in electrical potential that occurs with the passage of an impulse along a nerve or muscle fibre when it is stimulated. *A. research* a method of undertaking social research that incorporates the researcher's involvement as a direct and deliberate part of the research process, i.e. the researcher acts as a change agent. *Cumulative a.* the sudden and markedly increased action of a drug after administration of several doses. *Reflex a.* an involuntary response to a stimulus conveyed to the nervous system and reflected to the periphery, passing below the level of consciousness (*see also* REFLEX).

activator (ˌaktəˈvaytə) a substance, hormone or enzyme that stimulates a chemical change, although it may not take part in the change. In chemistry, a catalyst. For example, yeast is the activator in the process by which sugar is converted into alcohol; the digestive secretions are activated by hormones to carry out normal digestion.

active (ˈaktiv) causing change; energetic. *A. immunity* an immunity in which individuals have been stimulated to produce their own antibodies. *A. labour* the normal progress of the birth process, including uterine contractions, dilation of the cervix to at least 3–4 cm, and the descent of the fetus into the birth canal. *A. listening* the act of alert, intentional hearing and demonstration of an interest in what a person has to say through verbal signs, non-verbal gestures and body language. *A. movements* movements made by the patient, as distinct from passive movements. *A. principle* the ingredient in a drug that is primarily responsible for its therapeutic action. *A. transport* the movement of ions or molecules across the cell membranes and epithelial layers, usually against a concentration gradient, resulting directly from the expenditure of metabolic energy. Under normal circumstances more potassium ions are present within the cell and more sodium ions extracellularly. The process of maintaining these normal differences in electrolytic composition between the intracellular fluids is active transport. The process differs from simple diffusion or osmosis in that it requires the expenditure of metabolic energy.

activities of daily living (ADL) (akˈtivəteez ov dayleeˈ living) those activities usually performed in the course of a person's normal daily self-care routine, such as eating, cleaning teeth, washing and dressing. Assessing a person's ability to perform ADLs is part of a nursing health assessment.

activities of living (AL) (ˌakˈtivəteez ov living) those activities which meet the physical, psychological and social needs of the individual, e.g. eating, elimination, communication, breathing, expressing sexuality, working, play, etc.

activity theory (ˌakˈtivətee ˌthiəree) describes a psychosocial process whereby ageing people disengage from some activities of their earlier life and replace these with other hobbies and pastimes, according to their changing physical abilities and economic situation.

activity tolerance (ˌakˈtivətee ˈtolərəns) the amount of physical activity tolerated by a patient. It may be assessed in patients with cardiac or chronic respiratory disease. Graded exercise, including walking, cycling and going up and down stairs, may be used to rebuild confidence during the convalescent phase after any serious illness or injury as an important part of any rehabilitation program.

acuity (ə'kyooətee) sharpness. *A. of hearing* an acute perception of sound. *A. of vision* clear focusing ability.

acupressure ('akyə͵preshə) a system of complementary medicine in which pressure is applied to various points on the body with the aim of stimulating the innate self-healing capacity of the individual. *See* ACUPUNCTURE; SHIATSU.

acupuncture ('akyə͵pungchə) a Chinese medical system which aims to diagnose illness and promote health by stimulating the body's self-healing powers. The insertion of special needles into specific points along the 'meridians' of the body is used for the production of anaesthesia, the relief of pain and the treatment of certain conditions.

acute (ə'kyoot) a term applied to a disease or illness in which the attack is sudden, severe and of short duration. *A. respiratory distress syndrome (ARDS)* a severe form of acute lung function failure which occurs after an event such as trauma, inhalation of a toxic substance or septic shock. There is severe breathlessness and a dangerous reduction in the supply of oxygen to the blood. *A. stress disorder* an anxiety disorder that is usually transient, which occurs within 4 weeks following exposure or involvement to a traumatic event, such as witnessing a death or traumatic accident.

acute physiology and chronic health evaluation (͵ə'kyoot ͵fizee'oləjee and 'kronik helth ee͵valyoo'ayshən) *see* APACHE.

acyclic (ay'sieklik) occurring independently of a natural cycle of events such as the menstrual cycle.

adactylia (͵aydak'tili·ə) congenital absence of fingers or toes.

Adam's apple ('adəmz 'apuhl) the laryngeal prominence, a protrusion of the front of the neck formed by the thyroid cartilage.

adamantine (͵adə'manteen, -tien) pertaining to the enamel of the teeth.

adaptation (͵adəp'tayshən) 1. the process of modification that a living organism undergoes when adjusting itself to new surroundings or circumstances. 2. a function of the stimulus to which the individual is exposed and of the individual's adaptation to the situation. The adaptation response may relate to physiological needs, role, 'self' concept and interdependence. 3. the process of overcoming difficulties and adjusting to changing circumstances. Neuroses and psychoses are often associated with failure of adaptation. 4. used in ophthalmology to mean the adjustment of visual function according to the ambient illumination. *Colour a.* 1. changes in visual perception of colour with prolonged stimulation. 2. adjustment of vision to degree of brightness or colour tone of illumination. *Dark a.* adaptation of the eye to vision in reduced illumination. *Light a.* adaptation of the eye to vision in bright illumination (photopia), with reduction in the concentration of the photosensitive pigments of the eye.

addict ('adikt) a person exhibiting addiction.

addiction (ə'dikshən) 1. the taking of drugs or alcohol leading to physiological and psychological dependence with a tendency to increase use. 2. the state of being devoted to a particular activity or interest, e.g. gambling, exercise or computer games to the exclusion of the normal activities of daily living. *See* DEPENDENCE and DRUG ADDICTION.

Addison's anaemia (ˈadəsənz əˈneemi·ə) *Thomas Addison, British physician, 1793–1860*. Pernicious anaemia.

Addison's disease (ˈadiˌsənz diˈzeez) deficiency disease caused by inadequate secretion of hormones by the adrenal cortex; characterised by progressive anaemia, low blood pressure, weakness and brown pigmentation of the skin. Also known as primary adrenal insufficiency.

Addisonian crisis (ˈadiˌsohni·ən ˈkriesəs) *see* ADRENAL CRISIS.

additives (ˈadiˌtivz) substances added to improve, enhance or preserve something. *Food a.* used in the food industry to preserve and make the food look more attractive; these are given serial numbers, e.g. E102 (tartrazine), E200 (sorbic acid) and E621 (Monosodium L-glutamate or MSG). Some additives may produce an allergic reaction in some people, and a few are thought to be implicated in behavioural problems in children.

adducent (əˈdyoosənt) leading towards the midline. *A. muscle* the medial rectus muscle of the eye, which turns it inwards.

adductor (əˈduktə) a muscle that draws a limb towards the midline of the body. The opposite of abductor.

adenine (ˈadəˌneen) one of the purine bases found in DNA.

adenitis (ˌadəˈnietəs) inflammation of a gland, also referred to as LYMPHADENITIS.

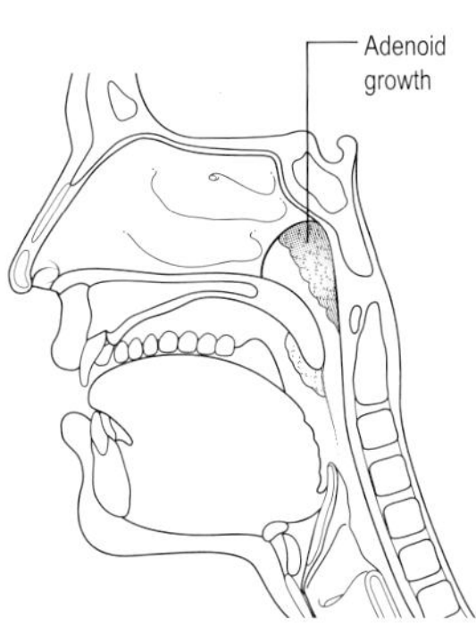

Adenoid growth.

adenohypophysis (ˈadənoh·hie-ˈpofəsəs) the anterior lobe of the pituitary gland.

adenoid (ˈadəˌnoyd) 1. having a glandular appearance, particularly lymphoid. 2. pharyngeal tonsil or nasopharyngeal tonsil. *See* TONSIL. (*see* figure above).

adenoidectomy (ˌadənoyˈdektəmee) the surgical removal of adenoid tissue from the nasopharynx.

adenoma (ˌadəˈnohmə) a benign tumour of glandular tissue.

adenomyoma (ˌadənohmieˈohmə) benign tumour of the endometrium of the uterus, composed of a mass of smooth muscle containing endometrial tissue and glands.

adenomyosis (ˌadənohmieˈohsis) a condition in which the endometrium of the uterus breaks through the muscle wall of the uterus, usually resulting in painful and profuse periods.

adenopathy (ˌadəˈnopəthee) enlargement of any gland, especially those of the lymphatic system.

adenosarcoma (ˌadənohsahˈkohmə) a malignant tumour of connective and glandular tissue. *Embryonal a.* *see* NEPHROBLASTOMA.

adenosine (a'denə͵seen) a nucleoside consisting of adenine and D-ribose (a pentose sugar). *A. triphosphate (ATP)* a compound containing three phosphoric acids. It is present in all cells and serves as a store for energy.

adenovirus (͵adənoh'vierəs) a virus of the Adenoviridae family. Many types have been isolated, some of which cause respiratory tract infections, while others are associated with conjunctivitis, epidemic keratoconjunctivitis or gastrointestinal infections.

ADH antidiuretic hormone. Vasopressin. *See also* ANTIDIURETIC.

adhesion (əd'heezhən) union between two surfaces normally separated. Usually the result of inflammation when fibrous tissue forms, e.g. peritonitis may cause adhesions between organs. A possible cause of intestinal obstruction.

adhesive capsulitis (əd'heesiv͵ kapsyəalietəs) *See* FROZEN SHOULDER.

adipose ('adə͵pohs, -z) of the nature of fat. Fatty.

adiposity (͵adə'posətee) the state of being too fat. Obesity.

adiposogenital dystrophy (͵adə'poso͵jenit'əl'distrəfee) a condition occurring in adolescent boys with increased body fat accompanied by underdevelopment of the genitalia and altered secondary sexual characteristics caused by damage to the HYPOTHALAMUS usually as a result of a tumour or infection. *See also* FRÖHLICH'S SYNDROME.

aditus ('adətəs) an opening or passageway; often applied to that between the middle ear and the mastoid antrum.

adjustment (ə'justmənt) in psychology, the ability of a person to adapt to changing circumstances or environment.

adjuvant ('ajəvənt) 1. any treatment used in conjunction with another to enhance its efficacy. 2. a substance administered with a drug to enhance its effect.

ADL *see* ACTIVITIES OF DAILY LIVING.

Adler's theory ('adləz ͵thiəree) *Alfred Adler, Austrian psychiatrist, 1870–1937.* The theory that neuroses develop as a compensation for feelings of inferiority, either social or physical.

adolescence (͵adə'lesəns) the period between puberty and maturity. In the male, 14–25 years. In the female, 12–21 years.

adopt (͵a'dopt) 1. to take a person, especially another's child, into a legal relationship as one's own. 2. to choose to follow a course of action.

adoption (͵a'dopshən) the legal procedure by which a child is transferred from his or her birth parents to adopting parents. Adoption legislation is different in each jurisdiction in Australia and it is necessary to refer to each state and territory for particular information, rules and regulations.

adrenal (ə'dreenəl) 1. near the kidneys. 2. a triangular endocrine gland situated above each kidney. *A. cortex* the outer and greater portion of the adrenal gland. *A. crisis* an acute life-threatening state of profound adrenocortical insufficiency requiring immediate therapy. Also called Addisonian crisis.

adrenalectomy (əˈdreenəˌlektəmee) surgical excision of an adrenal gland.

adrenaline (əˈdrenələn) a hormone secreted by the medulla of the adrenal gland. Has an action similar to normal stimulation of the sympathetic nervous system: (a) causing dilatation of the bronchioles; (b) raising the blood pressure by constriction of surface vessels and stimulation of the cardiac output; and (c) releasing glycogen from the liver. It is therefore used to treat such conditions as asthma, collapse and hypoglycaemia. It acts as a haemostat in local anaesthetics.

adrenergic (ˌadrəˈnərjik) pertaining to nerves that release the chemical transmitter noradrenaline in order to stimulate the muscles and glands they supply.

adrenocortical (əˌdreenohˈkawtikəl) pertaining to the adrenal cortex.

adrenocorticotrophin (əˌdreenohˌkawtikohˈtrohfən) adrenocorticotrophic hormone (ACTH) secreted by the anterior lobe of the pituitary body. Stimulates the adrenal cortex to produce cortisol. *See* CORTICOTROPHIN.

adrenogenital (əˌdreenohˈjenət'l) relating to both the adrenal glands and the gonads. *A. syndrome* a condition of masculinisation caused by overactivity of the adrenal cortex, resulting in precocious puberty in the male infant and masculinisation in the female. Both genders are liable to Addisonian crises.

adrenolytic (əˈdreenohˈlitik) a drug that inhibits the stimulation of the sympathetic nerves and the activity of adrenaline.

adsorbent (ədˈsawbənt, -ˈzawb-) a substance that has the power of attracting gas or fluid to itself, e.g. charcoal.

adsorption (ədˈsawpshən, -ˈzawp-) the power of certain substances to attach gases or other substances in solution to their surface and so concentrate them there. This is made use of in chromatography.

adult (əˈdult, ˈadult) mature. A mature person.

adulteration (əˈdultəˈrayshən) addition of an impure, cheap or unnecessary ingredient to cheat with, cheapen or falsify a preparation.

advance care directive or statement (ˌadˈvans kair directiv aw ˈstaytˌmənt) a written declaration made by a mentally competent person that sets out their wishes with regard to life-prolonging medical interventions if they are incapacitated by an irreversible disease or are terminally ill and prevented from making their wishes known to health professionals at the time. Also referred to as advance health directive or advanced care plan or living will.

advanced life support (ALS) (ˌadˈvanst lief ˌsəˈpawt) resuscitation techniques used during a cardiac arrest that follows on from basic life support. They include defibrillation and the administration of appropriate drugs. Paediatric advanced life support (PALS) is a structured and algorithmic method of life support for children with severe medical emergencies.

advanced trauma life support (ATLS) (ˌadˈvanst trawmə lief ˌsəˈpawt) a set of protocols recommended for use by doctors and paramedics when dealing with seriously injured people at the scene of an accident. The immediate treatment of shock from reduced blood volume by the infusion of fluids is an integral component of the life support regimen.

advancement (əd'vahnsmənt, əd'vans-) in surgery, an operation to detach a tendon or muscle and reattach it further forward. Used in the treatment of strabismus and plastic surgery.

adventitia (ˌadvən'tish·ə, -'tishə) the outer coat of an artery or vein.

advocacy ('advəkəsee) the process whereby a nurse or another healthcare professional provides a patient and/or the patient's family with information to enable them to make informed decisions relating to the care situation. The nurse is then able to support the patient's decision vis-à-vis other professionals and also to incorporate the informed decisions into care planning.

aeration (air'rayshən) supplying with air. Used to describe the oxygenation of blood, which takes place in the lungs.

aerobe ('air·rohb) an organism that can live and thrive only in the presence of oxygen.

aerobic exercise (ˌair'ohbik 'eksəˌsiez) physical exercises for which the degree of effort is such that it can be maintained for long periods without undue breathlessness. The aim of this form of exercising is to increase the effectiveness of the heart and lungs and the supply of oxygen to the tissues of the body.

aeropathy (air'ropəthee) any illness caused by a change in atmospheric pressure, e.g. decompression sickness.

aerophagy (air'rofajee) the excessive swallowing of air.

aerosol ('air·rəˌsol) finely divided particles or droplets. *A. sprays* used in medicine to humidify air or oxygen, or for the administration of drugs by inhalation.

aetiology (ˌayti'oləjee) the science of the causes of disease.

afebrile (ay'feebriel) without fever.

affect (ə'fekt) in psychiatry, the feeling experienced in connection with an emotion or mood.

affection (ə'fekshən) 1. a morbid condition or disease state. 2. a warm feeling for someone or something.

affective (ə'fektiv) pertaining to the emotions or moods. *A. psychoses* major mental disorders in which there is grave disturbance of the emotions.

afferent ('afə·rənt) conveying towards the centre. *A. nerves* the sensory nerve fibres that convey impulses from the periphery towards the brain. *A. paths* or *tracts* the course of the sensory nerves up the spinal cord and through the brain. *A. vessels* arterioles entering the glomerulus of the kidney, or lymphatics entering a lymph gland. *See* EFFERENT.

affiliation (ˌa'fileeˌayshən) the judicial decision about the paternity of a child with a view to the issue of a maintenance order.

affinity (ə'finətee) in chemistry, the attraction of two substances to each other, e.g. haemoglobin and oxygen.

afibrinogenaemia (ˌayfiebrinəjə-'neemi·ə) the absence of fibrinogen in the blood. The clotting mechanism of the blood is impaired as a result.

African tick fever ('afrikən tik 'feevə) a disease caused by a spirochaete, *Borrelia duttonii*. Transmitted by ticks. *See* RELAPSING FEVER.

afterbirth ('ahftəˌbərth) a lay expression used to describe the placenta, cord and membranes expelled after childbirth.

aftercare (ˈahftəˌkair) social, medical or nursing care provided after a period of hospital treatment.

afterimage (ˈahftəˌimij) a visual impression that remains briefly after the cessation of sensory stimulation.

afterpains (ˈahftəˌpaynz) pains due to uterine contraction after childbirth.

agammaglobulinaemia (ayˌgamə ˌglobyuhləˈneemi·ə) a condition in which there is a lack of gamma-globulin in the blood. The patients are therefore susceptible to infections because of an inability to form antibodies.

aganglionosis (ayˈgang·glee·ənˈoh-səs) *see* HIRSCHSPRUNG'S DISEASE.

agar (ˈaygah) a gelatinous substance prepared from seaweed. Used as a culture medium for bacteria and as a laxative because it absorbs liquid from the digestive tract and swells, so stimulating peristalsis.

age (ˈayj) 1. the duration of or the measure of time of the existence of a person or object. 2. to undergo change as a result of the passage of time. *Achievement a. see* DEVELOPMENTAL MILESTONES. *A. spots* with increasing age, skin blemishes appear; most commonly they are seborrhoeic keratoses, which are brown or yellow and can occur anywhere on the body. Also common with increasing age are freckles, red pinpoint blemishes on the trunk and solar keratoses due to overexposure to the sun. Treatment is usually unnecessary except occasionally for solar keratoses, which may eventually progress to skin cancer. *Chronological a.* the actual measure of time elapsed since a person's birth. *Gestational a.* an expression of age of a developing fetus, usually given in weeks. It is measured from the date of the mother's last menstrual period and so is approximately 2 weeks longer than time from conception. *Mental a.* the age level of intellectual ability of a person as gauged by standard intelligence tests.

age-associated memory impairment (ˈayj aˈsohseeayted ˈmemə·ree imˈpairmənt) with age, short-term memory declines; most older people learn to overcome and compensate for this deficit. However, for some it may be a considerable problem in daily living. Memory loss associated with dementia is often due to Alzheimer's disease or cerebral vascular disease. *See* DEMENTIA and ALZHEIMER'S DISEASE.

aged care (ˈayj'd kair) those services provided to people over the age of 65 years; normally refers to residential aged care services.

ageing (ˈayjing) the structural changes that take place with time and that are not caused by accident or disease. Heredity is an important determinant of life expectancy, but factors such as smoking, an excessive intake of alcohol, obesity, poor diet and insufficient exercise can all contribute to physical and mental deterioration. *A. population* a phenomenon that occurs when the median age of a country or region rises due to rising life expectancy and/or declining birth rates. As the number of older people increases, the demand for healthcare increases.

ageism (ˈayjizəm) the systematic discrimination against people on the grounds of age, based on stereotyping of the elderly as helpless, infirm, confused and requiring healthcare and supportive social services.

agenesis (ay'jenəsəs) the failure of a structure to develop properly.

agent ('ayjənt) any substance or force capable of producing a physical, chemical or biological effect. *Alkylating a.* a cytotoxic preparation. *Chelating a.* a chemical compound that binds metal ions. *Wetting a.* a substance that lowers the surface tension of water and promotes wetting.

agglutination (ə,glootə'nayshən) the collecting into clumps, particularly of cells suspended in a fluid and of bacteria affected by specific immune serum. *A. test* a means of aiding diagnosis and identification of bacteria. If serum containing known agglutinins comes into contact with the specific bacteria, clumping will take place (*see* WIDAL REACTION). *Cross a.* a simple test to decide the group to which a blood belongs (*see* BLOOD GROUPS).

agglutinin (ə'glootənən) any substance causing agglutination (clumping together) of cells, particularly a specific antibody formed in the blood in response to the presence of an invading agent. Agglutinins are proteins (*see* IMMUNOGLOBULIN) and function as part of the immune mechanism of the body. When the invading agents that bring about the production of agglutinins are bacteria, the agglutinins produced bring about agglutination of the bacterial cells.

agglutinogen (,agluh'tinəjən) any substance which, when present in the bloodstream, can cause the production of specific antibodies or agglutinins.

aggregation (,agrə'gayshən) the massing together of materials, as in clumping. *Familial a.* the increased incidence of cases of a disease in a family compared with that in control families. *Platelet a.* the clumping together of platelets which may be induced by a number of agents, such as thrombin and collagen.

aggression (ə'greshən) animosity or hostility shown towards another person or object as a response to opposition or frustration.

agitation (ajə'tayshən) 1. shaking. 2. mental distress causing extreme restlessness.

aglutition (,aygloo'tishən) difficulty in the act of swallowing. Dysphagia.

agnosia (ag'nohzi·ə) an inability to recognise objects because the sensory stimulus cannot be interpreted, in spite of the presence of a normal sense organ.

agonist ('agənəst) the prime mover. A muscle opposed in action by another (the antagonist).

agony ('agənee) extreme suffering, either mental or physical.

agoraphobia (,agə·rə'fohbi·ə) a type of anxiety disorder in which there is a fear of being in an open, crowded or public places. Exposure to the feared situation may cause anticipatory anxiety or panic and avoidance of the places feared.

agranulocyte (ay'granyələ,siet) a white blood cell without granules in its cytoplasm. The term includes monocytes and lymphocytes.

agranulocytosis (ay,granyəlohsie-'tohsəs) a condition in which there is a marked decrease or complete absence of granular leucocytes in the blood, leaving the body defenceless against bacterial invasion. May result from: (a) the use of toxic drugs; (b) irradiation. Characterised by a sore throat, ulceration of the mouth and pyrexia.

It may result in severe prostration and death.

agraphia (ayˈgrafi·ə) an absence of the power of expressing thought in writing. It arises from a lack of muscular coordination or as a result of a motor dysfunction.

AHF antihaemophilic factor (clotting factor VIII).

AHG antihaemophilic globulin (clotting factor VIII). *See also* ANTIHAEMOPHILIC.

AHPRA Australian Health Practitioner Regulation Agency. This organisation is responsible for the implementation of the National Registration and Accreditation Scheme across Australia. AHPRA came into operation on 1 July 2010.

AID artificial insemination of a woman with donor semen.

AIDS (aydz) acquired immunodeficiency syndrome. The late symptomatic stage of chronic disease caused by human immunodeficiency virus (HIV) infection, which progressively impairs the body's cell-mediated immune responses to infections and cancers. This results in serious 'opportunistic infections' caused by microorganisms that do not usually cause illness in people with a healthy immune system, e.g. *Pneumocystis carinii* pneumonia (PCP), or cancers such as Kaposi's sarcoma (KS) and lymphoma. Additionally, this late stage of HIV disease is characterised by a high and rising level (viral load) of HIV and a progressively decreasing number (less than 200 cells/mm^3) of CD4$^+$ T lymphocytes in the plasma. Prior to AIDS, many HIV-infected people experience a variety of recurrent signs and symptoms, including lymphadenopathy, night sweats, diarrhoea, weight loss, malaise, oropharyngeal or vaginal candidiasis (thrush) and herpes zoster (shingles). Formerly known as the AIDS-related complex, this stage is now generally referred to as early symptomatic HIV disease (as opposed to AIDS, which is also known as late symptomatic HIV disease).

AIH artificial insemination by husband or partner is a fertility treatment that involves placing the partner's sperm inside the woman's uterus.

ailment (ˈaylment) any minor disorder of the body.

AIN *see* ASSISTANT IN NURSING.

air (air) a mixture of gases that make up the earth's atmosphere. It consists of: non-active nitrogen 79%; oxygen 21%, which supports life and combustion; traces of neon, argon, hydrogen, etc.; and carbon dioxide 0.03%, except in expired air, when 6% is exhaled as a result of diffusion that has taken place in the lungs. Air has weight and exerts pressure, which aids in syphonage from body cavities. *A. bed* a rubber mattress inflated with air. *A. embolism* an embolism caused by air entering the circulatory system. *A. hunger* a form of dyspnoea in which there are deep sighing respirations, characteristic of severe haemorrhage or acidosis. *Residual a.* air remaining in the lungs after deep expiration. *Stationary a.* air retained in the lungs after normal expiration. *Supplemental a.* the extra air forced out of the lungs with expiratory effort. *Tidal a.* air that passes in and out of the lungs in normal respiratory action.

airway (ˈairˌway) the passage by which the air enters and leaves the lungs. *Oropharyngeal a.* a medical device or tube to maintain or open

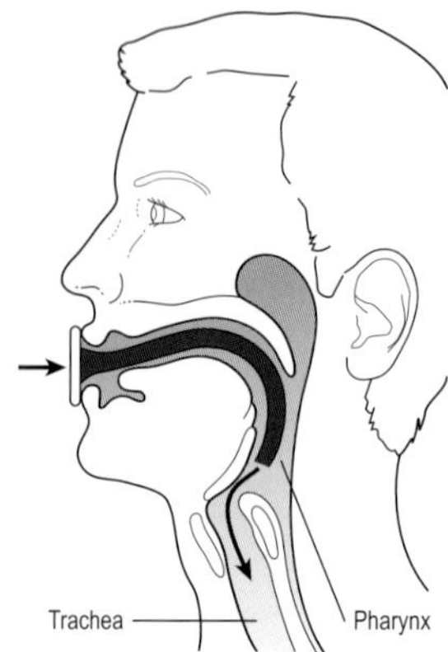

Oropharyngeal airway.

an airway. Also used for securing unobstructed respiration during general anaesthesia or on other occasions when the patient is not ventilating or exchanging gases properly. It may be passed through the mouth or nose. The tube prevents a flaccid tongue from resting against the posterior pharyngeal wall and causing obstruction of the airway (*see* figure above).

akinesia (ˌaykəˈneezi·ə) loss of muscle power. This may be the result of a brain or spinal cord lesion or, temporarily, due to anaesthesia.

akinetic (ˌaykəˈnetik) relating to states or conditions where there is lack of movement.

alacrima (ayˈlakrəmə) a deficiency or absence of secretion of tears.

alalia (əˈlayli·ə) loss or impairment of the power of speech due to muscle paralysis or a cerebral lesion.

alanine (ˈaləˌneen, -nien) an amino acid formed by the ingestion of dietary protein.

albinism (ˈalbəˌnizəm) a condition in which there is congenital absence of pigment in the skin, hair and eyes. It may be partial or complete.

albino (alˈbeenoh) a person affected with albinism.

Albright's syndrome (ˈawlbriets ˈsinˌdrohm) *Fuller Albright, American physician, 1900–1969.* Condition in which there is abnormal development of bone, excessive pigmentation of the skin and, in females, precocious sexual development.

albumin (ˈalbyəmən) 1. any protein that is soluble in water and moderately concentrated salt solutions and is coagulable by heat, e.g. egg white. 2. the most abundant serum-binding protein, formed principally in the liver and constituting about 60% of the 6–8% protein concentration in the plasma. Albumin is a very important factor in regulating the exchange of water between the plasma and the interstitial compartment (space between the cells). A drop in the amount of albumin in the plasma results in an increase in tissue fluid, which, if severe, becomes apparent as oedema. Albumin also serves as a transport protein.

albuminuria (alˌbyooməˈnyoo·ri·ə) the presence of albumin in the urine, occurring, e.g. in renal disease, in most feverish conditions and, sometimes, in pregnancy. *Orthostatic* or *postural a.* a non-pathological form that affects some individuals after prolonged standing, but disappears after bed rest for a few hours.

alcohol (ˈalkəˌhol) a volatile liquid distilled from fermented saccharine liquids and forming the basis of wines and spirits. The official British Pharmacopoeia (BP) preparation of ethyl alcohol (ethanol) contains 95% alcohol and 5% water. Used: (a) as an antiseptic; (b) in the preparation of tinctures; and (c) as a preservative for anatomical specimens. Taken internally, it acts as a temporary heart stimulant and, in large quantities, as a depressant poison. It has some value as a food, with 30 mL brandy producing about 400 J. *Absolute a.* that which contains not more than 1% by weight of water. *A. fast* pertaining to bacteria that, once having been stained, are resistant to decolourisation by alcohol. *A. related disorders* a variety of physical and mental disorders associated with prolonged and excessive consumption of alcohol including hepatitis, cirrhosis and some cancers, e.g. of the oesophagus, larynx and throat. Heavy alcohol consumption in pregnancy increases the risk of miscarriage and fetal alcohol syndrome. Alcoholics are more likely to suffer from personality changes, depression and the development of dementia. Many alcoholics suffer from a poor diet and are prone to nutritional deficiency. *See* WERNICKE–KORSAKOFF SYNDROME. *A. withdrawal syndrome* a group of symptoms that develop in a person suffering from alcoholism within 6–24 hours of taking the last drink of alcohol. The symptoms include restlessness, tremors, loss of appetite, nausea, vomiting, insomnia, disorientation, seizures and delirium tremens. Treatment involves sedation, improving nutrition, counselling and social support.

alcoholic (ˌalkəˈholik) 1. pertaining to alcohol. 2. a person addicted to excessive, uncontrolled alcohol consumption. This results in loss of appetite and vitamin B deficiency, leading to peripheral neuritis with eye changes and cirrhosis of the liver, and to progressive deterioration in the personality.

alcoholism (ˈalkəhoˌlizəm) the state of poisoning resulting from alcoholic addiction.

aldosterone (ˌaldohˈstiə·rohn, alˈdostəˌrohn) a compound, isolated from the adrenal cortex, that aids the retention of sodium and the excretion of potassium in the body, and by so doing aids the maintenance of electrolyte balance. *A. antagonists* a group of drugs which block the action of aldosterone.

aldosteronism (alˈdostə·rəˌnizəm) an excess secretion of aldosterone caused by an adrenal neoplasm. The serum potassium is low, and the patient has hypertension and severe muscular weakness.

aleukaemia (ˌaylooˈkeemi·ə) an acute condition in which there is an absence or deficiency of white cells in the blood.

Alexander technique (aləks·ˈandəˌtekˈneek) *Frederick M. Alexander, Australian actor and physiotherapist, 1869–1955.* A process of psychophysical postural re-education. Body posture is believed to affect physical and psychological wellbeing and the postural re-education process aims to assist individuals in monitoring how they consciously use their bodies to promote good health.

alexia (əˈleksi·ə, ay-) a form of aphasia in which there is an inability to recognise written or printed words. Word blindness.

algorithm (ˈalgəˌrithəm) a process or set of rules used in calculations, e.g.

of medications, or for other problem-solving. Computer programs are the most familiar examples of algorithms in everyday use.

alienation (ˌayli·əˈnayshən) a feeling of estrangement or separation from others or from self. A symptom of schizophrenia. Sufferers often believe that they are under the control of someone else. *See* DEPERSONALISATION.

alignment (əˈlienmənt) the state of being arranged in a line, i.e. in the correct anatomical position.

aliment (ˈaləmənt) food or nourishment.

alimentary (ˌaləˈmentə·ree, -tree) relating to the system of nutrition. *A. canal* or *tract* the passage through which food passes, from mouth to anus. *A. system* the alimentary tract together with the liver and other organs concerned in digestion and absorption.

alimentation (ˌalə mənˈtayshən) the giving or receiving of nourishment. The process of supplying the patient's need for nutrition.

alkalaemia (ˌalkəˈleemi·ə) an increase in the alkali content of the blood. *See* ALKALOSIS.

alkali (ˈalkəˌlie) a substance capable of uniting with acids to form salts, and with fats and fatty acids to form soaps. Alkaline solutions turn red litmus paper blue. *A. reserve* the ability of the combined buffer systems of the blood to neutralise acid. The pH of the blood is normally slightly on the alkaline side, between 7.35 and 7.45. The principal buffer in the blood is bicarbonate; the alkali reserve is essentially represented by the plasma bicarbonate concentration.

alkaline (ˈalkəˌlien) having the reactions of an alkali. *A. phosphatase* an enzyme localised on cell membranes that hydrolyses phosphate esters, liberating inorganic phosphate, and has an optimal pH of about 10.0. Serum alkaline phosphatase activity is elevated in obstructive jaundice and bone disease.

alkalinity (ˌalkəˈlinətee) 1. the quality of being alkaline. 2. the combining power of a base, expressed as the maximum number of equivalents of acid with which it reacts to form a salt.

alkaloid (ˈalkəˌloyd) one of a group of active nitrogenous compounds that are alkaline in solution. They usually have a bitter taste and are characterised by powerful physiological activity. Examples are morphine, cocaine, atropine, quinine, nicotine and caffeine. The term is also applied to synthetic substances that have structures similar to plant alkaloids, such as procaine.

alkalosis (ˌalkəˈlohsəs) an increase in the alkali reserve in the blood. It may be confirmed by estimation of the blood carbon dioxide content and treated by giving normal saline or ammonium chloride intravenously to encourage the excretion of bicarbonate by the kidneys.

alkylating agent (ˈalkəˌlayting ˈayjənt) a drug that damages the deoxyribonucleic acid (DNA) molecule of the nucleus of the cell. Many are nitrogen mustard preparations and may be termed 'chromosome poisons'; they are used in cancer chemotherapy.

all-or-none law (awl aw nun law) a principle stating that in individual cardiac and skeletal muscle fibres, there are only two possible reactions to a stimulus: either there is no reaction at all or there is a full reaction, with no gradation of response according to the strength of the stimulus. Whole muscles can grade their response by increasing or decreasing the number of fibres involved.

allantois (əˈlantoh·s) a membranous sac projecting from the ventral surface of the fetus in its early stages. It eventually helps to form the placenta.

allele (ˈaleel, əˈleel) allelomorph. One of a pair of genes that occupy the same relative positions on homologous chromosomes and produce different effects on the same process of development.

allelomorph (əˈleeləˌmawf) allele.

Allen test (ˈalən ˌtest) used to test the blood supply to the hand, specifically for the patency of the radial and ulnar arteries. It is performed prior to radial arterial sampling or cannulation.

allergen (ˈaləˌjən) a substance that may produce an allergy or manifestation of an immune response.

allergic rhinitis (ˈaləˌjik rieˈnietəs) a common condition where there is inflammation of the inside of the nose caused by an allergen such as pollen, dust, mould or animal skin. *See also* HAY FEVER.

allergy (ˈaləjee) a hypersensitivity to some foreign substances that are normally harmless but which produce a violent reaction in the patient. Asthma, hay fever, angioneurotic oedema, migraine and some types of urticaria and eczema are allergic states. *See* ANAPHYLAXIS.

allied health (ˈalied helth) a group of healthcare services distinct from nursing, medicine and dentistry, such as occupational therapy, speech pathology and physiotherapy, provided by licensed professionals.

allocate (ˈaləˌkayt) to assign for a particular purpose.

allocation (ˌaləˈkayshən) the act of allocating. *Clinical a.* a period of time spent in a ward/department/unit where there are patients/clients. *Patient a.* one nurse is designated as responsible for the care of one patient or a group of patients for a spell of duty. *Task a.* patient care in a ward/unit is provided by a group of nurses. Each nurse is allocated specific nursing activities.

allograft (ˈalləˌgrahft) an organ or tissue transplanted from one person to another of a dissimilar genotype but of the same species. *Non-viable a.* skin, taken from a cadaver, which cannot regenerate. *Viable a.* living tissue transplanted. *See* HOMOGRAFT.

alloimmunisation (ˈalləˌimyənieˈ-zayshən) the immune response to donated blood, bone marrow or transplanted organ; Rh-negative pregnant women with an Rh-positive fetus can become alloimmunised following a sensitising event, e.g. antepartum haemorrhage or miscarriage, through the development of antibodies that target the foreign material, causing haemolytic disease of the newborn.

allopathy (ˌaloˈpəthee) the practice of conventional medicine, i.e. with drugs having opposite effects to the symptoms.

alopecia (ˌaləˈpeeshi·ə) baldness. Loss of hair. The cause of simple baldness is not yet fully understood, although it is known that the tendency to become bald is limited almost entirely to males, runs in certain families and is more common in certain racial groups than in others. Baldness is often associated with ageing. *A. areata* hair loss in sharply defined areas, usually the scalp or beard. *Cicatricial a., a. cicatrisata* irreversible loss of hair associated with scarring, usually on the scalp. Also known as scarring alopecia. *Male-pattern a.* loss of scalp hair, genetically determined and androgen dependent, beginning with frontal recession and progressing symmetrically to leave, ultimately, only a sparse peripheral rim of hair.

alpha (ˈalfə) the first letter of the Greek alphabet, a. *A. cells* cells found in the islet of Langerhans in the pancreas. They produce the hormone glucagon. *A. fetoprotein (AFP)* a plasma protein originating in the fetal liver and gastrointestinal tract. The serum AFP level is used to monitor the effectiveness of cancer treatment; the amniotic fluid AFP level is used in the prenatal diagnosis of neural tube defects. *A. receptors* tissue receptors associated with the stimulation (contraction) of smooth muscle.

alternative medicine (awlˈtərnətiv ˌmedəsən) a form of medicine differing from conventional healthcare. Consists of a range of treatments essentially based on a holistic approach to health and wellbeing, including homeopathy, aromatherapy, hypnosis, naturopathy, acupuncture and others. These therapies fall into three categories: (a) touch and movement; (b) medicinal; and (c) psychological. Commonly called complementary therapies. *See* COMPLEMENTARY.

altitude sickness (ˌaltəˌtyood ˈsiknəs) a condition caused by hypoxia that occurs as a result of lower oxygen pressure at high altitudes before acclimatisation to the increased altitude.

altruism (ˈaltrooˌizəm) a sense of unconditional concern for the welfare of others.

aluminium (ˌalyəˈmini·əm, ˌalə-) symbol Al. A silver-white metal with a low specific gravity, compounds of which are astringent and antiseptic. *A. hydroxide* compound used as an antacid in the treatment of gastric conditions.

alveolar (ˌalviˈohlə) concerning an alveolus, or air sac of the lung. *A. air* air found in the alveoli.

alveolitis (ˌalviohˈlietəs) inflammation of the alveoli. *Extrinsic allergic a.* inflammation of the alveoli caused by inhalation of an antigen, such as pollen.

Alzheimer's cells (ˈalts·hieməz ˌsels) *Aloysius Alzheimer, German neurologist, 1864–1915.* 1. giant astrocytes with large prominent nuclei found in the brain in hepatolenticular degeneration and hepatic comas. 2. degenerated astrocytes.

Alzheimer's disease (ˈalts·hieməz diˈzeez) a progressive form of neuronal degeneration in the brain and the most common cause of dementia in people of all ages. It is more common in older than younger people and is not just a form of presenile dementia, as was originally thought. The degeneration of neurones is accompanied by changes in the brain's biochemistry. At present this condition is irreversible and there is no effective treatment. The most important aspect of treatment is the provision of appropriate nursing and social care for sufferers, together with ongoing support for their families.

amalgam (ə'malgəm) a compound of mercury and other metals. *Dental a.* now rarely used for filling teeth.

amaurosis (ˌamaw'rohsəs) loss of vision resulting from a systemic cause, such as disease of the optic nerve or brain, diabetes or renal disease. The visual loss may be partial or complete, temporary or permanent.

ambidextrous (ˌambi'dekstrəs) equally skilful with either hand.

ambivalence (am'bivələns) the existence of contradictory emotional feelings towards an object, commonly of love and hate for another person. If these feelings occur to a marked degree, they lead to psychological disturbance.

amblyopia (ˌambli'ohpi·ə) dimness of vision without any apparent lesion of the eye. Uncorrectable by optical means.

ambulant ('ambyələnt) able to walk.

ambulatory (ˌambyə'laytə·ree) having the capacity to walk. *A. treatment* or *care* health services provided on an outpatient or day care basis.

amelioration (əˌmeelyə'rayshən) improvement of symptoms; a lessening of the severity of a disease.

amenorrhoea (aˌmenə'reeə, ayˌ-men-) the absence of menstruation. *Primary a.* the non-occurrence of the menses. *Secondary a.* the cessation of the menses after they have been established, owing to disease or pregnancy.

Ames test (aymz ˌtest) a biological assay to assess the mutagenic potential of chemical compounds. A positive test indicates that the chemical is mutagenic and therefore may act as a carcinogen, since cancer is often linked to mutation.

Essential Amino Acids
1. Threonine
2. Lysine
3. Methionine
4. Valine
5. Phenylalanine
6. Leucine
7. Tryptophan
8. Isoleucine
9. Histidine

ametropia (ˌaymə'trohpi·ə) defective vision. A general word applied to incorrect refraction.

amino acid (ə'meenoh 'asəd) a chemical compound containing both NH_2 and COOH groups. The end product of protein digestion. *Essential a. a.* one required for replacement and growth but which cannot be synthesised in the body in sufficient amounts and which must therefore be obtained in the diet (*see* table). Histidine is also essential in childhood. *Non-essential a. a.* one necessary for proper growth but that can be synthesised in the body and is therefore not specifically required in the diet. (*See* table above.).

aminoglycoside (ə'meenoh'gliekəˌsied) any of a group of bacterial antibiotics, derived from various species of *Streptomyces*, that interfere with the function of bacterial ribosomes. The aminoglycosides include gentamicin, netilmicin, streptomycin, tobramycin, amikacin, kanamycin and neomycin. They are used to treat infections caused by Gram-negative organisms and are classified as bactericidal agents because of their interference with bacterial replication. All the aminoglycoside antibiotics are highly toxic, requiring monitoring of blood serum levels and careful observation of the patient for early signs of toxicity, particularly ototoxicity and nephrotoxicity.

amitosis (ˌaməˈtohsəs) multiplication of cells by simple division or fission.

ammonia (əˈmohni·ə) NH_3. A naturally occurring compound of nitrogen and hydrogen formed by the decomposition of proteins and amino acids. Converted into urea by the liver.

amnesia (amˈneezi·ə, amˈneezha) partial or complete loss of memory. *Anterograde a.* loss of memory of events that have taken place since an injury or illness. *Retrograde a.* loss of memory for events prior to an injury or illness. It often applies to the time immediately preceding an accident.

amniocentesis (ˌamneeohsənˈteesəs) the withdrawal of fluid from the uterus through the abdominal wall by means of a syringe and needle and ultrasound (*see* figure below). It is primarily used in the diagnosis of chromosome disorders in the fetus and in cases of hydramnios. Mothers who are Rh-negative should be given a reduced dose of anti-D immunoglobulin after the procedure to prevent them making antibodies.

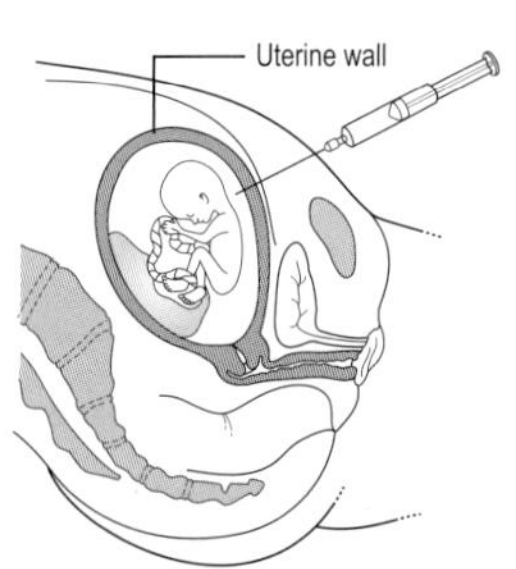

Amniocentesis.

amniography (ˌamneeˈogrəfee) radiography of the gravid uterus.

amnion (ˈamni·ən) the innermost membrane enveloping the fetus and enclosing the liquor amnii, or amniotic fluid.

amniotic (ˌamneeˈotik) pertaining to the amnion. *A. fluid* the albuminous fluid contained in the amniotic sac, liquor amnii.

amoeba (əˈmeebə) a minute unicellular protozoon. It is able to move by pushing out parts of itself (called pseudopodia). Capable of reproduction by amitotic fission. Infection of the intestines by *Entamoeba histolytica* causes ‘amoebic dysentery’.

amoebiasis (ˌamiˈbieəsəs) infection with amoeba, particularly *Entamoeba histolytica*.

amoebic (əˌmeebik) pertaining to, caused by, or of the nature of an amoeba. *A. abscess* an abscess cavity of the liver resulting from liquefaction necrosis due to entrance of *Entamoeba histolytica* into the portal circulation in amoebiasis; amoebic abscesses may affect the lung, brain and spleen. *A. dysentery* a form of dysentery caused by *Entamoeba histolytica* and spread by contaminated food, water and flies; also called amoebiasis. Amoebic dysentery is mainly a tropical disease, but many cases occur in temperate countries. Symptoms are diarrhoea, fatigue and intestinal bleeding. Complications include involvement of the liver, liver abscess and pulmonary abscess.

amoeboid (əˈmeeboyd) resembling an amoeba in structure or movement.

amorphous (əˈmawfəs) without definite shape. The term may be applied to fine powdery particles, as opposed to crystals.

amphiarthrosis (ˌamfeeahˈthrohsəs) a form of joint in which the bones are joined together by fibrocartilage, e.g. the junctions of the vertebrae.

amphoric (amˈfor·ik) pertaining to a bottle. Used to describe the sound sometimes heard on auscultation over cavities in the lungs, which resembles that produced by blowing across the mouth of a bottle.

ampoule (ˈampyool) a small glass or plastic phial in which sterile saline, water or drugs of specified dose for injection are sealed.

ampulla (amˈpuhlə) the flask-like dilatation of a canal, e.g. of a uterine tube.

amputation (ˌampyəˈtayshən) the surgical removal of a limb or other part of the body, e.g. the breast.

amputee (ˌampyəˈtee) a person who has had one or more limbs amputated.

amylase (ˈaməˌlayz) an enzyme that reduces starch to maltose. Found in saliva (ptyalin) and pancreatic juice (amylopsin).

amyloid (ˈaməˌloyd) 1. pertaining to starch. 2. a waxy starch-like material that is a complex protein forming in tissues and organs leading to disturbances of function called amyloidosis.

amylopsin (ˌaməˈlopsən) an enzyme found in the pancreas. *See* AMYLASE.

amylum (ˈamələm) [L.] starch.

amyotonia (ayˌmieohˈtohni·ə) atonic condition of the muscles. *A. congenita* any of several rare congenital diseases marked by general hypotonia of the muscles. Also called Oppenheim's disease or floppy baby syndrome.

anabolic (ˌanəˈbolik) relating to anabolism. *A. compound* a substance that aids in the repair of body tissue, particularly protein. Androgens may be used in this way. *A. steroid* a synthetic steroid hormone derived from testosterone or prepared synthetically to promote general body growth. Used in medicine to treat some forms of weight loss, to increase appetite or to promote muscle growth. Also known as anabolic–androgenic steroids (AAS).

anabolism (əˈnabəˌlizəm) the building up or synthesis of cell structure from digested food materials. See METABOLISM.

anacidity (ˌanəˈsidətee) a decrease in normal acidity.

anaclitic (ˌanəˈklitik) denoting the dependence of the infant on the mother or mother-substitute for its sense of wellbeing. *A. choice* a psychoanalytical term for the adult selection of a loved one who closely resembles one's mother (or another adult on whom one depended as a child). *A. depression* severe and progressive depression found in children who have lost their mothers and have not found a suitable substitute.

anacrotism (əˈnakrəˌtizəm) an abnormal pulse evidenced by the presence of a prominent notch on the ascending limb of the pulse wave tracing.

anaemia (əˈneemi·ə) a deficiency in either quality or quantity of red corpuscles in the blood that reduces the oxygen-carrying capacity of the blood, giving rise especially to symptoms of anoxaemia. There is pallor, breathlessness on exertion with palpitations, lassitude, headache, giddiness and often a history of poor resistance to infection. Anaemia may be due to many different causes. Increasingly, with the advent of electronic cell counters, anaemia is now classified according to the morphological characteristics of the erythrocytes. *Aplastic a.* the bone marrow is unable to produce red blood corpuscles. A rare condition. *Deficiency a.* any type that is due to the lack of the necessary factors for red cell formation, e.g. hormones or vitamins. *Haemolytic a.* a variety in which there is excessive destruction of red blood corpuscles caused by antibody formation in the blood (*see* RH FACTOR) by drugs or by severe toxaemia, as in extensive burns. *Iron-deficiency a.* the most common type of anaemia; due to a lack of absorbable iron in the diet. It may also be due to excessive or chronic blood loss, or to poor absorption of dietary iron. *Macrocytic a.* a type in which the cells are larger than normal; present in pernicious anaemia. *Microcytic a.* a variety in which the cells are smaller than normal, as in iron deficiency. *Pernicious a.* a variety caused by the inability of the stomach to secrete the intrinsic factor necessary for the absorption of vitamin B_{12} from the diet. *Sickle-cell a.* a hereditary haemolytic anaemia seen most commonly in people living in or originating from the Caribbean islands, Africa, Asia, the Middle East and the Mediterranean. The red blood cells are sickle shaped. *Splenic a.* a congenital, familial disease in which the red blood cells are fragile and easily broken down.

anaerobe (ˈanəˌrohb) a microorganism that can live and thrive in the absence of free oxygen. These organisms are found in body cavities or wounds where the oxygen tension is very low. Examples are the bacilli of tetanus and gas gangrene.

anaesthesia (ˌanəsˈtheezi·ə) loss of feeling or sensation in a part or in the whole of the body, usually induced by drugs. *Basal a.* basal narcosis. Loss of consciousness, although supplemental drugs have to be given to ensure complete anaesthesia. *Epidural a.* injection into the extradural space between the vertebral spines and beneath the ligamentum flavum. *General a.* unconsciousness produced by inhalation or injection of a drug. *Inhalation a.* drugs or gas are administered by a face mask or endotracheal tube to cause general anaesthesia. *Intravenous a.* unconsciousness is produced by the introduction of a drug into a vein. *Local a.* local analgesia. Nerve conduction is blocked by injection of a local anaesthetic, by freezing with ethyl chloride or by topical application. *Spinal a.* injection of an anaesthetic agent into the spinal subarachnoid space.

anaesthetic (ˌanəsˈthetik) a drug causing anaesthesia.

anaesthetist (əˈneesthətist) a person who is medically qualified to administer an anaesthetic and in the techniques of life support for the critically ill or injured.

anal (ˈaynˈl) pertaining to the anus. *A. eroticism* sexual pleasure derived from anal functions. *A. fissure see* FISSURE. *A. fistula see* FISTULA. *A. stage* the second stage of a child's psychosexual development, characterised by the child's sensual interest in the anal area and the passing or retention of faeces.

analeptic (ˌanəˈleptik) a drug that stimulates the central nervous system.

analgesia (ˌanəlˈjeezi·ə) insensibility to pain, especially the relief of pain without causing unconsciousness. *Patient controlled a.* a preset dose of analgesic, which the patient controls according to need. In-built safety measures prevent accidental overdose.

analgesic (ˌanəlˈjeezik, -sik) 1. relating to analgesia. 2. a remedy that relieves pain. *A. cocktail* an individualised mixture of drugs used to control pain.

analogue (ˈanəˌlog) 1. an organ with a different structure and origin to, but the same function as, another organ. 2. a compound with a similar structure to another but differing in respect of a particular element.

analysis (əˈnaləsəs) 1. the act of determining the component parts of a substance. 2. in psychiatry, a method of trying to understand the complex mental processes, experiences and relationships with other individuals or groups of individuals to determine the reasons for an individual's behaviour. *A. of covariance (ANCOVA)* a statistic that measures differences among group means and uses a statistical technique to equate the groups under study in relation to another given variable. *A. of variance (ANOVA)* a statistic that tests whether groups differ from each other, rather than testing each pair of means separately. ANOVA considers the variation among all groups.

anaphase (ˈanəˌfayz) part of the process of mitosis or meiosis.

anaphylaxis (ˌanəfəˈlaksəs) anaphylactic shock. A severe reaction, often fatal, occurring in response to drugs, e.g. penicillin, but also to bee stings and food allergy, e.g. nuts in sensitive individuals. The symptoms are severe dyspnoea, rapid pulse, profuse sweating and collapse.

anaplasia (ˌanəˈplayzi·ə) a change in the character of cells, seen in tumour tissue.

anarthria (anˈahthri·ə) the inability to articulate speech sounds owing to a brain lesion or damage to peripheral nerves innervating articulatory muscles.

anastomosis (əˌnastəˈmohsəs) in surgery, any artificial connection of two hollow structures, e.g. gastroenterostomy. In anatomy, the joining of the branches of two blood vessels.

anatomy (əˈnatəmee) the science of the structure of the body.

Ancylostoma (ˌansiˈlostəmə) hookworm. A genus of nematode roundworms which may inhabit the duodenum and cause extreme anaemia and malnutrition. *A. duodenale* a hookworm, very widespread in tropical and subtropical areas.

androgen (ˈandrəˌjən) one of a group of hormones secreted by the testes and adrenal cortex. They are steroids which can be synthesised and produce the secondary male characteristics and the building up of protein tissue. *A. insensitivity syndrome (AIS)* a rare genetic condition that affects the development of a child's genitals and reproductive organs.

android (ˈandroyd) resembling a man. *A. pelvis* a female pelvis shaped like a male pelvis with a wedge-shaped entrance and narrow anterior segment.

anencephaly (ˌanənˈkefəlee, -ˈsef-) congenital absence of the cranial vault, with the cerebral hemispheres completely missing or reduced to small masses.

anergy (ˈanˌəjee) 1. a specific immunological tolerance in which T-cells fail to respond normally. The state can be reversed. 2. tiredness, lethargy, lack of energy.

aneurine (ˈanyəˌreen) thiamine. An essential vitamin involved in carbohydrate metabolism. The main sources are unrefined cereals and pork, vitamin B_1.

aneurysm (ˈanyəˌrizəm) a local dilatation of a blood vessel, usually an artery (*see* figure below). Atherosclerosis is responsible for most arterial aneurysms; any injury to the arterial wall may predispose to the formation of a sac. Aneurysms are common in the aorta, but may also occur in peripheral vessels. A sign of a large aneurysm is a pulsating swelling that produces a blowing murmur on auscultation. *Dissecting a.* a condition in which longitudinal splitting occurs between the outer and middle layers of the vascular wall. Most commonly seen in the aorta and is a result of bleeding into the weakened wall separating the layers of the wall. *Fusiform a.* a spindle-shaped arterial aneurysm. *Saccular a.* a dilatation of only a part of the circumference of an artery.

angina (anˈjienə) 1. a tight strangling sensation or pain. 2. an inflammation of the throat causing pain on swallowing. *A. cruris* intermittent claudication; severe pain in the leg after walking. *A. pectoris* cardiac pain that occurs on exertion owing to insufficient blood supply to the heart muscles. *Vincent's a.* infection and ulceration of the tonsils by a spirochaete, *Borrelia vincentii*, and a bacillus, *Fusobacterium fusiformis*.

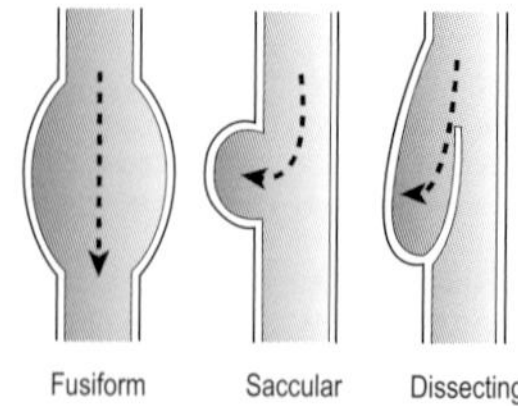

Types of aneurysm.

angiocardiography (ˌanjeeohˌkahdeeˈogrəfee) the radiological examination of the heart and large blood vessels by means of cardiac catheterisation and an opaque contrast medium.

angio-oedema (ˈanjeeoh ohˈdeemə) a type of reaction; most commonly caused by an allergy, characterised by well-defined swellings or wheals of sudden and rapid onset in the skin, throat, mouth, eyes and other areas. Fatal oedema of the glottis may occur, resulting in a medical emergency. *See* OEDEMA.

angiography (ˌanjeeˈogrəfee) the radiological examination of the blood vessels using an opaque contrast medium.

angioma (ˌanjeeˈohmə) a benign tumour composed of dilated blood vessels.

angioneurosis (ˌanjeeohnyəˈrohsəs) a neurosis affecting the blood vessels, which may produce paralysis.

angioneurotic (ˌanjeeohnyəˈrotik) pertaining to angioneurosis. *A. oedema see* OEDEMA.

angioplasty (ˌanjeeohˌplastee) surgery of a narrowed artery to promote the normal flow of blood. *Balloon a.* a technique in which a catheter with an elastic, flexible (balloon-like) tip that can be inflated is used to widen the narrowed blood vessel, e.g. in the heart. Usually a stent is inserted to keep the artery open. Stents have now been developed coated in slow-release drugs that reduce further risk of arterial narrowing. *See* STENT.

angiosarcoma (ˌanjeeohsahˈkohmə) a malignant vascular growth.

angiospasm (ˈanjeeohˌspazəm) a spasmodic contraction of an artery, causing cramping of the muscles.

angiotensin (ˌanjeeohˈtensən) a substance that raises the blood pressure. It is a polypeptide produced by the action of renin on plasma globulins.

angle of Louis (angəl ov luəs) *see* STERNAL ANGLE OF LOUIS.

anhidrosis (ˌanhəˈdrohsəs) a marked deficiency in the secretion of sweat.

anhidrotic (ˌanhəˈdrotik) an agent that decreases perspiration. An adiaphoretic.

anhydraemia (ˌanhieˈdreemi·ə) a deficiency of water in the blood.

aniline (ˈanəˌleen, -lən) a chemical compound derived from coal tar, used for making antiseptic dyes. It is an important cause of serious industrial poisoning associated with bone marrow depression as well as methaemoglobinaemia.

anima (ˈanimə) 1. the soul. 2. Jung's term for the unconscious or inner being of the individual, as opposed to the personality presented to the world (persona). In Jungian psychoanalysis, the more feminine soul or feminine component of a man's personality.

aniridia (anˈi·ridee·ə) lack of part or the whole of the iris.

anisocoria (anˌiesohˈkoh·ri·ə) inequality of diameter of the pupils of the two eyes.

anisocytosis (anˌiesohsieˈtohsəs) inequality in the size of the red blood cells.

anisometropia (anˌiesohməˈtrohpi·ə) a marked difference in the refractive power of the two eyes.

ankle (ˈangkəl) the joint between the leg and foot, formed by the tibia and fibula articulating with the talus.

ankle–brachial pressure index (ABPI) (ˈankəl ˈbrakee'l preshə indeks) the measurement of the ratio of systolic blood pressure at the ankle, measured by a Doppler ultrasound probe, to that measured at the brachial artery to quantify the degree of arterial occlusion in the leg. Forms an important part of a leg ulcer assessment regarding the patient's suitability for compression bandaging.

ankyloblepharon (ˌangkəlohˈblefə-·ron) adhesions and scar tissue on the ciliary borders of the eyelids, giving the eye a distorted appearance.

ankylosing spondylitis (ˌangkəˈlohzˈhing ˌspondəˈlohetəs) a chronic condition in which there is inflammation of the spine and other areas of the body leading to back pain and stiffness, pain and swelling of other parts of the body and extreme tiredness. The cause is unknown, but there may be a genetic link.

ankylosis (ˌangkəˈlohsəs) consolidation, immobility and stiffness of a joint as a result of disease.

ANMAC *see* AUSTRALIAN NURSING AND MIDWIFERY ACCREDITATION COUNCIL.

annular (ˈanyələ) ring-shaped.

anoci-association (aˌnohseeə-ˌsohseeˈayshən, -ˌsohshi-) the exclusion of pain, fear and shock in surgical operations, brought about by means of local anaesthesia and basal narcosis.

anodyne (ˈanəˌdien) 1. pain-relieving or relaxing. 2. a drug or other treatment that relieves pain.

anomaly (əˈnoməlee) considerable variation from the normal.

anomie (ˈanəmee) a feeling of hopelessness and lack of purpose.

Anopheles (əˈnofəˌleez) a genus of mosquito. Many are carriers of the malarial parasite and their bite can infect humans. Other species transmit FILARIASIS.

anophthalmia (ˌanofˈthalmee·ə) the congenital absence of one or both eyes.

anorchism (anˈawkizəm) a condition in which the testicles have failed to develop or to descend.

anorexia (ˌanəˈreksee·ə) loss of appetite for food. *A. nervosa* a condition in which there is complete lack of appetite, with extreme emaciation. It is due to psychological causes and most commonly occurs in young women with poor self-esteem or fear of obesity associated with a distorted body image, leading them to perceive themselves as fat and to take extreme forms of dietary control in order to lose weight.

anosmia (anˈozmi·ə) loss of the sense of smell.

ANOVA *see* ANALYSIS OF VARIANCE.

anovular (anˈovyələ) applied to the absence of ovulation. Usually refers to uterine bleeding when there has been no ovulation, the result of taking contraceptive pills.

anoxaemia (ˌanokˈseemi·ə) a complete lack of oxygen in the blood.

anoxia (anˈoksi·ə) lack of oxygen to an organ or tissue.

antacid (antˈasəd) a substance neutralising acidity, particularly of the gastric juices.

antagonist (anˈtagənəst) 1. a muscle that has an opposite action to another, e.g. the biceps to the triceps. 2. in pharmacology, a drug that inhibits the action of another drug or enzyme, e.g. methotrexate is a folic acid antagonist. 3. in dentistry, a tooth in one jaw opposing one in the other jaw.

antecubital (ˌanteeˈkyoobətəl) at the bend of the elbow.

anteflexion (ˌanteeˈflekshən) a bending forward, as of the body of the uterus. *See* RETROFLEXION.

antenatal (ˌanteeˈnayt'l) before birth. *A. care* care provided by midwives, general practitioners and obstetricians during pregnancy. Deviations from normal can be detected and treated early. The mother and support person can be prepared for labour and parenthood and health education offered. WHO recommends that during pregnancy a mother should receive antenatal care on at least four occasions. In Australia, National Clinical Practice Guidelines on Pregnancy Care provide evidence-based recommendations to support high quality, safe antenatal care in all settings. The guidelines also cover core practices in antenatal care and also provides specific approaches on improving the experience of antenatal care for Aboriginal and Torres Strait Islander women, migrants and refugee women and women with severe mental illness.

antepartum (ˌanteeˈpahtəm) shortly before birth, i.e. in the last 3 months of pregnancy. *A. haemorrhage* bleeding from the uterus during pregnancy that occurs before the onset of labour. *See* PLACENTA PRAEVIA.

anterior (anˈtiə·ri·ə) situated at or facing towards the front. The opposite of posterior. *A. capsule* the anterior covering of the lens of the eye. *A. chamber of the eye* the space between the cornea in front and the iris and lens behind. *A. fontanel* a diamond-shaped unossified area between the frontal and two parietal bones just above an infant's forehead at the junction of the coronal and sagittal sutures. *See* FONTANEL.

anterograde (ˈantə·roh͵grayd) extending or moving forwards.

anteversion (͵anteeˈvərzhən) the forward tilting of an organ, e.g. the normal position of the uterus. *See* RETROVERSION.

anthelmintic (anthelminthic) (͵ant-helˈmintik, ͵anthel-) 1. destructive to worms. 2. an agent destructive to worms.

anthracosis (͵anthrəˈkohsəs) a disease of the lungs, caused by inhalation of coal dust; a form of pneumoconiosis. Also known as Miner's lung.

anthrax (ˈanthraks) an acute, notifiable, infectious disease due to *Bacillus anthracis*, acquired through contact with infected animals or their by-products.

anthropoid (ˈanthrə͵poyd) resembling a human. *A. pelvis* female pelvis in which the anteroposterior diameter exceeds the transverse diameter.

anthropology (͵anthrəˈpoləjee) the study of human beings that focuses on origins, historical and cultural development, and races. *Cultural a.* that branch of anthropology concerned with individuals and their relationship to others and to their environment. *Medical a.* biocultural discipline concerned with both the biological and the sociocultural aspects of human behaviour, and the ways in which the two interact to influence health and disease. *Physical a.* that branch of anthropology that concerns the physical and evolutionary characteristics of human beings.

anthropometry (͵anthrəˈpomətree) the science that deals with the comparative measurement of parts of the human body, such as height, weight, body fat, etc.

anti-D gamma globulin (͵anteeˈdee ˈgamə ˈglobyələn) an antibody that is given by intramuscular injection to an Rh-negative woman within 72 hours of delivery of her infant or following termination of her pregnancy, miscarriage or invasive investigations such as AMNIOCENTESIS, to prevent haemolytic disease of the newborn in the next pregnancy. Anti-D is also available to all Rh-negative women as antenatal prophylaxis. Also called Rhesus factor. *See* RH FACTOR.

anti-inflammatory (͵anteeˈinflamətree) a drug that reduces or acts against inflammation. May belong to one of several groups.

antiarrhythmic (͵antee·ayˈrithmik) an agent used to treat cardiac arrhythmias.

antibacterial (͵anteebakˈtiə·ri·əl) a substance that destroys or suppresses the growth of bacteria.

antibiotic (͵anteebieˈotik) substances (e.g. penicillin), produced by certain bacteria and fungi, that prevent the growth of, or destroy, other bacteria. *A. resistance* the evolution and survival, as a result of worldwide antibiotic misuse, of bacteria undergoing the process of natural selection, despite the use of antibiotics to which they were once sensitive.

antibody (ˈantee͵bodee) also known as immunoglobulin, an antibody is one of a group of these glycoprotein molecules found either on the cell surface of B lymphocytes (membrane antibody), where they act as antigen receptors, or produced and secreted by B lymphocytes that have been stimulated and transformed by an antigen into plasma cells. Secreted antibodies are found in blood, serum and in other body fluids and tissues.

Antibodies react and combine with specific antigens during humoral immune responses, forming immune complexes. Antibodies are an important component of acquired (learned) immunity. There are five different types or classes of antibody, each named by the abbreviation for immunoglobulin (Ig) and a letter of the alphabet, i.e. IgM, IgG, IgA, IgD and IgE. IgG (also called GAMMA GLOBULIN) is the most abundant of the five classes of antibody and is the major immunoglobulin in the secondary humoral immune response.

anticholinergic (ˌanteeˌkohlinˈərjik) a drug that inhibits the action of acetylcholine.

anticholinesterase (ˌanteeˌkohlə-ˈnestəˌrayz) an enzyme that inhibits the action of the enzyme acetylcholinesterase, thereby potentiating the action of acetylcholine at postsynaptic receptors in the parasympathetic nervous system, thus allowing return of normal muscle contraction.

anticoagulant (ˌanteekohˈagyələnt) a substance that prevents or delays blood from clotting, e.g. warfarin or heparin. New anticoagulants are available and becoming increasingly common, requiring less frequent blood monitoring.

anticonvulsant (ˌanteekənˈvulsənt) a substance that arrests or prevents convulsions. Anticonvulsant drugs such as phenytoin are used in the treatment of epilepsy and other conditions in which convulsions occur.

antidepressant (ˌanteedəˈpresənt) one of a group of drugs which elevate mood, often diminish anxiety and increase coping behaviour. Tricyclic antidepressants and selective serotonin reuptake inhibitors (SSRIs) are most commonly used in the treatment of depression. These drugs are usually successful in relieving the symptoms of depression, but may take 2–3 weeks before any improvement is noted. Antidepressant drugs are not addictive, but abrupt withdrawal may result in physical symptoms and should be avoided.

anti-discriminatory practice (antee dəsˈkrimənətəri ˈpraktis) the professional policies, practice and provisions that actively seek to reduce institutional discrimination experienced by individuals and groups, particularly on the grounds of age, race, gender, disability, social class or sexual orientation. Anti-discriminatory practice can utilise particular legislation, such as the *Sex Discrimination Act 1984 (Cwlth)* and the *Disability Discrimination Act 1992 (Cwlth)* to challenge discrimination.

antidiuretic (ˌanteeˌdieyəˈretik) a substance that reduces the volume of urine excreted. *A. hormone (ADH)* a hormone which is secreted by the posterior pituitary gland. vasopressin.

antidote (ˈantəˌdoht) an agent that counteracts the effect of a poison.

antiembolic (ˌantee·emˈbolik) against embolism. Antiembolic hose/stockings are worn to prevent the formation or decrease the risk of deep vein thrombosis, especially in patients after surgery or those confined to bed.

antiemetic (ˌantee·əˈmetik) a drug that prevents or overcomes nausea and vomiting.

antifungal (ˌantiˈfungˈgəl) a preparation effective in treating fungal infections.

antigen (ˈantəˌjen, -jən) any substance, bacterial or otherwise, which in suitable conditions may stimulate the production of an immune response.

antiglobulin (ˌanteeˈglobyələn) an antibody against human globulin.

antihaemophilic (ˌanteeˌheemohˈfilik) 1. effective against the bleeding tendency in HAEMOPHILIA. 2. an agent that counteracts the bleeding tendency in haemophilia. *A. factor (AHF)* one of the clotting factors, deficiency of which causes classic, sex-linked haemophilia; also called Factor VIII and antihaemophilic globulin (AHG). It is available in a preparation for preventive and therapeutic use.

antihistamine (ˌanteeˈhistəˌmeen, -min) any one of a group of drugs which block the tissue receptors for histamine. They are used to treat allergic conditions, e.g. drug rashes, hay fever and serum sickness, and include promethazine.

antihypertensive (ˌanteeˌhiepəˈtensiv) 1. effective against hypertension. 2. an agent that reduces high blood pressure.

antimalarial (ˌanteeˈmalairee'l) against malaria. Drugs that are used both in the treatment of an attack and for prophylaxis. All visitors to countries where malaria is rife should take preventative antimalarial drugs. Expert advice should be sought regarding the appropriate drug and dose. *See* MALARIA.

antimetabolite (ˌanteemeˈtabəliet) one of a group of chemical compounds which prevent the effective utilisation of the corresponding metabolite, and interfere with normal growth or cell mitosis if the process requires that metabolite.

antimycotic (ˌanteemieˈkotik) a preparation effective in treating fungal infections.

antineoplastic (ˌanteeˌneeohˈplastik) effective against the multiplication of malignant cells.

antiperistalsis (ˌanteeˌperiˈsta lsəs) contrary contractions which propel the contents of the intestines backwards and upwards.

antiperspirant (anteˈepərspərənt) a substance applied to the body as a lotion, cream or spray to reduce sweating. Use can sometimes result in irritation, especially if the skin is broken.

antiphospholipid syndrome (APS) (anteeˌfosfəˈlipəd ˈsindrohm) also known as Hughes syndrome, is an immune disorder causing increase risk of blood clots.

antipruritic (ˌanteeˌprooˈritik) an external application or drug that relieves itching.

antipyretic (ˌanteepieˈretik) an agent that reduces fever.

antisepsis (ˌanteeˈsepsəs) the prevention of infection by destroying or arresting the growth of harmful microorganisms.

antiseptic (ˌantəˈseptik) 1. preventing sepsis. 2. any substance that inhibits the growth of bacteria, in contrast to a germicide, which kills bacteria outright.

antiserum (ˌanteeˈsiə·rəm) animal or human blood serum which contains antibodies to infective organisms or to their toxins. The serum donor must have previously been infected with the identified organism.

antisocial (ˌanteeˈsohshəl) against society. *A. behaviour* in psychiatry, the refusal of an individual to accept the normal obligations and restraints imposed by the community upon its members.

antispasmodic (ˌanteespazˈmodik) any measure used to prevent or relieve the occurrence of muscle spasm.

antitoxin (ˌanteeˈtoksən) a substance produced by the body cells as a reaction to invasion by bacteria, which neutralises their toxins. *See* IMMUNITY.

antitussive (ˌanteeˈtusiv) 1. effective against cough. 2. an agent that suppresses coughing.

antivenin (ˌanteevəˈneen) an antitoxic serum to neutralise the poison injected by the bite of a snake or insect.

antiviral (anteevierəl) 1. acting against viruses. 2. a drug that is effective against viruses causing disease, e.g. aciclovir.

antrum (ˈantrəm) a cavity in bone. *Mastoid a.* the tympanic antrum, which is an air-conditioning cavity in the mastoid portion of the temporal bone. *Maxillary a.* antrum of Highmore; the air sinus in the upper jawbone.

anuria (əˈnyoo·ri·ə) cessation of the secretion of urine.

anus (ˈaynəs) the extremity of the alimentary canal, through which the faeces are discharged. *Imperforate a.* one where there is no opening because of a congenital defect.

anxiety (angˈzieətee) a chronic state of tension, which affects both mind and body. *A. neurosis see* NEUROSIS.

anxiolytic (ˌanksee·ohˈlitik) a substance, such as diazepam, used for relief of anxiety. Anxiolytics may quickly cause dependence and are not suitable for long-term administration.

aorta (ayˈawtə) the large artery rising out of the left ventricle of the heart and supplying blood to all the body. *Abdominal a.* that part of the artery lying in the abdomen. *Arch of the a.* the curve of the artery over the heart. *Thoracic a.* that part which passes through the chest.

aortic (ayˈawtik) pertaining to the aorta. *A. incompetence* owing to previous inflammation the aortic valve has become fibrosed and is unable to close completely, thus allowing backward flow of blood (*a. regurgitation*) into the left ventricle during diastole. *A. stenosis* a narrowing of the aortic valve. *A. valve* the valve between the left ventricle of the heart and the ascending aorta, which prevents the backward flow of blood through the artery.

aortography (ay·awˈtogrəfee) radiographic examination of the aorta. A radio-opaque contrast medium is injected into the blood to render visible lesions of the aorta or its main branches.

APACHE (əˈpachee) abbreviation for acute physiology and chronic health evaluation. A classification system for indicating severity of illness in intensive care patients.

apathy (ˈapəthee) an appearance of indifference, with no response to stimuli or display of emotion.

aperient (əˈpiəri·ənt) a drug that produces an action of the bowels. A laxative.

aperistalsis (ˌayperiˈstalsəs) lack of peristaltic movement of the intestines.

Apert's syndrome (aˈpairz ˈsinˌdrohm) *Eugène Apert, French paediatrician, 1868–1940.* A congenital abnormality in which there is fusion at birth of all the cranial sutures, in addition to syndactyly (webbed fingers).

apex (ˈaypeks) the top or pointed end of a cone-shaped structure. *A. beat* the beat of the heart against the chest wall which may be felt during systole. *A. of the heart* the end closing the left ventricle. *A. of the lung* the extreme upper part of the organ.

Apgar score (ˈapgah skaw) *Virginia Apgar, American anaesthetist, 1909–1974.* A system used in the assessment of the newborn: skin colour, respiratory effort, heart rate, reflex irritability and muscle tone. The Apgar score is assessed 1 minute after birth and again at 5 minutes. Most healthy infants score 9 at birth. A score below 7 would indicate cause for concern (*see* table below).

APH *see* ANTEPARTUM HAEMORRHAGE.

aphagia (əˈfayji·ə, ay-) loss of the power to swallow.

aphakia (ay-, əˈfayki·ə, -ˈfak-) absence of the lens of the eye; aphacia.

aphasia (əˈfayzi·ə, ay-) a communication disorder due to brain damage; characterised by complete or partial disturbance of language comprehension, formulation or expression. Partial disturbance is also called dysphasia. *Broca's a.* disorder in which verbal output is impaired, and in which verbal communication may be affected as well. Speech is slow and laboured, and writing is often impaired. *Developmental a.* a childhood failure to acquire normal language when deafness, learning difficulties, motor disability or severe emotional disturbance are not causes.

aphonia (əˈfohni·ə, ay-) inability to produce sound. The cause may be organic disease of the larynx or may be purely functional.

aphrodisiac (ˌafrəˈdiziak) a drug which excites sexual desire.

aphthae (ˈapthie) small ulcers surrounded by erythema on the inside of the mouth (aphthous ulcers).

apical (ˈaypikəl) pertaining to the apex of a structure.

apicectomy (ˈaypeeˈsektəmee) excision of the root of a tooth. Root resection.

aplasia (əˈplayzi·ə, ay-) incomplete development of an organ or tissue or absence of growth.

Apgar Score			
Sign	*Score*		
	0	1	2
Appearance	Blue/pale	Body pink, extremities blue	Pink
Pulse rate	Absent	Below 100	Above 100
Grimace	None	Grimace (on stimulation)	Cries
Activity	Limp	Some (flexion of extremities)	Active
Respiration	Absent	Weak cry, hypoventilation	Strong cry

aplastic (ayˈplastik) without power of development. *A. anaemia see* ANAEMIA.

apnoea (ˈapni·ə) cessation of respiration. *A. mattress* mattress designed to sound an alarm if the infant lying on it ceases breathing. *A. monitors* designed to give an audible signal when a certain period of apnoea has occurred. *A. of prematurity* apnoeic periods occurring in the respiration of newborn infants in whom the respiratory centre is immature or depressed. *Cardiac a.* the temporary cessation of breathing caused by a reduction of the carbon dioxide tension in the blood, as seen in Cheyne-Stokes respiration. *Sleep a.* transient attacks of failure of autonomic control of respiration, becoming more pronounced during sleep.

apocrine (ˈapəkrien, -krin) pertaining to modified sweat glands that develop in hair follicles, such as are mainly found in the axillary, pubic and perineal areas.

aponeurosis (aˌpohnyəˈrohsəs) a sheet of tendon-like tissue which connects some muscles to the parts that they move.

apophysis (əˈpofəsəs) a prominence or excrescence, usually of a bone.

apoplexy (ˈapəˌpleksee) a sudden fit of insensibility, usually caused by rupture of a cerebral blood vessel or its occlusion by a blood clot producing coma and paralysis of one side of the body. Rarely used term for a stroke.

apparition (ˌapəˈrishən) a hallucinatory vision, usually the phantom appearance of a person. A spectre.

appendectomy (ˌapənˈdektəmee) *see* APPENDICECTOMY.

appendicectomy (əˌpendəˈsektəmee) removal of the vermiform appendix.

appendicitis (əˌpendəˈsietəs) inflammation of the vermiform appendix.

appendix (əˈpendiks) a supplementary or dependent part. *A. epiploicae* small tag-like structures of peritoneum containing fat, which are scattered over the surface of the large intestine, especially the transverse colon. *Vermiform a.* a worm-like tube with a blind end, projecting from the caecum in the right iliac region. It may be from 2.5 to 15 cm long.

apperception (ˌapəˈsepshən) conscious reception and recognition of a sensory stimulus.

appetite (ˈapəˌtiet) the desire for food. It is stimulated by the sight, smell or thought of food, and is accompanied by the flow of saliva in the mouth and gastric juice in the stomach. The stomach wall receives extra blood supply in preparation for its digestive activity. Appetite is psychological, dependent on memory and associations, as compared with hunger, which is physiologically aroused by the body's need for food. Appetite can be discouraged by unattractive food, surroundings or company, and by emotional states such as anxiety, irritation, anger and fear.

apposition (ˌapəˈzishən) the bringing into contact of two structures, e.g. fragments of bone in setting a fracture.

appraisal (ˌaˈprayzəl) a formal review, usually annually, of a healthcare professional's performance by a trained appraiser in order to provide feedback on past performance, identifying progress made and agreeing together on future goals and objectives.

apprehension (ˌaprəˈhenshən) a feeling of dread or fear.

apraxia (əˈpraksi·ə) the inability to perform correct movements because of a brain lesion and not because of sensory impairment or loss of muscle power in the limbs. *Oral a.* inability to perform volitional movements of the tongue and lips in the absence of paralysis or paresis. Involuntary movements may, however, be observed, e.g. the patient might purse their lips in order to blow out a match.

aptitude (ˈaptəˌtyood) the natural ability or capacity to acquire mental and physical skills. *A. test* the evaluation of a person's ability for learning certain skills or carrying out specific tasks.

apyrexia (ˌaypieˈreksi·ə) the absence of fever.

aqua (ˈakwə) [L.] water. *A. destillata* distilled water.

aqueduct (ˈakwəˌdukt) a canal for the passage of fluid. *A. of Sylvius* the canal connecting the third and fourth ventricles of the brain.

aqueous (ˈakwi·əs, ˈay-) watery. *A. humour* the fluid filling the anterior and posterior chambers of the eye.

Arachis (ˈarəkis) a genus of leguminous plants used in various preparations such as earwax softeners and skin medications.

arachnodactyly (əˌraknəˈdaktəlee) abnormally long and thin fingers and toes. A congenital condition.

arachnoid (əˈraknoyd) 1. resembling a spider's web. 2. a web-like membrane covering the central nervous system between the DURA MATER and the PIA MATER.

arborisation (ˌahbə·rieˈzayshən) the branching terminations of many nerve fibres and processes.

arbovirus (ˌahbohˈvierəs) one of a large group of viruses transmitted by insect vectors (arthropod-borne), e.g. mosquitoes, sandflies or ticks. The diseases caused include many types of encephalitis, also yellow, dengue, sandfly and Rift Valley fevers.

arcus (ˈahkəs) [L.] bow, arch. *A. senilis* an opaque circle appearing round the edge of the cornea in old age.

ARDS adult respiratory distress syndrome.

areola (əˈreeohlə) 1. a space in connective tissue. 2. a ring of pigmentation, e.g. that surrounding the nipple.

arginase (ˈahjəˌnayz) an enzyme of the liver that splits arginine into urea and ornithine.

arginine (ˈahjəˌneen, -ˌnin) an essential amino acid produced by the digestion of protein. It forms a link in the excretion of nitrogen, being hydrolysed by the enzyme arginase.

Argyll Robertson pupil (ahˈgiel ˈrobətsən ˈpyoopəl) *D. Argyll Robertson, British ophthalmologist, 1837–1909. See* PUPIL.

arm (ˈahm) each of the upper limbs of the body between the shoulder and wrist.

Arnold-Chiari malformation (ˌahnəld ˌkeeˈahree ˌmalfawˈmayshən) *Julius Arnold, German pathologist, 1835–1915*; *Hans Chiari, German pathologist, 1851–1916.* Herniation of the cerebellum and elongation of the MEDULLA OBLONGATA; occurs in HYDROCEPHALUS associated with spina bifida. *See also* CHIARI MALFORMATION.

aromatherapy (ərohməˈtherəpee) the therapeutic use of specially prepared essential or aromatic oils obtained from the different parts of plants, including the flowers, leaves, seeds, wood, roots and bark. The oils may be diluted for use in massage, baths or infusions.

arousal (ə'rowzəl) a state of alertness and increased response to stimuli.

arrector pili (ə'rektə pi'li) small muscle attached to the hair follicle of the skin. When contracted, it causes the hair to become erect, producing the appearance known as gooseflesh or goosebumps.

arrest (ə'rest) a cessation or stopping. *Cardiac a.* cessation of ventricular contractions. *Developmental a.* discontinuation of a child's mental or physical development at a certain stage. *Respiratory a.* cessation of breathing.

arrhythmia (ə'rithmi·ə, ay-) variation from the normal rhythm, e.g. in the heart's action. *Sinus a.* an abnormal pulse rhythm due to disturbance of the sinoatrial node, causing quickening of the heart on inspiration and slowing on expiration.

art therapy ('aht 'therəpee) the use of the creative arts as a medium to encourage patients to express their feelings when unable to do so verbally.

artefact ('ahtə,fakt) something that is man-made or introduced artificially.

arterial blood gases (ABGs) (ah'tiəriəl blud gases) normally present in arterial blood and include oxygen, carbon dioxide and nitrogen. Measurements of the partial pressures of oxygen and carbon dioxide together with the blood's pH provide important information on the oxygen saturation of the haemoglobin and acid–base state of the blood, indicating the adequacy of ventilation in critical care situations.

arteriectomy (ah,tiə·ri'ektəmee) the removal of a portion of artery wall, usually followed by anastomosis or a replacement graft. *See* ARTERIOPLASTY.

arteriography (ah'tiə·ree'ografee) radiography of arteries after the injection of a radio-opaque contrast medium.

arteriole (ah'tiə·ree,ohl) a small artery.

arterioplasty (ah'tiə·reeoh,plastee) the reconstruction of an artery by means of replacement or plastic surgery.

arteriorrhaphy (ah'tiə·ree,o·rəfee) ligature of an artery.

arteriosclerosis (ah,tiə·reeohsklə-'rohsəs) a gradual loss of elasticity in the walls of arteries due to thickening and calcification. It is accompanied by high blood pressure, and precedes the degeneration of internal organs associated with old age or chronic disease.

arteriotomy (ah,tiə·ree'otəmee) an incision or puncture into an artery.

arteriovenous (ah,tiə·reeoh'veenəs) both arterial and venous; pertaining to both artery and vein, e.g. an arteriovenous aneurysm, fistula or shunt for HAEMODIALYSIS.

arteritis (,ahtə'rietəs) inflammation of an artery. *Giant cell a.* a variety of polyarteritis resulting in partial or complete occlusion of a number of arteries. The carotid arteries are often involved. *Temporal a.* occlusion of the extracranial arteries, particularly the carotid arteries.

artery (ahtə·ree) a tube of muscle and elastic fibres, lined with endothelium, which distributes blood from the heart to the capillaries throughout the body.

arthralgia (ah'thralji·ə) neuralgic pains in a joint.

arthrectomy (ahˈthrektəmee) excision of a joint.

arthritis (ahˈthrietəs) inflammation of one or more joints. Movement in the joint is restricted, with pain and swelling. *Acute rheumatic a.* *See* RHUMATIC FEVER. *Osteo-a.* a degenerative condition attacking the articular cartilage and aggravated by an impaired blood supply, previous injury or overweight, mainly affecting weight-bearing joints and causing pain. *Rheumatoid a.* a chronic inflammation, usually of unknown origin. The disease is progressive and incapacitating, owing to the resulting ankylosis and deformity of the bones. Usually affects older adults.

arthroclasia (ˌahthrəˈklayzi·ə) the breaking down of adhesions in a joint to produce freer movement.

arthrodesis (ˌahthrəˈdeesəs) the fixation of a movable joint by surgical operation.

arthrography (ahˈthrografee) the examination of a joint by means of X-rays. An opaque contrast medium may be used.

arthrogryposis (ˌahthrohgrieˈpohsəs) 1. a congenital abnormality in which fibrous ankylosis of some or all of the joints in the limbs occurs. 2. a tetanus spasm.

arthroplasty (ˈahthrəˌplastee) the surgical reconstruction or replacement of a painful, degenerated joint. *Charnley's a.* *see* MCKEE FARRAR A. *Cup a.* reconstruction of the articular surface, which is then covered by a vitallium cup. *Excision a.* excision of the joint surfaces affected, so that the gap thus formed then fills with fibrous tissue or muscle. *Girdlestone a.* an excision arthroplasty of the hip. *McKee Farrar a.* replacement of both the head and the socket of the femur. *Replacement a.* partial removal of the head of the femur and its replacement by a metal prosthesis.

arthroscope (ˈahthrəˌskohp) an endoscope for examining the interior of a joint.

arthroscopy (ˈahthrəˌskopee) keyhole surgery used to diagnose and treat joint problems.

articular (ahˈtikyələ) pertaining to a joint.

articulation (ahˈtikyəˈlayshən) 1. a junction of two or more bones. 2. the enunciation of words.

artificial (ˌahtəˈfishəl) not natural. *A. feeding* 1. the giving of food other than by placing it directly in the mouth. It may be provided via the mouth, using an oesophageal tube, or may be introduced into the stomach through a fine tube via the nostril (the nasogastric route). An opening through the abdominal wall into the stomach (i.e. a gastrostomy) may allow direct introduction, or food may be injected intravenously (*see* PARENTERAL). 2. in reference to the feeding of infants, giving food other than human milk. *A. insemination* the insertion of sperm into the uterus by means of syringe and cannula instead of coitus. The husband's, partner's or donor semen may be used. *A. kidney* a dialysis machine to remove unwanted waste materials from the patient with acute or chronic renal failure. *See* HAEMODIALYSIS. *A. respiration* a means of resuscitation from asphyxia. *A. tears* sterile solutions designed to maintain the moisture of the cornea when the latter is abnormally dry due to inadequate tear production. Methylcellulose is a common ingredient.

arytenoid (ˌarəˈteenoyd) resembling the mouth of a pitcher. *A. cartilages* two cartilages of the larynx; their function is to regulate the tension of the vocal cords attached to them.

asbestos (asˈbestos, -təs) a fibrous non-combustible silicate of magnesium and calcium that is a good non-conductor of heat. There are three types of asbestos fibre (white, brown and blue) that were widely used in the building industry. White fibre was the most commonly used and blue and brown fibre the most dangerous to health. In many countries there are now strict regulations controlling the use of asbestos (which has declined), including its removal from buildings. Contact with asbestos over a prolonged period may result in asbestosis, bronchial and laryngeal cancer and mesothelioma.

asbestosis (ˌasbesˈtohsəs) a form of pneumoconiosis (chronic lung disease), due to the inhalation of asbestos fibres causing scarring of the lung tissue. It results in breathlessness and leads to respiratory failure. It may be latent for many years. *See* MESOTHELIOMA.

ascariasis (ˌaskəˈrieəsəs) the condition in which roundworms are found in the gastrointestinal tract. Treatment is with anthelmintic drugs to eliminate the infestation.

ascites (əˈsieteez) abnormal accumulation of fluid in the peritoneal cavity. It may be the result of local inflammation or venous obstruction, or be part of a generalised oedema. It is a complication, for example, of cirrhosis of the liver, malignant neoplastic disease or congestive heart failure.

ascorbic acid (əsˈkawbik ˈasəd) vitamin C. This acid is found in many vegetables and fruits and is an essential dietary constituent for humans. Vitamin C is destroyed by heat and deteriorates during storage. It is necessary for connective tissue and collagen fibre synthesis, and promotes the healing of wounds. Deficiency causes scurvy.

asemia (ayˈseemi·ə) inability to understand or to use speech or signs as a result of a cerebral lesion. Aphasia.

asepsis (ayˈsepsəs) freedom from pathogenic microorganisms.

aseptic (ayˈseptik) free from sepsis. *A. technique* a method of carrying out sterile procedures so that there is the minimum risk of introducing infection. Achieved by the sterility of equipment and a non-touch technique.

asexual (ayˈseksyooəl, aˈsek-) without sex. *A. reproduction* the production of new individuals without sexual union, e.g. by cell division or budding.

asparaginase (əˈsparəjəˌnayz) an enzyme that catalyses the deamination of asparagine; used as an antineoplastic agent against cancers, e.g. acute lymphocytic leukaemia, in which the malignant cells require exogenous asparagine for protein synthesis.

aspartame (əˈspahtaym) a synthetic compound of two amino acids (L-aspartyl-L-phenylalanine methyl ester) used as a low calorie sweetener. It is 180 times as sweet as sucrose (table sugar); the amount equal in sweetness to a teaspoon of sugar contains 0.1 calorie (4.2 J). Aspartame does not promote the formation of dental caries. It should be avoided by patients with phenylketonuria.

aspartate transaminase (AST) (ə'spahtayt tran'zamə,nayz) or aspartate aminotransferase an enzyme released when the liver or muscles are damaged. Levels of AST are measured as markers of liver health.

aspect ('aspekt) that part of a surface facing in a particular direction. *Dorsal a.* that facing and seen from the back. *Ventral a.* that facing and seen from the front.

aspergillosis (,aspəjə'lohsəs) a bronchopulmonary disease in which the mucous membrane is attacked by the fungus *Aspergillus*.

Aspergillus (,aspə'jiləs) a genus of fungi. *A. fumigatus* a common cause of aspergillosis, found in soil and manure.

aspermia (ay'spərmi·ə) absence of sperm.

asphyxia (as'fiksi·ə) a deficiency of oxygen in the blood and an increase in carbon dioxide in the blood and tissues. Symptoms include irregular and disturbed respirations, or a complete absence of breathing, and pallor or cyanosis. Asphyxia may occur whenever there is an interruption in the normal exchange of oxygen and carbon dioxide between the lungs and the outside air. Common causes are drowning, electric shock, lodging of a foreign body in the air passages, inhalation of smoke and poisonous gases and trauma to, or disease of, the lungs or air passages. Treatment includes immediate remedy of the situation (*see* RESPIRATION ARTIFICIAL and Appendix 6) and removal of the underlying cause whenever possible.

aspiration (,aspə'rayshən) 1. the act of inhaling. 2. the drawing off of fluid from a cavity by means of suction.

assault (,a'solt) unlawful personal attack or trespass upon another person, even if only with threatening words. It is both a crime and a tort and, therefore, may result in either criminal or civil liability.

assay ('asay, ə'say) a quantitative examination to determine the amount of a particular constituent of a mixture, or of the biological or pharmacological potency of a drug.

assertiveness (ə'sərtivnəs) a form of behaviour characterised by a confident declaration or affirmation of a statement without need of proof. To assert oneself is to compel recognition of one's rights or position without either aggressively transgressing the rights of another and assuming a position of dominance, or submissively permitting another to deny one's rights or rightful position. *A. training* instruction and practice in techniques for dealing with interpersonal conflicts and threatening situations in an assertive manner, avoiding the extremes of aggressive and submissive behaviour.

assessment (ə'sesmənt) 1. the critical analysis and valuation or judgement of the status or quality of a particular condition, situation or other subject of appraisal. In the nursing process, assessment involves the gathering of information about the health status of the patient/client, analysis and synthesis of the data and the making of a clinical nursing judgement (*see* NURSING PROCESS). The outcome of the nursing assessment is the establishment of a nursing diagnosis, the identification of the nursing problems and establishing a nursing care plan. 2. an examination set by an examining authority to test a candidate's skills and knowledge.

assimilation (ə͵simə'layshən) the process of transforming food so that it can be absorbed and utilised as nourishment by the tissues of the body.

Assistant in Nursing (AIN) (͵a'sistənt in nərsing) an employee in a healthcare facility who essentially works under the direction and supervision of a registered nurse and assists with patient care. Most AIN positions require a TAFE qualification at Certificate III level.

association (ə͵sohsi'ayshən, -͵soh-shi-) coordination of function of similar parts. *A. fibres* nerve fibres linking different areas of the brain. *A. of ideas* a mental impression in which a thought or any sensory impulse will call to mind another object or idea connected in some way with the former. *Free a.* a method employed in psychoanalysis in which the patient is encouraged to express freely whatever comes to mind. This method may allow material that is in the unconscious to be recalled.

associative play (ə͵sohsee·ətiv play) a form of play in which a group of children participate in similar activities without formal organisation or direction.

asthenia (as'theni·ə) lack of strength or energy. Debility. Loss of tone.

asthenic (as'thenik) description of a type of body build: a pale, lean, narrowly built person with poor muscle development.

asthenopia (͵asthe'nohpi·ə) eyestrain likely to arise in long-sighted people when continual effort of accommodation is required for close work.

asthma ('asmə) is a chronic lung condition characterised by wheezing, coughing, tightness in the chest and shortness of breath. The illness often commences in childhood, but can commence at any age; in about half of the children affected, it may be outgrown. Asthma symptoms may be precipitated by indoor or outdoor pollution, including mould, gases, chemicals, particles, chest infections, cold air, vigorous exercise or cigarette smoke, or associated with emotional upset. There is often a family history of asthma or other allergic conditions. Management involves avoidance of known allergens and treatment is with relievers such as bronchodilators, with or without preventers such as corticosteroids. Other drug therapies used include cromons (mast cell stabilisers) useful in preventing exercise-induced asthma and inhaled anticholinergic drugs that may also be used to assist bronchodilation. A person experiencing an acute attack that does not respond to initial drug therapy should be referred or go to hospital for immediate assessment and treatment. *A. action plan* assists a person with asthma and/or their carer to take early action to prevent or reduce the severity of an asthma episode. Undertaking a regular review of the asthma action plan is important as the level of asthma severity or control may change over time. *Cardiac a.* attacks of dyspnoea and palpitation, arising most often at night, associated with left-sided heart failure and pulmonary congestion. Treatment is with diuretic therapy.

astigmatism (ə'stigmə͵tizəm) inequality of the refractive power of an eye, due to curvature of its corneal meridians. The curve across the front of the eye from side to side is not quite the same as the curve from above downwards. The focus on the retina is then not a point but a diffuse and indistinct area. May be congenital or acquired.

astringent (ə'strinjənt) an agent causing contraction of organic tissues, thereby checking secretions, e.g. silver nitrate.

astrocytoma (ˌastrohsie'tohmə) a malignant tumour of the brain or spinal cord. It is slow growing. A GLIOMA.

asymmetry (ay'simətree, a-) inequality in size or shape of two normally similar structures or of two halves of a structure that are normally the same.

asymptomatic (ˌaysimptə'matik, a-) without symptoms.

asynclitism (ay'sin'klit'izm) occurs when the fetal head is not in the same longitudinal axis as the fetal vertebral column with the result that the head of the baby is presenting first and is tilted to the shoulder. Many babies enter the pelvis in an asynclitic presentation, and most asynclitism corrects spontaneously as part of the normal birthing process. The major problem of asynclitism is that it causes the fetal head to present a larger diameter to the maternal pelvis than it would in an occiput-anterior (OA) position. Persistent asynclitism can cause a difficult or dysfunctional labour and may be associated with caesarean birth.

asynergy (ay'sinəˌjee) lack of coordination of structures which normally act in harmony.

asystole (ay'sistəlee) absence of heartbeat; cardiac arrest.

at risk (ət 'risk) whereby an individual or population may be vulnerable to a particular disease, hazard or injury. At risk situations are those involving possible problems that may be preventable with appropriate intervention, or, if they should occur, treatment.

ataraxia (ˌatə'raksi·ə) a state of detached serenity with depression of mental faculties or impairment of consciousness.

ataxia, ataxy (ə'taksi·ə) failure of muscle coordination, resulting in irregular jerky movements and unsteadiness in standing and walking from a disorder of the controlling mechanisms in the brain, or from inadequate input to the brain from joints and muscles. *Hereditary a.* Friedreich's ataxia.

atelectasis (ˌatə'lektəsəs) a collapsed or airless state of the lung, which may be acute or chronic and may involve all or part of the lung: (a) from imperfect expansion of pulmonary alveoli at birth (*congenital a.*); and (b) as the result of disease or injury.

atheroma (ˌathə'rohmə) an abnormal mass of fatty or lipid material with a fibrous covering, existing as a discrete, raised plaque within the intima of an artery.

atherosclerosis (ˌathə·rohsklə'rohsəs) a condition in which the fatty degenerative plaques of atheroma are accompanied by arteriosclerosis, a narrowing and hardening of the vessels.

athetosis (ˌathee'tohsəs) a recurring series of slow, writhing movements of the hands, usually associated with several neurological disorders, such as CEREBRAL PALSY.

athlete's foot ('athleets fuht) a fungal infection between the toes, easily transmitted to other people. *See* TINEA.

atlas ('atləs) the first cervical vertebra, articulating with the occipital bone of the skull.

atmosphere (ˈatməsˌfiə) 1. the gases that surround the earth, extending to an altitude of 16 km. 2. the air or climate of a particular place, e.g. a smoking atmosphere. 3. mental or moral environment, tone or mood.

atmospheric pressure (ˌatməsˈferik preshə) pressure exerted by the air in all directions. At sea level it is about 100 kPa.

atom (ˈatəm) the smallest particle of an element that retains all the properties of that element. It is made up of a central positively charged nucleus and, moving around it in orbit, negatively charged electrons.

atomiser (ˈatəˌmiezə) an instrument by which a liquid is divided to form a fine spray or vapour (nebuliser).

atony (ˈatənee) lack of tone, e.g. in the muscle detrusor of the bladder resulting in incontinence.

atopy (ˈatəpee) a state of hypersensitivity to certain antigens. There is an inherited tendency that includes asthma, eczema and hayfever.

ATP *see* ADENOSINE TRIPHOSPHATE.

atresia (əˈtreezi·ə) absence of a natural opening or tubular structure, e.g. of the anus or vagina; usually a congenital malformation.

atrial (ˈaytri·əl) relating to the atrium. *A. fibrillation* over-stimulation of the atrial walls, so that many areas of excitation arise and the atrioventricular node is bombarded with impulses, many of which it cannot transmit, resulting in a highly irregular pulse. *A. flutter* rapid, regular action of the atria. The atrioventricular node transmits alternate impulses or one in three or four. The atrial rate is usually about 300 beats per minute. *A. septal defect* the non-closure of the foramen ovale at the time of birth, giving rise to a congenital heart defect.

atrioventricular (aytreeohvenˈtrikyələ) pertaining to the atrium and ventricle. *A. bundle see* BUNDLE OF HIS. *A. node* a node of neurogenic tissue situated between the atrium and ventricle and transmitting impulses. *A. valves* the bicuspid and tricuspid valve on the left and right sides of the heart respectively.

atrium (ˈaytree·əm) *pl.* atria. 1. *a cavity*, entrance or passage. 2. one of the two upper chambers of the heart. Formerly called auricle.

atrophy (ˈatrəfee) wasting of any part of the body, due to degeneration of the cells from disuse or lack of nourishment or nerve supply. *Progressive muscular a.* a rare subtype of motor neurone disease with degeneration of the lower motor neurones with wasting of muscle tissue.

atropine (ˈatrəˌpeen, -pin) an alkaloid which inhibits respiratory and gastric secretions, relaxes muscle spasm and dilates the pupil.

attack (əˈtak) an episode or onset of illness. *A. rate* number of cases of a disease in a particular group, e.g. a school, over a given period, related to the population of that group. *Transient ischaemic a.* brief attack (a few hours or less) of cerebral dysfunction of vascular origin with STROKE-like symptoms, without lasting neurological deficit.

attention deficit disorder (ADD) (əˈtenshən ˈdeˌfəsət ˌdəˈsawdə) *see* ATTENTION DEFICIT HYPERACTIVITY DISORDER.

attention deficit hyperactivity disorder (ADHD) (əˈtenshən ˈdeˌfəsət ˌhiepə·rakˈtivətee ˌdəˈsawdə) a disorder of childhood characterised by patterns of behaviour, including marked failure of attention, impulsiveness and increased motor activity that impact on social, educational or work performance. ADHD affects more boys than girls and can continue through adulthood for some people. Treatment involves medication, behaviour therapy and social support. Also known as attention deficit disorder (ADD).

attenuation (əˈtenyooˈayshən) a bacteriological process by which organisms are rendered less virulent by culture in artificial media through many generations, exposure to light, air, etc.; it is used for vaccine preparations.

attitude (ˈatəˌtyood) 1. a posture or position of the body; in obstetrics, the relation of the various parts of the fetal body to one another. 2. a pattern of mental views established by cumulative prior experience.

atypical (ayˈtipikəl) irregular; not conforming to type.

audiogram (ˈawdeeohˌgram) a graph produced by an audiometer.

audiologist (ˌawdeeˈoləjist) an allied health professional specialising in audiology, who provides services that include: (a) evaluation of hearing function to detect hearing impairment and, if there is a hearing disorder, to determine the anatomical site involved and the cause of the disorder; (b) selection of appropriate hearing aids; and (c) training in lip reading, use of hearing aids and maintenance of normal speech.

audiology (ˌawdeeˈoləjee) the science concerned with the sense of hearing, especially the evaluation and measurement of impaired hearing and the rehabilitation of those with impaired hearing.

audiometer (ˌawdeeˈomətə) an instrument for testing hearing, whereby the threshold of the patient's hearing can be measured.

audit (ˈawdət) systematic review and evaluation of records and other data to determine the quality of the services or products provided in a given situation. *A. trail* the process in which careful documentation of the research process makes it possible for students and other researchers to understand how any particular finding was reached. *Concurrent a.* audit conducted at the time the care is being provided to clients/patients. It may be conducted by means of observation and interview of clients/patients, review of open charts or conferences with groups of consumers and providers of nursing care. *Medical a.* the systematic critical analysis of the quality of medical treatment and care, including the procedures for diagnosis and treatment, the use of resources, outcomes, and the resultant quality of life for the patient. *Nursing a.* an evaluation of structure, process and outcome as a measurement of the quality of nursing care. *Retrospective a.* audit conducted after the patient's discharge. Methods include the study of a closed patient's chart and nursing care plan, questionnaires, interviews and surveys of patients and families.

augmentation (ˌawg·mənˈtayshən) 1. enhancement of labour after it has begun. 2. breast enlargement through mammoplasty.

aura (ˈawrə) the premonition, peculiar to an individual, which often precedes an epileptic fit.

aural (ˈawrəl) referring to the ear.

auricle (ˈawrikəl, ˈor-) 1. the external portion of the ear. 2. obsolete term for the atrium.

auriscope (ˈawrəˌskohp, ˈor-) an instrument for examining the drum of the ear. An otoscope.

auscultation (ˌoskəlˈtayshən) examining the internal organs by listening to the sounds that they give out. In *direct* or *immediate a.* the ear is placed directly against the body. In *mediate a.* a stethoscope is used.

Australian Nursing and Midwifery Accreditation Council (ANMAC) (əsˈtrayli·ən nərsing and midˈwifə·ree əkˌredəˈtayshən kownsəl) established in 1992 as a forum for considering the regulation of nursing in Australia within a national focus. ANMAC is a peak national nursing and midwifery body concerned with standards and processes for the regulation of nursing and midwifery within Australia. ANMAC also undertakes assessment programs for international nurses and midwives who wish to practise in Australia.

autism spectrum disorders (ASD) (ˈawtizəm spekˈtrum disawdəs) complex neurodevelopmental disability with onset of symptoms shown from early childhood and characterised by impairments in reciprocal social interactions, impairment in communication skills and rigid, repetitive behaviours. Symptoms of people with ASD fall on a continuum, with some individuals showing mild symptoms and others having much more severe symptoms. There are three types of ASD: autistic disorder, Asperger syndrome and developmental disorder.

autistic (awˈtistik) pertaining to autism.

autoagglutination (ˈawtoh·əˌglootiˌnayshən) 1. clumping or agglutination of cells by an individual's own serum, as in autohaemagglutination. Autoagglutination occurring at low temperatures is called cold agglutination. 2. agglutination of particulate antigens, e.g. bacteria, in the absence of specific antigens.

autoantibody (ˈawtohˈanteeˌbodee) an antibody formed in response to, and reacting against, an antigenic constituent of the individual's own tissues.

autoantigen (ˌawtohˈantəjən) a tissue constituent that stimulates production of autoantibodies in the organism in which it occurs.

autoclave (ˈawtəˌklayv) a steam-heated sterilising apparatus in which the temperature is raised by reducing the air pressure inside; steam is injected under pressure, bringing about efficient sterilisation of instruments and dishes treated in this way.

autodigestion (ˌawtohdieˈjeschən, -di-) dissolution of tissue by its own secretions.

autoeroticism (ˌawtoh·əˈrotəˌsizəm) sexual pleasure derived from self-stimulation of erogenous zones (mouth, anus, genitals and skin). *See* MASTURBATION.

autogenic therapy (awˈtojənˌik therəpee) a complementary therapy combining self-hypnosis and relaxation.

autogenous (awˈtojənəs) generated within the body and not acquired from external sources.

autograft (ˈawtəˌgrahft) the transfer of skin or other tissue from one part of the body to another to repair some deficiency.

autoimmune disease (ˌawtoh·əˈmyoon diˈzeez) condition in which the body develops antibodies to its own tissues, e.g. in autoimmune thyroiditis (HASHIMOTO'S DISEASE).

autoimmunisation (ˌawtohˈimyə-nieˈzayshən) the formation of antibodies against the individual's own tissue.

autoinfection (ˌawtoh·inˈfekshən) self-infection, transferred from one part of the body to another by fingers, towels, etc.

autoinoculation (ˌawtoh·əˌnokyə-ˈlayshən) inoculation with a microorganism from the body itself.

autointoxication (ˌawtoh·inˌtoksəˈ-kayshən) poisoning by toxins generated within the body itself.

autologous (awˈtoləgəs) related to self; belonging to the same organism. *A. blood transfusion (ABT)* the patient donates blood before elective surgery for transfusion postoperatively. ABT may also be obtained as a blood salvage procedure during operation or postoperatively. Avoids cross-matching, compatibility and transfusion infection problems.

autolysis (awˈtoləsəs) a breaking up of living tissues, e.g. as may occur if pancreatic ferments escape into surrounding tissues. It also occurs after death.

automated auditory brainstem response (AABR) (ˈawtohˈmaytəd awˈdətawrˈee ˈbraynˌstem rəˈspons) a hearing test that records brain activity in response to clicking sounds via sensors placed on the infant's head. Used for newborn hearing screening.

automatic (ˌawtəˈmatik) performed without the influence of the will.

automatism (awˈtoməˌtizəm) performance of non-reflex acts without apparent volition, and of which the patient may have no memory afterwards, as in somnambulism. *Post-epileptic a.* automatic acts following an epileptic fit.

autonomic (ˌawtəˈnomik) self-governing. *A. nervous system* the sympathetic and parasympathetic nerves that control involuntary muscles and glandular secretion, over which there is no conscious control.

autonomy (awˈtonəmee) the right of personal freedom of action, which is regarded as one of the hallmarks of a profession.

autoplasty (ˈawtohˌplastee) 1. replacement of missing tissue by grafting a healthy section from another part of the body. 2. in psychoanalysis, instinctive modification within the psychic systems in adaptation to reality.

autopsy (awˈtopsee, ˈawtəp-) postmortem examination of a body to determine the cause of death.

autosome (ˈawtohˌsohm) any chromosome other than the sex chromosomes. In humans there are 22 pairs of autosomes and one pair of sex chromosomes.

autosuggestion (ˌawtohsəˈjesjən) suggestion arising in one's self. Uncritical acceptance of an idea arising in the individual's own mind.

autotransfusion (ˌawtohtrans-ˈfyoozhən, -trahns-) reinfusion of a patient's own blood.

autotransplantation (ˌawtohˌtrans-plahnˈtayshən) transfer of tissue from one part of the body to another part.

avascular (ayˈvaskyuhlə) not vascular. Bloodless. *A. necrosis* death of bone owing to deficient blood supply, usually following an injury.

average (ˈavˌrəj) 1. the value or score that is typical of a group.

The result is obtained by adding several amounts together and then dividing the total by the number of amounts. Sometimes also referred to as the mean. 2. a colloquial term used to mean 'usual' or 'ordinary'.

aversion (ə'vərzhən) intense dislike. *A. therapy* a method of treating addictions by associating the craving for what is addictive with painful or unpleasant stimuli. It is rarely used.

avian influenza ('ayvee'n ˌinfloo'enzə) commonly known as bird flu, a disease of poultry and other birds caused by strains of the influenza virus that can occasionally infect people who are in close contact with infected birds. The severity of the disease depends on the strain of the virus involved; the strain caused by the H5N1 virus is particularly virulent. At the present time, normal influenza vaccines do not protect against the H5N1 virus. *See* ORTHOMYXOVIRUS and SWINE INFLUENZA.

aviation medicine ('ayveeˌayshən ˌmedəsən) the medical speciality concerned with the effects of air travel and with the causes and treatment of health problems that may occur in flight.

avitaminosis (ayˌvitəmə'nohsəs) a condition resulting from an insufficiency of vitamins in the diet. A deficiency disease.

avoidance (ə'voydəns) a conscious or unconscious defence mechanism whereby an individual seeks to escape or avoid certain situations, feelings or conflicts.

avulsion (ə'vulshən) the tearing away of one part from another. *Phrenic a.* a tearing away of the phrenic nerve. It paralyses the diaphragm on the affected side.

axilla (ak'silə) an armpit.

axiom (acksee'm) a statement or proposition that can be accepted without evidence as it is obviously true.

axis ('aksəs) 1. a line through the centre of a structure. 2. the second cervical vertebra.

axon ('akson) the process of a nerve cell along which electrical impulses travel. The nerve fibre.

axonotmesis (ˌaksonət'meesəs) nerve injury characterised by disruption of the axon and myelin sheath but with preservation of the connective tissue fragments, resulting in degeneration of the axon distal to the injury site; regeneration of the axon is spontaneous.

azoospermia (ˌayzoh·oh'spərmi·ə) absence of spermatozoa in the semen.

azygous ('azəˌgos, ə'ziegəs) something that is unpaired. *A. vein* an unpaired vein that ascends the posterior MEDIASTINUM and enters the superior VENA CAVA.

Bb

Ba symbol for *barium*.

Babinski's reflex or sign (bə'binskeez 'reefleks or sien) *Joseph Babinski, French neurologist, 1857–1932*. On stroking the sole of the foot, the great toe bends upwards instead of downwards (dorsal instead of plantar flexion). Present in disease or injury to the spinal cord or brain. Babies who have not walked react in the same way, but normal flexion develops later.

baby ('baybee) an infant or young child who is not yet walking. *B. blues* the transient feelings of unhappiness and tearfulness that affect many women after the birth of their baby. *B. Friendly Health Initiative (BFHI)* part of a global campaign by the United Nations International Children's Emergency Fund (UNICEF) to implement practices that protect, promote and support breastfeeding. Within Australia the governance of BFHI was passed from UNICEF to the Australian College of Midwives in 1995. *B. talk* the speech pattern and sounds of young children learning to talk. *Battered b.* one suffering from the result of continued violence; extensive bruising, fractures of limbs, ribs and skull, or an internal trauma may be found. *Blue b.* one suffering from cyanosis at birth as a result of atelectasis or congenital heart malformation.

Bach flower remedies (bahk 'flowə 'remedəz) a system of complementary medicine based on homeopathic principles, devised by *Edward Bach, British physician and homeopath, 1886–1936*. Flower remedies aim to treat emotional and psychological disorders. There are 38 flower remedies. *See also* HOMEOPATHY.

Bachelor of Nursing (BN) (bachələ ov nərsing) an academic degree awarded on satisfactory completion of a 3-year course of study in a college or university. The course length may vary, e.g. with recognition of prior learning. The recipient is eligible to apply for registration with the Australian Health Practitioner Regulation Agency (AHPRA) to become a registered nurse.

bacillaemia (ˌbasəl'leemi·ə) the presence of bacilli in the blood.

bacilluria (ˌbasə'lyoo·ri·ə) the presence of bacilli in the urine.

Bacillus (bə'siləs) a genus of aerobic, spore-bearing Gram-positive bacteria. *B. anthracis* the causative agent of anthrax.

bacillus (bə'siləs) loosely, the cause of any bacterial infection by a rod-shaped microorganism, e.g. *Escherichia coli*, the colon bacillus.

back (bak) dorsum [L]. Posterior trunk from neck to pelvis. *B. bone* the vertebral column. *B. slab* plaster or plastic splint in which a limb is supported. *Hunchback* KYPHOSIS.

backache ('bakˌayk) any pain in the back, usually the lower part. The pain is often dull and continuous, but sometimes sharp and throbbing.

Backache, or lumbago, can range in intensity from mild to severe, is one of the most common ailments, and may be caused by a variety of disorders. Healthcare workers are at particular risk of work-related back problems and one in six nurses are thought to experience back pain.

bacteraemia (ˌbaktəˈreemi·ə) the presence of bacteria in the bloodstream.

bacteria (bakˈtiə·ri·ə) a general name given to minute vegetable organisms which may live on organic matter. There are many varieties, only some of which are pathogenic to humans, animals and plants. Each bacterium consists of a single cell and, given favourable conditions, multiplies by subdivision. Bacteria are classified according to their shape: (a) *bacilli*, rod-shaped;

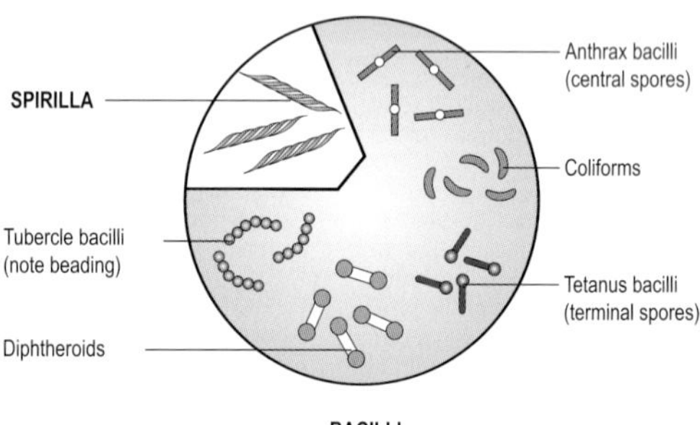

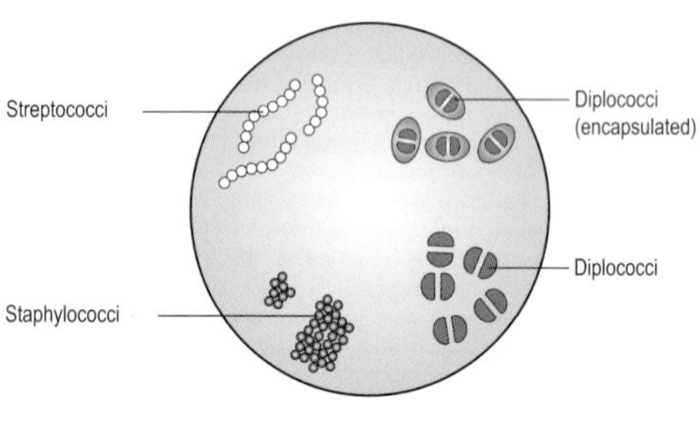

Bacteria: bacilli (rod-shaped) and cocci (spherical).

(b) *cocci*, spherical (*see* figure, p. 50) subdivided into (i) streptococci (in chains), (ii) staphylococci (in groups), (iii) diplococci (in pairs); and (c) *spirilla*, *spirochaetes*, spiral. *Pathogenic b.* those whose growth in the body gives rise to disease, either by destruction of tissue or by formation of toxins, which circulate in the blood. Pathogenic bacteria thrive on organic matter in the presence of warmth and moisture.

bacterial (bak'tiə·ri·əl) pertaining to bacteria.

bactericidal (bak,tiə·ri'sied'l) capable of killing bacteria; e.g. disinfectants, great heat, intense cold or sunlight.

bactericide (bak'tiə·rə'sied) an agent that kills bacteria.

bacteriologist (bak,tiə·ree'oləjəst) one who is qualified in the science of bacteriology.

bacteriology (bak,tiə·ree'oləjee) the scientific study of bacteria.

bacteriolysin (bak,tiə·ree'oləsən, -rioh'liesin) an antibody produced in the blood to assist in the destruction of bacteria. The action is specific.

bacteriolysis (bak,tiə·ree'oləsəs) the dissolution of bacteria by a bacteriolytic agent.

bacteriophage (bak'tiə·ree·ə,fayj, -fahzh) a virus that infects only bacteria. Many strains exist, some of which are used for identifying types of STAPHYLOCOCCI and salmonellae.

bacteriostat (bak,tiə·reeoh'stat) an agent that inhibits the growth of bacteria.

bacteriostatic (bak,tiə·reeoh'statik) inhibiting the growth of bacteria.

bag (bag) a sac or pouch. *Ambu b.* a bag valve mask (BVM). It is a handheld device used to provide positive pressure ventilation to a patient who is not breathing or who is breathing inadequately. Use of the Ambu bag to ventilate a patient is frequently called 'bagging'. *B. of waters* the membranes enclosing the amniotic fluid and the developing fetus in utero. *Colostomy b.* following a colostomy, a receptacle worn over the stoma by the patient, to receive the faecal discharge. *Douglas b.* a receptacle for the collection of expired air, permitting measurement of respiratory gases. *Ileostomy b.* receptacle worn over the stoma for the collection of waste products after ILEOSTOMY. *Politzer b.* a soft bag of rubber for inflating the pharyngotympanic (eustachian, also known as the auditory) tube. *Urine b.* a receptacle used for urine by ambulatory patients with urinary incontinence.

bagging ('baging) the artificial ventilation performed with a ventilator or respirator bag, such as an Ambu bag or reservoir bag on an anaesthesia machine.

baker's cyst ('baykerz sist) *see* POPLITEAL CYST.

Bainbridge reflex ('baynbrij 'reefleks) *Francis Bainbridge, British physiologist, 1874–1921.* An increase in the heart rate caused by an increase in right atrial pressure.

balance ('baləns) the ability to remain upright and to move without falling over. In physiological terms the harmonious relationship between parts and organs of the body and their functions or between substances in the body. *See* ACID–BASE BALANCE. *B. of probabilities* the standard of proof required in civil proceedings.

balanced diet ('balənst 'dieət) a varied diet that contains all the nutritional elements in the correct quantities required for growth and repair of body tissues.

balanced salt solution (BSS) (ˈbalənst solt səˈlooshən) a solution that is made to a physiological pH with appropriate concentrations of salts and electrolytes. Used during intraocular surgery to replace intraocular fluids.

balanitis (ˌbaləˈnietəs) inflammation of the glans penis and of the prepuce, usually associated with PHIMOSIS. Balanoposthitis.

baldness (ˈbawldnəs) an absence of hair, especially from the scalp. *See* ALOPECIA.

ballottement (bəˈlotmənt) [Fr.] a palpatory technique for detecting an organ or floating object not near the surface of the body, e.g. abdominal palpation of the uterus when testing for pregnancy. The uterus is pushed upwards by a finger in the vagina and, if a fetus is present, it will fall back again like a heavy body in water.

bandage (ˈbandij) 1. a strip or roll of gauze or other material for wrapping or binding any part of the body. 2. to cover by wrapping with such material. Bandages may be used to stop the flow of blood, to provide a safeguard against contamination or to hold a dressing in place. They may also be used to hold a splint in position or otherwise immobilise an injured part of the body to prevent further injury and to facilitate healing.

banding (ˈbanding) placing a band around a vessel to restrict the flow from it. *Pulmonary arterial b.* a palliative operation used in treating infants with ventricular septal defects.

bank (bank) an institution offering services, or a store of donated human tissues for use in the future by other individuals, e.g. *blood b.*, *human milk b.*, *sperm b. Nurse b.* a group of nurses who are known to the employing authority and available for employment on an on-call basis.

Bankart's operation (ˈbangkhahtz ˌopəˈrayshən) *Arthur Bankart, British orthopaedic surgeon, 1879–1951.* An operation to repair a defect in the glenoid cavity that causes repeated dislocation of the shoulder joint.

barbiturates (bahˈbityə·rəts, -ˈrayts) a large group of sedative and hypnotic drugs derived from barbituric acid, e.g. phenobarbitone, amylobarbitone. Prolonged use may lead to addiction.

bariatric (ˌbareeˈatrik) a branch of medicine that deals with obesity, its effects, treatment and control. *See* OBESITY. *B. surgery* surgical procedures to help weight loss. Common procedures include gastric banding, gastric bypass, biliopancreatic division and gastric stapling. Bariatric surgical procedures are only considered for people with severe obesity, not for individuals with a mild weight problem.

barium (ˈba·ree·əm) *symbol* Ba. A soft, silvery, metallic element. *B. sulfate* a heavy mineral salt that is comparatively impermeable to X-rays and therefore can be used as a contrast medium, given as a meal or as an enema. Used to demonstrate abnormality in the stomach or intestines, and to show peristaltic movement. *B. sulfide* the chief constituent of depilatory preparations, i.e. those which remove hair.

baroreceptors (ˌbarohreeˈseptərz) the sensory branches of the glossopharyngeal and vagus nerves that influence the blood pressure. The receptors are situated in the walls of the carotid sinus and aortic arch.

barotrauma (ˌbarohˈtrawmə) injury due to pressure, such as to structures of the ear, owing to differences between atmospheric and intratympanic pressures. May affect air travellers or scuba divers.

Barr body (bah bodee) *Murray Barr, Canadian anatomist, 1908–1995*. Small, dark-staining area underneath the nuclear membrane of female cells. Represents an inactive X chromosome.

Barré-Guillain syndrome (baray-ˌgiyanh ˈsinˌdrohm) *see* GUILLAIN-BARRÉ SYNDROME.

barrier (ˈbaree·ə) an obstruction. *B. contraceptive* mechanical barrier preventing sperm from entering the cervical canal, e.g. diaphragm, sheath. *B. cream* a cream used to protect the skin against irritant substances and water, e.g. hand cream. *B. nursing* method of preventing the spread of infection from one patient to other patients and/or staff. This normally involves nursing the patient in a separate room or cubicle and the use of isolation techniques. (*See* Appendix 10.) *Blood–brain b.* the selective barrier which separates the circulating blood from the cerebrospinal fluid. *Placental b.* semipermeable membrane between maternal and fetal blood. *Protective b.* radiation-absorbing shield, e.g. lead, concrete, to protect the body against ionising radiations. *Reverse b. nursing* an isolation technique used to prevent the transmission of infection to the patient who may be especially vulnerable, e.g. the immunosuppressed patient. *See* UNIVERSAL PRECAUTIONS.

Bartholin's glands (ˈbahtəlinz glandz) *Caspar Bartholin, Danish anatomist, 1655–1738*. Two glands situated in the LABIA MAJORA, with ducts opening inside the vulva. *B. cyst* a small fluid filled swelling on one of the glands, usually painless, but if infected will lead to pyrexia, pain and discomfort.

basal (ˈbaysəl) 1. fundamental. 2. referring to a base. *B. cell* any one of the cells in the deepest layer of the stratified epithelium; the base. *B. cell carcinoma* a common type of skin cancer. Generally occurs in later life, most usually on the face, scalp or neck, and is caused by skin damage from the ultraviolet irradiation in sunlight over many years. Without treatment, the carcinoma invades and destroys the surrounding tissues, but rarely invades other parts of the body. Treatment is usually with surgery. People who have had a basal cell carcinoma should be alert to any changes in their skin as they may develop new tumours. The risk of further tumours is also further reduced by avoiding overexposure to sunlight, wearing protective clothing and a sunscreen preparation on the skin. Also known as a rodent ulcer or BCC. *B. ganglia* the collections of nerve cells or grey matter in the base of the cerebrum. They consist of the caudate nucleus and putamen, forming the corpus striatum, and the GLOBUS PALLIDUS. Such cells are concerned with modifying and coordinating voluntary muscle movements. *B. metabolic rate (BMR)* an indirect method of estimating the rate of metabolism in the body by measuring the oxygen intake and carbon dioxide output on breathing. The age, sex, weight and size of the patient have to be taken into account.

base (bays) 1. the lowest part or foundation. 2. the main constituent of a compound. 3. an alkali or other substance that can unite with an acid to form a salt.

baseline (ˈbaysˌlien) a known quantity with which an unknown is compared when measured or assessed.

basement membrane (ˈbaysmənt ˈmembrayn) a thin layer of modified connective tissue supporting layers of cells, found at the base of the epidermis and underlying mucous membranes.

basic life support (BLS) (ˈbaysik lief ˌsəˈpawt) a protocol of resuscitation of a collapsed patient which comprises initial assessment, airway maintenance, expired air ventilation and chest compression. BLS implies that no equipment is available to be used. Its purpose is to maintain adequate ventilation and circulation until further means are available to reverse the underlying condition. (*See* Appendix 6.)

basilar (ˈbasələ) situated at the base. *B. artery* midline artery at the base of the skull, formed by the junction of the vertebral arteries.

basilic (bəˈsilik) prominent. *B. vein* a large vein on the inner side of the arm.

basophil (ˈbaysəˌfil) (*adj.* basophilic) 1. any structure, cell or histological element staining readily with basic dyes. 2. a granular leucocyte with an irregularly shaped, relatively pale-staining nucleus that is partially constricted into two lobes, and with cytoplasm containing coarse bluish-black granules of variable size. 3. a beta cell of the adenohypophysis.

basophilia (ˌbaysəˈfili·ə) 1. an affinity of cells or tissues for basic dyes. 2. the reaction of relatively immature erythrocytes to basic dyes whereby the stained cells appear blue, grey or greyish-blue, or bluish granules appear. 3. abnormal increase of basophilic leucocytes in the blood. 4. basophilic leucocytosis.

bath (bahth) 1. a medium (e.g. water, vapour, sand or mud) with which the body is washed or in which the body is wholly or partially immersed for therapeutic or cleansing purposes; application of such a medium to the body. 2. the equipment or apparatus in which a body or object may be immersed. *Bed b.* washing a patient in bed. *Emollient b.* a bath in a soothing and softening liquid, used in various skin disorders. It is prepared by adding soothing agents such as gelatin or similar emollient substances to the bath water, for the purpose of relieving skin irritation and pruritus. The skin should be dried by patting rather than rubbing after the bath. Care must be taken to avoid chilling. *Hot b.* one taken in water at 36–44°C. Care must be taken to avoid faintness. *Sponge b.* one in which the patient's body is not immersed, but is wiped with a wet cloth or sponge. Sponge baths are most often employed for reduction of body temperature in the presence of a fever, in which case the water used is tepid and may contain alcohol to increase evaporation of moisture from the skin. *Tepid b.* one taken in water at 30–33°C. *Warm b.* one taken in water at 32–40°C. *Whirlpool b.* one in which the water is kept in constant motion by mechanical means. It has a gentle massaging action that promotes relaxation.

battered baby syndrome *see* CHILD ABUSE.

B-cell (beeˌsel) *see* IMMUNITY.

BCG vaccine (ˌbeecee'gee 'vakseen) bacillus Calmette-Guérin vaccine, a tuberculosis vaccine prepared from an artificially weakened strain of bovine tubercle bacillus (*Mycobacterium bovis*). The vaccine is given to those at risk of tuberculosis and for whom a tuberculin test is negative. This includes some healthcare workers, close contacts of people with tuberculosis and immigrants and their families from countries with a high rate of tuberculosis.

bearing down (ˌbair·ing'down) 1. the expulsive pains in the second stage of labour. 2. a feeling of heaviness and downward strain in the pelvis, present with some uterine growths or displacements.

beat (beet) pulsation of the heart or an artery. *Apex b.* pulsation of the heart felt over its apex. The beat of the heart is felt against the chest wall. *Dropped b.* the occasional loss of a ventricular beat. *Ectopic b.* one that originates somewhere other than the sinoatrial node.

Beck Depression Inventory (BDI) (bek də'preshən in'ventəree) a self-scoring system used to determine the presence and severity of depression.

Beck Scale for Suicide ideation (BSS) (bek skayl faw 'sooəsied 'iedeeˌayshən) an assessment tool used to identify the potential and risk of suicide in vulnerable patients.

becquerel ('bekərəl) (Bq) the SI unit of radioactivity equal to the quantity of material undergoing one disintegration per second; 3.7×10^{10} becquerels is equal to 1 curie.

bed (bed) 1. a supporting structure or tissue. 2. a couch or support for the body during sleep. *B. cradle* a frame placed over the body of a bed patient. See CRADLE. *Capillary b.* the capillaries of a tissue, area or organ considered collectively, and their volume capacity. *Fracture b.* a bed for the use of patients with broken bones. *Nail b.* the area of modified epidermis beneath the nail over which the nail plate slides as it grows.

bed board ('bed bawd) a rigid board placed beneath the mattress of a bed to give firm support to the patient lying on it.

bedbug ('bedˌbug) a bug of the genus *Cimex*, a flattened, oval, reddish insect that inhabits houses, furniture and neglected beds, and feeds on humans, usually at night.

bed pan ('bed pan) a shallow vessel used for defecation or urination by patients confined to bed.

bed rest ('bed rest) limiting the patient to staying in bed for a prescribed period for therapeutic reasons.

bedsore ('bed'saw) an ulcer-like sore caused by prolonged pressure, shear, friction or a combination of the factors usually over a bony prominence. Also called pressure (decubitus) ulcer or, more recently, pressure injury. *See* PRESSURE INJURY.

bed-wetting ('bedˌweting) involuntary voiding of urine. *See* ENURESIS.

bee sting (bee sting) injury caused by the venom of a bee. Symptoms of a severe allergic reaction, such as collapse or swelling of the body, indicate ANAPHYLAXIS and require that medical help be sought.

behaviour (bee'hayvyə, bə-) the way in which an organism reacts to an internal or external stimulus. *B. disorders* may take many forms, such as truancy, stealing, temper tantrums. *B. modification* an approach to correction of undesirable behaviour that focuses on changing observable actions. Modification of the behaviour is accomplished through systematic manipulation of the environmental and behavioural variables related to the specific behaviour to be changed. *B. therapy* a therapeutic approach in which the focus is on positive behaviour change (*see also Cognitive behavioural therapy*). *Incongruous b.* behaviour that is out of keeping with the person's normal reaction or has the opposite effect to that consciously desired.

behavioural sciences (ˌbəˈhayvyəˌ-ruhl ˈsieənsəs) the application of scientific principles to the study of the behaviour of organisms, e.g. sociology, psychology, anthropology.

behaviourism (beeˈhayvyəˌrizəm, bə-) the purely objective study and observation of the behaviour of individuals.

Behçet's syndrome (bayˈsetz ˈsinˌdrohm) *Hulusi Behçet, Turkish dermatologist, 1889–1948.* A rare chronic condition that is a form of systemic vasculitis, resulting in painful, recurring mouth and genital ulcers, arthritis, skin lesions and inflammation of the eyes.

bejel (ˈbayjəl) a non-venereal but infectious form of syphilis caused by a TREPONEMA, indistinguishable from that causing syphilis. Occurs mainly in children of Africa and the Middle East. The primary lesion is on the mouth, spreading to the trunk, arms and legs. Treated with penicillin.

belching (ˈbelching) the noisy expulsion of gas from the stomach through the mouth. *See* ERUCTATION.

beliefs (ˌbəˈleefs) thoughts, ideas and concepts developed by an individual over a period of time from cultural influences, education, religion, parents and family. *Health b.* those beliefs held by an individual regarding the maintenance of their physical and mental wellbeing, which may be at variance with those beliefs held by the healthcare practitioner, possibly leading to conflict and non-compliance with prescribed treatment.

belle indifference (ˌbel inˈdifə·ronhs) [Fr.] an indication of conversion hysteria, in which the patient describes symptoms, appearing not to be distressed by them.

Bell's palsy (belz ˈpawlzee) *Charles Bell, British physiologist, 1774–1842.* Facial paralysis due to oedema of the facial nerve.

benchmarking (ˈbenchˌmahking) comparing 'like with like' in order to identify the best practice; a process whereby organisations identify the best performers in order to improve their own performance. A scoring system is used that enables one hospital, department or other healthcare facility to compare their practices and services with another similar to their own. A quality assurance technique.

bends (bendz) a colloquial term for DECOMPRESSION SICKNESS.

beneficence (bənˈifisəns) the duty to do good, to avoid harm to other people and to protect the weak and the vulnerable. In the healthcare setting, this involves staff acting in the best interests of their patients and, if necessary, acting as an advocate for them.

benign (bəˈnien) 1. the opposite to malignant. 2. describes a non-invasive condition or illness that is not usually serious, even though treatment may be required for health or cosmetic reasons.

bereavement (bə'reev·mənt) the experience of suffering loss, usually of a loved one by death or separation, but may also include the loss of previous good health, position or wealth. Produces a psychological reaction that has recognised stages that may overlap; these include anger, denial, disbelief and, finally, acceptance. Collectively recognised as mourning or grieving.

beriberi ('beree,beree) a deficiency disease due to insufficiency of vitamin B_1 (thiamine) in the diet. The disease is more common in areas where refined rice is the main staple in the diet. It is a form of neuritis, with pain, paralysis and oedema of the extremities.

berry aneurysm (bəree 'anyə,rizəm) small, saccular dilation of the wall of a cerebral artery.

berylliosis (bə,rilee'ohsəs) an industrial lung disease due to inhalation of the metallic element beryllium. Interstitial fibrosis arises, impairing lung function.

beta ('beetə) the second letter in the Greek alphabet, β. *B. blockers* drugs used to block the action of adrenaline on beta-adrenergic receptors in cardiac muscle, thus decreasing the workload of the heart. *B. cells* insulin-producing cells found in the ISLETS OF LANGERHANS in the pancreas. *B. rays* electrons used therapeutically for treatment of lesions of the eye and bone. *B. receptors* associated with the inhibition (relaxation) of smooth muscle. They also bring an increase in the force of contraction and rate of the heart.

bezoar ('beezaw) a mass of hair, fruit or vegetable fibres sometimes found in the stomach or intestines.

bias (bieəs) in research, any tendency for results to differ from the true value in some consistent way. It is always associated with some systematic, non-random and usually undesirable phenomenon.

bicarbonate (bie'kahbə,nayt, -nət) any salt containing the HCO_3 anion. *Blood b., plasma b.* the bicarbonate of the blood plasma, an important parameter of ACID–BASE BALANCE measured in blood gas analysis.

bicellular (bie'selyələ) composed of two cells.

biceps ('bieseps) a muscle with two heads; a flexor of the arm; one of the hamstring muscles of the thigh.

biconcave (bie'konkayv) pertaining to a lens or other structure with a hollow or depression on each surface (*see* figure).

biconvex (bie'konveks) pertaining to a lens or other structure that protrudes on both surfaces (*see* figure).

bicornuate (bie'kawnyooət) having two horns. *B. uterus* a congenital malformation in which there is a partial or complete vertical division into two parts of the body of the uterus.

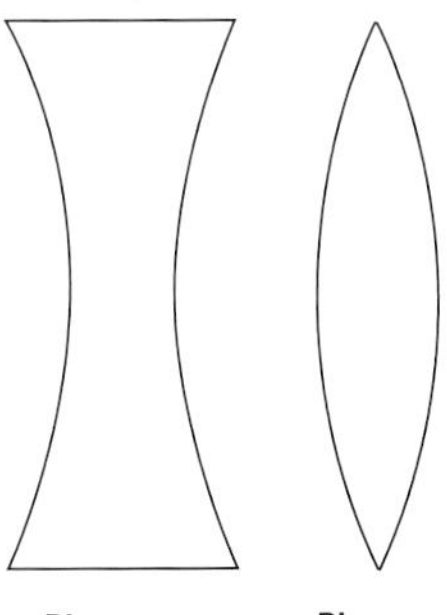

Biconcave. **Biconvex.**

bicuspid (bie'kuspəd) having two cusps or projections. *B. teeth* the premolars. *B. valve* the mitral valve of the heart between the left atrium and left ventricle.

bidet ('beeday) a low narrow basin on a stand, for washing the perineum and genitalia.

bifid ('biefəd) divided or cleft into two parts.

Bifidus factor ('bifi,dus 'fak,tə) present in human milk; promotes growth of Gram-positive bacteria in gut flora, particularly *Lactobacillus bifidus*. This microorganism reduces the pH in the gut, preventing the multiplication of pathogens.

bifocal (bie'fohkəl) having two foci, as with spectacles in which each of the lenses has two different foci.

bifurcate (bie'fərkayt) to divide into two branches; arteries bifurcate frequently, thereby getting smaller.

bifurcation (,bie'fəkayshən) the junction where a vessel divides into two branches, e.g. where the aorta divides into the right and left iliac vessels.

bigeminal (,bie'jemən'l) double. *B. pulse* two pulse beats which occur together, regular in time and force. A regular irregularity.

biguanides (bie'gwahniedz) oral hypoglycaemic agents for treating diabetes. They exert their effect by decreasing GLUCONEOGENESIS in muscle tissue. Effective only in those people with diabetes who have functioning ISLET OF LANGERHANS cells. Most commonly used in type 2 diabetes mellitus, especially for individuals who are overweight.

bilateral (bie'latə·rəl) pertaining to both sides.

bile (biel) a secretion of the liver, greenish-yellow to brown in colour. It is concentrated in the gallbladder and passes into the small intestine, where it assists digestion by emulsifying fats and stimulating peristalsis. *B. ducts* the canals or passageways that conduct bile. The hepatic and cystic ducts join to form the common bile duct. *B. pigments* bilirubin and biliverdin, produced by haemolysis in the spleen. Normally these colour the faeces only, but in jaundice the skin and urine may also become coloured. *B. salts* sodium taurocholate and sodium glycocholate, which cause the emulsification of fats.

Bilharzia (bil'hahtsi·ə) *Theodor Bilharz, German physician, 1825–1862*. A genus of blood fluke now known as *Schistosoma*.

bilharziasis (,bilhaht'sieəsəs) *see* SCHISTOSOMIASIS.

biliary ('bilyə·ree) pertaining to bile, the bile ducts and gallbladder. *B. colic* spasm of muscle walls of the bile duct, causing excruciating pain when gallstones are blocking the tube. Pain is usually in the right upper quadrant of the abdomen and referred to the shoulder. *B. fistula* an abnormal opening between the gallbladder and the surface of the body.

biliousness ('bileeəs,nəs) a symptom complex comprising nausea, abdominal discomfort, headache and constipation.

bilirubin (,bilee'roobən) an orange bile pigment produced by the breakdown of haem and reduction of biliverdin. It normally circulates in plasma and is taken up by liver cells and conjugated to form diglucuronide, the water-soluble pigment excreted in the bile. Bilirubin may be classified as indirect ('free' or unconjugated) while en route to the liver from its site of formation by reticuloendothelial cells, and direct (bilirubin diglucuronide) after its conjugation in the liver with glucuronic acid. Normally the body produces a total of about 260 mg of bilirubin per day. Almost 99% of this is excreted in the faeces; the remaining 1% is excreted in the urine as UROBILINOGEN. The typical yellowness of jaundice is caused by the accumulation of bilirubin in the blood and body tissues.

bilirubinaemia (ˌbileeˌroobəˈnee-mi·ə) the presence of bilirubin in the blood.

biliuria (ˌbileeˈyoo·ri·ə) bile or bile salts in the urine.

Billings method (ˈbilingz ˈmethuhd) a method of estimating ovulation time by observing changes in the cervical mucus that occur during the menstrual cycle.

bimanual (bieˈmanyooəl) using both hands. *B. examination* examination with both hands. Used chiefly in gynaecology, when the internal genital organs are examined between one hand on the abdomen, and the other hand or a finger within the vagina.

binary (ˈbienə·ree) made up of two parts. *B. fission* the multiplication of cells by division into two equal parts. *B. scale* one used in calculating, in which only two digits, 0 and 1, are used. Computer programming techniques use this scale.

binaural (bieˈnawrəl) pertaining to both ears. *B. stethoscope see* STETHOSCOPE.

Binet's test (ˈbeenayz ˌtest) *Alfred Binet, French physiologist, 1857–1911.* A method of ascertaining the mental age of children or young persons by using a series of questions standardised on the capacity of normal children at various ages.

Bing test (bing ˌtest) *Albert Bing, German otologist, 1844–1922.* A vibrating tuning fork is held to the mastoid process and the auditory meatus is alternately occluded and left open; an increase and decrease in loudness (positive Bing) is perceived by the normal ear and in sensorineural hearing impairment, but in conductive hearing impairment no difference in loudness is perceived (negative Bing).

binge eating disorder (BED) (binj ˈeeting disawdə) an eating disorder characterised by regular episodes of binge eating without purging, which is accompanied by feelings of being out of control and highly distressed.

binge–purge syndrome (binj pərj ˈsinˌdrohm) an alternative term for BULIMIA.

binocular (bəˈnokyələ, bie-) relating to both eyes.

binovular (bəˈnovyələ) derived from two ova. *B. twins* twins, who may or may not be of different sexes.

bioassay (ˌbieohˈasay) biological assay. The use of animals or an isolated organ preparation to determine the effect of the active power of a sample of a drug. Comparison is made with the effect of a standard preparation.

bioavailability (ˌbieohˈəvayləˌbilətee) the proportion of a drug that reaches the target organs of the body. Bioavailability depends on metabolism, diet and administrative route. Intravenous administration results in 100% bioavailability. Orally administered drugs have a much lower bioavailability.

biochemical screening (ˌbieohˈkemikəl ˌskreening) tests in pregnancy, when the maternal serum is analysed for biochemical markers that identify babies with fetal Down syndrome or inherited metabolic disorders. The newborn blood-spot screening test also relies on biochemical markers to identify genetic conditions and disorders of the metabolism such as PKU and cystic fibrosis.

biochemistry (ˌbieohˈkemәstree) the chemistry of living matter.

biofeedback (ˌbieohˈfeedˌbak) visual or auditory evidence provided to an individual of the satisfactory performance of an autonomic body function (e.g. sounding a tone when blood pressure is at a satisfactory level) so that, through conditioning, the patient may assert control over that function.

biogenesis (ˌbieohˈjenәsәs) 1. the origin of life. 2. the theory that living organisms can originate only from those already living and cannot be artificially produced.

biohazard (ˈbieohˌhazәd) any hazard arising from inadvertent human biological processes, e.g. accidental inoculation, needlestick injury.

biology (bieˈolәjee) the science of living organisms, dealing with their structure, function and relations with one another.

biomechanical engineering (ˌbieohˈmәkanәk'l ˌenjәˈneerәng) the application of engineering knowledge and methods to the functions of the body. Used both as a means of explanation of bodily function and in the treatment of disorders of the body. Practical applications include the use of artificial joints, electronic hearing aids and pacemakers.

biometrics, biometry (ˌbieәˈmetriks; bieˈomәtree) 1. anthropometry. 2. the use of statistics in biological science.

biomicroscopy (ˌbieohmieˈkroskә-pee) a microscopic examination of living tissues, e.g. of the structures of the anterior of the eye during life. *See* SLIT LAMP.

biophysical profile (BPP) (ˌbieohˈ-fizәk'l ˈprohˌfiel) a non-invasive test of fetal wellbeing using ultrasound to measure fetal heart rate, fetal tone, somatic movements, breathing movements and amniotic fluid volume. Each factor is scored to obtain a total biophysical score, which is an accurate predictor of fetal death in high-risk pregnancies. The score may be affected by gestation, maternal illness, therapeutic medication, substance abuse or fetal abnormality.

bioplasm (ˈbieohˌplazәm) protoplasm. The active principle in matter which produces living organisms.

biopsy (ˈbieopsee) the removal of some tissue or organ from the living body, e.g. a lymph gland, for examination to establish a diagnosis. *Core needle b.* a procedure similar to a fine needle biopsy except a larger core (hollow) needle is inserted into the breast to remove a small sample of tissue from an area of concern. Usually done using guidance of ultrasound. A small inert titanium marker may by inserted and left inside the breast to mark the area that was sampled for future reference. *Aspiration b.* biopsy in which the tissue is obtained by suction through a needle and syringe. *Cone b.* biopsy in which an inverted cone of tissue is excised, as from the uterine cervix. *Excisional b.* removal of an entire lesion and significant portion of normal-looking tissue for examination. *Needle b.* tissue obtained by the puncture of a lesion with a needle. Rotation of the needle removes tissue within the lumen of the needle.

biorhythm (ˈbieohˌrithəm) any cyclic, biological event, e.g. sleep cycle and menstrual cycle, affecting daily life.

biosensors (ˈbieohˌsensəz) non-invasive instruments that measure the result of biological processes, e.g. body temperature.

biostatistics (ˌbieohstəˈtistiks) that branch of biometry that deals with the data and laws of human mortality, morbidity, natality and demography. Also called vital statistics.

biosynthesis (ˌbieohˈsinthəsəs) the creation of a compound within a living organism.

biotin (ˈbieətən) formerly termed vitamin H, now part of the vitamin B complex and present in all normal diets.

biparietal (biepəˈrieət'l) pertaining to both parietal eminences or bones.

biparous (bieˈparəs) giving birth to two infants at a time.

bipolar (bieˈpohlə) with two poles. *B. disorder* formerly known as manic-depressive illness, characterised by swings in mood between opposite extremes of severe depression and mania or overexcitability. Initially, the mood disturbance may consist of depression or excitability, but eventually it alternates between the two. Often accompanied by grandiose ideas or negative delusions. *B. nerve cells* cells having two nerve fibres, e.g. ganglionic cells.

birth (ˈbərth) the act of being born. *B. centre* a home-like health facility where antenatal care, intrapartum and postnatal care is provided by midwives, in consultation with other health professionals, for women judged to be at minimum risk for obstetric complications. Also called a birthing centre. *B. certificate* statement issued by the Registrar for births, marriages and deaths for the particular state or territory in which the baby is born, which certifies details of parentage, name and sex of child, and date and place of birth. It gives legal status to the child and is necessary before any government child benefit can be paid. A birth certificate is issued to any baby born alive, irrespective of the period of gestation. *B. control* limiting the size of the family by abstention from sexual intercourse or the use of contraceptives. *B. mark* a naevus present from birth. *B. plan* a plan prepared by the expectant mother, usually in conjunction with her partner and midwife, which records her preferences for care during and after labour. *B. rate* the proportion of the number of live births in a specific area during a given period of the total population of that area, usually expressed as the number of births per 1000 of population. *Premature b.* one taking place before term. *B. registration* in Australia is compulsory (it is required by law). The relevant legislation in each state and territory specifies that registration of all births and stillbirths must occur within a specified time period.

birthing chair (ˈbərthing chair) a specially designed chair for use in labour and delivery to promote greater mobility for the mother.

birthing pool (ˈbərthing pool) a specially designed pool allowing mothers to give birth under water.

bisexual (ˌbieˈsekshyooəl) 1. having gonads of both sexes. 2. hermaphrodite. 3. having both active and passive sexual interests or characteristics. 4. capable of the function of both sexes. 5. both heterosexual and homosexual. 6. an individual who is both heterosexual and homosexual. 7. of, relating to or involving both sexes, as in bisexual reproduction.

bite (biet) 1. to seize with the teeth. 2. a wound made by biting from either a human or an animal. Treatment for both types of bite is through cleansing and, if necessary, a dressing. Consideration should be given to the immunisation status of the person as there is a risk of tetanus. For human bites, there is also a risk of transmission of hepatitis B, hepatitis C, herpes simplex and HIV infection. With animal bites, preventive antibiotics may be prescribed together with anti-rabies vaccine and immunoglobulin, if the person's history indicates that the animal is infected with the rabies virus. 3. an impression made by the teeth on a thin sheet of malleable material such as wax.

Bitot's spots (ˈbeetohz spotz) *Pierre Bitot, French physician, 1822–1888.* Collections of dried epithelium, microorganisms, etc., forming shiny, greyish spots on the cornea. A sign of vitamin A deficiency.

bivalve (bieˌvalv) 1. having two valves, as the shells of molluscs such as oysters. 2. to cut a plaster cast into an anterior and a posterior section. *B. speculum* a vaginal speculum with two blades that can be adjusted for easy insertion.

blackhead (ˈblakˌhed) *see* COMEDO.

blackout (ˈblakowt) momentary failure of vision and unconsciousness due to cerebral circulatory insufficiency.

blackwater fever (ˈblakˌwawtəˌfeevə) a form of malignant malaria in which severe haemolysis causes a dark discolouration of the urine. *See* MALARIA.

bladder (ˈbladə) a membranous sac for holding fluid or gas. *Atonic b.* a condition in which there is lack of tone in the urinary bladder wall, which may be the result of incomplete emptying over a long period. *B. retraining* a process of education used by nurses to reduce the urgency of micturition and episodes of urinary incontinence by increasing the time intervals between emptying the bladder. *B. worm* a cysticercus. *Irritable b.* a condition in which there is a frequent desire to micturate. *Urinary b.* the reservoir for urine.

Blalock-Taussig operation (ˌblaylok ˈtawsig ˌopəˈrayshən) *Alfred Blalock, American surgeon, 1899–1964; Helen Taussig, American paediatrician, 1898–1986.* A surgical procedure to construct a shunt to overcome insufficient pulmonary blood flow in malformations such as TETRALOGY OF FALLOT.

blanch test (blahnch test) a test of blood circulation in the fingers or toes. Pressure is applied to the fingernail or toenail until normal colour is lost. The pressure is then removed. If the circulation is normal, colour should return almost immediately or within 2 seconds. The time may be prolonged by a compromise of circulation, such as arterial occlusion, hypovolaemic shock or hypothermia. Also known as capillary nail test or nail blanch test.

bland (bland) non-stimulating. *B. fluids* mild and non-irritating fluids such as barley water and milk.

blast (blahst) 1. an immature cell. 2. a wave of high air pressure caused by an explosion.

blastocyst (ˈblastəˌsist) *see* BLASTULA.

blastoderm (ˈblastəˌderm) the germinal cells of the embryo, consisting of three layers: ectoderm, mesoderm and entoderm.

blastolysis (blaˈstoləsəs, ˌblastəˈ-liesəs) the destruction of germ substance.

blastomycosis (ˌblastohmieˈkohsəs) a fungal infection which, after invasion of the skin, may cause granulomatous lesions in the mouth, pharynx and lungs.

blastula (ˈblastyələ) an early stage in the development of the fertilised ovum. This stage precedes the gastrula. Also called blastocyst.

bleb (bleb) *see* BLISTER.

bleeder (ˈbleedə) 1. a colloquial name for one who suffers from haemophilia. 2. a vessel that is difficult to seal at operation.

bleeding (ˈbleeding) 1. escape of blood from an injured vessel. 2. venesection. *B. gums see* GINGIVITIS *B. time* the time taken for oozing to cease from a sharp prick of the finger or ear lobe. The normal value is 1–3 minutes. *Functional b.* bleeding from the uterus when no organic lesion is present.

blennorrhagia (ˌblenəˈrayji·ə) 1. an excessive discharge of mucus, e.g. LEUCORRHOEA. 2. GONORRHOEA.

blennorrhoea (ˌblenəˈreeə) normal discharge of mucus. *See* BLENNORRHAGIA.

blepharitis (ˌblefəˈrietəs) inflammation of the eyelids. *Allergic b.* that associated with response to drugs or cosmetics applied to the eye or eyelids. *Squamous b.* that associated with dandruff of the scalp.

blepharon (ˈblefə·ron) the eyelid.

blepharophimosis (ˌblefə·rohfie-ˈmohsəs) abnormal narrowing of the aperture between the eyelids. Usually congenital but may arise from chronic inflammation.

blepharospasm (ˌblefə·rohˈspazəm) prolonged spasm of the orbicular muscles of the eyelids.

blind (bliend) without sight. *B. spot* the point where the optic nerve leaves the retina, which is insensitive to light.

blind loop syndrome (bliend ˈloop ˈsinˌdrohm) a condition of stasis in the small intestine, which aids bacterial multiplication, leading to diarrhoea and salt deficiencies. The cause may be intestinal obstruction or surgical ANASTOMOSIS.

blindness (ˈbliendnəs) lack or loss of ability to see; lack of perception of visual stimuli. Blindness is defined as less than 6/60 vision with glasses (vision of 6/60 is the ability to see only at 6 metres what the normal eye can see at 60 metres). A person with this level of vision may be registered as 'legally blind'. A person may also be registered as having vision impairment or low vision when they have permanent vision loss that cannot be corrected with glasses and affects many aspects of daily life.

blister (ˈblisˈtə) a bleb or vesicle. A collection of serum between the epidermis and the skin. *Blood b.* a blister containing blood, usually caused by a pinch or bruise.

block (blok) a stoppage or obstruction. The term is used to describe: (a) various forms of regional anaesthesia, e.g. epidural block; (b) obstruction to the passage of a nervous impulse due to disease, e.g. heart block (*see* HEART); and (c) an interruption of mental function.

blood (blud) the fluid that circulates through the heart and blood vessels, supplying nutritive material to all parts of the body and carrying away waste products. Blood is a red viscid fluid and consists of plasma in which are suspended erythrocytes (red blood cells), LEUCOCYTES (white blood cells) and lymphocytes, and platelets or thrombocytes. (a) The red corpuscles or ERYTHROCYTES contain haemoglobin, which combines with oxygen in passing through the lungs. This oxygen is released into the tissues from the capillaries and oxidation takes place. (b) The white corpuscles or leucocytes defend against invading microorganisms, which they have power to destroy. (c) Blood platelets or THROMBOCYTES are concerned with the clotting of blood. Plasma also contains many other specialised substances with important roles to play in immunity and blood clotting.

blood bank (blud bank) 1. a place of storage for blood. 2. an organisation that collects, processes, stores and transfuses blood.

blood-borne viruses ('blud bawn 'vierəsəs) viruses that are transmitted by blood and some other body fluids (e.g. semen, amniotic fluid), such as hepatitis B virus, hepatitis C virus and human immunodeficiency viruses (HIV-1, HIV-2).

blood–brain barrier (BBB) (blud brayn 'bareeə) membranous barrier separating the blood from the brain. It is permeable to water, oxygen, carbon dioxide, glucose, alcohol, general anaesthetics and some drugs.

blood casts (blud kahsts) casts of coagulated red blood cells formed in the renal tubules and found in urine.

blood clotting, coagulation (blud 'klotəng, ˌkoh'agyoolayshən) the formation of a jelly-like substance over the ends or within the walls of a blood vessel, with resultant stoppage of the blood flow. Clotting is one of the natural defence mechanisms of the body when injury occurs. A clot will usually form within 5 minutes of a blood vessel being damaged. The exact process of clotting or coagulation is triggered by exposure of coagulation factors in the blood plasma to tissue factor that is expressed beneath the surface of the blood vessel wall lining (called endothelium) when trauma occurs or pathology exists in the patient such as infection, inflammation or cancer. This exposure of tissue factor activates one of the most important coagulation factors called factor VII (7), which then activates the rest of the extrinsic coagulation cascade. This results in the formation of thrombin factor XI (11) which converts fibrinogen to fibrin. Normal levels of functioning platelets are required for the coagulation factors to work as they are used as a lipid platform or scaffold. Fibrin, platelets and embedded red and white cells then form this mesh or clot. Factor XIII (13) then crosslinks the fibrin to stabilise it further. Von Willebrand factor and platelets also help to repair traumatised vessels and prevent bleeding. Plasma coagulation factors are:

I Fibrinogen
II Prothrombin
Tissue factor
IV Calcium ions
VII Factor VII (7)
VIII Factor VIII (8)
IX Christmas factor
X Stuart factor (Power factor)
XI Factor XI (11)
XII Hageman factor or contact factor
XIII Fibrin stabilising factor

blood count (blud kownt) the number of blood cells in a given sample of blood, usually expressed as the number of cells per litre of blood (as the red blood cell, white blood cell or platelet count). A differential white cell count determines the number of various types of leucocyte in a sample of blood. (*See* Appendix 4.)

blood dyscrasia (blud dis'krayzyə) any abnormality of the blood cells or of the clotting elements.

blood gas (blud gas) gas dissolved in the liquid part of the blood, including oxygen, carbon dioxide and nitrogen.

blood gas analysis (blud gas ə'naləsis) laboratory studies of arterial and venous blood for the purpose of measuring oxygen and carbon dioxide levels and pressure or tension, and hydrogen ion concentration (pH). Analyses of blood gases provide the following information: PaO_2—partial pressure (P) of oxygen (O_2) in the arterial blood (a); SaO_2—percentage of available haemoglobin that is saturated (Sa) with oxygen (O_2); $PaCO_2$—partial pressure (P) of carbon dioxide (CO_2) in arterial blood (a); pH—an expression of the extent to which the blood is alkaline or acidic; HCO_3—the level of plasma bicarbonate; an indicator of the metabolic acid–base status.

blood glucose (blud 'glukohs) the amount of glucose present in the blood. The normal range is 3.5–5.5 mmol/L. When the amount exceeds 10 mmol/L, glucose is excreted in the urine, as in DIABETES MELLITUS.

blood groups ('blud groops) ABO system (*see* table). In clinical practice, there are four main blood types: A, B, O and AB. In addition to this major grouping, there is a rhesus (Rh) system that is important in the prevention of haemolytic disease of the newborn resulting from incompatibility of blood groups in mother and fetus. In determining a blood group, a sample of blood is taken and mixed with specially prepared sera. One serum, anti-A agglutinin, causes blood of group A to agglutinate; another serum, anti-B agglutinin, causes blood of group B to agglutinate. Thus, if anti-A serum alone causes clumping, the blood is group A; if anti-B serum alone causes clumping, the blood group is B. If both cause clumping, the blood group is AB, and if it is not clumped by either, it is identified as group O. Transfusion with an incompatible ABO group causes severe haemolytic reaction and death may occur.

blood pressure (BP) ('blud preshə) the pressure exerted on the artery walls by the blood as it flows through them. It can be measured in milligrams of mercury using a sphygmomanometer. Two

ABO system

Group	Antigen present in red cell	Antibody present in plasma
AB	A and B	—
A	A	Anti-B (β)
B	B	Anti-A (α)
O	—	Anti-A and Anti-B (α and β

readings are made. Arterial pressure fluctuates with each heartbeat and one measure records the pressure while the heart is in SYSTOLE (when the heart is ejecting blood into the arteries) and is the higher, or systolic, pressure. The other measure records the pressure while the heart is in diastole (when the aortic and pulmonary valves are closed and the heart is relaxed); this is the lower, or diastolic, pressure. The range of normal blood pressure recording varies according to age and body size, but in the normal young adult is approximately 100–120/70–80 mmHg.

blood sugar (blud ˈshuhgə) *see* BLOOD GLUCOSE.

blood transfusion (blud tranzˈfyoo-shən) introduction of blood from the vein of one person (donor) or from a blood bank into the vein of another (recipient) in cases of severe loss of blood, trauma, septicaemia, etc. It is used to supplement the volume of blood and to introduce constituents, such as clotting factors or antibodies that are deficient in the patient. *Autologous b. t.* the use of a person's own blood donated earlier for transfusion. The patient's blood may also be salvaged during surgery, filtered and returned to the circulation, thus reducing the need for donated blood transfusion.

blood urea (blud yooreeə) excretory product of protein present in the blood. The normal range is 3.1–8.1 mmol/L; this increases in renal failure when the kidneys cease to function normally.

blue baby (blu ˈbaybee) a child born with a very blue colour. The colour may be due to ATELECTASIS or to a defect in the heart, in consequence of which arterial and venous blood become mixed. *See* FALLOT'S TETRALOGY.

blush (blush) growing redness of the face, usually a reaction to emotion or heat.

BMI *see* BODY MASS INDEX.

BMR *see* BASAL METABOLIC RATE.

body (ˈbodee) 1. the trunk, or animal frame, with its organs. 2. the largest and most important part of any organ. 3. any mass or collection of material.

body dysmorphic disorder (ˈbodee ˌdisˈmorˈfik ˈdisˈawdə) an anxiety disorder that causes a person to have a distorted view of how they look and worry excessively about their appearance.

body image (ˈbodee imij) the person's perception of their physical self and the thoughts and feelings that result from that perception. These feelings can be positive, negative or both and are influenced by individual and environmental factors.

body language (ˈbodee ˈlanˌgwij) the expression of thoughts or emotions by means of posture or gestures. Body language may include unintended 'signs' as well as intended communication.

body mass index (BMI) (bodee mas indeks) the weight (kg) divided by the square of the height (m). A BMI of 18.5–24.9 indicates an ideal weight; below 18.4 is underweight; a BMI of 25–29.9 is overweight, a BMI of 30–39.9 is classified as obese and over 40 very obese. These figures apply to adults under the age of 60 years only and are not applicable to children, people over 60 years, those with chronic health problems, athletes or pregnant or breastfeeding women.

Body Substance Isolation (BSI) (bodee ˈsubstəns uysuhˈlayshən) an INFECTION CONTROL system, developed in 1987, that further elaborated UNIVERSAL PRECAUTIONS and focused on the isolation of all moist and potentially infectious body substances (blood, faeces, urine, sputum, saliva, wound drainage and other body fluids) from all patients, regardless of their presumed infection status, primarily through the use of gloves. This concept has now been further developed and is known by the terms STANDARD PRECAUTIONS and TRANSITION-BASED PRECAUTIONS. (*See* Appendix 10.)

boil (boyl) an acute staphylococcal inflammation of the skin and subcutaneous tissues around a hair follicle. It causes a painful swelling with a central core of dead tissue (slough), which is eventually discharged. A FURUNCLE.

bolus (ˈbohləs) 1. a large pill. 2. a rounded mass of masticated food immediately before being swallowed or one passing through the intestines. 3. a quantity of a drug injected directly to raise its concentration in the blood to a therapeutic level.

bonding (ˈbonding) the attachment process that occurs between an infant and his or her parents, especially the mother, during the first hours and days following birth. Bonding is a reciprocal process and is considered a biological need for the future development, both physical and emotional, of the infant. *Dental b.* the use of bonding agents to restore or improve the appearance of damaged or defective teeth.

bone (bohn) the dense connective tissue forming the skeleton. It is composed of cartilage or membrane impregnated with mineral salts, chiefly calcium phosphate and calcium carbonate. This is arranged as an outer hard compact tissue and an inner network of cells (cancellous tissue), in the spaces of which is red bone marrow. In the shaft of long bones is a medullary cavity containing yellow marrow. Microscopically, the bone tissue is perforated with minute HAVERSIAN CANALS containing blood vessels and lymphatics for the maintenance and repair of the cells (*see* figure, p. 68). Bone is covered by a fibrous membrane, the PERIOSTEUM, containing blood vessels and by which the bone grows in girth. *B. age* a measure of skeletal development in assessing physical maturity in children by using X-rays to show how much the bones have grown in a particular body area. *B. density testing* a dual-energy X-ray absorptiometry (DEXA) machine is used to determine bone density or strength. It can identify osteopenia (a mild form of bone loss) or osteoporosis (decreased bone density). *B. graft* transplantation of a healthy piece of bone to replace missing or repair defective bone. *B. marrow* substance which fills the marrow cavities of bones. Basically there are two types: yellow and red marrow. The red marrow, consisting mainly of haematopoietic tissue, is responsible for producing the red blood cells, platelets and most white blood cells. The yellow is mostly fatty connective tissue. *B. marrow transplantation* a procedure used to treat aplastic anaemia, acute leukaemia, lymphoma, myeloma and some rare congenital disorders, with varying success. Healthy stem cells are taken from the donor and infused into the bloodstream of the recipient, whose own bone marrow is no longer able to produce healthy blood cells.

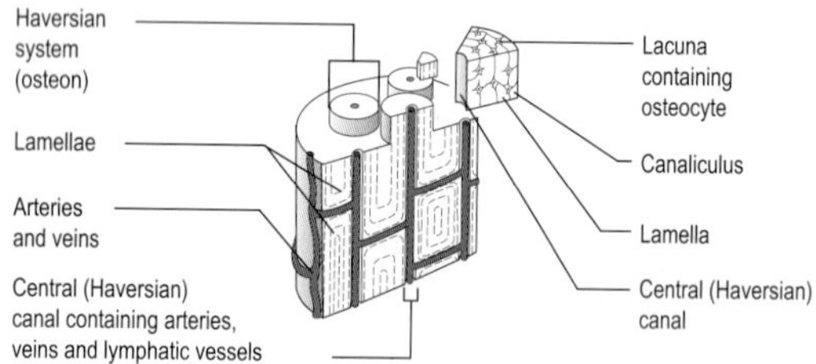

Structure of compact bone.

bong (bong) a water pipe used for smoking CANNABIS and other drugs.

borborygmus (ˌbawbəˈrigməs) a rumbling sound caused by gas in the intestines.

Bordetella (ˌbawdəˈtelə) a genus of bacteria. *B. pertussis* the causal agent of whooping cough.

Bornholm disease (ˈbawnˌholm diˈzeez) an epidemic myalgia with pleural pain and fever due to Coxsackie virus infection. It is named after the Danish island of Bornholm, where there was an outbreak in 1930.

botulism (ˈbotyəˌlizəm, ˈbochə-) an extremely severe form of food poisoning due to a neurotoxin (botulin) produced by *Clostridium botulinum*, sometimes found in improperly canned or preserved foods. The symptoms include vomiting, abdominal pain, headache, weakness, constipation and nerve paralysis, which causes difficulty in seeing, breathing and swallowing. Death is usually due to paralysis of the respiratory organs.

bougie (ˈboozhee, booˈzhee) a flexible cylindrical instrument used to dilate a stricture, as in the oesophagus or urethra.

bovine (ˈbohvien) relating to the cow or ox. *B. spongiform encephalopathy (BSE)* commonly known as 'mad cow disease', is a fatal, neurodegenerative disease of cattle. BSE has attracted wide attention because it seems possible to transmit the disease to humans and it is believed to be the cause of variant CREUTZFELDT-JAKOB DISEASE (VCJD), a human brain-wasting disease. *B. tuberculosis* that caused by infection from infected cows' milk, usually affecting glands and bones.

bowel (ˈbowəl) the intestine. *B. sounds* relatively high-pitched abdominal sounds caused by the propulsion of the intestinal contents through the lower alimentary canal.

Bowen's disease (ˈbohənz diˈzeez) a very early form of skin cancer affecting the squamous cells. The main symptom is a red, scaly patch on the skin.

bowleg (ˈbohˌleg) deformity where there is an outward curvature of one or both legs near the knee. This results in a gap between the knees on standing. Also called genu varum.

Bowman's capsule (ˈbohmənz ˈkapsyool) *Sir William Bowman,*

British physician, 1816–1892. The expanded end of the kidney tubule, which surrounds the GLOMERULUS.

brace (brays) 1. a support used in orthopaedics to hold parts of the body in their correct positions. 2. an orthodontic appliance to correct the alignment of teeth.

brachial (ˈbrayki·əl, ˈbrak-) relating to the arm. *B. artery* the continuation of the axillary artery along the inner side of the upper arm. *B. plexus* a network of nerves at the root of the neck supplying the upper limb.

brachytherapy (ˌbrakiˈtherəpee) radiotherapy delivered into or adjacent to a tumour by means of an intracavitary or interstitial radioactive source.

Braden scale (ˌbraydən ˈskayl) *see* PRESSURE INJURY RISK ASSESSMENT SCALES.

bradycardia (ˌbradeeˈkahdi·ə) abnormally low rate of heart contractions and consequent slow pulse (fewer than 60 beats per minute).

bradycephaly (ˌbradeeˈkefəlee) a common condition affecting babies, also known as flat head syndrome, where the back of the head is flattened as a result of spending a lot of time lying on their backs. The head widens and the forehead may bulge. The head shape will generally improve over time. *See also* PLAGIOCEPHALY.

bradykinesia (bradeeˌkəneezi·ə) excessive slowness of voluntary movements and speech; a characteristic of Parkinsonism and some other nervous system disorders.

bradykinin (ˌbradeeˈkienən) peptide formed from the degradation of protein by enzymes. It is a powerful vasodilator that also causes contraction of smooth muscle.

Braille (brayl) a method of printing developed by *Louis Braille, 1809–1852* for people with a visual impairment. Letters of the alphabet are represented by patterns of raised dots. These dots are read by passing the fingertips over them.

brain (brayn) that part of the central nervous system contained in the skull. It consists of the CEREBRUM, MIDBRAIN, CEREBELLUM, MEDULLA OBLONGATA and PONS VAROLII.

brainstem (ˈbraynˌstem) the lower part of the brain which links with the spinal cord and controls the automatic functions of the body, e.g. heart and respiratory rate. This consists of the MIDBRAIN, PONS VAROLII and MEDULLA OBLONGATA.

brainstorming (ˈbraynˌstawming) an approach to problem-solving through the encouragement of intensive discussion in a group, generating ideas and solutions about an issue.

bran (bran) the husk of grain, i.e. the coarse outer coat of cereals. High in roughage and vitamins of the B complex, bran is frequently recommended as a dietary component both for those with alimentary disorders and for those in normal health.

branchial (ˈbrangki·əl) relating to the clefts (branchia) that are present in the neck and pharynx in the developing embryo. Normally they disappear. *B. cyst* a cystic swelling arising from a branchial remnant in the neck. *B. sinus* (lateral cervical sinus) a tract leading from the posterior cervical region which opens in the lower neck in front of the sternomastoid muscle.

Braun's frame (ˈbrawnz fraym) *Heinrich Braun, German surgeon, 1862–1934*. A metal frame that incorporates one or more pulleys and is used to elevate the lower limb and to apply skeletal traction for a compound fracture of the tibia and fibula.

Braxton Hicks contractions (ˈbrakstən hiks konˈtrakshənz) *J. Braxton Hicks, British gynaecologist, 1823–1897.* Painless uterine contractions occurring during pregnancy, becoming increasingly rhythmic and intense during the third trimester. Sometimes called 'false labour'.

BRCA gene (ˈbrakˈah jeen) (BReast CAncer gene) $BRCA_1$ and $BRCA_2$ are two different genes that produce tumour suppressor proteins. When either gene is faulty DNA damage may not be repaired properly and cells are more likely to develop additional alterations that can lead to cancer, particularly of the breast and ovary. A harmful $BRCA_1$ or $BRCA_2$ mutation can be inherited from either parent.

breast (brest) 1. the anterior or front region of the chest. 2. the mammary gland. *B. abscess* formation of pus in the mammary gland. *B. bone* the sternum. *B. cancer* the breast is a common site of cancer in women and occurs occasionally in men. Although the survival rates for breast cancer continue to increase, the incidence of the disease in the Western world is also increasing. Improvement in these survival rates has come from increased public awareness, breast self-examination, breast cancer screening programs and improved methods of treatment. It is recommended that women perform a simple self-examination of the breasts each month (*see* figure, p. 71). The best time for this is just after menstruation when the breasts are normally soft, but should also be continued after the menopause on a regular basis. If any lump in the breast can be felt, a doctor should be consulted immediately. More than 90% of breast cancers are discovered by the patients themselves. *B. pump* an apparatus for removal of milk from the breast. *Pigeon b.* prominent sternum, a deformity resulting from rickets.

breastfeeding (ˈbrestˌfeeding) the method of feeding a baby with milk directly from the mother's breasts. Midwives and paediatricians agree that breastfeeding is usually better for the baby and the mother, both physically and emotionally. In Australia, the Baby Friendly Health Initiative (BFHI) aims to encourage healthcare services to promote and support breastfeeding. Developed by UNICEF and the World Health Organisation (WHO), the initiative provides a framework called the *Ten Steps to Successful Breastfeeding* (*see* table, p. 72) for accredited Baby Friendly hospitals to operate within. These standards ensure all mothers and babies receive appropriate support and contemporary information during the antenatal and postnatal period regarding infant feeding.

breath (breth) the air taken in and expelled by the expansion and contraction of the thorax. *B. holding* when a young child cries, holds its breath and goes blue. *B. sounds* the sounds heard when a stethoscope is placed over the lungs during respiration. *B. test* 1. using a breathalyser to analyse a person's breath in order to determine the level of alcohol consumed within a certain period of time. Used to test drivers to assess if the person is within or above the legal limit

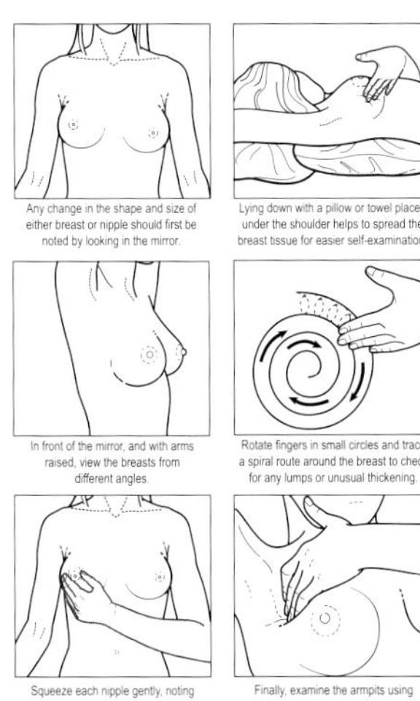

Any change in the shape and size of either breast or nipple should first be noted by looking in the mirror.

Lying down with a pillow or towel placed under the shoulder helps to spread the breast tissue for easier self-examination.

In front of the mirror, and with arms raised, view the breasts from different angles.

Rotate fingers in small circles and trace a spiral route around the breast to check for any lumps or unusual thickening.

Squeeze each nipple gently, noting any discharge or bleeding.

Finally, examine the armpits using the spiral technique and note any unusual findings.

Breast self-examination or breast awareness.

There is no one method recommended over another for women to use when checking their breasts. Some women may feel more comfortable with a structured way (see figure above) while others may prefer another pattern, such as feeling their breast using up and down lines or working in circles or moving in and out in a wedge-like fashion, ensuring all the breast is covered, as well as between the breasts and the underarms. The main point to remember is that women (and men) of all ages need to become familiar with the normal look and feel of their breasts.

Breast changes to look/feel for include:

• a lump or lumpiness, especially if it is only in one breast or dimpling of the skin or redness.

• any changes to the shape of the nipple, for example the nipple is pulled in (inverted).

• discharge from the nipple particularly if it contains blood.

• any pain that is unusual and does not go away.

• a swelling in the armpit or around the collarbone.

Undertaking regular breast self-examination lets women know what is normal for their breasts. If changes are detected they need to be reported to their general practitioner without delay.

For more information on how to be breast aware, visit the Breast Cancer Network Australia, Cancer Australia or Cancer Council Australia websites or relevant organisations related to the country of your practice.

Breast self-examination.

Ten Steps to Successful Breastfeeding

- Have a written breastfeeding policy that is routinely communicated to all healthcare staff
- All healthcare staff trained to implement the policy
- All pregnant mothers informed of the benefits and management of breastfeeding
- Mothers assisted to commence breastfeeding within half an hour of delivery
- Show mothers how to breastfeed and maintain lactation, even if they are separated from their infants
- Neonates to be given nothing other than breast milk unless medically necessary
- Practise rooming-in, i.e. allow mothers and infants to remain together 24 hours a day
- Encourage breastfeeding on-demand
- No teats or pacifiers to be given to breastfeeding infants
- Establishment of breastfeeding support groups and refer mothers to them on discharge from hospital or clinic.

Source: UNICEF Australia, Baby Friendly Health Initiative.

of alcohol consumption. 2. widely used to explore pathophysiology of functional gastrointestinal (GI) disorders, such as small intestinal bacterial overgrowth, ileal disease, lactose deficiency, steatorrhoea and *Helicobacter pylori.*

breathing (ˈbreeˈthing) the alternate inspiration and expiration of air into and out of the lungs. *See also* RESPIRATION.

breech (breech) the buttocks. *B. presentation* a position of the fetus in the uterus such that the buttocks present.

bregma (ˈbregmə) the anterior fontanel. The membranous junction between the coronal and sagittal sutures.

bridge (brij) in dentistry, an irremovable prosthesis carrying false teeth that bridges gaps left when natural teeth are extracted.

broad ligaments (brawd ˈligəməntz) folds of peritoneum extending from the uterus to the sides of the pelvis, and supporting the blood vessels to the uterus and uterine tubes.

Broca's area of speech (ˈbrohkəz ˈairi·ə ov speech) *Pierre Paul Broca, French surgeon, 1824–1880.* The motor centre associated with speech, situated in the left cerebral hemisphere. Damage to the nerve cells contained in it can impair speech.

Brodie's abscess (ˌbrohdeez ˈabsəs) *Sir Benjamin Brodie, British surgeon, 1783–1862. See* ABSCESS.

bromhidrosis (ˌbromhəˈdrohsəs) offensive and fetid sweat.

bronchi (ˈbrongkee) plural of bronchus.

bronchiectasis (ˌbrongkeeˈektəsəs) chronic dilatation of the bronchi and bronchioles with secondary infection, usually involving the lower lobes of the lung. The condition may occur as a congenital malformation of the alveoli with resultant dilatation of the terminal bronchi and is associated with cystic fibrosis. Most often it is an acquired disease secondary to partial obstruction of the bronchi with necrotising infection. The symptoms include a chronic cough and purulent sputum. May lead to respiratory failure.

bronchiole (ˈbrongkeeˈohl) one of the smallest of the subdivisions of the bronchi.

bronchiolitis (ˌbrongkeeohˈlietəs) inflammation of the bronchioles.

bronchitis (ˌbrongˈkietəs) inflammation of the bronchi. *Acute b.* a short-lived infection, common in young children and the elderly. It is a descending infection from the common cold, influenza, measles and other upper respiratory conditions. *Chronic b.* a persisting infection of the larger airways characterised by daily mucus production for at least three months and lasting two or more consecutive years. It is one of a number of lung conditions, including emphysema, that are collectively known as chronic obstructive pulmonary disease (COPD).

bronchoadenitis (ˌbrongkohˌadəˈnietəs) inflammation of the bronchial glands.

bronchodilator (ˌbrongkohdieˈlaytə) any agent that causes dilatation of the bronchi.

bronchography (brongˈkografee) radiography of the bronchial tree after introduction of a radio-opaque medium.

bronchomycosis (ˌbrongkohmieˈkohsəs) a general term used to cover a variety of fungal infections of the bronchi: aspergillosis and pulmonary candiasis.

bronchophony (brongˈkofənee) resonance of the voice as heard in the chest over the bronchi on auscultation.

bronchopneumonia (ˌbrongkohnyooˈmohni·ə) a descending infection starting around the bronchi and bronchioles. *See* PNEUMONIA.

bronchopulmonary (ˌbrongkohˈpulmənə·ree, -ˈpuhl) relating to the lungs, bronchi and bronchioles. *B. dysplasia (BPD)* a chronic respiratory condition occurring in babies who have been ventilated for long periods or have needed prolonged oxygen therapy. It results in serious disruption of lung growth. Examination of radiographs and lung specimens reveals patches of collapse and fibrosis. Following ventilation, these babies usually require supplementary oxygen for several weeks or even months to keep the arterial oxygen tension above 55 kPa.

bronchorrhoea (ˌbrongkəˈreeə) an excessive discharge of mucus from the bronchi.

bronchoscope (ˈbrongkohˌskohp) an endoscope that enables the operator to see inside the bronchi. It can also be used to wash out the bronchi, remove foreign bodies or take a biopsy.

bronchoscopy (brongˈkoskəˌpee) examination of the bronchi by means of a bronchoscope.

bronchospasm (ˌbrongkohˌspazəm) difficulty in breathing caused by the sudden constriction of smooth muscle in the walls of the bronchi. This may arise in asthma or chronic bronchitis.

bronchospirometer (ˌbrongkohspieˈromətə) an instrument used to measure the capacity of one lung or of one lobe of the lung, or of each lung separately.

bronchotracheal (ˌbrongkohˈtrakeeəl, ˌbrongkohtrəˈkeeəl) relating to both the trachea and the bronchi. *B. suction* the removal of mucus with the aid of suction.

bronchus (ˌbrongkəs) (*pl.* bronchi), any of the larger passages conveying air to (right or left principal bronchus) and within (lobar and segmental bronchi) the lungs.

brow (brow) the forehead. *B. presentation* a position of the fetus such that the forehead appears at the cervix first.

brown fat (brown fat) a special type of adipose tissue found in the newborn infant, and which is widely distributed throughout the body. The tissue is highly vascular and owes its colour to the large number of mitochondria found in the cytoplasm of its cells. It allows the infant to increase its metabolic rate and thus its heat production when subjected to cold. At the same time the fat itself is used up.

browser (browzə) a computer program used to access and navigate the internet.

Brucella (broo'selə) a genus of bacteria primarily pathogenic in animals but which may affect humans.

brucellosis (ˌbroosə'lohsəs) a rare generalised infection involving primarily the reticuloendothelial system, marked by remittent undulant fever, malaise, headache and anaemia. It is caused by various species of *Brucella* and is transmitted to humans from domestic animals such as pigs, goats and cattle, especially through infected milk or contact with the carcass of an infected animal. The disease is also called undulant fever because one of the major symptoms in humans is a fever that fluctuates widely at regular intervals. Prevention is best accomplished by the pasteurisation of milk and a program of testing, vaccination and elimination of infected animals. Also called Malta fever, abortus fever and Mediterranean fever.

Brudzinski's sign (broo'jinskeez sien) *Josef Brudzinski, Polish physician, 1874–1917.* 1. passive flexion of one thigh causing spontaneous flexion of the opposite thigh. 2. flexion of the neck causing bilateral flexion of the hips and knees. These signs are indicative of meningeal irritation.

Brugada syndrome (broo'gah'dah 'sinˌdrohm) *Pedro and Josep Brugada.* A rare but serious hereditary condition resulting in cardiac arrhythmias that can be life threatening.

bruise (brooz) a superficial injury to tissues produced by sudden impact in which the skin is unbroken. A contusion.

bruit ('brooee) [Fr.] an abnormal sound or murmur heard on auscultation of the heart and large vessels.

bruxism ('brooksizəm) teeth clenching, particularly during sleep. This occurs in persons under tension and may cause headaches as a result of muscle fatigue.

BSE *see* BOVINE SPONGIFORM ENCEPHALOPATHY.

bubo ('byooboh) inflammation of the lymphatic glands of the axilla or groin. Typical of bubonic plague (*see* PLAGUE) and is sexually transmitted.

buccal ('bukəl) pertaining to the cheek or to the mouth.

buccinator ('buksəˌnaytə) a muscle of the cheek, between the mandible and the maxilla.

Budd-Chiari syndrome (ˌbud kee'ah·ree 'sinˌdrohm) *George Budd, British physician, 1808–1882*; *Hans Chiari, Austrian pathologist, 1851–1916.* A condition in which thrombosis of the hepatic vein causes vomiting, jaundice, enlargement of the liver and ascites.

Buerger's disease ('bərgəz di'zeez) *Leo Buerger, American physician, 1879–1943. See* THROMBOANGIITIS OBLITERANS.

buffer ('bufə) 1. a physical or physiological system that tends to oppose change within that system, e.g. the reflexes involved in blood pressure homeostasis. 2. a chemical system that acts to prevent change in the concentration of another chemical substance. Sodium bicarbonate is the chief buffer of the blood and tissue fluids. 3. anything that is used to reduce shock or jarring upon contact.

buggery ('bugə·ree) anal intercourse, either heterosexual or homosexual. In law the term also includes sexual contact with an animal (bestiality). Also known as sodomy.

bulbar ('bulbə) pertaining to the MEDULLA OBLONGATA. *B. paralysis see* PARALYSIS.

bulbourethral (ˌbulbohyə'reethrəl) relating to the bulb of the urethra (bulb of the penis). *B. glands* small glands opening into the male urethra. Cowper's glands.

bulimia (byoo'limi·ə) abnormal increase in the sensation of hunger. *B. nervosa* a pattern of 'binge eating' controlled by self-induced vomiting or use of laxatives or episodes of uncontrolled and compulsive overeating occurring in response to stress. Bulimic 'binges' often occur in anorexia nervosa.

bulk-forming agent ('bulk fawming 'ayjənt) an antidiarrhoeal agent that makes the faeces less fluid by absorbing water.

bulla ('bulə) a large, fluid-containing blister.

bullying (booleeing) the tormenting of others through verbal harassment, physical assault or other subtle methods of coercion such as manipulation or sending hurtful or scary messages or phone calls, SMS texts, emails or other social media messages. Bullying is widespread and occurs in settings where people interact. This includes schools and workplaces. These settings have a responsibility to create an environment where children and adults feel safe. In recent years, steps have been taken to develop policies against bullying. *See also* HARASSMENT.

bundle ('bund'l) a collection of nerve fibres all running in the same direction. *B. branch block* the delay in conduction along either branch of the atrioventricular bundle of the heart. The abnormality is detected by an ECG recording.

bundle of His ('bund'l ov 'his) *Wilhelm His Jr, German physiologist, 1863–1934.* The band of neuromuscular fibres which, passing through the spectrum of the heart, divides at the apex into two parts, these being distributed into the walls of the ventricles. The impulse of contraction is conducted through the structure. Atrioventricular bundle.

bunion ('bunyən) a prominence of the head of the metatarsal bone at its junction with the great toe, caused by inflammation and swelling of the bursa at that joint. Usually due to shoes that distort the natural shape of the foot. Also known as HALLUX VALGUS.

buphthalmos (buf'thalməs) abnormal enlargement of the eyes in congenital glaucoma.

Burkitt's lymphoma (bərkitsˌ lim'fohmə) *Dennis Burkitt, Irish surgeon, 1911–1993.* African lymphoma. A cancer of the lymphatic system frequently in the jaw, occurring almost exclusively in children living in low-lying moist areas. Occurs in New Guinea and Central Africa. The Epstein–Barr virus (EB virus), a herpes virus, has been isolated from Burkitt's lymphoma cells in culture, and has been implicated as a causative agent.

burn (bərn) an injury to tissues caused by: (a) physical agents, the sun, excess heat or cold, friction, nuclear radiation; (b) chemical agents, acids or caustic alkalis; (c) electrical current. Burns are described as being partial thickness (involving only the epidermis) or full thickness (involving the dermis and underlying structures). Clinically, emphasis is placed on the percentage of the body affected by the burn. The treatment of shock and prevention of infection and malnutrition need special attention. *See* LUND AND BROWDER CHART.

burnout (bərnowt) a term used to describe a state of emotional, mental and physical exhaustion as a result of excessive and prolonged stress among workers and, commonly, in members of the health professions. Burnout is characterised by chronic fatigue, insomnia, impaired concentration, anxiety, depression and anger. Other signs may include cynicism and detachment that can lead to ineffectiveness and lack of accomplishment in the work situation.

burr (bər) a bit for a surgical drill, used for cutting bone or teeth. *B. hole* a circular hole drilled in the cranium to permit access to the brain or to release raised intracranial pressure.

bursa (ˈbərsə) a small sac of fibrous tissue, lined with synovial membrane and containing synovial fluid. It is situated between parts that move upon one another at a joint to reduce friction.

bursitis (bərˈsietəs) inflammation of the bursa. It produces pain and may impede movement of the joint. *Prepatellar b.* HOUSEMAID'S KNEE.

buttock (ˈbutək) either of the two prominences formed by the flesh-covered gluteal muscles at either side of the lower spine.

bypass (ˈbieˌpahs) diversion of flow. Formation of a shunt. *Aortocoronary b.* diversion of flow from the aorta to the coronary arteries via a saphenous vein or artificial graft. *Femoropopliteal b.* diversion of flow from the femoral to the popliteal artery to overcome an occlusion.

byssinosis (ˌbisəˈnohsəs) an industrial disease caused by inhalation of cotton or linen dust in the workplace. A type of PNEUMOCONIOSIS.

byte (biet) the storage space in the memory of a computer allocated to one character or letter, usually composed of a sequence of 8 bits.

Cc

C symbol for *carbon*, *Celsius* or *centigrade*, and *cytosine*.

© symbol for copyright.

Ca symbol for *calcium*.

cachexia (kəˈkeksi·ə) a condition of extreme debility. The patient is emaciated, the skin being loose and wrinkled from rapid wasting, but shiny and tense over bone. The eyes are sunken, the skin yellowish, and there is a grey, 'muddy' complexion. The mucous membranes are pale and anaemia is extreme. The condition is typical of the late stages of chronic diseases.

cadaver (kəˈdavə, -ˈdah-) a corpse. The dead body used for dissection.

caecum (ˈseekəm) the blind pouch forming the beginning of the large intestine. The vermiform appendix is attached to it.

caesarean section (səˈzairi·ən ˈsekshən) delivery of a fetus by an incision through the abdominal wall and uterus. Performed for the safety of either the mother or the infant. Tradition has it that Julius Caesar was born in this way.

caesium (ˈseezi·əm) *symbol* Cs. A metallic element. *C.-137* radioactive caesium; a fission product from uranium.

café-au-lait spot (ˈkafay oh lay spot) pigmented macules of a distinctive light-brown colour, like coffee with milk, as in NEUROFIBROMATOSIS and ALBRIGHT'S SYNDROME.

caffeine (ˈkafeen) an alkaloid of tea and coffee which acts as a nerve stimulant and diuretic.

caffeinism (kafˌee·ənizəm) an agitated state due to excessive ingestion of caffeine.

caisson disease (ˈkaysən diˈzeez) *see* DECOMPRESSION SICKNESS and BENDS.

calamine (ˈkaləˌmien) preparation of zinc carbonate or zinc oxide coloured pink with ferric oxide. It is an astringent and antipruritic used in lotion or ointment form for skin diseases.

calcaneum (kalˈkayni·əm) the heel bone. Calcaneus.

calcareous (kalˈkair·ri·əs) chalky. Containing lime.

calciferol (kalˈsifə·rol) the chemical name for vitamin D.

calcification (ˌkalsifəˈkayshən) 1. the deposit of lime in any tissue, e.g. in the formation of callus. 2. the deposit of lime salts in cartilage as part of the normal process of bone formation. *Dystrophic c.* the deposition of calcium in abnormal tissue, such as scar tissue or atherosclerotic plaques, without abnormalities of blood calcium.

calcitonin (ˌkalsəˈtohnən) a polypeptide hormone, produced by the parafollicular or C cells of the thyroid gland, which regulates blood calcium levels.

calcium (ˈkalsi·əm) *symbol* Ca. A metallic element necessary for the normal development and functioning of the body. Calcium is the most abundant mineral in the body; it is a constituent of bones and teeth. Deficiency or excess of serum calcium causes nerve and muscle dysfunction and abnormalities in blood clotting. The correct concentration is regulated by hormones. *C. carbonate* chalk. *C. gluconate* used as an antacid; a compound that is easily absorbed and can be given by intramuscular or intravenous route to raise the blood calcium. *C. lactate* a compound that increases the coagulability of blood; used orally as a calcium supplement.

calculus (ˈkalkyələs) [L] *little stone* 1. a stony concretion which may be formed in any of the secreting organs of the body or their ducts. *Arthritic c.* gouty deposits in or near joints. *Biliary c.* gallstone. *Coral c.* a large stone in the kidney, with branches resembling coral. *Mulberry c.* a gallstone made of calcium oxalate and shaped like a mulberry. *Renal c.* one formed in the kidney. *Salivary c.* stone in a salivary duct. *Staghorn c.* a many-branched stone sometimes found in the renal pelvis. *Urinary c.* one found anywhere in the urinary tract. *Vesical c.* stone formed in the urinary bladder. 2. a calcified deposit that forms on the surface of the teeth leading to tooth decay and gum disease.

calibrator (ˌkaləˈbraytə) 1. an instrument for measuring the size of openings. 2. an instrument used to dilate a tube, e.g. in urethral stricture.

caliper (ˈkaləpə) a two-pronged instrument that may be used to exert traction on a part. *Walking c.* an appliance fitted to a boot or shoe to give support to the lower limb. It may be used when the muscles are paralysed or in the repair stage of fractures.

calipers (ˈkaləpəz) a compass for measuring diameters and curved surfaces. *Skinfold c.* an instrument used in nutritional assessment for determining the amount of body fat. A fold of skin and subcutaneous tissue, usually over the triceps muscle, is pinched away from the underlying muscle using the thumb and forefinger.

callisthenics (ˌkaləsˈtheniks) mild gymnastics for developing the muscles and producing a graceful carriage.

callosity (kəˈlosətee) the plaques of thickened skin often seen on the soles of the feet or the palms of the hand; areas subject to friction.

callous (ˈkaləs) hard and thickened.

callus (ˈkaləs) 1. a callosity. 2. the tissue that grows round fractured ends of bone and develops into new bone to repair the injury.

calor (ˈkalə) [L.] heat; one of the signs of inflammation.

caloric (kəˈlor·ik, ˈkalə·rik) pertaining to heat or calories.

calorie (ˈkalə·ree) *symbol* cal. A unit of heat. Used to denote physiological values of various food substances, estimated according to the amount of heat they produce on being oxidised in the body. *See* OXIDISATION. A Calorie (with an uppercase initial letter) (or kilocalorie) represents the heat required to raise the temperature of 1 kg (1000 g) of water by 1°C. A calorie (with a lowercase initial letter) represents the heat required to raise the temperature of 1 g of water by 1°C. In the SI system the calorie is replaced by the joule (1 cal = 4.18 kJ).

calorific (ˌkaləˈrifik) heat-producing.

calorimeter (ˌkaləˈrimətə) an apparatus for measuring the heat that is produced or lost during a chemical or physical change.

calyx (ˈkayliks, ˈkal-) any cup-shaped vessel or part. *C. of kidney* the cup-like terminations of the ureter in the renal pelvis surrounding the pyramids of the kidney.

Campylobacter (ˈkampəlohˌbaktə) a genus of bacteria, family *Spirillaceae*, made up of Gram-negative, non-spore-forming, motile, spirally curved rods. Causes an acute intestinal illness lasting several days. Usually associated with unpasteurised milk, partially cooked meat and poultry.

canal (kəˈnal) a tubular passage. *Alimentary c.* the passage along which the food passes on its way through the body. *C. of Schlemm* that which drains the aqueous humour. *Cervical c.* the passage through the cervix of the uterus. *Semicircular c.* one of the three canals in the middle ear responsible for maintenance of balance.

canaliculus (ˌkanəˈlikyələs) a small channel or canal.

cancellous (ˈkansələs) being porous or spongy. Applied to the honeycomb type of bone tissue in the ends of long bones and in flat and irregular bones.

cancer (ˈkansə) a general term to describe malignant growths in tissue, of which CARCINOMA is of epithelial and SARCOMA of connective tissue origin, as in bone and muscle. The basic aetiology of cancer remains unknown, but many potential causes are now recognised, e.g. cigarette smoking, ionising radiation, exposure to certain chemicals and overexposure to the sun. Hereditary factors also play an important part in its development. A cancerous growth is one that is not encapsulated, but infiltrates into surrounding tissues, the cells of which it replaces by its own. It is spread by the lymph and blood vessels and causes metastases in other parts of the body. Death is caused by destruction of organs to a degree incompatible with life, by extreme debility and anaemia, or by haemorrhage. For early warning signs of cancer, *see* table, p. 80. *C. care pathway* describes the key steps in a patient's cancer journey and expected standards of care at each stage. *C. centre* offers a focused and integrated program of work that is multidisciplinary and provides clinical care including surgery, radiotherapy and/or chemotherapy, cancer research and education. Other services may include complementary therapies and psychosocial support. The centres aim to accelerate the control and cure cancer. *C. journey* an individual's experience of cancer, from detection and screening, diagnosis and treatment, to relapse, recovery and/or palliative care. *C. phobia* an irrational fear of cancer. *C. staging* a measure of how much a cancer has grown and spread. A common method of cancer staging is based on the measurement of the primary tumour (T), any spread to lymph nodes (N) and rate of metastases (M), and is known as the TNM classification. There are also other staging systems, some using a number system such as stage 1, 2, 3 or 4 (or stage I, II, III or IV). *C. screening see* SCREENING. *C. survivor* anyone who has finished their active cancer treatment. *C. units* specialist wards and clinics in general hospitals that provide services for the treatment and care of patients with cancer.

Early Warning Signs of Cancer

- Changes in bowel or bladder habits.
- A sore that does not heal, particularly around the mouth, tongue or lips, or anywhere on the skin.
- Unusual bleeding or discharge; blood in the urine or bowel movements; blood or bloody discharge from the nipple or any body opening; unexplained vaginal bleeding or discharge, or any bleeding after the menopause.
- Thickening or lump in the breast, testicles or elsewhere on the body.
- Indigestion or difficulty swallowing.
- Obvious change in the size, colour, shape or thickness of a wart, mole, birthmark or mouth sore.
- Nagging cough, hoarseness or difficulty in swallowing.
- Unexpected weight loss, night sweats or fever.

Special note: Pain is not usually an early warning sign of cancer.

cancrum oris (ˌkangkrəm ˈorəs) *See* NOMA.

Candida (ˈkandədə) a genus of small fungi, formerly called *Monilia. C. albicans* the variety that causes CANDIDIASIS.

candidiasis (ˌkandəˈdieəsəs) infection by the *Candida* fungus. Occurs particularly in moist areas, such as the mouth, vagina and skinfolds. Popularly known as 'thrush'. Candidiasis can occur as a result of a debilitating illness or immuno-suppressive therapy and/or cytotoxic drugs. The infection may also occur as a result of disturbed intestinal flora, and in pregnancy. Oral infection may be due to poor hygiene, carious teeth or badly fitting dentures.

canine (ˈkaynien) 1. pertaining to a dog. 2. an ˈeye tooth'. There is one on each side of both the upper jaw and the lower jaw between the incisors and the molars. *See* DENTITION.

cannabis (ˈkanəbəs) a drug derived from the hemp plant, *Cannabis sativa.* It may be swallowed or smoked and produces a temporary sense of wellbeing or euphoria, often followed by lethargy. Cannabis is a highly regulated drug in Australia and its use and supply is controlled by a number of Australian, state and territory laws. Alternative terms for cannabis include marijuana, dope, hashish, hash, grass, pot, spliff, weed, ganja, reefer and bhang. *Medicinal c.* In 2016, amendments were made to the scheduling of medicinal cannabis products. This involved Schedule 9 (S9) Prohibited Substances being down-regulated to Schedule 8 (S8) Controlled Drugs for certain medicinal cannabis products such as raw cannabis, which can be vaporised, cannabis extracts in oils, solvent extracts, gels and creams. These products can be used in the treatment of certain conditions such as epilepsy, multiple sclerosis and Crohn's disease. It may also be used to counter the nausea and vomiting associated with chemotherapy and in palliative care. For the current status of medicinal cannabis check individual state and territory laws.

cannula (ˈkanyələ) a hollow tube for insertion into the body by which fluids are introduced or removed. Usually a TROCAR is fitted into it to facilitate its introduction.

canthus (ˈkanthəs) the angle formed by the junction of the upper and lower eyelids.

CAPD *see* CONTINUOUS AMBULATORY PERITONEAL DIALYSIS.

capeline bandage (ˈkayplien ˈbandij) a cap-like covering of two interwoven bandages used for protecting the head or a limb stump.

capillarity (ˌkapəˈlarətee) the action by which a liquid will rise upwards in a fibrous substance or in a fine tube. Capillary attraction.

capillary (kəˈpilə·ree) 1. hair-like. 2. a minute vessel connecting an arteriole and a venule. 3. a minute vessel of the lymphatic system.

capitellum (ˌkapəˈteləm) capitulum. 1. the small rounded head at the elbow end of the humerus. 2. the bulb of a hair.

capsular (ˈkapsyələ) relating to a capsule. *C. ligaments* those that completely surround a movable joint, forming a capsule that loosely encloses the bones and is lined with synovial membrane, which secretes a fluid for lubrication of the articular surfaces. Also called articular capsule.

capsule (ˈkapsyool) 1. a fibrous or membranous sac enclosing an organ. 2. a small soluble case of gelatin in which a nauseous medicine may be enclosed. 3. the gelatinous envelope that surrounds and protects some bacteria.

capsulitis (ˌkapsyəˈlietəs) inflammation of the capsule of a joint.

capsulotomy (ˌkapsyəˈlotəmee) the incision of a capsule, particularly that of a joint or of the lens of the eye.

caput (ˈkapuht) head. *C. succedaneum* a transient soft swelling on an infant's head, due to pressure during labour, which disappears within the first few days of life.

carbaminohaemoglobin (kahˌbamə-nohˌheeməˈglohbən) a compound of carbon dioxide and haemoglobin, present in the blood.

carbohydrate (ˌkahbohˈhiedrayt) a compound of carbon, hydrogen and oxygen. Carbohydrates are classified into mono-, di-, tri-, poly- and heterosaccharides. In food they are an important and immediate source of energy for the body: 1 g of carbohydrate yields 17 kJ (4 cal). They are synthesised by all green plants. In the body they are absorbed immediately or stored in the form of glycogen.

carbon (ˈkahbən) *symbol* C. A non-metallic element. *C. dioxide* a gas which, when dissolved in water, forms weak carbonic acid. As a product of metabolism by the oxidation of carbon, it leaves the body via the lungs. It can be compressed until it freezes, and then forms a solid (carbon dioxide snow, also known as dry ice), used as an escharotic in various skin conditions. Inhalations of the gas in a 5–7% mixture with oxygen are useful for stimulating the depth of respiration. *C. monoxide* a colourless gas that is very poisonous. It is a major constituent of coal gas and is usually present in the exhaust gases of petrol and diesel engines. In poisoning, there is vertigo, flushed face with very red lips, loss of consciousness and convulsions. The blood is bright red because of the formation of carboxyhaemoglobin. *C. tetrachloride* a powerful anthelmintic used in treating hookworm and whipworm. Also used in cleaning fluids; the inhalation of its vapours in solvent abuse can depress central nervous system activity and cause degeneration of the liver and kidneys.

carbonic anhydrase (kah'bonik an'hiedrayz) an enzyme that catalyses the decomposition of carbonic acid into carbon dioxide and water, facilitating transfer of carbon dioxide from tissues to blood and from blood to alveolar air.

carboxyhaemoglobin (kah'boksee-ˌheemə'glohbən) the combination of carbon monoxide with haemoglobin in the blood in carbon monoxide poisoning.

carbuncle ('kahbungkəl) an acute staphylococcal inflammation of subcutaneous tissues, which causes local thrombosis in the veins and death of tissue with several discharging sinuses. In appearance it resembles a collection of boils.

carcinogen ('kahsənə'jən, kah'-sinəjən) any substance or agent that can produce a cancer.

carcinogenic (ˌkahsinoh'jenik) pertaining to substances or agents that produce or predispose to cancer.

carcinoid syndrome ('kahsə'noyd 'sinˌdrohm) a rare condition associated with certain bowel tumours, which spread to other parts of the body. Marked by attacks of severe cyanotic flushing of the skin and by diarrhoea, bronchoconstrictive attacks, pain, serious heart damage, sudden drops in blood pressure, oedema and ascites. Symptoms are caused by serotonin, prostaglandins and other biologically active substances secreted by the tumour.

carcinoma (ˌkahsə'nohmə) a malignant growth of epithelial tissue. Microscopically the cells resemble those of the tissue in which the growth has arisen. *Basal cell c.* a rodent ulcer (*see* ULCER). *Epithelial c.* EPITHELIOMA. *Squamous cell c.* one arising from the squamous epithelium of the skin.

carcinomatosis (ˌkahsə'nohmə-'tohsəs) the condition in which a carcinoma has given rise to widespread metastases.

cardia ('kahdi·ə) the area immediately surrounding the opening from the oesophagus into the stomach. The cardia sphincter helps reduce reflux of stomach contents back up into the oesophagus.

cardiac ('kahdeeˌak) 1. pertaining to the heart. 2. pertaining to the cardia. *C. arrest* the cessation of the heartbeat. *C. arrhythmia* an abnormal rate or rhythm of myocardial conduction. *C. asthma see* ASTHMA. *C. atrophy* fatty degeneration of the heart muscle. *C. bed* one that can be manipulated to form a chair shape for those who are comfortable only when sitting up. *C. catheterisation* a procedure whereby a radio-opaque catheter is passed to the heart, usually from the femoral or radial artery, jugular vein or femoral vein. Its passage through the heart can be watched on a screen. Also blood pressure readings and specimens can be taken, thus aiding diagnosis of heart abnormalities. Once in place, the catheter can be used to perform a number of procedures, including coronary angiography and cardiac ablation. *C. cycle* the sequence of events, lasting about 0.8 seconds, during which the heart completes one contraction. *C. failure see* HEART FAILURE. *C. massage* rhythmic compression of the heart performed in order to re-establish circulation of the blood in cardiac arrest. *C. monitor* equipment used to monitor and visually record the cardiac cycle. *C. pacemaker* an electrical device that stimulates the heart muscle to maintain myocardial contractions. *See* PACEMAKER. *C. stimulant* a pharmacological agent that increases the action of the heart. Cardiac glycosides, e.g. digoxin and digitalis, increase myocardial contractions and decrease the heart rate and conduction velocity, thus allowing more time for the ventricles to relax and fill with blood. *C. tamponade* compression of the heart by a collection of fluid or blood in the pericardial sac.

cardialgia (ˌkahdeeˈalji·ə) pain in the region of the heart. Cardiodynia.

cardiogenic (ˌkahdeeohˈjenik) originating in the heart. *C. shock* shock caused by disease or failure of heart action.

cardiography (ˌkahdeeˈogrəfee) the recording of the force and movements of the heart producing a tracing on paper (cardiogram) or monitor.

cardiologist (ˌkahdeeˈoləjəst) a medically qualified person skilled in the diagnosis of heart disease.

cardiology (ˌkahdeeˈoləjee) the study of the heart: how it works and its diseases.

cardiomegaly (ˌkahdeeohˈmegəlee) enlargement of the heart.

cardiomyopathy (ˌkahdeeohmieˈ-opəthee) a chronic disorder of the heart muscle not resulting from atherosclerosis.

cardiopulmonary (ˌkahdeeoh-ˈpulmənəree) relating to the heart and lungs. *C. bypass* the use of a heart–lung machine to oxygenate and pump the blood around the body while a surgeon operates on the heart.

cardiopulmonary resuscitation (CPR) (ˌkahdeeohˈpulmənəree rəˈsusə·tayshən) an emergency procedure including chest compressions that is performed when a person's breathing or heartbeat has stopped; designed to pump the heart to get blood circulating and deliver oxygen to the brain until definitive treatment can stimulate the heart to start working again. (*See* Appendix 6.)

cardioscope (ˈkahdeeohˌskohp) a flexible instrument with a lens and illumination attachment; used for examining the inside of the heart.

cardiospasm (ˈkahdeeohˌspazəm) spasm of the sphincter muscle at the cardiac end of the stomach. It may result in dilatation of the oesophagus, difficulty in swallowing solids and liquids and regurgitation of undigested food. ACHALASIA.

cardiothoracic (ˌkahdeeohˈthə·rasik) pertaining to the heart and thoracic cavity. A specialised branch of surgery.

cardiotocography (ˌkahdeeoh-tə·kogrəfee) the simultaneous recording of the fetal heart rate, fetal movements and uterine contractions in order to discover possible lack of oxygen (hypoxia) to the fetus. Also known as fetal heart monitoring.

cardiotomy (ˌkahdeeˈotəmee) surgical incision into the heart or the cardia. *C. syndrome* an inflammatory reaction after heart surgery. There is PYREXIA, PERICARDITIS and pleural effusion.

cardiotoxic (ˌkahdeeohˈtoksik) anything that has a deleterious or poisonous effect on the heart.

cardiovascular (ˌkahdeeohˈvaskyələ) concerning the heart and blood vessels. *C. system* the heart together with the two chief networks of blood vessels: the systemic circulation and the pulmonary circulation.

cardioversion (ˌkahdeeohˈvərshən) a method of restoring an abnormal heart rhythm to normal (e.g. atrial fibrillation) by means of an electric shock.

carditis (kah'dietəs) inflammation of the heart.

care (kair) the provision of welfare and protection to children, older people in need, the sick and other vulnerable people. An important component of nursing practice (and that of other healthcare professionals) that extends the concept to include psychosocial and physical care interventions. *C. pathway* an integrated approach or pathway which determines and utilises locally agreed multidisciplinary practice based on guidelines and evidence for a specific patient or client group. It may form part or all of the clinical record; it documents the care given and facilitates the evaluation of outcomes. *C. plan* an individualised plan for the care of a patient. Nursing information in this document includes data from the patient assessment regarding the patient's needs and nursing diagnosis, and the specific nursing interventions are outlined, the desired goals stated and the priorities set. *See* NURSING CARE PLAN. *Person-centred c.* puts the person, their experiences, wellbeing, needs and feelings at the centre of the caring process. Most of all, person-centred care is about seeing the person first and the disease or illness second. It is about ensuring that the care provided is always focused on the person and not on the fact that they have a disease or illness. Encompassed in the concept of person-centred care is a partnership where a collaborative, respectful and trusting relationship develops between the healthcare professional and the person.

carer (kairə) an unpaid non-professional who provides care for someone in need at home; most commonly a member of the individual's family or partner.

caries ('kair·eez) suppuration and subsequent decay of bone, corresponding to ulceration in soft tissues. In caries, the bone dissolves; in necrosis, it separates in large pieces and is thrown off. *Dental c.* decay of the teeth due to penetration of bacteria through the enamel to the dentine. *Spinal c.* tuberculosis of the spine. Pott's disease.

carneous ('kahnee·əs) fleshy. *C. mole* a tumour of organised blood clot surrounding a dead fetus in the uterus. *See* ABORTION.

carotene ('karə·teen) the colouring matter in carrots, tomatoes and other yellow foods and in fats. It is a provitamin capable of conversion into vitamin A in the liver.

carotid (ka'rotəd) the principal artery on each side of the neck. *C. bodies* chemoreceptors in the bifurcation of both carotid arteries which monitor the oxygen content of the blood. *C. sinuses* dilated portions of the internal carotids containing the baroreceptors that monitor blood pressure.

carpal ('kahpəl) relating to the carpus or wrist. *C. tunnel syndrome* compression of the median nerve at the wrist, causing numbing and tingling in the fingers and thumb.

carpopedal (ˌkahpə·ped'l) relating to the wrist and foot. *C. spasm* spasm of the hands and feet such as occurs in tetany.

carpus ('kahpəs) the eight bones forming the wrist and arranged in two rows: (a) scaphoid, lunate, triquetral, pisiform; (b) trapezium, trapezoid, capitate, hamate.

carrier (ˈkari·ə) 1. a person who harbours the microorganisms of an infectious disease but is not necessarily affected by it, although the person may infect others. 2. one who carries and passes on a hereditary abnormality.

cartilage (ˈkahtəlij) a specialised, fibrous connective tissue present in adults and forming most of the temporary skeleton in the embryo. The three most important types are hyaline cartilage, elastic cartilage and fibrocartilage. Also, a general term for a mass of such tissue in a particular site in the body. *Elastic c.* cartilage containing elastic fibres and forming the pinna of the ear, the epiglottis and part of the nasal septum. *Fibro c.* cartilage in which bundles of white fibres predominate, forming the intervertebral discs and costal cartilages. *Hyaline c.* flexible, somewhat elastic, semitransparent cartilage with an opalescent bluish tint, composed of a basophilic fibril-containing substance with cavities in which the CHONDROCYTES occur.

cartilaginous (ˈkahtə·lajənəs) of the nature of cartilage.

caruncle (ˈkarəngkəl) a small fleshy swelling. *Lacrimal c.* a small reddish body situated at the medial junction of the eyelids. *Urethral c.* a small fleshy growth occurring at the urinary orifice in females and giving rise to great pain on micturition.

case (kays) a particular instance of disease, as in 'a case of leukaemia'; sometimes used incorrectly to designate the patient with the disease. *C. conference* a meeting of professionals involved in the care of a particular person (sometimes including relatives or the nominated carer of the patient), to agree on patterns of action and to monitor progress. *C. control study* an epidemiological study in which the characteristics of cases of disease are compared with a matched control group of persons without the disease. Also called retrospective study or case referent study. *C. fatality rate* the number of persons dying of a particular disease expressed as a proportion of the total contracting the disease; usually expressed as a percentage. *C. history* the collected data concerning an individual, and his or her family and environment, including the medical history and any other information that may be useful in analysing and diagnosing the health issues or for instructional or research purposes. *C. load* a system of care whereby a nurse, midwife or health visitor is responsible for a group of patients or clients. *C. mix* a system of classification of patients and associated procedures into groups based on the type and mix of the patients treated. Provides a useful measure for audit and performance comparisons. *C. mix database* a computerised record system which combines all the data received from patient administration systems and operational systems to provide a comprehensive set of information about all the treatment and services received by each patient/client during an episode of care. The information helps to develop normal care profiles for different groups, to analyse and compare different treatment regimens, to produce comparative costings for different treatments, etc. It may also be used as part of the medical audit process. *C. studies* the study of a selected phenomenon that provides in-depth description of its dimensions and processes.

caseation (ˌkaysee'ayshən) degeneration of diseased tissue into a cheesy mass.

casein ('kayseeən, -seen) the chief protein of milk. It forms a curd from which cheese is made. *C. hydrolysate* a pre-digested concentrated protein; a useful supplement for a high-protein diet.

cast (kahst) 1. a tiny structure formed by deposits of secretions, minerals or other substances in the lumen of renal tubules, bronchioles or other organs. Casts often appear in samples of urine or blood collected for laboratory examination. 2. a positive copy of the tissues of the jaws, made in an impression, over which denture bases or other restorations may be fabricated. 3. to form an object in a mould. 4. a stiff dressing or casing, usually made of plaster of Paris, used to immobilise body parts. 5. STRABISMUS.

castration (ka'strayshən) the removal of the testes in the male or the ovaries in the female.

CAT computerised axial tomography. *See* COMPUTED AXIAL TOMOGRAPHY.

cat-scratch disease (fever) (katskrach di'zeez (ˌfeeva)) a benign, subacute, regional lymphadenitis with fever, resulting from a scratch or bite of a cat or a scratch from a surface contaminated by a cat. Three-quarters of all cases occur in children. The fever is due to a small bacterium called *Rochalimaea henselae*.

catabolism (kə'tabə·lizəm) the chemical breakdown of complex substances in the body to form simpler ones, with a release of energy. *See* METABOLISM.

catalase ('katə·layz) an enzyme found in body cells, including red blood cells and liver cells.

catalyst ('katələst) a substance that hastens or brings about a chemical change without itself undergoing alteration; e.g. enzymes act as catalysts in the process of digestion.

cataract ('katə·rakt) opacity of the crystalline lens of the eye, causing partial or complete blindness. It may be congenital or may be due to degenerative changes, injury or diabetes.

catarrh (kə'tah) chronic inflammation of a mucous membrane accompanied by an excessive discharge of mucus.

catatonia (ˌkatə'tohni·ə) a syndrome of motor abnormalities occurring in schizophrenia, but less commonly in organic cerebral disease, characterised by stupor and the adoption of strange postures, or outbursts of excitement and hyperactivity. The patient may change suddenly from one of these states to the other.

catecholamines (ˌkatəkolə·meenz) a group of compounds that have the effect of sympathetic nerve stimulation. They have an aromatic and an amine portion and include DOPAMINE, ADRENALINE and NORADRENALINE (norepinephrine).

catgut ('katˌgut) a substance used in surgery for sutures and ligatures. It becomes absorbed gradually in the body at a variable rate, according to the preparation. Catgut has largely been replaced by synthetic absorbable sutures.

catharsis (kə'thahsəs) 1. a cleansing or purgation. 2. the bringing into consciousness and the emotional reliving of a forgotten (repressed) painful experience as a means of releasing anxiety and tension.

catheter ('kathətə) a tubular, flexible instrument, passed through body channels for withdrawal of fluids from (or introduction of fluids into) a body cavity. Catheters are made of a variety of materials, including plastic, metal, rubber and gum-elastic. *Angiographic c.* one through which a contrast medium is injected for visualisation of the vascular system of an organ. *Arterial c.* one inserted into an artery and used as part of a catheter–transducer–monitor system to continuously observe the BLOOD PRESSURE of critically ill patients. An arterial catheter also may be inserted for radiological studies of the arterial system and for delivery of chemotherapeutic agents directly into the arterial supply of malignant tumours. *Cardiac c.* a long, fine catheter especially designed for passage, usually through a peripheral blood vessel, into the chambers of the heart under fluoroscopic control. *Central venous c.* a long, fine catheter inserted into a vein for the purpose of administering, through a large blood vessel, parenteral fluids (as in parenteral nutrition), antibiotics and other therapeutic agents. This type of catheter is also used in the measurement of central venous pressure. *Self-retaining c.* a catheter made in such a way that, after introduction, the blind end expands so that it can remain in the bladder. Useful for continuous or intermittent drainage or where frequent specimens are required. *Ureteric c.* a fine gum-elastic catheter passed up the ureter to the renal pelvis and used to insert a contrast medium in retrograde urography.

catheterisation (ˌkathətə·rieˈzay-shən) the insertion of a catheter into a body cavity.

cation (ka·tai·ən) an ion or group of ions having a positive charge and moving towards the negative electrode in electrolysis.

cauda (ˈkawdah) a tail-like appendage. *C. equina* the bundle of coccygeal, sacral and lumbar nerves with which the spinal cord terminates.

caudal (ˈkawd'l) referring to a cauda. *C. block* a local anaesthetic agent injected into the sacral canal so that operations may be carried out in the peritoneal area without a general anaesthetic.

caul (kawl) the amnion, which occasionally does not rupture but envelops the infant's head at birth.

causalgia (kawˈzalji·ə) an intense burning pain which persists after peripheral nerve injuries.

caustic (ˈkostik, ˈkaw-) a substance, usually a strong acid or alkali, capable of burning organic tissue. Silver nitrate (*lunar c.*), carbolic acid and carbon dioxide snow are those most commonly used, e.g. silver nitrate to destroy warts.

cauterisation (ˌkawtə·rieˈzayshən) the destruction of tissue with CAUTERY.

cautery (ˈkawtə·ree) 1. the application of searing heat by a hot instrument, an electric current, or other means such as a laser. 2. an agent so used. *Cold c.* cauterisation by carbon dioxide, also called cryocautery.

cavernoma (ˈkavəˈnohmə) a cluster of abnormal blood vessels usually found in the brain or spinal cord, which resemble a raspberry. Cavernomas are also known as cavernous angioma, cavernous haemangioma or cerebral cavernous malformation (CCM).

cavernous (ˈkavənəs, kəˈvərnəs) having caverns or hollows. *C. breathing* sounds heard on auscultation over a pulmonary cavity. *C. sinus* a venous channel lying on either side of the body of the sphenoid bone through which pass the internal carotid artery and several nerves. *C. sinus thrombosis* a serious complication of any infection of the face, the veins from the orbit draining into the sinus and carrying the infection into the cranium.

cavitation (ˌkavəˈtayshən) the formation of cavities, e.g. in the lung in tuberculosis.

cavity (ˈkavətee) a confined space or hollow or potential hollow within the body or one of its organs, e.g. the abdominal cavity or a decayed hollow in a tooth.

CCU critical care unit; coronary care unit.

cell (sel) 1. the basic structural unit of living organisms (*see* figure). A microscopic mass of protoplasm consisting of a nucleus surrounded by cytoplasm and enclosed in a cell membrane from which all organic tissues are constructed. Each cell may reproduce itself by mitosis. 2. a small, more or less enclosed, space. *C. division* the processes by which cells multiply. *See* MITOSIS and MEIOSIS.

cellulitis (ˌselyəˈlietəs) a diffuse inflammation of connective tissue, especially of subcutaneous tissue, which causes a typical brawny, oedematous appearance of the part; local abscess formation is not common.

cellulose (ˈselyəˌlohs, -ˌlohz) a carbohydrate forming the covering of vegetable cells, i.e. vegetable fibres. Not digestible in the alimentary tract of humans but gives bulk and, as 'roughage', stimulates peristalsis.

Celsius scale (ˈselsi·əs ˌskayl) *Anders Celsius, Swedish astronomer, 1701–1744.* A temperature scale with the melting point of ice set at 0° and the boiling point of water at 100°. The normal temperature of

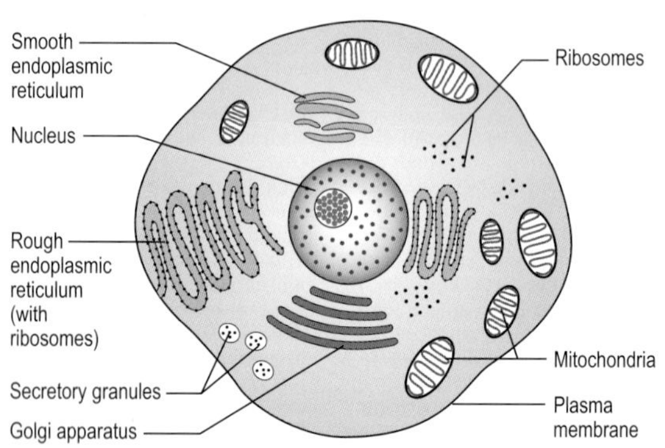

Major parts of the cell.

the human body is 36.9°C. Formerly known as the Centigrade scale. *See* FAHRENHEIT SCALE.

cementum (sə'mentəm) cement. Connective tissue with a bone-like structure which covers the root of a tooth and supports it within the socket.

censor (ˌsensə) 1. a member of a committee on ethics or for critical examination of a medical or other society. 2. the psychic influence that prevents unconscious thoughts and wishes coming into consciousness.

censorship ('sensəˌship) in psychiatry, the process of selecting, accepting or rejecting conscious ideas, memories and impulses arising from the individual's subconscious.

census ('sensəs) enumeration of a population. A national census usually records name, address, age, sex, occupation, marital status and other social information.

Centigrade ('sentəˌgrayd) *see* CELSIUS SCALE.

centile (sentiel) *see* PERCENTILE.

central ('sentrəl) pertaining to the centre or midpoint. *C. nervous system (CNS)* the brain and spinal cord. *C. sulcus* a deep groove in each of the hemispheres of the brain separating the frontal and parietal lobes. *C. venous pressure* the pressure recorded by the introduction of a catheter into the right atrium in order to monitor the condition of a patient after a major operative procedure, such as heart surgery.

Centre of Excellence (sentə ov eksələns) a tertiary healthcare provider that has been identified as the most expert and cost effective and produces the best outcomes for the patient. Can also relate to research centres of excellence.

Central Sterile Supplies and Disinfection Unit (CSSD) ('sentrəl 'steriel sə'pliz and ˌdisin'fekshən 'yoohnət) a hospital sterilisation and disinfection unit or department.

central venous catheter/line ('sentrəl 'veenəs 'kathətə/lien) a special catheter that is inserted into a large central vein through either a peripheral vein or a skin tunnel for the administration of drugs, the infusing of hypertonic fluids and to measure pressures. The catheter/line also allows long-term access for the administration of medications, nutritional support and blood products.

centrifugal (sentrə'fyoogəl) 1. denoting a force that is directed outwards, away from a central point or axis. 2. a direction away from the head. Efferent; the reverse of centripetal.

centrifuge ('sentrəˌfyooj) an apparatus that rotates at high speed. If a test tube, for example, is filled with a fluid such as blood or urine and rotated in a centrifuge, any bacteria, cells or other solids in it are precipitated.

centripetal (sen'tripət'l, 'sentrəˌpeet'l) conveying from the periphery to the centre. Afferent; the reverse of centrifugal.

centromere ('sentrəˌmiə) the region(s) of the chromosomes which become(s) allied with the spindle fibres at MITOSIS and MEIOSIS.

centrosome ('sentrəˌsohm) a body in the cytoplasm of most animal cells, close to the nucleus. It divides during mitosis, one half migrating to each daughter cell.

centrosphere ('sentrəˌsfiə) the cell centre, in an area of clear cytoplasm near the nucleus.

cephalhaematoma (ˌkefəlˌheemə'tohmə, sef-) a swelling beneath the pericranium, containing blood, which may be found on the head of the newborn infant. Caused by pressure during labour. Gradually reabsorbed within the first few days of life.

cephalic (kə'falik, sə-) relating to or situated near the head.

cephalocele ('kefəloh,seel, 'sef-) cerebral hernia. *See* HERNIA.

cephalography (,kefə'logrəfee, ,sef-) radiographic examination of the contours of the head.

cephalometry (,kefə'lomətree, ,sef-) measurement of the dimensions of the head of a living person either directly or by radiography. *See also* PELVIMETRY.

cerclage (sər'klahzh) [Fr.] encircling of a part with a ring or loop, as for correction of an incompetent cervix uteri or fixation of the adjacent ends of a fractured bone. *See* SHIRODKAR'S OPERATION.

cerebellum (,serə'beləm) the portion of the brain below the cerebrum and above the medulla oblongata. Its functions include the coordination of fine voluntary movements and posture.

cerebral ('serəbrəl) relating to the cerebrum. *C. cortex* the outer layer of the cerebrum, composed of neurones. *C. haemorrhage* rupture of a cerebral blood vessel. Likely causes are aneurysm and hypertension. *See* APOPLEXY. *C. hernia see* HERNIA. *C. irritation* a condition of general nervous irritability and abnormality, often with photophobia, which may be an early sign of meningitis, tumour of the brain, etc. It is also associated with trauma. *C. palsy* a condition caused by injury to the brain during or immediately after birth. Coordination of movement is affected, and may cause the child to be flaccid or athetoid, in which condition there is constant random and uncontrolled movement. *See* SPASTIC.

cerebration (,serə'brayshən) mental activity.

cerebrospinal (,serəbroh'spien'l) relating to the brain and spinal cord. *C. fluid (CSF)* the fluid made in the choroid plexus of the ventricles of the brain and circulating from them into the subarachnoid space around the brain and spinal cord.

cerebrovascular (,serəbroh'vaskyələ) pertaining to the arteries and veins of the brain. *C. accident* a disorder (also called stroke) arising from an embolus, thrombus or haemorrhage in the cerebrum; may vary in severity from a transient weakness or tingling in a limb to profound paralysis, coma and death. *C. disease* any disorder of the blood vessels of the brain and its meninges.

cerebrum ('serəbrəm) the largest part of the brain, occupying the greater portion of the cranium and consisting of the right and left hemispheres divided by the longitudinal fissure

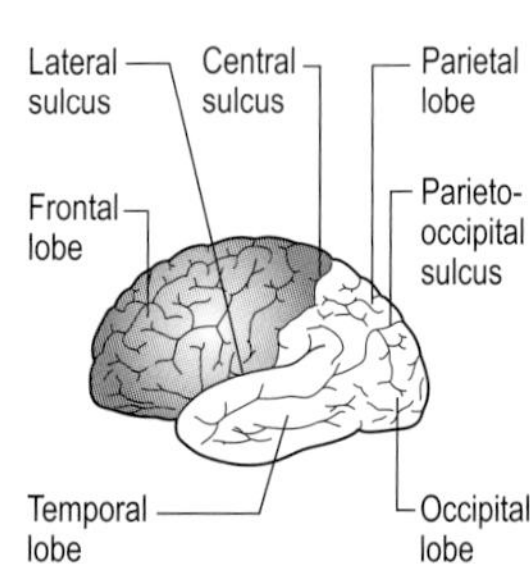

Cerebrum.

(*see* figure, p. 90). Each hemisphere contains a lateral ventricle. The internal substance is white and the convoluted surface is grey. It is the centre of the higher functions of the brain.

cerumen (sə'roomən) a waxy substance secreted by the ceruminous glands of the auditory canal. Ear wax.

cervical ('sərvikəl, sə'vie-) pertaining to the neck or the constricted part of an organ, e.g. uterine cervix. *C. canal* the passage through the uterine cervix. *C. cancer* cancer of the uterine cervix. *C. collar* a rigid or semi-rigid immobilising support for the neck. *C. dilatation* the opening of the diameter of the cervix during labour, miscarriage or gynaecological surgery. In labour the opening is measured on vaginal examination. The opening is expressed in centimetres or finger breadths; one finger breadth is approximately 2 cm. At full dilatation the diameter of the cervical opening is 10 cm. *C. rib* a short extra rib, often bilateral, which sometimes occurs on the seventh cervical vertebra and may cause pressure on an artery or nerve. *C. smear* a test for disorders of the cervical cells; material is scraped from the uterine cervix and examined microscopically. *C. spondylosis* a degenerative disease of the intervertebral joints and discs of the neck. *C. vertebra* one of the seven bones forming the neck portion of the spinal column. Also known as cervical dilation.

cervicitis (ˌservə'sietəs) inflammation of the neck of the uterus.

cervix ('sərviks) a constricted portion or neck. *C. uteri* the neck of the uterus; it is about 2 cm long and projects into the vagina. Capable of wide dilatation during childbirth.

cestode ('sestohd) TAPEWORM.

CFS *see* CHRONIC FATIGUE SYNDROME.

chafe (chayf) irritation of the skin as caused by friction between skinfolds. Occurs particularly in moist areas.

chalazion (kə'lazi·ən) a MEIBOMIAN or tarsal cyst. A swollen sebaceous gland in the eyelid. A small, hard tumour may develop.

chancre ('shangkə) 1. the initial lesion of syphilis developing at the site of inoculation. 2. a papular lesion occurring at the site of infection in tuberculosis or in sporotrichosis.

chancroid ('shangkroyd) soft chancre. A venereal ulceration, due to *Haemophilus ducreyi*, accompanied by inflammation and suppuration of the local glands.

character ('karəktə) 1. the combination of traits and qualities distinguishing the unique nature of the individual. 2. a letter, mark or numeral seen on a computer screen or printed. *C. change* indicates alteration in a person's recognised behaviour to one alien to the person's normal manner of conduct. *C. disorder* a chronic state in which the person exhibits maladaptive and unacceptable forms of behaviour and social response.

Charcot's disease or joint (shah'kohz di'zeez or joynt) *Jean-Martin Charcot, French neurologist, 1825–1893.* A chronic progressive, degenerative disease of the stress-bearing portion of one or more joints. The disease is the result of an underlying neurological disorder (e.g. diabetic neuropathy), tabes dorsalis from syphilis, or leprosy.

Charcot's triad ('shahˌkohz trieəd) nystagmus, intention tremor and scanning speech. A trio of signs of disseminated SCLEROSIS.

chart (ˈchaht) a record in graphic or tabular form. *Genealogical c.* a graph showing various descendants of a common ancestor, used to indicate those affected by genetically determined disease. *Reading c.* a chart with material printed in gradually increasing type sizes, used in testing acuity of near vision. *Reuss' c.* chart with coloured letters printed on coloured backgrounds, used in testing colour vision. *Snellen's c.* a chart printed with block letters in gradually decreasing sizes, used in testing visual acuity.

charting (ˈchahting) the keeping of clinical charts or records of the important facts about patients and the progress of their illness. It usually involves recording or collecting data related to the medical and nursing history, results of physical examinations, laboratory reports, results of special diagnostic tests and the observations of the nursing staff. Medical treatments, medications, nursing approaches to problems and the patient's response to treatment are also recorded on the charts.

cheilosis (kieˈlohsəs) maceration at the angles of the mouth; fissures may also occur. It may be associated with general debility or riboflavin deficiency.

chelating agent (keeˈlayting ˈayjənt) a drug that has the power of combining with certain metals and so aiding excretion, to prevent or overcome poisoning.

chemical change (ˈkemikəl ˈchaynj) this differs from physical change in that a profound alteration in properties results, usually permanently and usually accompanied by use of energy in a new substance, e.g. hydrogen (two atoms) plus oxygen produces water.

chemical compound (ˈkemikəl ˈkompownd) any substance produced by chemical change which may then be broken up into its components only by chemical means, unlike a mixture, which can usually be separated mechanically.

chemistry (ˈkeməstree) the science that deals with the elements, the atoms which compose them and the compounds that they form.

chemoprophylaxis (ˌkeemoˈprofəlaksis) the prevention of an acute or recurrent attack of a specific disease by the administration of chemotherapeutic agents, e.g. antibiotics to treat infections or the use of antitubercular drugs for tuberculosis.

chemoreceptor (ˌkeemohreeˈseptə, ˌkem-) a sensory nerve ending or group of cells that are sensitive to chemical stimuli in the blood.

chemosis (keeˈmohsəs) swelling of the conjunctiva due to the presence of fluid; an oedema of the conjunctiva.

chemotaxis (ˌkeemohˈtaksəs, ˌkem-) the reaction of living cells to chemical stimuli. These are either attracted (*positive c.*) or repelled (*negative c.*) by acids, alkalis or other substances.

chemotherapy (ˌkeemohˈtherəpee, ˌkem-) the specific treatment of disease by the administration of chemotherapeutic agents prescribed to delay or arrest growth of cancer cells. Administered by oral, intramuscular and intravenous routes and occasionally directly into a body cavity, e.g. the bladder. Used to arrest the progress of, or eradicate, a specific pathological condition in the body without causing irreversible harm to healthy tissue.

chest (chest) the thorax. *Barrel c.* one more rounded than usual, with raised ribs and, usually, KYPHOSIS. It is often present in emphysema. *C. leads* leads applied to the chest during the course of an electrocardiographic recording. *Flail c.* where part of the chest wall moves in opposition to respiration as a result of multiple fractures of the ribs. *Pigeon c.* a chest with the sternum protruding forwards.

Cheyne-Stokes respiration (chayn stohks ˌrespəˈrayshən) *John Cheyne, British physician, 1776–1836; William Stokes, British physician, 1804–1878.* Tidal respiration. A form of irregular but rhythmic breathing with temporary cessations (apnoea). It is likely to be present in cerebral tumour, narcotic poisoning and advanced cases of ARTERIOSCLEROSIS and URAEMIA.

Chiari malformations (khi·ahˈreeˌ malfawˈmayshənz) structural defects in the cerebellum, sometimes causing hydrocephalus as a result of obstruction of the cerebral spinal fluid. These malformations can also cause headaches, difficulty in concentrating and thinking and a range of other symptoms.

chiasma (kieˌazmə) a crossing point. *Optic c.* the crossing point of the optic nerves.

chickenpox (ˈchikənˌpoks) *see* VARICELLA.

chilblain (ˈchilˌblayn) a condition resulting from defective circulation when exposure to cold causes localised swelling and inflammation of the hands or feet, with severe itching and burning sensations.

child (chield) the human young, from infancy to puberty. *C. abuse* the non-accidental use of physical force or the non-accidental act of omission by a parent or other custodian responsible for the care of a child. Child abuse encompasses malnutrition and other kinds of neglect through ignorance, as well as deliberate withholding from the child of necessary basic physical and emotional care, including medical and dental care necessary for the child to grow. Examples of physical abuse range from burns and exposure to extreme cold, to beating, poisoning, strangulation, and withholding food and water, and fabricating illness so that the child is subject to unnecessary medical intervention (also known as Munchausen syndrome). Legislation in Australian states and territories provides for the protection of children from abuse through voluntary and/or mandatory reporting. In Australia it is an offence to fail to notify the appropriate authorities when child abuse is suspected. *C. sexual abuse* the subjection of a child to a sexual experience that is inappropriate for his or her emotional or developmental level and that is coercive in nature. Sexual abuse can occur with or without physical contact taking place. Non-contact child sexual abuse includes grooming, exploitation, persuading children to perform sexual acts over the internet and flashing. *Deprived c.* a vague term usually implying that the child in question has been raised in a situation lacking in love, affection and consistent parenting responses from adults. Sometimes used to suggest that the child has experienced a generalised deficit of life opportunities, both interpersonal and social.

childbirth (ˈchieldˈbərth) the act or process of giving birth to a child. PARTURITION. *See also* NATURAL CHILDBIRTH.

child development (chield dəˈveləpˌ-mənt) the stages of physical, psychological and social growth and attainment that occur from birth to adulthood.

Chinese medicine (chieˈneez medəsən) traditional system based on the principles of YIN AND YANG, combining acupuncture with a range of medications from herbal and animal sources.

chiropody (kiˈropədee, shi-) the study and care of the feet and the treatment of foot diseases.

chiropractic (ˌkierəˈpraktik) a system of treatment employing manipulation of the spine and other bony structures.

chi-squared test (kie skwaird ˌtest) (χ^2) a statistical test to determine whether two or more groups of observations differ significantly from one another, i.e. more than would be expected by chance.

Chlamydia (kləˈmidi·ə) a genus of bacteria comprising three species: *C. psittacosis*, the cause of psittacosis (parrot fever); *C. pneumoniae* which causes *Chlamydia* pneumonia (especially in children and in young adults); and *C. trachomatis* which includes 15 serotypes and causes many illnesses, including pneumonia acquired through maternal transmission, acute and chronic conjunctivitis (e.g. adult and neonatal inclusion conjunctivitis), trachoma and adult pharyngitis. *Chlamydia* is a sexually transmitted infection (STI); it affects both men and women and is the most commonly reported STI in Australia. Spread can be prevented through safe sex practices and treatment is with antibiotics

chloasma (klohˈazmə) a condition in which there is brown, blotchy discolouration of the skin of the face, especially during pregnancy.

chlorine (ˈklaw·reen) *symbol* Cl. A yellow, irritating poisonous gas. A powerful disinfectant, bleach and deodorising agent. Used in hypochlorites for sterilisation purposes.

cholangiography (kəˌlanjiˈogrəfee) radiography of the hepatic, cystic and bile ducts after the insertion of a radio-opaque contrast medium.

cholangitis (ˌkohlanˈjietəs) inflammation of the bile ducts.

cholecystectomy (ˌkohləsiˈstek-təmee) excision of the gallbladder.

cholecystitis (ˌkohləsiˈstietəs) inflammation of the gallbladder.

cholecystoduodenostomy (ˌkohləˌ-sistohˌdoo·ohdəˈnostəmee) an anastomosis between the gallbladder and the duodenum.

cholecystography (ˌkohləsiˈ-stogrəfee) radiography of the gallbladder after administration of a radio-opaque contrast medium.

cholecystolithiasis (ˌkohləˌsistohli-ˈthieəsəs) the presence of stones in the gallbladder.

cholecystostomy (ˌkohləˌsistostəmee) an incision into the gallbladder, usually to remove gallstones.

choledocholithiasis (ˌkohləˌ-dohkohləˈthieəsəs) the presence of stones in the bile duct.

cholelithiasis (ˌkohləliˈthieəsəs) the presence of gallstones in the gallbladder or bile ducts.

cholera (ˈkolə·rə) an acute, notifiable, infectious enteritis which is endemic and epidemic in Asia and also in Africa. Caused by *Vibrio cholerae*, it is associated with faecal contamination of water supplies, overcrowding and poor hygienic conditions. It is marked by profuse diarrhoea, muscle cramp, suppression of urine with severe dehydration; it is often fatal, but with the early administration of rehydration, together with salts and sugar solution as soon as possible, affected people make a full recovery. Oral cholera vaccination is available to travellers to areas where cholera is endemic. For travellers, the local drinking water should be boiled or sterilised and uncooked foods avoided.

cholestasis (ˌkohlə'staysəs) arrest of the flow of bile due to obstruction of the bile ducts.

cholesteatoma (ˌkohləˌsteeə'tohmə) a rare, small tumour containing cholesterol. It may occur in the middle ear or in the meninges, central nervous system or bones of the skull.

cholesterol (kə'lestəˌrol) a sterol found in nervous tissue, red blood cells, animal fat and bile. It is a precursor of bile acids and steroid hormones, and occurs in the most common type of gallstone, in ATHEROMA of the arteries, in various cysts and in carcinomatous tissue. Most of the body's cholesterol is synthesised, but some is obtained in the diet. Blood cholesterol levels are influenced by diet, weight, heredity and metabolic diseases, e.g. diabetes mellitus, and can be measured by blood tests. Dietary measures to lower cholesterol include reducing the saturated fat intake and increasing exercise.

choline ('kohleen) an essential amine, found in the blood, cerebrospinal fluid and urine, which aids fat metabolism. Formerly classified as a vitamin of the B complex.

cholinergic (ˌkohlə'nərjik) pertaining to nerves that release acetylcholine, as the chemical stimulator, at their nerve endings. *C. drugs* drugs that inhibit CHOLINESTERASE and so prevent the destruction of acetylcholine.

cholinesterase (ˌkohlə'nestəˌrayz) an enzyme that rapidly destroys acetylcholine.

chondral ('kondrəl) pertaining to cartilage.

chondritis (kon'drietəs) inflammation of cartilage.

chondroblast ('kondrəˌblast) an embryonic cell that forms cartilage.

chondrocyte ('kondrəˌsiet) a mature cartilage cell.

chondroma (kon'drohmə) an innocent new growth arising in cartilage.

chondromalacia (ˌkondrohmə'lay-shi·ə) a condition of abnormal softening of cartilage.

chorda ('kawdə) a sinew or cord.

chordee (kaw'dee) downward curvature of the penis caused by congenital anomaly (common in HYPOSPADIAS) or urethral infection.

chorditis (kaw'dietəs) inflammation of the vocal or spermatic cords.

chordotomy (kaw'dotəmee) an operation on the spinal cord to divide the anterolateral nerve pathways for relief of intractable pain. Cordotomy.

chorea (ko'reeə) a symptom of disease of the basal ganglia whereby the individual suffers from spasmodic, involuntary, rapid movements of the face, shoulders and hips. Chorea may also be a side effect of certain drugs. *Huntington's c.* (or Huntington's disease) a rare hereditary disorder which manifests itself in early middle age. The individual also suffers from progressive dementia, which often precedes a premature death. *Sydenham's c.* may occur in childhood or pregnancy. Characterised by rapid, irregular voluntary movement. Recovery may take some time, but most children will recover completely.

choreiform (koˈree·əfawm) resembling chorea.

choriocarcinoma (ˌko·riohˌkahsəˈnohmə) formerly known as chorioepithelioma. A highly malignant NEOPLASM usually arising from the trophoblast of a hydatidiform mole (*see* HYDATIDIFORM MOLE). It may develop after an abortion or the evacuation of a hydatidiform mole or even in normal pregnancy. Metastases usually develop rapidly, but the disease normally carries a good prognosis if early treatment is given.

chorion (ˈko·reeən, ˈkaw·ri·ən) the outer membrane enveloping the fetus; the placenta.

chorionic (ˌko·reeˈonik) pertaining to the chorion. *C. gonadotrophin* human chorionic gonadotrophin (HCG). *C. villi* small protrusions on the chorion from which the placenta is formed. They are in close association with the maternal blood and, by diffusion, interchange of nutriment, oxygen and waste matters is effected between the maternal and the fetal blood. *C. villus biopsy* tissue removed from the gestational sac early in pregnancy so that chromosomal and other inherited disorders can be identified. Can be carried out at an earlier stage than AMNIOCENTESIS.

chorioretinitis (ˌko·reeohˌretəˈnietəs) inflammation of the choroid and retina of the eye.

choroid (ˈko·royd) the pigmented and vascular coat of the eyeball, continuous with the iris and situated between the sclera and retina. It reduces the amount of light that falls upon the retina. *C. plexus* specialised cells in the ventricles of the brain that produce cerebrospinal fluids. There is one choroid plexus in each ventricle.

choroiditis (ˌko·royˈdietəs) inflammation of the choroid.

choroidoretinitis (koˌroydohˌretəˈnietəs) an inflammatory condition of both the choroid and the retina of the eye.

Christmas disease (ˈkrisməs diˈzeez) a hereditary bleeding disease similar to haemophilia but due to a deficiency of clotting factor IX; also called haemophilia B. The name is derived from that of the first patient to be studied.

chromatography (ˌkrohməˈtogrəfee) a method of chemical analysis by which substances in solution may be separated as they percolate down a column of powdered absorbent or ascend an absorbent paper by capillary traction. A definite pattern is produced and substances may be recognised by the use of appropriate colour reagents. Amino acids can be identified in this way.

chromatometry (ˌkrohməˈtomətree) the measurement of colour perception.

chromosome (ˈkrohməˌsohm) in animal cells, a structure in the nucleus, containing a linear thread of DEOXYRIBONUCLEIC ACID (DNA), which transmits genetic information and is associated with RIBONUCLEIC ACID (RNA) and histones. During cell division, the material composing the chromosome is compactly coiled. Each organism of a species is normally characterised by the same number of chromosomes in its somatic cells, 46 being the number usually present in humans: 22 pairs of autosomes, and two sex chromosomes (XX or XY), which determine the sex of the organism. In the mature GAMETE (ovum or spermatozoon) the number of chromosomes is halved as a result of MEIOSIS.

chronic (ˈkronik) (of a disease or disorder) persisting for a long period, often for the remainder of a person's lifetime; the opposite of acute. *C. fatigue syndrome (CFS)* extreme fatigue for the person over a long period, often years. The cause of this condition is not fully understood, although some cases have been reported following recovery from a viral infection. Most commonly affects women between 25 and 45 years of age. The main symptom is constant tiredness, but other symptoms may include poor concentration, sore throat, tender lymph nodes, and muscle and joint pain. Also known as myalgic encephalomyelitis (ME). *C. obstructive pulmonary disease (COPD)* a combination of chronic bronchitis and emphysema in which there is disruption of air flow into or out of the lungs. Dyspnoea, wheezing and cough predominate, often made worse by any exertion or pollution in the environment. Patients may be severely disabled and require oxygen for long periods. *C. kidney disease (CKD)* progressive loss of kidney function over a period of months or years.

chronological (kronəlojikəl) the recording of a number of events starting with the earliest and following the order in which they occurred. *C. age* the age of an individual expressed as a period of time that has elapsed since birth. In infants this may be given in hours, days or weeks, but for children and adults it is expressed in years.

Chvostek's sign (ˌvosteks sien) *Frantisek Chvostek, Austrian surgeon, 1835–1884.* A spasm of the facial muscles which occurs in tetany. It can be elicited by tapping the facial nerve.

chyle (kiel) digested fats which, as a milky fluid, are absorbed into the lymphatic capillaries (lacteals) in the villi of the small intestine.

chylothorax (ˌkielohˈthor·raks) the presence of effused chyle in the pleural cavity.

chyme (kiem) the semi-liquid, acid mass of food that passes from the stomach to the intestines.

chymotrypsin (ˌkiemohˈtripsən) an enzyme secreted by the pancreas. It is activated by trypsin and assists in the breakdown of proteins.

Ci symbol for *curie*, a unit of radioactivity.

cicatrix (ˈsikətriks) the scar of a healed wound (*see* KELOID).

cilia (ˈsili·ə) 1. the eyelashes. 2. microscopic filaments projecting from some epithelial cells, known as ciliated membranes, as in the bronchi, where cilia wave the secretion upwards.

ciliary (ˈsili·əˌree) hair-like. *C. body* a structure just behind the corneoscleral margin, composed of the ciliary muscle and processes. *C. muscle* the circular muscle surrounding the lens of the eye. *C. processes* the fringed part of the choroid coat arranged in a circle in front of the lens.

Cimex (ˈsiemeks) a genus of blood-sucking bugs. *C. lectularius* the common bedbug.

CINAHL *see* CUMULATIVE INDEX TO NURSING AND ALLIED HEALTH LITERATURE.

circadian (sər'kaydi·ən) denoting a period of 24 hours. *C. rhythm* the rhythm of certain biological activities that take place daily.

circinate (ˌsərsəˌnayt) having a circular outline. *Tinea circinata* ringworm.

circle of Willis ('serkəl ov 'wiləs) *Thomas Willis, British physician and anatomist, 1621–1675.* An anastomosis of arteries at the base of the brain, formed by the branches of the internal carotid and the basilar arteries.

circulation (ˌsərkyə'layshən) movement in a circular course, as of the blood. *Collateral c.* enlargement of small vessels establishing adequate blood supply when the main vessel to the part has been occluded. *Coronary c.* the system of vessels that supplies the heart muscle itself. *Extracorporeal c.* 1. removal of the blood by intravenous cannulae, passing it through a machine to oxygenate it, and then pumping it back into circulation. 2. the 'heart–lung' machine or pump respirator, used in cardiac surgery. *Lymph c.* the flow of lymph through lymph vessels and glands. *Portal c.* the passage of blood from the alimentary tract, pancreas and spleen, via the portal vein and its branches through the liver and into the hepatic veins. *Pulmonary c.* passage of the blood from the right ventricle via the pulmonary artery through the lungs and back to the heart by the pulmonary veins. *Systemic c.* the flow of blood throughout the body. The direction of flow is from the left atrium to the left ventricle and through the aorta, with its branches and capillaries. Veins then carry it back to the right atrium, and so into the right ventricle (*see* figure).

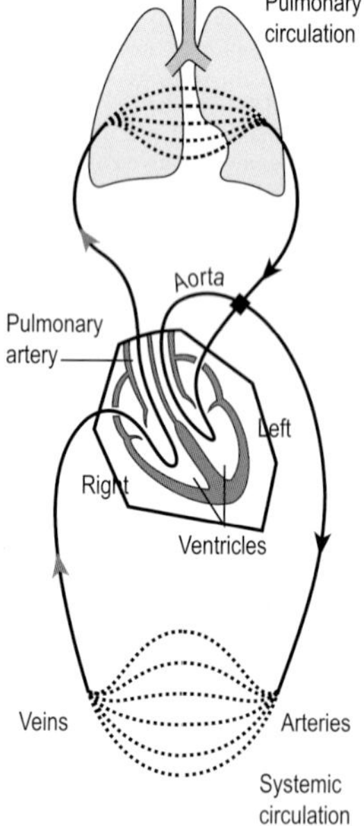

Circulation.

circumcision (ˌsərkəmˌsizhən) excision of the prepuce or foreskin of the penis. An operation performed for religious reasons, or sometimes for phimosis or paraphimosis. *Female c. see* FEMALE GENITAL MUTILATION.

circumduction (ˌsərkəm'dukshən) moving in a circle, e.g. the circular movement of the upper limb (*see* figure, p. 99).

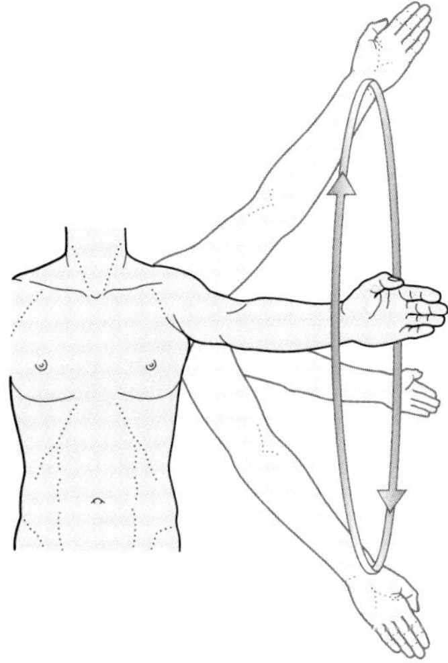

Circumduction.

circumoral (ˌsərkəmˈo·rəl) around the mouth. *C. pallor* a pale area around the mouth contrasting with the flushed cheeks, e.g. in scarlet fever.

cirrhosis (səˈrohsəs) a degenerative change that can occur in any organ, but especially in the liver. May be due to viruses, microorganisms or toxic substances (*portal c.*). Fibrosis results and interferes with the working of the organ. In the liver it causes portal obstruction, with fatigue, muscle cramps and weight loss. Consequent developments may include ascites, jaundice, splenomegaly, oesophageal varices and episodes of bleeding and bruising. Clinical features may vary considerably. Digital clubbing may be present.

cisterna (siˈstərnə) a space or cavity containing fluid. *C. chyli* the dilated portion of the thoracic duct containing CHYLE. *C. magna* the subarachnoid space between the cerebellum and the MEDULLA OBLONGATA.

cisternal (siˈstərnəl) concerning the cisterna. *C. puncture* insertion of a hollow needle into the cisterna magna to withdraw cerebrospinal fluid.

citric acid (ˈsitrik ˈasəd) acid found in the juice of lemons, limes, etc.; an antiscorbutic.

CJD *see* CREUTZFELDT-JAKOB DISEASE.

Cl symbol for chlorine.

clamp (klamp) a metal surgical instrument used to compress any part of the body.

clang association (klang ə'sohsee'ayshən) rhyming speech. A way of speaking where words are associated that are similar in sound. Observed in some mental disorders.

clapping ('klaping) in physiotherapy, rhythmic beating with cupped hands. Frequently used over the chest to aid expectoration.

class action (klahs akshən) a proceeding in a civil court whereby a number of individuals jointly claim compensation for similar damage, e.g. due to a faulty product.

classification ('klahsifik'ayshun) a process in which ideas and objects are grouped and understood according to predetermined characteristics. *C. scheme* a system of organising data or information, usually involving categories of items with similar characteristics into groups. Examples include North American Nursing Diagnoses Association (NANDA) and Diagnostic and Statistical Manual of Mental Disorders (DSM-5).

claudication (ˌklawdə'kayshən) lameness. *Intermittent c.* limping, accompanied by severe pain in the legs on walking, which disappears with rest; a sign of occlusive arterial disease.

claustrophobia (ˌklostrə'fohbi·ə, ˌklaw-) fear of confined spaces, such as small rooms.

clavicle ('klavikəl) the collarbone. A long bone, part of the shoulder girdle.

clavus ('klayvəs) a corn.

clawfoot (ˌklaw'fuht) a deformity of the foot in which the longitudinal arch is abnormally raised. *See* PES CAVUS.

clawhand (ˌklaw'hand) a deformity of the hand in which the fingers are bent and contracted, giving a claw-like appearance.

cleft (kleft) a fissure or longitudinal opening. *C. lip* a congenital fissure in the upper lip, often accompanied by cleft palate. *C. palate* a congenital defect in the roof of the mouth due to failure of the medial plates of the palate to meet. Often associated with cleft lip.

client ('klieənt) 1. recipient of a professional service. 2. a recipient of healthcare, regardless of the person's state of health and where the service is delivered. 3. a patient.

climacteric (klie'maktə·rik, ˌkliemək'terik) the period of the menopause in women. Also used to denote a decline in sexual drive in men.

climax ('kliemaks) 1. the stage when a disease is at its greatest intensity. 2. the stage in sexual intercourse when orgasm occurs.

clinic ('klinik) 1. instruction of students at the bedside. 2. a department of a hospital devoted to the treatment of a particular type of disease or a place that patients attend for a consultation with a medical or nurse practitioner.

clinical ('klinikəl) relating to bedside observation and the treatment of patients. *C. audit* a cyclical measurement and evaluation by health professionals of the clinical standards they are achieving. *C. governance* a framework through which health organisations are accountable for continuously improving the quality of their services and for safeguarding high standards of care by creating an environment in which excellence in care will flourish. *C. judgement* an application of information based on actual observation of a patient combined with subjective and objective data and clinical experience that leads to a decision. *C. nurse consultant (CNC)* an advanced practice nurse who provides leadership and a consultancy service to other clinicians in their field of expertise. Criteria for classification vary according to industrial awards. *C. nurse specialist* a qualified nurse who has acquired advanced knowledge and skills in a specific area of clinical nursing. *C. pathway* a description of practice likely to result in favourable outcomes for a particular diagnosis that uses prospectively defined resources to minimise costs. It may be based on research, literature or common practice. *C. risk management* the means by which adverse events occurring in organisations and usually related to the delivery of patient care are systematically assessed and reviewed in order to seek ways for prevention of future incidents. *C. skills* skills required by clinicians (doctors, nurses, dentists and other clinical professions). Clinical skills vary depending on specialty but core skills remain constant, e.g. communication, history-taking, record-keeping, basic physical examination. *C. supervision* an exchange between practising professionals to enable the development of professional skills. Has a vital role in sustaining and developing professional practice in nursing and midwifery. *C. trial* a research investigation designed to provide objective information on the therapeutic efficacy of a particular drug or therapy.

Clinical Research Centre (klinikəl ˈreeˌsərch sentə) an organisation, often associated with a nursing, medical or allied health school or teaching hospital, that studies, analyses, correlates and describes healthcare processes to improve patient outcomes in Australia and internationally.

clip (klip) a metal device for holding the two edges of a wound together or for controlling the flow of liquid through a tube.

clitoridectomy (ˌklitə·rəˈdektəmee) excision of the clitoris. *See* CIRCUMCISION.

clitoris (ˈklitə·rəs, ˈkliet-) a small organ, formed of erectile tissue, situated at the anterior junction of the labia minora in the female.

clone (klohn) cells which are genetically identical to each other and have descended by asexual reproduction from the parent cell, to which they are also genetically identical.

clonic (ˈklonik) having the character of clonus. The second stage of a grand mal fit; also referred to as a tonic–clonic seizure. Previously called grand mal and also termed convulsion or fit. *See* EPILEPSY.

clonus (ˈklohnəs) spasmodic muscle rigidity and relaxation which occurs spasmodically. *Ankle c.* spasmodic movements of the calf muscles when the foot is suddenly pushed upwards, the leg being extended.

close-ended item (kloz endəd ietəm) survey question that the respondent may answer with only one of a fixed number of choices.

Clostridium (kloˈstridi·əm) a genus of anaerobic spore-forming bacteria, found as commensals of the gut of animals and humans and saprophytes of the soil. Pathogenic species include *C. botulinum* (botulism), *C. tetani* (tetanus) and *C. perfringens* (also known as *C. welchii*) (gas gangrene).

Clostridium difficile (*C. difficile*) (klo'stridi·əm ˌdifis'ilee) a spore-forming bacterium that is present in the gut of some adults and children and normally does not cause any problems in healthy people. However, sometimes antibiotics are given to a patient to treat an infection that can interfere with the balance of the 'good bacteria' present in the gut. When this happens, *C. difficile* bacteria can multiply and cause symptoms such as diarrhoea and pyrexia. Most cases occur in a healthcare environment, such as a hospital or care home. Generally, people with *C. difficile* infection make a full recovery, but the infection can sometimes be fatal, especially in frail older people or the very young. A particularly virulent form of *C. difficile*, known as type 027, is associated with severe hospital outbreaks. The risks of transmitting *C. difficile* among patients during healthcare episodes can be minimised by prudent antimicrobial prescribing, the isolation of those with *C. difficile* diarrhoea with enhanced environmental cleansing, and especially hand hygiene. Care should be taken not to rely on alcohol hand gels, which do not destroy bacterial spores. (*See* Appendix 10.)

clot (klot) a semisolid mass formed in a liquid, such as blood or lymph, by coagulation.

clotting ('kloting) coagulation. The formation of a clot (*see* BLOOD CLOTTING). *C. time* coagulation time; the length of time taken for shed blood to coagulate.

clubbing ('klubing) broadening and thickening of the tips of the fingers (and toes) due to bad circulation. It occurs in chronic diseases of the heart and respiratory system, such as congenital cardiac defect and tuberculosis.

clubfoot (ˌklub'fuht) TALIPES. A congenital deformity of the foot.

clumping ('klumping) collecting together into clumps. The reaction of bacteria and blood cells when agglutination occurs.

cluster headache (klusˌtah 'hedˌayk) a painful and rare chronic disease that affects men more than women at a ratio of 4:1. The headaches typically occur as clusters of attacks, short-acting, very painful, affecting one side of the head. There is no specific cause, but it appears to be a disorder of an 'internal clock' in the hypothalamus.

CMV *see* CYTOMEGALOVIRUS.

Co symbol for COBALT.

coagulase (koh'agyə·layz) an enzyme formed by pathogenic staphylococci that causes coagulation of plasma. Such bacteria are termed *c. positive*.

coagulation (kohˌagyu'layshən) clotting (*see* BLOOD CLOTTING).

coagulum (koh'agyələm) the mass of fibrin and cells formed when blood clots. The mass formed when other masses coagulate, e.g. milk curd.

coal tar (kohl tah) a by-product obtained in the destructive distillation of coal; used in ointment or solution in treatment of eczema and psoriasis.

coarctation (ˌkoh·ahk'tayshən) a condition of contraction or stricture. *C. of aorta* a congenital malformation characterised by deformity of the aorta, causing narrowing, usually severe, of the lumen of the vessel. Surgical resection of the stricture may be performed.

cobalt ('kohbawlt) *symbol* Co. A metallic element, traces of which are necessary in the diet to prevent anaemia. *Radioactive c.* cobalt 60, used as a source of gamma irradiation in radiotherapy.

cocaine (koh'kayn) a colourless alkaloid, obtained from coca leaves, which has a powerful but brief stimulant action. Formerly used as a local anaesthetic, cocaine has been replaced by less addictive preparations such as procaine, lignocaine and amethocaine. It is now a major recreational drug, producing euphoria with many undesirable behavioural and social effects. It is highly addictive and usually taken by snorting. Regular inhaling of the drug can damage the lining of the nose. Overdose can cause seizures and cardiac arrest. Also known, in its various forms, as 'crack', 'coke', 'blow', 'snow', 'Charlie' or 'c'.

cocainism (koh'kaynəzəm) addiction to cocaine. Long-term abuse is associated with a toxic psychosis.

coccus ('kokəs) a bacterium of spheroidal shape.

coccydynia (ˌkoksə'dini·ə) persistent pain in the region of the coccyx.

coccyx ('koksiks) the terminal bone of the spinal column, in which four rudimentary vertebrae are fused together to form a triangle.

cochlea ('kokli·ə) the spiral canal of the internal ear.

cochlear implant ('kokli·ə ˌimplahn't) a surgically implanted electronic device that is inserted into the inner ear to provide sound to the profoundly deaf. The implant stimulates the hearing nerve and provides sound signals directly to the brain. Cochlear implants are also known as 'bionic ears'.

Cochrane database (kokrən daytəbays) *Archibald Cochrane, Scottish epidemiologist, 1909–1988.* Database of systematic reviews of published research; an international multidisciplinary collaboration of health professionals, consumers and researchers who review randomised controlled clinical trials.

code (kohd) 1. a set of rules governing one's conduct. 2. a system by which information can be communicated. *Genetic c.* the arrangement of nucleotides in the DNA of the chromosomes and in the RNA of the protein transcription apparatus of the cell. *C. of conduct* a code of conduct for nurses and for midwives. Revised periodically, these codes are intended to provide definite standards of practice and conduct that are essential to the ethical discharge of the nurse's and midwife's responsibility and to inform the public, other health professionals and employers of the standard of professional conduct expected of a registered practitioner. (*See* Appendix 8.)

coeliac ('seeleeˌak) relating to the abdomen. *C. disease* an inflammatory condition of the gastrointestinal tract due to a hypersensitivity to gluten (found in barley, wheat, oats and rye) in the diet. Damage to the gut causes malabsorption, leading to weight loss and vitamin and mineral deficiencies that may cause anaemia and ill health. Diagnosis is made by blood, urine and faecal testing together with jejunal biopsies. Treatment involves a lifelong gluten-free diet. Coeliac disease can affect all ages and runs in some families. *C. plexus* nerve complex that supplies the abdominal organs.

coenzyme (koh'enziem) an organic molecule activator to a larger protein enzyme.

cognition (kog'nishən) the action of knowing.

cognitive (kog'ni·tiv) pertaining to cognition. *C. abilities and skills* relates to brain-based skills and mental processes needed to carry out any task. It also involves the mechanisms of how you learn, remember and pay attention rather than any actual knowledge you have learnt. *C. behavioural therapy (CBT)* a method of treating psychological disorders based on the approach that the client's problems arise from a faulty way of looking at the world and oneself. In cognitive behavioural therapy, the client is helped to identify negative or false cognitions and then encouraged to try out new thought strategies in daily living. *Mild c. impairment (MCI)* a disorder that causes a slight but noticeable decline in cognitive abilities, such as memory, or other thinking skills such as processing visual and spatial information, complex thinking functions. In MCI these problems are less severe than those experienced by people with dementia.

cohabit (ˌkoh'habət) 1. to live together and have a relationship without being married. 2. to coexist.

cohort ('kohˌhawt) a group of people possessing a common characteristic, such as being born in the same year or of the same sex, used in research to make generalisations derived from quantitative data. *C. study* concerning a specific group or subpopulation in a research study.

coil ('koy'l) *see* INTRAUTERINE CONTRACEPTIVE DEVICE.

coitus ('koytəs, 'koh·itəs) sexual intercourse between male and female. *C. interruptus* a method of contraception in which the erect penis is removed from the vagina before ejaculation occurs.

cold (kohld) 1. of low temperature. 2. a viral infection affecting the membranes of the nose and throat and the bronchial tubes. *C. sore* herpes simplex. *See* HERPES.

colectomy (koh'lektəmee) the surgical excision of a portion or all of the colon.

colic ('kolik) acute paroxysmal abdominal pain. *Biliary c.* pain due to the presence of a gallstone in a bile duct. *Infantile c.* excessive crying due to pain and distress; most common in the first 3 months of life. The infant may pull up his or her legs and expel gas from the anus or 'belch'. May be due to air swallowing, milk intolerance or natural hyperactivity. *Intestinal c.* severe, griping, spasmodic abdominal pain which may be a symptom of food poisoning or of intestinal obstruction. *Renal c.* pain due to the presence of a stone in the ureter. *Uterine c.* spasmodic pain originating in the uterus, as in DYSMENORRHOEA.

coliform ('kohliˌfawm) resembling the bacillus *Escherichia coli*.

colitis (kə'lietəs, koh-) inflammation of the colon. It may be due to a specific organism, as in dysentery. *Ulcerative c.* a chronic disease, often of unknown cause, in which there are attacks of diarrhoea, with the passage of blood and mucus.

collagen ('koləjən) a fibrous structural protein that constitutes the protein of the white (collagenous) fibres of skin, tendon, bone, cartilage and all other connective tissues. It also occurs dispersed in a gel to provide stiffening, as in the vitreous humour of the eye. *C. diseases* a group of diseases having in common certain clinical and histological features that are manifestations of involvement of connective tissues (*see* CONNECTIVE TISSUES).

collapse (kə'laps) 1. a state of extreme prostration due to defective action of the heart, severe shock or haemorrhage. 2. falling in of a structure.

collarbone ('kolə·bohn) the CLAVICLE.

collateral (kə'latə·rəl) accessory to. *C. circulation see* CIRCULATION.

Colles' fracture ('koliz frakchə) *Abraham Colles, Irish surgeon, 1773–1843.* Fracture of the lower end of the radius at the wrist following a fall on the outstretched hand. Typically, it produces a 'dinner fork' deformity.

colloid ('koloyd) 1. glue-like. 2. translucent, yellowish, gelatinous substance resulting from colloid degeneration. 3. a chemical system composed of a continuous medium of small particles which do not settle out under the influence of gravity and will not pass through a semipermeable membrane, as in DIALYSIS.

coloboma (ˌkoloh'bohmə) a congenital fissure of the eye affecting the choroid coat and the retina.

colon ('kohlon) the large intestine, from the caecum to the rectum. *Ascending c.* that part rising up to the right of the abdomen to in front of the liver. *Descending c.* that part running down from in front of the spleen to the sigmoid colon. *Giant c.* megacolon. *Irritable c.* (*see* IRRITABLE BOWEL SYNDROME). *Pelvic c., sigmoid c.* that part lying in the pelvis and connecting the descending colon with the rectum. *Transverse c.* that part lying across the upper abdomen connecting the ascending and descending portions.

colonic (kə'lonik) pertaining to the colon. *C. irrigation* colonic lavage (*see* LAVAGE).

colonoscope (koh'lonəˌskohp) a fibreoptic instrument, passed through the anus, for examining the interior of the colon.

colony ('kolənee) a mass of bacteria formed by multiplication of cells when bacteria are incubated under favourable conditions.

colostomy (kə'lostəmee) an artificial opening (stoma) in the large intestine brought to the surface of the abdomen for the purpose of evacuating the bowel.

colostrum (kə'lostrəm) the fluid secreted by the breasts in the last few weeks of pregnancy and for the first 3 or 4 days after delivery, until lactation begins. Colostrum is high in protein and initially low in lactose; its fat content is equivalent to breast milk. It is an important source of passive antibody.

colour index ('kulə ˌindeks) an index of the amount of haemoglobin in red blood cells. In normal blood the figure is 1, in iron deficiency anaemia it is less than 1 and in megaloblastic anaemia it is more than 1. *See* BLOOD.

colour vision deficiency ('kulə 'vizhən də'fishənsee) any abnormality in colour vision that causes difficulty distinguishing between certain colours. The most common types of colour vision deficiency are reduced discrimination between red and green. A total absence of colour vision is very rare. *See* ACHROMATOPSIA.

colpitis (kol'pietəs) inflammation of the vagina.

colpocele ('kolpohˌseel) a hernia of either bladder or rectum into the vagina.

colpohysterectomy (ˌkolpohˌhistəˈrektəmee) removal of the uterus through the vagina.

colpoperineorrhaphy (ˌkolpohˌperineeˈo·rəfee) the repair by suturing of an injured vagina and torn perineum.

colpopexy (ˈkolpohˌpeksee) suture of a prolapsed vagina to the abdominal wall.

colporrhaphy (kolˈpo·rəfee) repair of the vagina. *Anterior c.* repair for CYSTOCELE. *Posterior c.* repair for rectocele.

colposcope (ˈkolpəˌskohp) a speculum for examining the vagina and cervix by means of a magnifying lens; used for the early detection of malignant changes.

coma (ˈkohmə) a state of unconsciousness from which the patient cannot be aroused. It is characterised by an absence of both spontaneous eye movements and response to painful stimuli. *See* GLASGOW COMA SCALE.

comatose (ˌkohməˌtohs, -ˌtohz) in the condition of coma.

comedo (koˈmeedoh) a blackhead. A plug of keratin and sebum within the dilated orifice of a hair follicle.

comfort (kumfət) to provide relief of, or freedom from, pain, depression or anxiety. *C. eating* eating at inappropriate times or eating unusual amounts for the relief of distress or anxiety. *C. measure* a specific action taken to promote the comfort of the patient, e.g. rearranging pillows or providing a change of position.

comforter (kumfətə) a baby's dummy or pacifier.

commensal (kəˈmensəl) living on or within another organism, and deriving benefit without harming or benefiting the host individual.

comminuted (ˈkoməˌnyootəd) broken into small pieces, as in a comminuted fracture. *See* FRACTURE.

commissure (ˈkomisˌyooə) a site of union of corresponding parts, as the angle of the lips or eyelids.

commode (ˌkəˈmohd) a bedside chair with a cutaway seat that allows a receptacle to be fitted underneath for the collection of urine and faeces. Used by a patient who is unable to reach or use the nearest toilet.

communicable disease (kəˈmyoonikəbəl diˈzeez) an infectious disease caused by a microorganism that may be transmitted from a person, animal or the environment to susceptible persons, either directly or indirectly.

communication skills (komyoonikayshən skils) in the broadest sense involve listening, speaking, writing and reading. In the context of healthcare, they generally focus on listening and giving information to patients. Communication skills cover both verbal and non-verbal forms of communication. They may extend to communicating with other clinicians, communicating at conferences or formal meetings and presenting material in class settings.

community (kəˈmyoonətee) a group of individuals living in an area, having a common interest or belonging to the same organisation. *C. care* the care of individuals within the community, by healthcare professionals and carers as an alternative to institutional or long-stay residential care. *C. nurse* a nurse who is based within the community with a responsibility for providing nursing services within the patient's own home or environment. Community nurses have a strong commitment to health promotion and the prevention of ill health. *Therapeutic c.* any treatment setting (usually psychiatric) which provides a living–learning situation through group processes emphasising social, environmental and personal interactions.

compartment syndrome (kəm-ˈpahtmənt ˈsinˌdrohm) muscle ischaemia caused by increased pressure in an osteofascial compartment. May be caused by oedema or bleeding following trauma or excessive muscle use.

compatibility (kəmˌpatəˈbilətee) mutual suitability. The mixing together of two substances without chemical change or loss of power. *See* BLOOD GROUPS.

compensation (ˌkompənˈsayshən) 1. making good a functional or structural defect. 2. mental mechanism (unconscious) by which a person covers up a weakness by exaggerating a more desirable characteristic.

compensatory techniques (ˈkom-pənˌsaytəree ˌtekˈneeks) assistance for patients/clients in developing new skills to compensate for a recognised handicap or deficit.

competence (kompətəns) a set of professionally agreed deliverables, outputs and roles that the healthcare professional must be able to perform in a particular post.

competency (kompətənsee) a set of behaviour patterns, knowledge and skills that the holder needs to bring to a position in order to perform the required role and functions with competence.

complaint (ˌkəmˈplaynt) an act of expressing dissatisfaction with a service or individual; may be written or verbal. *C. management* the policies and procedures in place within a health service to respond to and learn from complaints received from patients, their families and members of the community regarding care, treatment and services.

complement (ˈkompləmənt) a substance present in normal serum which combines with an antigen–antibody complex (*c. fixation*) to destroy bacteria. *C. fixation test* measurement of the amount of complement with antigen–antibody complex. Complement fixation tests are used to detect antibodies for infectious diseases. *C. system* a series of small inactive plasma proteins that are an important part of the innate immune response to infection. When stimulated by the presence of either an antibody–antigen complex or certain microbial products or antigens, complement proteins act as a biochemical cascade, with one protein activating the next. This results in the formation of activated complement which, by various means, attacks and destroys pathogenic microorganisms and dissolves and removes immune complexes.

complementary (ˌkompləˈmentə·ree) pertaining to that which completes or makes perfect. *C. feed* feed given to infants to supplement breastfeeding if the mother has insufficient milk. *C. therapies* a range of treatments, including yoga, reflexology, homeopathy, acupuncture and others, which may be combined with traditional medicine.

complete androgen insensitivity syndrome (ˈkompleet ˈandrəˌjən inˈsensəˈtivətee ˈsinˌdrohm) a condition that affects sexual development before birth and during puberty. People with the condition are genetically male but do not respond to male hormones and as a result have female external genitalia and breasts.

complex (ˈkompleks) a grouping of various things, as of signs and symptoms, forming a syndrome. In psychology, a grouping of ideas of emotional origin which are completely or partially represented in the unconscious mind. *Inferiority c.* a feeling of inadequacy; responses may vary from assertiveness or aggression (as compensation or cover) to passivity and withdrawal (because of feelings of inadequacy). *See* ELECTRA COMPLEX and OEDIPUS COMPLEX. *C. regional pain syndrome* is a uncommon chronic pain in which the patient experiences persistent, severe and debilitating pain often triggered by an injury, but which persists after healing has taken place.

compliance (komplieˈəns) the degree to which a person follows professional advice regarding their therapy.

complication (kompləˈkayshən) an accident or second disease process arising during the course of or following the primary condition; may be fatal.

compos mentis (ˈkompəs ˈmentəs) [L.] of sound mind.

compound (ˈkompownd) composed of two or more parts or substances. *C. fracture* a fracture in which the broken end or ends of the bone have torn through the skin; also called an open fracture.

comprehension (ˌkomprəˈhenshən) mental grasp of the meaning of a situation.

compress (ˈkompres) folded material, e.g. lint (wet or dry), applied to a part of the body for the relief of swelling and pain.

compression (kəmˈpreshən) 1. the act of pressing upon or together; the state of being pressed together. 2. in embryology, the shortening or omission of certain developmental stages. *C. bandages* used in the treatment of leg ulcers to improve venous return and reduce venous hypertension. Following successful healing of the leg ulcer, compression hose are worn to prevent reoccurrence. *C. garments* may be fitted and used following burns or for a patient with lymphoedema. They work by exerting pressure on the tissues thus preventing the build-up of fluid in the tissues.

compulsion (kəmˈpulshən) an overwhelming urge to perform an irrational act or ritual.

computed axial tomography (CAT or CT) scan (kəmˈpyooˌtəd akˈseeəl təˈmogrəfee skan) a computerised technique to examine a cross-section of the entire body. A CT scanner produces an image of tissue density in a complete cross-section of the part of the body being scanned.

conation (kohˈnayshən) a striving in a certain direction.

computerised records (kəmˈpyooˌtərˈiesəd ˈreˌkordz) health records held on computer systems, which are required by law to be secure and maintain confidentiality, usually achieved by limiting access and by controlling data sharing.

concept (ˈkonˌsept) an image or idea held in the mind.

conception (kənˈsepshən) 1. the act of becoming pregnant by the fertilisation of an ovum. 2. a concept.

conceptual framework (kənˈsept-yooəl, kənˈsepshooəl fraymwərk) a group of concepts that are broadly defined and organised to provide a rationale or structure for the interpretation of information.

concussion (kən'kushən) a violent jarring shock. *C. of the brain* temporary loss of consciousness produced by a fall or a blow on the head. There may be amnesia, slow respiration and a weak pulse.

conditioned response (kən'dishənd rə'spons) a response that does not occur naturally but may be developed by regular association of a physiological function with an unrelated outside event, such as the ringing of a bell or flashing of a light. Eventually, the physiological function starts whenever the outside event occurs. Also called conditioned reflex. *See also* UNCONDITIONED RESPONSE.

conditioning (kən'dishəning) a form of learning in which a response is elicited by a neural stimulus that had previously been repeatedly presented in conjunction with the stimulus that originally elicited the response. Also called classical and respondent conditioning.

condom ('kondəm) a contraceptive sheath worn during sexual intercourse and affording some protection for both partners against sexually transmitted diseases, available for both males and females.

conductive deafness (kən'duktiv 'def͵nəs) deafness caused by the faulty conduction of sound from the outer to the inner ear.

conductor (kən'duktə) 1. a substance through which electricity, light, heat or sound can pass. 2. any part of the nervous system that conveys impulses.

condyle ('kondiel, -dil) a rounded eminence occurring at the end of some bones and articulating with another bone.

condyloma (͵kondə'lohmə) *pl.* condylomata. An elevated wart-like lesion of the skin. *C. acuminata* small, pointed PAPILLOMA of viral origin, usually occurring on the skin or mucous surfaces of the external genitalia or perianal region; genital wart. *C. lata* wide, flat, syphilitic condyloma occurring on moist skin, especially about the genitals and anus.

cone (kohn) a solid figure with a rounded base, tapering upwards to a point. *C. biopsy* the removal of a cone-shaped section from the cervix of the uterus. It is performed for confirmation of the diagnosis when a cervical smear test result suggests the presence of pre-cancerous cells. *Retinal c.* the cone-shaped end of a light-sensitive cell in the retina, used for acute vision and for distinguishing colours.

confabulation (kən͵fabyə'layshən) the production of fictitious memories and the relating of experiences which have no relation to truth, to fill in the gaps due to loss of memory. A symptom of KORSAKOFF'S SYNDROME.

confidence ('konfədəns) self-assurance arising from the belief in one's own ability to achieve. *C. interval* in statistics, a range of values that has some specified probability. It quantifies the uncertainty of a statistic or the probable value range within which a population parameter is expected to lie.

confidentiality (͵konfə͵denshee'-alətee) the non-disclosure of information except to another authorised person, or assurance that a research participant's identity cannot be linked to the information that was provided to the researcher.

conflict (ˈkonflikt) a mental state arising when two opposing wishes or impulses cause emotional tension and often cannot be resolved without repressing one of the impulses into the unconscious. Conflict situations may be associated with an anxiety neurosis.

confluent (ˈkonflooənt) running together.

confusion (kənˈfyoozhən) disturbed orientation in regard to time, place, person or situation, sometimes accompanied by disordered consciousness.

congenital (kənˈjenətˈl) existing and present at the time of birth. *C. adrenal hyperplasia (CAH)* a group of inherited enzyme deficiencies that impair normal corticosteroid synthesis by the adrenal cortex. The most common enzyme deficiency is 21-hydroxylase deficiency, which accounts for over 90% of cases. Females may present with ambiguous genitalia at birth. Treatment involves hormone replacement including hydrocortisone therapy. *C. cataracts* present at birth, seen in children with certain genetic conditions or following infection during pregnancy. *C. dislocation of the hip* also known as *C. dysplasia of the hip*, *C. subluxation of the hip* a condition where the femoral head and ACETABULUM are misshaped, resulting in an abnormal articulation. *C. heart defect* a structural defect of the heart or great vessels or both; present at birth. *C. infection* an infection which takes place in utero. The most important congenital infections are RUBELLA, CYTOMEGALOVIRUS, HERPES SIMPLEX, HUMAN IMMUNODEFICIENCY VIRUS (HIV), SYPHILIS and TOXOPLASMOSIS.

congestion (kənˈjeschən) an abnormal accumulation of blood in any part. *Pulmonary c.* congestion of the lung, as in pneumonia and congestive heart failure.

conjunctiva (ˌkonjungkˈtəvə) the mucous membrane covering the front of the eyeball and lining the eyelids.

conjunctivitis (kənˌjungktəˈvietəs) inflammation of the conjunctiva. 'Pink eye' ophthalmia. *Catarrhal c.* a mild form, usually due to cold or irritation. *Granular c.* trachoma. *Phlyctenular c.* marked by small vesicles or ulcers on the membrane. *Purulent c.* caused by virulent organisms, with discharge of pus.

connective (kəˈnektiv) joining together. *C. tissues* those that develop from the mesenchyme and are formed of a matrix containing fibres and cells. Areolar tissue, cartilage and bone are examples.

consanguinity (ˌkonsang·gwinətee) blood relationship.

conscious (konshəs) the state of being awake or aware. Levels of consciousness are loosely defined states of awareness of, and response to, stimuli, essential for the assessment of an individual's neurological status. The level of consciousness is an accurate indicator of the degree of brain (dys)function.

consent (kənˈsent) in law, voluntary agreement with an action proposed by another. Consent is an act of reason; the person giving consent must be of sufficient mental capacity and be in possession of all essential information in order to give valid and informed consent. It is a legal requirement that doctors or researchers inform patients about to undergo surgery or invasive tests or to be a subject involved in a clinical trial of the risks and probable outcomes of the treatment or research. *C. forms* in non-emergency situations, written informed consent is generally required before many clinical procedures, such as surgery (including biopsies), endoscopy and radiographic procedures involving catheterisation. The doctor or the health professional concerned must explain to the patient the diagnosis, the nature of the procedure, including the risks involved and the chances of success, and the alternative methods of treatment that are available. A signed declaration that the doctor has explained the nature of the procedure to the patient in non-technical words should be included. Nurses or other members of the healthcare team may be involved in filling out the consent form and witnessing the signature of the patient. If the patient is a minor, or incapable of giving informed consent, the next-of-kin or guardian must sign the consent form. *Informed c.* a process whereby patients, parents or guardians and research participants are kept fully informed of the procedures that they will be undertaking; enabling them to make an informed choice for consent. Ensuring informed consent is a moral and legal duty for all healthcare professionals.

conservative treatment (kən'sərvətiv 'treetmənt) the use of non-radical methods to restore health and preserve function.

consolidation (kən,solə'dayshən) a state of becoming solid. *C. of lung* in pneumonia, the infected lobe becomes solid with exudate.

constipation (,konstə'payshən) incomplete or infrequent action of the bowels, with consequent filling of the rectum with hard faeces. *Atonic c.* constipation due to lack of muscle tone in the bowel wall. *Spastic c.* a form of constipation where spasm of part of the bowel wall narrows the canal.

consultation (kən,sol'tayshən) a process in which the assistance of a specialist healthcare practitioner is sought to identify ways to treat problems or issues related to patient management or in the planning of healthcare programs.

consumer (,kən'syoomə) in healthcare, may be the user, client, patient or carer, in terms of the services being provided.

consumption (kən'sumpshən) 1. the act of consuming, or the process of being consumed. 2. a wasting away of the body; once applied to pulmonary tuberculosis.

contact ('kontakt) 1. a mutual touching of two bodies or persons. 2. an individual known to have been in association with an infected person or animal or a contaminated environment. *C. dermatitis* a skin rash marked by itching, swelling, blistering, oozing and scaling. It is caused by direct contact between the skin and a substance to which the person is allergic or sensitive. *C. lens* a glass or plastic lens worn under the eyelids in the front of the eye. It may be worn for therapeutic or for cosmetic reasons.

contagion (kən'tayjən) 1. the communication of disease from one person to another by direct contact. 2. an infectious disease.

containment (kən'taynmənt) a term used in communicable disease control, meaning prevention of spread of disease from a focus of infection.

contamination (kən͵tamə'nayshən) being soiled or exposed to harmful agents.

content analysis ('kontent ə'naləsəs) a research technique for the objective, systematic and quantitative description of communications and documentary evidence.

continent ('kon͵tənənt) 1. able to control urination and defecation. 2. exercising self-restraint, especially abstaining from sexual activity.

continuing healthcare (kən'tinyooing helthkair) ongoing care of the physically, mentally and emotionally handicapped, and those suffering from chronic incapacitating illness.

continuing education (͵kən'tinyooing ͵edyoo'kayshən) further study and learning after the attainment of basic qualifications. This is vital for all professional practitioners so that they may keep up to date within their field and is accomplished in the form of organised study days or courses, or by individual reading and study.

continuing professional development (CPD) (͵kən'tinyooing ͵prə'feshənəl ͵də'veləpmənt) in Australia, the *Health Practitioner Regulation National Law (2009)* (the National Law) requires nurses and midwives on the register to participate in at least 20 hours of professional development per year. One hour of active learning will equal 1 hour of CPD. The CPD must be relevant to the nurse or midwife's context of practice. A written record must be kept of CPD activity per year.

continuity of care (͵kontən'yooətee ov kair) the concept of a healthcare provider (general practitioner, nurse, midwife, etc.) being continually involved with a person throughout treatment over a period which may extend over years.

continuous ambulatory peritoneal dialysis (CAPD) (͵kən'tinyooəs ͵amb'yoolaytəree ͵perətoh'neeəl ͵die'aləsis) treatment in which the patient is ambulant while receiving peritoneal dialysis.

continuous positive airway pressure (CPAP) (͵kən'tinyooəs 'posətiv airway preshə) a process whereby medical gas is delivered to the patient at positive pressure to hold open alveoli that would normally close at the end of expiration, thereby increasing oxygenation and reducing the work of breathing.

contraception (͵kontrə'sepshən) the prevention of conception and pregnancy.

contraceptive (͵kontrə'septiv) an agent used to prevent conception, e.g. condom, cap that occludes the cervix, spermicidal pessary or cream, hormone skin patches, subdermal implants, intrauterine device (IUD) and oral contraceptives (hormone pills).

contract (͵kən'trakt) 1. to make or to enter into an agreement with a person, authority or company to deliver services or goods. ('kontrakt) 2. in healthcare, an agreement, usually written, between two people with differing interests and concerns.

contraction (kən'trakshən) a shortening or drawing together, especially applied to muscle action. *Uterine c.s* those occurring during labour.

contracture (kən'trakchə) fibrosis causing permanent contraction. *Dupuytren's c.* See DUPUYTREN'S CONTRACTURE and figure p. 148. *Volkmann's ischaemic c.* contraction resulting from impairment of the blood supply. May occur in upper or lower limbs.

contraindication (͵kontrə͵ində-'kayshən) any condition that makes a particular line of treatment impracticable or undesirable.

contralateral (ˌkontrəˈlatə·rəl) occurring on the opposite side.

contrast medium (ˈkontrahst ˈmeedi·əm) a substance used in radiography to make certain organs visible or more visible.

contrecoup (ˌkontrəˈkoo) [Fr.] an injury occurring on the opposite side or at a distance from the site of the blow, e.g. brain damage on the opposite side of the skull to the blow.

control (kənˈtrohl) 1. restraint or command of objects or events. 2. a standard for testing where the procedure is identical in all respects to the experiment but the factor being studied is absent. *Birth c.* contraception. *C. group* a group of subjects who in the course of an experimental research project do not experience the factor under consideration. This enables the researcher to make a comparison with the effects produced on the experimental group. *Infection c.* standard and transmission-based precautions, and procedures within the healthcare service that provide guidelines for all staff to control infection within hospitals and in all healthcare facilities, e.g. ambulances and the community. *See* INFECTION.

controlled trial (ˌkənˈtrohld trie'l) a research method in which one group of subjects in a trial are not exposed to the experimental treatment or investigation, in an attempt to decrease the possibility of error and increase the possibility that the findings of the study are an accurate reflection of reality. *See* RANDOMISED CONTROLLED TRIAL.

contusion (kənˈtyoozhən) a bruise.

convalescence (ˌkonvəˈlesəns) period of recovery following illness, injury or operation. Also referred to as REHABILITATION.

convection (kənˈvekshən) a method of transmission of heat by the circulation of warmed molecules of a liquid or a gas.

conversion (kənˈvərshən) 1. the act of changing into something of different form or properties. 2. the transformation of emotions into physical manifestations. 3. manipulative correction of malposition of a fetal part during labour.

convolution (ˈkonvəˈlooshən) a fold or coil, e.g. of the cerebrum or renal tubules.

convulsion (kənˈvulshən) involuntary contractions of the voluntary muscles. Convulsive seizures are symptomatic of some neurological disorders; they are not in themselves a disease entity. *Clonic c.* a convulsion marked by alternate contracting and relaxing of the muscles. *Febrile c.* a convulsion occurring almost exclusively in children aged 6 months to 5 years of age, and associated with a fever of 40°C or higher. *Tonic c.* prolonged contraction of the muscles, as a result of an epileptic discharge. *See* EPILEPSY.

Coombs' test (koomz ˌtest) *Robin Coombs, British immunologist, 1921–2006.* A test to detect the presence of any antibody on the surface of the red blood cell. Used to detect Rh antibodies in maternal or fetal blood and in the diagnosis of haemolytic anaemia.

coordination (kohˌawdəˈnayshən) harmony of movement between several muscles or groups of muscle so that complicated manoeuvres can be made.

COPD *see* CHRONIC OBSTRUCTIVE PULMONARY DISEASE.

coping (ˈkohping) the process of contending with life difficulties in an effort to overcome or work through them. *C. mechanisms* conscious or unconscious strategies or mechanisms that a person uses to cope with stress or anxiety.

copper (ˈkopə) *symbol* Cu. A metallic element, traces of which are present in all human tissues.

coprolalia (ˈkoprəˈlayli·ə) the uncontrolled use of obscene speech. *See* TOURETTE'S SYNDROME.

coprolith (ˈkoprəlith) a faecalith. A hard mass of faeces in the rectum or colon.

copulation (ˌkopyəˈlayshən) coitus. Sexual intercourse.

cord (kawd) a long, cylindrical, flexible structure. *Spermatic c.* that which suspends the testicle in the scrotum, and contains the spermatic artery and vein and VAS DEFERENS. *Spinal c.* the part of the central nervous system enclosed in the spinal column. *Umbilical c.* the connection between the fetus and the placenta, through which the fetus receives nourishment. *Vocal c.s* folds of mucous membrane in the larynx, which vibrate to produce the voice.

cordotomy (kawˈdotəmee) *see* CHORDOTOMY.

corn (kawn) a local hardening and thickening of the skin from pressure or friction, occurring usually on the feet. CLAVUS.

cornea (ˈkawni·ə) the transparent portion of the anterior surface of the eyeball continuous with the sclerotic coat. *Conical c.* keratoconus.

corneal (ˈkawni·əl) pertaining to the cornea. *C. graft* a means of restoring sight by grafting healthy transparent cornea from a donor in place of diseased tissue. KERATOPLASTY.

corneoscleral (ˌkawniohˈskliə·rəl) relating to both the cornea and the sclera. *C. junction* the point where the edge of the cornea joins the sclera. The LIMBUS.

cornu (ˈkawnyoo) a horn. *C. of the uterus* one of the two horn-shaped projections where the uterine tubes join the uterus at the upper pole on either side.

coronal (kəˈrohnˈl) relating to the crown of the head. *C. suture* the junction of the frontal and parietal bones.

coronary (ˈko·rənə·ree) encircling. Crown-like. *C. arteries* the vessels that supply the heart. *C. artery bypass graft (CABG)* an operation carried out to bypass a coronary artery narrowed by atheroma using a graft from a healthy saphenous vein or an internal mammary artery. *C. care unit* a ward or unit within a hospital which provides for the monitoring and intensive care, by a specialist team of staff, of patients who have suffered an attack of coronary thrombosis and of those who are in the immediate postoperative period following heart surgery. *C. circulation see* CIRCULATION. *C. thrombosis see* THROMBOSIS.

coronaviruses (ˌkərˈohnəˌvierəsəs) members of a family (*Coronaviridae*) of large, enveloped, positive-stranded RNA viruses, including types 229E, NL63, OC43, and HKU1, which cause illnesses in humans that can range from the common cold to more severe diseases, such as pneumonia or bronchitis. Most people get infected with one or more of these viruses at some point in their lives; infection is more common in people with co-morbidities or weakened immune systems and infants or older adults. Occasionally coronaviruses that infect animals can evolve and become a new human coronavirus, such as MERS-CoV (the beta coronavirus that causes Middle East Respiratory

Syndrome) and SARS-CoV (the beta coronavirus that causes SEVERE ACUTE RESPIRATORY SYNDROME or SARS). A more recently identified coronavirus (COVID-19), first reported in December 2019 in Wuhan City in China, is causing an outbreak of respiratory illnesses in a growing number of countries outside China, including Australia. There is preliminary evidence to suggest that the virus spreads from person-to-person through close contact with an infected person, through droplets produced from an infected person's coughs and sneezes or through touching contaminated surfaces. The incubation period for COVID-19 is between 2 and 14 days and symptoms include fever, cough, sore throat, fatigue and dyspnoea. Prevention is through the systematic implementation of standard and transmission-based precautions including PPE (see Appendix 10). Also known as SARS-CoV-2 or 2019-nCoV.

coroner (ˈko·rənə) a public official (appointed at a state level with powers to delegate at a local level) who holds inquests concerning unexpected, sudden, violent or suspicious deaths.

corpse (kawps) a dead body. Cadaver.

corpulent (ˈkawpyələnt) obese.

corpus (ˈkawpəs) a body. *C. albicans* the scar tissue on the surface of the ovary which replaces the CORPUS LUTEUM before the recommencement of menstruation. *C. callosum* the mass of white matter that joins the two cerebral hemispheres together. *C. cavernosum* either of the two columns of the erectile tissue forming the body of the clitoris or the penis. *C. luteum* the yellow body left on the surface of the ovary and formed from the remains of the Graafian follicle after the discharge of the ovum. If it retrogresses, menstruation occurs, but it persists for several months if pregnancy supervenes. *C. striatum* a mass of grey and white matter in the base of each cerebral hemisphere.

corpuscle (ˈkawpusəl) a small protoplasmic body or cell, as of blood or connective tissue. *See* BLOOD.

correlation (ˌko·rəˈlayshən) the degree of association between two variables. *C. study* a type of non-experimental research design that examines the relationship between two or more variables.

corrosive (kəˈrohsiv, -ziv) a substance that erodes and destroys.

cortex (ˈkawteks) [L.] an outer layer, as the bark of the trunk or root of a tree, or the outer layer of an organ or other structure, as distinguished from its inner substance. *Adrenal c.* the tissue surrounding the medulla or core of the adrenal gland. *Cerebral c.* the grey matter covering the two cerebral hemispheres. *Renal c.* the outer covering of the kidney.

corticospinal (ˌkawtikohˈspien'l) relating to the cerebral cortex and the spinal cord. *C. tract* the pyramidal tract; the nerve fibres making up the main pathway for rapid voluntary movement.

corticosteroid (ˌkawtikohˈstiə·royd) any of the hormones produced by the adrenal cortex or their synthetic substitutes. Glucocorticoids are responsible for metabolism of carbohydrate, fat and protein. They have powerful anti-inflammatory properties. Mineralocorticoids, e.g. aldosterone, are responsible for salt and water regulation.

corticotrophin (ˌkawtikohˈtrohfən) adrenocorticotrophic hormone (ACTH).

cortisol (ˈkawtəˌsol) the naturally occurring hormone of the adrenal cortex.

cortisone (ˈkawtəˌzohn, -ˌsohn) a naturally occurring corticosteroid. Inactive in humans until converted into cortisol.

Corynebacterium (koˌrienibak-ˈtie·ri·əm) a genus of slender, rod-shaped, Gram-positive and non-motile bacteria. *C. diphtheriae* Klebs-Löffler bacillus, the causative agent of diphtheria.

coryza (kəˈriezə) acute infection of the upper respiratory tract, characterised by profuse discharge from nasal mucous membranes, sneezing and watering of the eyes. The medical name for the common cold.

cosmetic (ˌkozˈmetik) 1. improving something outwardly. 2. relating to treatment intended to improve a person's appearance. *C. dentistry* treatment to improve the appearance of the teeth or to prevent further damage to teeth or gums, e.g. the whitening of teeth or fitting a crown to a damaged tooth. *C. surgery* an operation to improve a person's appearance, e.g. mammoplasty to reduce or enhance the breasts or the removal of skin blemishes or excess body fat and tissue.

cost effectiveness (ˌkost əˈfektiv-nəs) a concept which relates cost to the effectiveness of a service and thus provides value for money, e.g. screening programs to detect cervical cancer, rate of detection, and cost of the service and of treatment.

costal (ˈkost'l) relating to the ribs. *C. cartilages* those that connect the ribs to the sternum directly or indirectly.

costochondritis (ˌkostˈohˈkənˌ-driˈtietəs) inflammation of the cartilage that joins the ribs to the sternum. It will usually resolve after a few weeks.

cot death (kot deth) *see* SUDDEN INFANT DEATH SYNDROME.

cotyledon (ˌkoteeˈleedən) a cup-shaped depression. Applied to the subdivisions of the placenta.

cough (kof) voluntary or reflex explosive expulsion of air from the lungs. Its purpose is usually to expel a foreign body or accumulations of mucus. *Dry c.* one where no expectoration occurs. *Wet c.* one where expectoration of mucus or foreign body occurs. *Whooping c.* infectious disease caused by *Bordetella pertussis*.

counselling (ˈkownsəling) a process of consultation and discussion in which one individual (the counsellor) listens actively and offers guidance to another who is experiencing difficulties (the client). The counsellor does not direct or make decisions for the client. The general aim is to solve problems and increase awareness. The emphasis is on clients finding their own solutions. *Disaster c.* specialised counselling offered to victims of a major disaster (e.g. an aircraft crash or terrorist attack) or a natural event (e.g. an earthquake). The survivors of such disasters often experience psychological problems and POST-TRAUMATIC STRESS DISORDER, resulting in ill health.

counterextension (ˌkowntərək-ˈstenshən) 1. the holding back of the upper fragment of a fractured bone while the lower is pulled into position. 2. the raising of the foot of the bed in such a way that the weight of the body counteracts the pull of the extension apparatus on the lower part of the limb. Used especially for fracture of the femur.

counterirritant (ˌkowntəˈirətənt) a substance that produces mild inflammation of the skin when applied to it, but relieves pain and congestion.

countertraction (ˌkowntəˌtrakshən) the reduction of fractures by traction from two opposing directions at once.

coupling (ˈkupling) in cardiology, the frequent occurrence of a normal heartbeat followed by an extraventricular one. May occur as a result of digitalis overdose.

couvade (kooˈvahd) the experiencing of the symptoms of pregnancy and childbirth by the father. This psychosomatic phenomenon is common in many societies.

coxa (ˈkoksə) the hip joint. *C. valga* a deformity of the hip in which there is an increase in the angle between the neck and the shaft of the femur. *C. vara* a deformity in which the angle between the neck and the shaft of the femur is smaller than normal.

Coxiella (ˌkokseeˈelə) a genus of microorganisms of the order Rickettsiales. *C. burnetii* the causative agent of Q fever.

Coxsackie virus (kokˈsakee vierəs) one of a group of enteroviruses that may give rise to a variety of illnesses, including meningitis, pleurodynia, acute MYOCARDITIS and acute PERICARDITIS.

CPAP *see* CONTINUOUS POSITIVE AIRWAY PRESSURE.

CPD *see* CONTINUING PROFESSIONAL DEVELOPMENT.

CPR cardiopulmonary resuscitation. (*See* Appendix 6.)

crab louse (ˈkrab ˌlows) *Phthirus pubis*. *See* LOUSE.

crack (krak) purified form of cocaine, produced by a technique known as 'freebasing'. *See* COCAINE.

cradle (ˌkraydˈl) 1. a frame placed over the body or limb of a bed patient for protecting injured parts and preventing them from coming into contact with the bedclothes. 2. infant's bed with protective sides and, in the past, often on rockers. 3. to support, hold, comfort in the arms. *C. cap* an oily crust sometimes seen on the scalp of infants; also called milk crust (crusta lactea). Caused by excessive secretions from the sebaceous glands in the scalp.

cramp (kramp) a painful, spasmodic, muscular contraction which may result from fatigue. *Occupational c.* painful muscle spasms usually in the arm or hand; occurs in professions such as surgeons, writers, musicians, miners and machine operators.

cranial (ˈkrayni·əl) relating to the cranium. *C. nerves* the 12 pairs of nerves arising directly from the brain.

craniopharyngioma (ˌkrayneeohfaˌrinjeeˈohmə) a cerebral tumour arising in the craniopharyngeal pouch just above the SELLA TURCICA.

craniosacral therapy (ˌkrayneeohˈsaykrəl ˈtherəpee) a form of osteopathic treatment in which very gentle manipulation of the cranium attempts to release tensions within the skull which are thought to be the cause of various problems. The therapy has been successfully used to treat babies that are fractious after difficult forceps or vacuum extraction deliveries, colic and hyperactivity in older infants.

craniostenosis (ˌkrayneeohstəˈnohsəs) premature closure of the suture lines of the skull in an infant. Surgery may be required to relieve raised intracranial pressure.

craniosynostosis (ˌkrayneeohsiˈnostəsəs) premature closure of the cranial sutures.

craniotabes (ˈkrayneeohˈtaybeez) a patchy thinning of the bones of the vault of the skull of an infant; associated with rickets and OSTEOGENESIS IMPERFECTA (brittle bones).

craniotomy (ˌkraynee'otəmee) a surgical opening of the skull made to relieve pressure, arrest haemorrhage or remove a tumour.

cranium ('krayni·əm) 1. the skull. 2. the bony cavity that contains the brain.

creatine ('kreeəˌteen, -tin) a nitrogenous compound present in muscle. It is also found in the urine in conditions in which muscle is rapidly broken down, e.g. acute fevers and starvation. *C. phosphate* a high-energy phosphate stored in muscle.

creatinine (kree'atəˌneen) a normal constituent of urine; a product of protein metabolism.

creatinuria (kreeˌatəˌnyoo·ri·ə) increased concentration of creatine in the urine.

credentialling (krə'denshəling) review and examination of the credentials of healthcare professionals to ensure that they meet a set of educational or occupational criteria necessary to deliver care and support to the patient and the family.

credibility (ˌkredə'bilətee) a criterion for evaluating the data of a qualitative research study, referring to the amount of confidence in the truth of the given information.

crepitation (ˌkrepə'tayshən) 1. the grating sound caused by friction of the two ends of a fractured bone or on movement of an arthritic joint. 2. a similar sound heard in the lungs through a stethoscope. *See* RALE.

crepitus ('krepətəs) 1. *see* CREPITATION. 2. the noisy discharge of flatus from the bowels.

cretinism ('kretəˌnizəm) congenital hypothyroidism. An obsolete term.

Creutzfeldt-Jakob disease (CJD) (ˌkroytsfelt'yakob di'zeez) *Hans Gerhard Creutzfeldt, German physician, 1885–1964; Alfons Jakob, German physician, 1884–1931.* A progressive dementia transmissible through prion protein. A new variant of CJD that has been reported in young adults has a shorter incubation period and is usually fatal.

cribriform ('kribrəˌfawm) perforated like a sieve. *C. plate* part of the ethmoid bone. *See* ETHMOID.

cricoid ('kriekoyd) ring shaped. *C. cartilage* the ring-shaped cartilage at the lower end of the larynx.

cri du chat syndrome (kree doo sha 'sinˌdrohm) a hereditary congenital syndrome characterised by hypertelorism, microcephaly, severe mental deficiency and a plaintive cat-like cry; due to the deletion of part of the short arm of chromosome 5. Is often called 5p– (5p 'minus') syndrome.

crisis ('kriesəs) 1. a decisive point in acute disease; the turning point towards either recovery or death. *See* LYSIS. 2. a sudden paroxysmal intensification of symptoms in the course of a disease. 3. life crisis; a period of disorganisation that occurs when a person meets an obstacle to an important life goal, such as the sudden death of a family member or a difficult family conflict. *Addisonian c., adrenal c.* symptoms of fatigue, nausea and vomiting, and collapse accompanying an acute attack of adrenal failure. *Blast c.* a sudden, severe change in the course of chronic myelocytic leukaemia. The clinical picture resembles that seen in acute myelogenous leukaemia, with an increase in the proportion of myeloblasts. *C. intervention* counselling or psychotherapy for patients in a life crisis that is directed at supporting the patient through the crisis and helping the patient to cope with the stressful event that precipitated it. *Identity c.* usually occurring during adolescence, manifested by a loss of the sense of the sameness and historical continuity of one's self, and inability to accept the role the individual perceives as being expected of them by society.

criterion (krieˈtiə·ri·ən) the basis on which a decision is made, e.g. for drug dosage, treatment plans, research trials.

critical (ˈkritikəl) 1. arising from a crisis. 2. implying serious risk or uncertainty as to outcome. *C. appraisal* the process of objectively and critically evaluating a research report's content for scientific merit and relevance, e.g. relating the findings to practice, theory or education. *C. care unit* a unit within a hospital that supports and treats patients with critical disorders or diseases of the vital physiological systems. May also be called INTENSIVE CARE UNIT. *C. thinking* a purposeful, goal-directed approach based on scientific evidence rather than assumption or memorisation. Critical thinking is an organised approach to discovery that involves reflection and assimilation of information which enables the nurse or healthcare provider to arrive at an informed decision or to make a judgement.

Crohn's disease (krohnz diˈzeez) *Burrill Bernard Crohn, American physician, 1884–1983.* Regional ileitis. *See* ILEITIS.

Cronbach's alpha (kronˈbahks ˈalfə) *Lee Cronbach, American educational psychologist, 1916–2001.* In statistics, a test of internal consistency that simultaneously compares each item in a scale to all other items.

Crosby capsule (krosˈbee kapsyəl) *William Crosby, American physician, 1914–2005.* A capsule attached to the end of a flexible tube which is swallowed by the patient. When the capsule reaches the small intestine, as seen on radiological examination, a tissue biopsy of the small bowel mucosa can be taken.

cross-matching (kros matching) a test of the compatibility of donor blood to be transfused to a patient. *See* BLOOD GROUPS.

cross-sectional study (ˌkros ˈsek-shənəl studee) a non-experimental research design that looks at data at one point in time, i.e. in the immediate present.

croup (kroop) a condition resulting from acute obstruction of the larynx caused by allergy, foreign body, infection or new growth; occurs chiefly in infants and children. There is spasmodic DYSPNOEA, a harsh cough and stridor.

crown (krown) 1. that part of the tooth that appears above the gum. 2. the upper part of an organ or structure, such as the top of the head.

crowning (krowning) the stage in labour when the top of the infant's head becomes visible at the vulva.

cruciate (ˈkrooysheeayt) resembling a cross. *C. ligament see* LIGAMENT.

crus (krus) [L.] 1. the leg, from knee to foot. 2. a leg-like part.

crush syndrome (krutch ˈsindrohm) a severe life-threatening condition caused by extensive crushing trauma; the oedema, OLIGURIA and other symptoms of acute renal failure that follow crushing of a part, especially a large muscle mass, causing the release of MYOGLOBIN into the circulation.

crutch (krutch) appliance usually in the form of a light, tubular metal rod with hand grips and plastic loops for the forearms, to aid walking when the patient must not weight-bear (as in fractures of lower limbs) or when a lower limb is missing.

cryaesthesia (ˌkrieəsˈtheezi·ə) abnormal sensitivity to cold.
cryoanalgesia (ˌkrieohˌan'lˈjeezi·ə, -si·ə) the relief of pain by application of cold by CryoProbe to peripheral nerves.
cryobank (ˈkrieohˌbank) a facility for freezing and preserving semen at low temperatures (usually –196.5°C) for future use.
cryoprecipitate (ˌkrieohprəˈsipəˌ-tayt) any precipitate that results from cooling. Of particular therapeutic value is the cryoprecipitate from fresh plasma, which is rich in factor VIII and is used to treat haemophilia.
cryopreservation (ˌkrieohˌprezəˈ-vayshən) maintenance of the viability of excised tissue or organs by storing at very low temperatures.
cryosurgery (ˌkrieohˈsərjə·ree) the use of extreme cold to destroy tissue.
cryotherapy (ˌkrieohˈtherəpee) therapeutic use of cold.
cryptococcosis (ˌkriptohkokˈohsəs) infection caused by the yeast *Cryptococcus neoformans*, having a predilection for the brain and meninges but also invading the skin, lungs and other parts. It particularly affects persons immunocompromised by disease or therapy.
cryptorchidism (kripˌtawkəˌdizəm) failure of the testicles to descend into the scrotum; cryptorchism.
CT *see* COMPUTED AXIAL TOMOGRAPHY.
Cu symbol for COPPER.
cubitus (ˈkyoobətəs) 1. the forearm. 2. the elbow. *C. valgus* deformity of the elbow where the palm of the hand is abducted and thus faces outwards. *C. varus* deformity where there is adduction of the forearm.
cue (kyoo) something that gives a hint or idea of something else. A cue is a verbal or non-verbal signal in communication from one person to another. It is a remembered item which connects with further information or meaning.
cued recall (kyood ˈreeˌcawl) retrieval of information from memory with the help of cues, perhaps using the first letter of the word or name to be remembered.
culdoscope (ˈkuldəˌskohp) an endoscope used in CULDOSCOPY.
culdoscopy (kulˈdoskəpee) direct visual examination of the female viscera through an endoscope introduced into the pelvic cavity through the posterior vaginal FORNIX.
culture (ˈkulchə) 1. the propagation of microorganisms or of living tissue cells in special media conducive to their growth. 2. a collective noun for the symbolic and acquired aspects of human society, including convention, custom and language. 3. a singular noun for the customs and features of an ethnic (racial, religious or social) group. *C. shock* a feeling of alienation, often accompanied by feelings of depression and rejection, that results from a radical change in culture, e.g. as a result of migration from one country to another.
cultural safety (ˈkulchəˈral sayfˈtee) a concept of cultural safety drawn from the work of Māori nurses in New Zealand and represents a key philosophical shift from providing care regardless of difference, to care that takes account of a person's unique needs. In Australia, nurses and midwives are expected to provide culturally safe nursing and midwifery care by protecting the beliefs, practices and values of all cultures. In particular, nurses and midwives need to understand and acknowledge the historic factors, such as colonisation and power imbalance, how these factors impact on Aboriginal

and/or Torres Strait Islander people and how this group bears the burden of gross social, cultural and health inequality. *C. awareness* involves the appreciation of diversity and understanding of differences that exist between two cultures, e.g. being aware of the cultural values, beliefs and perceptions of other people. Externally visible cultural characteristics could include dress, music and physical characteristics. Also know as cultural competence. *C. safe care* an expectation that nurses and midwives engage with all people as individuals in a culturally safe and respectful way. Nurses and midwives will foster relationships that are open, honest and compassionate while providing respectful care to people from diverse cultural backgrounds. (*See* Appendix 8). *C. sensitivity* acknowledges the legitimacy of difference and then encourages self-reflection of cultural self-awareness as a way to ensure personal attitudes are not detrimental to an individual with a different background.

cumulative (ˈkyoomyələtiv) adding to. *C. action* occurs when a dose of a slowly released drug is given too frequently and accumulates in the system leading to the development of toxic symptoms, e.g. with some barbiturates and digoxin.

Cumulative Index to Nursing and Allied Health Literature (CINAHL) (ˈkyoomyələtiv ˈindeks too ˈnərsing and ˈalied ˈhelth litrachə) a computerised database of English-language nursing and allied health literature published bi-monthly with a yearly cumulation.

cupping (ˈkuping) 1. the formation of a cup-shaped depression with the hand: (a) to produce a skin erythema, thereby improving local circulation; and (b) to loosen excessive secretions from air passages, and perhaps induce coughing. 2. the use of a cupping glass to stimulate skin blood flow.

curative (ˈkyoo·rətiv) anything that promotes healing by overcoming disease.

curettage (ˈkyoo·rəˈtahzh, kyuhˈ-rettij) [Fr.] the scraping of a surface with a curette for therapeutic purposes or to obtain biopsy material.

curette (kyuhˈret) a spoon-shaped instrument used for the removal of unhealthy tissues by scraping.

Curling's ulcer (ˈkərlingz ˈulsə) *Thomas Curling, English surgeon, 1811–1888.* An ulcer of the duodenum developed after severe burns of the body.

cursor (kərsə) on the computer screen, a blinking character that indicates where the next character will appear.

curvature (ˈkərvəchə) the curving of a line, whether normal or abnormal. *Spinal c.* abnormal deviation of the vertebral column.

Cushing's disease (ˈkuhshingz diˈzeez) *Harvey Cushing, American surgeon, 1869–1939.* A condition of over-secretion by the adrenal cortex due to an adenoma of the pituitary gland. Symptoms include obesity, abnormal distribution of hair and atrophy of the genital organs.

cushingoid (ˈkuhshingˌoyd) referring to symptoms resembling those of Cushing's disease, e.g. the side effects of steroid therapy.

cusp (kusp) a pointed or rounded projection, such as on the crown of a tooth or a segment of a cardiac valve.

cutaneous (kyooˈtaynee·əs) pertaining to the skin.

cutdown (ˈkutˌdown) an incision into a vein with insertion of a catheter for intravenous infusion. It is performed when an infusion cannot be started by venepuncture. Also used with hyperalimentation therapy when concentrated solutions need to be given into the superior VENA CAVA.

cuticle (ˈkyootikəl) the narrow band of epidermis extending from the nail wall onto the nail surface; also called eponychium.

CVA *see* CEREBROVASCULAR ACCIDENT.

CVP *see* CENTRAL VENOUS PRESSURE.

cyanocobalamin (ˌsie·ənohkoh-ˈbaləmən) vitamin B_{12} (anti-anaemic factor) found in liver, eggs and fish. It combines with the intrinsic factor secreted in gastric juice for absorption, and is essential for erythrocyte maturation. Administered by injection in the treatment of PERNICIOUS ANAEMIA.

cyanosis (ˌsieəˈnohsəs) a bluish appearance of the skin and mucous membranes, caused by imperfect oxygenation of the blood. It indicates circulatory failure and is common in respiratory diseases. It is also seen in 'blue babies'.

cyberstalking (ˈsiebəˌstawking) internet harassment, e.g. repetitive unsolicited and/or inappropriate emails, including hate, obscene or threatening mail or live chat harassment. *See* HARASSMENT.

cycle (ˈsiekəl) a series of recurring events. *Cardiac c.* the events occurring between one heartbeat and the next. *Menstrual c.* the changes that occur each month in the female reproductive system.

cyclic (ˈsieklik) pertaining to or occurring in a cycle.

cyclodialysis (ˌsieklohdieˈaləsəs) an operation used in glaucoma to improve drainage from the anterior chamber of the eye at the corneoscleral junction.

cyclodiathermy (ˌsiekloh ˌdieəˈ-thərmee) a treatment for glaucoma without penetration of the eyeball. Diathermy is applied to the sclera to cause fibrosis around the ciliary body, so allowing the AQUEOUS HUMOUR to drain.

cycloplegia (ˌsieklohˈpleeji·ə) paralysis of the ciliary muscle of the eye.

cyclopropane (ˌsieklohˈprohpayn) a gas used for general anaesthesia. It is not irritating to the respiratory tract but is highly inflammable and is therefore potentially dangerous.

cyclothymia (ˈsieklohˈthiemi·ə) the marked swings of mood between depression and elation seen in BIPOLAR DISORDER.

cyesis (sieˈeesəs) pregnancy. *Pseudoc.* signs and symptoms suggestive of pregnancy arising when no fertilisation has taken place. 'Phantom pregnancy'.

cyst (sist) 1. a cavity or sac with epithelium, containing liquid or semisolid matter. 2. a stage in the life cycle of certain protozoan parasites when they acquire tough protective coats. *Branchial c.* one formed in the neck from non-closure of the branchial cleft during development. *Chocolate c.* an ovarian cyst occurring in ENDOMETRIOSIS. *Daughter c.* a small cyst that develops from a large one. *Dermoid c.* a congenital type containing skin, hair, teeth, etc. It is due to abnormal development of embryonic tissue. *Hydatid c.* the larval cyst stage of the tapeworm, usually found in the liver. *Meibomian c.* a swelling of a MEIBOMIAN GLAND caused by obstruction of its duct. *Multilocular c.* a cyst that is divided into compartments or locules. *Ovarian c.* a cyst of the ovary, usually non-malignant, but sometimes becoming very large and requiring surgical removal. *Retention c.* any cyst caused by blockage of a duct. *Sebaceous c.* a retention cyst caused by the blockage of a duct from a sebaceous gland so that the sebum collects. *Sublingual c.* a RANULA. *Thyroglossal c.* one in the thyroglossal tract near the hyoid bone at the base of the tongue.

cystadenoma (siˌstadəˈnohmə) a benign neoplasm made up of cysts containing secretions.

cystalgia (siˈstalji·ə) pain in the urinary bladder.

cystathioninuria (ˌsistəˌthieohnee-ˈnyoo·ri·ə) a hereditary disorder of cystathionine metabolism, marked by increased concentrations in the urine. May be associated with learning difficulties.

cystectomy (siˈstektəmee) complete or partial removal of the urinary bladder. The ureters are diverted into an isolated ileal segment (ileal conduit) or into the sigmoid colon.

cysteine (ˈsisˌteen, ˈsisˌtayn) a sulfur-containing amino acid formed by the ingestion of dietary proteins.

cystic duct (ˈsistik dukt) the duct between the gallbladder and the common bile duct.

cysticercosis (ˌsistisərˈkohsəs) a disease caused by infestation with the cysticercus (larval form) of *Taenia solium* (pork tapeworm).

cystic fibrosis (ˈsistik fieˈbrohsəs) a hereditary disorder associated with accumulation of excessively thick and tenacious mucus and abnormal secretion of sweat and saliva; also called cystic fibrosis of the pancreas and MUCOVISCIDOSIS. The disease is inherited as a recessive trait. The severity of cystic fibrosis varies widely. Although inherited, it may not manifest during the early weeks of life, or it may cause meconium ileus in the newborn. Most cases are detected soon after birth through newborn screening. Therapeutic management is long term, initially centring on replacement of pancreatic enzymes, physiotherapy and antibiotics. Even with prompt and vigorous treatment, permanent lung damage may occur. Lung or heart/lung transplants offer good results with an improved quality of life. Gene therapy is currently being developed. In those families with a history of the condition, amniocentesis can be used to determine if a fetus is affected. Diagnosis is by the serum immune reactive trypsin (IRT) test. Early diagnosis and treatment improves the long-term prognosis and life expectancy.

cystine (ˈsisteen, -tin) an amino acid closely related to cysteine. Sometimes excreted in urine in the form of minute crystals (cystinuria).

cystinosis (ˌsistəˈnohsəs) an inherited metabolic disorder in which cystine is deposited in the tissues.

cystitis (siˈstietəs) inflammation of the urinary bladder.

cystocele (ˈsistohˌseel) a prolapse of the bladder into the vagina.

cystodiathermy (ˌsistohˈdieəˌthərmee) the application of a high-frequency electric current to the bladder mucosa, usually for the removal of small lesions of the bladder.

cystography (siˈstogrəfee) radiography of the urinary bladder after the introduction of a radio-opaque contrast medium. *Micturating c.* radiographic examination during the act of passing urine.

cystolithiasis (ˌsistohliˈthieəsəs) stone or stones in the urinary bladder.

cystoscope (ˈsistə͵skohp) an endoscope for examining the interior of the urinary bladder.

cystostomy (siˈstostəmee) the operation of making a temporary or permanent opening into the urinary bladder.

cystotomy (siˈstotəmee) incision of the urinary bladder for removal of calculi, etc. *Suprapubic c.* incision above the pubes.

cystourethrography (͵sistoh͵yoo·rəˈthrogrəfee) radiography of the urinary bladder and urethra.

cytogenetics (͵sietohjəˈnetiks) the study of cells during mitosis in order to examine the chromosomes and the relationship between chromosome abnormality and disease.

cytology (sieˈtoləjee) the microscopic study of the form and functions of the cells of the body. *Exfoliative c.* an aid to the early diagnosis of malignant disease. Secretions or surface cells are examined for premalignant changes.

cytolysin (sieˈtoləsən) a substance that causes cytolysis. *See* BACTERIOLYSIN and HAEMOLYSIN.

cytolysis (sieˈtoləsəs) the destruction of cells.

cytomegalic inclusion disease (͵sietohˈmegəlik inˈkloozhən diˈzeez) an infection due to CYTOMEGALOVIRUS. In the congenital form, there is HEPATOSPLENOMEGALY with cirrhosis, and microcephaly with learning difficulties and developmental delay. Acquired disease may cause a clinical state similar to INFECTIOUS MONONUCLEOSIS.

cytomegalovirus (͵sietoh͵megəlohˈ-vierəs) a virus belonging to the herpes simplex group.

cytapheresis (ˈsietah͵fə͵reesəs) a technique to remove specific cellular components from the blood, e.g. white blood cells or platelets needed to treat a patient, or to remove abnormal constituents.

cytoplasm (ˈsietoh͵plazəm) the protoplasmic part of the cell surrounding the nucleus.

cytosine (ˈsietoh͵seen) one of the pyrimidine bases found in DEOXYRIBONUCLEIC ACID (DNA). *C. arabinoside* an antimetabolite used in the treatment of acute leukaemia. Cytarabine.

cytotoxic (͵sietohˈtoksik) 1. having a deleterious effect upon cells. 2. an agent or drug that damages or destroys cells. Used to treat various forms of cancer and sometimes other conditions. The handling of cytotoxic drugs is a health and safety issue. Healthcare workers should follow local guidelines and policies regarding administration of these drugs.

Dd

dacryolith (ˈdakreeoh͵lith) a calculus in a lacrimal duct.

dacryoma (͵dakreeˈohmə) a benign tumour that arises from the lacrimal epithelium.

dactyl (ˈdaktəl) a finger or toe; a digit.

dactylology (͵daktəˈloləjee) communication between individuals by signs made with the fingers and hands. Finger spelling.

daltonism (ˈdawltə͵nizəm) colour blindness; inability to distinguish red from green. *See* COLOUR VISION DEFICIENCY.

dander (ˈdandə) small scales from the hair or feathers of animals, which may be a cause of allergy in sensitive people.

dandruff (ˈdandrəf) white scales shed from the scalp. If moist from serous exudate, they have a greasy appearance.

Darwinism (ˈdahwə͵nizəm) *Charles Darwin, British naturalist, 1809–1882.* The theory of the evolution of species through natural selection.

data (ˈdaytə, dahtə) *sing.* datum; a collection of facts. *Continuous d.* data that have a continuous set of values, e.g. for variables such as height, weight and antibody titres in response to vaccination. *D. analysis* the phase of a study that includes inspecting, classifying, coding and tabulating information needed to perform quantitative or qualitative analysis. The process of data analysis includes various approaches and techniques and is dependent on the research design and what is appropriate for the data. *D. processing* the storage and analysis of data to produce statistical tabulations, often by computer. *D. protection.* Developments in technology and the ever-increasing volumes and flow of data have led to an increased focus on storage of personal information and cybersecurity. The *Privacy Act 1988* is an Australian law that regulates the handling of personal data/information about individuals regardless of how it is recorded. Health service providers need to be aware of their obligations under the *Privacy Act* and the amendments that take effect from 2018 under the Australian Notifiable Data Breaches (NDB) scheme with regard to the introduction of a mandatory notification procedure for data breaches. *D. saturation* a point in qualitative research when data collection may cease because no new information from participants is emerging; data from subsequent participants become repetitive and inclusion of more participants does not yield new ideas. *D. set* a collection of information made on a group and related to certain variables that are being investigated. *Discrete d.* data with a single value or characteristic, e.g. colour of hair.

database (ˈdaytəbays, dahtə-) information that is organised in a systematic way, so that it may easily be collected, stored, reviewed and updated. The information is most commonly stored in a computer, so that a computer program may consult it to answer queries. The information may be used for evaluation and audit; e.g. a patient care database.

day care (day kair) a specialised service for preschool children, either as a substitute for or as an extension to family life. A similar service may be provided for older people needing care and support and to provide respite for family carers. *See* DAY CENTRE.

day centre (day sentə) a specialised facility that offers care, treatment and a respite service for older people needing care or the mentally ill.

day nursery (day nərsree) a centre for the care, during the daytime, of children up to the age of 5 years. Provided by the social services department or by voluntary agencies. Priority is given to children from 'at-risk' families and to those with a mental or physical disability.

day patient care (day ˈpayshənt kair) a service provided either in a specialised ward or in a hospital ward for treatment/investigation/ minor surgery. The patient is admitted and discharged on the same day.

dB symbol for *decibel.*

D&C *see* DILATATION AND CURETTAGE.

DDT dichlorodiphenyltrichloroethane; dicophane. A powerful insecticide now rarely used because of its toxicity.

deafness (ˈdefˌnəs) complete or partial loss of hearing affecting about 10% of adults and more than 50% of people over 65 years of age. May be called 'hearing impairment' or 'hearing loss', especially when there is only partial loss of hearing. *Conduction* or *middle ear d.* deafness due to sound waves failing to reach the cochlea. *Perceptive* or *nerve d.* deafness due to damage to the cochlea or auditory nerve.

deamination (deeˌaməˈnayshən) a process of hydrolysis taking place in the liver, whereby amino acids are broken down and urea is formed.

death (deth) the cessation of all physical and chemical processes; occurs in all living organisms or their cellular components. *Brain d.* the diagnosis of clinical brainstem death. *Clinical d.* the absence of heartbeat (no pulse may be felt) and cessation of breathing. *Cot d.* SUDDEN INFANT DEATH SYNDROME (SIDS). *D. certificate* certificate issued by the registrar for deaths after receipt of a preliminary certificate completed and signed by an attending doctor, indicating the date and probable cause of death. Only after issue of this certificate, indicating that the death has been registered, can the body be disposed of. *D. instinct* a concept, introduced by Freud, proposing a self-destructive drive opposed by the sexual instinct which perpetually seeks a renewal of life. It may manifest as a repetition compulsion with the aim of annihilating oneself. *D. rate* the number of deaths per stated number of persons (100 or 10 000 or 100 000) in a certain region in a certain period.

death with dignity (deth with ˈdignuhtee) the philosophical concept that a terminally ill patient should be allowed to die peacefully, in a manner that is consistent with the patient's own beliefs and values, in the presence of loved ones, rather than experience a comatose, vegetative state with prolonged mechanical support systems.

debility (də'bilətee) a condition of weakness and lack of physical tone.

debridement (di'breedmonh, day-) [Fr.] the removal of foreign substances and injured tissues from the wound bed and surrounding tissue. Removal can be surgical, biological, enzymatic, autolytic or mechanical. The aim is to prepare the wound bed for healing.

decalcification (dee'kalsəfə'kayshən) removal of calcium salts, e.g. from bone in disorders of calcium metabolism.

decannulation (dee,kanyə'layshən) the removal of a cannula.

decapsulation (dee,kapsyə'layshən) removal of a fibrous capsule.

decay (dee'kay, də'kay) 1. the gradual decomposition of dead organic matter. 2. the process or stage of ageing of living matter. *Radioactive d.* the process by which an unstable atom loses energy by the emission of gamma rays or beta or alpha particles and is transformed to a more stable atom.

decerebrate (dee'serə,brayt) a person with brain damage whose neurological reactions are severely impaired and in whom cerebral functioning has ceased. A state of deep coma.

decibel ('desə,bel) *symbol* dB. A unit of intensity of sound, used particularly in estimating the degree of deafness.

decidua (də,sidyooə) the thickened lining of the uterus for the reception of the fertilised ovum to protect the developing embryo. It is shed when pregnancy terminates.

deciduous (də'sidyooəs) falling off; subject to being shed, as in deciduous teeth.

decision-making (,də'sizhən 'mayking) the act or process of choosing a preferred option or course of action from a set of alternatives. It forms the basis of almost all deliberate or voluntary behaviour. *D. rule* a formal or mechanical formula or principle for deciding on a course of action in response to input data. *D. theory* any theory that attempts to explain how decisions are reached. Most often applied to theories that use mathematical models to analyse human decision processes.

decompensation (,deekompən-'sayshən) failure to compensate. In particular, failure of the heart to overcome disability or increased workload.

decompression (,deekəm'preshən) return to normal environmental pressure after exposure to greatly increased pressure. *Cerebral d.* removal of a flap of the skull and incision of the DURA MATER for the purpose of relieving intracranial pressure. *D. sickness* a disorder characterised by joint pains, respiratory manifestations, skin lesions and neurological signs, occurring as a result of rapid reduction in air pressure. Aviators flying at high altitudes and people breathing compressed air in caissons and diving apparatus are particularly susceptible to this disorder. Also known as the bends, CAISSON DISEASE.

decongestant (,deekən'jestənt) 1. reducing congestion or swelling. 2. an agent that reduces congestion or swelling, usually of the nasal membranes. Decongestants may be inhaled, taken as spray or nose drops, or used orally in liquid or tablet form.

decontamination (,deekən,tamə'-nayshən) the freeing of a person or an object of some contaminating substance such as nerve gas, infective or radioactive material, etc. Decontamination involves a combination of processes including cleaning, disinfection and sterilisation. It is an important issue for public health in the prevention of hospital-acquired infection and minimising the risk of the iatrogenic transmission of other organisms.

decortication (dee ˌkawtə ˈkayshən) an operation to strip the outer layer of an organ, e.g. the removal of the thickened pleura in the treatment of chronic empyema.

decrement (ˈdekrəmənt) a decrease or stage of decline, as of a uterine contraction.

decrudescence (ˌdeekroo ˈdesəns) diminution or abatement of the intensity of symptoms.

decubitus (di ˈkyoobətəs) the position assumed when lying down. *D. ulcer* an ulcer due to interference with the local circulation from prolonged or severe pressure on the surface body tissue resulting in tissue anoxia and cell death; also called PRESSURE INJURY.

decussation (deekə ˈsayshən) a crossing, particularly of nerve fibres. A chiasma. *Pyramidal d.* the crossing of the pyramidal nerve fibres in the MEDULLA OBLONGATA.

deep breathing and coughing exercises (deep breedhing and ˌkoffing ˈeksə ˌsiez) a general term used for the use of respiratory manoeuvres which aim to alter the pattern of breathing, increasing lung volumes and facilitating the clearance of airway secretions. Commonly used for patients after prolonged inactivity or general anaesthesia.

deep venous thrombosis (DVT) (deep veenəs ˌthrəm ˈbohsəs) a blood clot that forms in the deep veins of the lower leg; may be symptomless or may cause redness, swelling, tenderness and fever. The clot can travel and lodge in the heart or lungs (*see* PULMONARY EMBOLISM), resulting in sudden death. The so-called 'economy class syndrome' is the formation of a clot occurring during or just after a long journey in an aeroplane, where the lack of space restricts leg movements. Other risk factors are obesity, smoking, previous DVT, pregnancy and being > 40 years of age. The condition has also been reported in travellers after a long road journey without any breaks.

defecation (ˌdefə ˈkayshən) the elimination of waste and undigested food, in the form of faeces, from the rectum.

defence (də ˈfens) behaviour directed to protection of the individual from injury. *Character d.* any character trait, e.g. a mannerism, attitude or affectation, which serves as a DEFENCE MECHANISM. *D. mechanism* in psychology, an unconscious mental process or coping pattern that lessens the anxiety associated with a situation or internal conflict and protects the person from mental discomfort. *Insanity d.* a legal concept that a person cannot be convicted of a crime if lacking criminal responsibility by reason of insanity at the time of commission of the crime.

defervescence (ˌdeefə ˈvesəns) the period of abatement of fever.

defibrillation (dee ˌfibrə ˈlayshən) the restoration of normal rhythm to the heart in ventricular or atrial fibrillation.

defibrillator (dee ˈfibrə ˌlaytə) an instrument by which normal rhythm is restored in the heart ventricular or atrial fibrillation by the application of a high-voltage electric current.

defibrination (dee͵fibrə'nayshən) the removal of fibrin from blood plasma to prevent clotting. Used in the preparation of sera.

deficiency disease (də'fishənsee di'zeez) a condition caused by dietary or metabolic deficiency, including all diseases due to an insufficient supply of essential nutrients.

deficit ('de͵fəsət) a deficiency or variation from that which is considered to be normal.

defined daily dose (DDD) (də'fuynd daylee 'dohs) the measure of the standard daily therapeutic dose of a drug. The World Health Organisation publishes a list of DDDs for various drugs.

deglutition (͵deegloo'tishən) the act of swallowing.

dehiscence (də'hisəns) separation of parts or sides, as of a wound.

dehydration (͵deehie'drayshən) excessive loss of fluid from the body by persistent vomiting, diarrhoea or sweating, or from the lack of intake. Severe dehydration is a serious condition that may lead to fatal SHOCK, ACIDOSIS and the accumulation of waste products in the body, as in URAEMIA.

déjà vu (͵dayzhah 'voo) [Fr.] an illusion that a new experience is a repetition of a previous experience.

deleterious (͵delə'tiə·ri·əs) harmful; injurious.

delinquency (də'lingkwənsee) criminal or antisocial conduct, especially among juveniles.

delirium (də'liə·ri·əm) 1. A state of mental excitement or wild enthusiasm. 2. Acute or subacute deterioration in mental functioning characterised by changes in mental functions, such as confusion, forgetfulness, agitation and inability to concentrate. Occurs more often in older people, especially when hospitalised. The cause is usually multifactorial and reversible, and may involve infection, dehydration, metabolic imbalance, hypoxia and medication toxicity. *D. tremens* an acute psychosis common in chronic alcoholism, usually following abstinence from alcohol. *Traumatic d.* a possible occurrence after severe head injury. There is much confusion and disorientation.

delivery (də'livə·ree) childbirth; parturition.

Delphi technique (d'elfee ͵tek'neek) the technique of collecting opinion on a particular research question. It is based on the premise that pooled intelligence enhances individual judgement and captures the collective opinion of a group of experts without them being physically assembled. It uses rounds or multiple stages of data collection, with each round using data from previous rounds.

deltoid ('deltoyd) triangular. *D. muscle* the triangular muscle of the shoulder arising from the clavicle and scapula, with insertion into the humerus.

delusion (də'loozhən) a false idea or belief held by a person which cannot be corrected by reasoning. *D. of grandeur* erroneous belief in one's own greatness, wealth or position. *D. of persecution* paranoia. *Depressive d.* a sense of unworthiness or sinfulness.

dementia (də'menshə) an umbrella term to describe a collection of symptoms caused by disorders affecting brain function. There is a progressive deterioration of the mental faculties which is irreversible and affects memory, intellect, judgement, personality and emotional control. *Frontotemporal d.* (including PICK'S DISEASE) dementia where the front and side parts of the brain are damaged. Clumps of abnormal proteins form inside brain cells, causing them to die. *Mixed d.* when someone has more than one type of dementia, and a mixture of the symptoms of those types. It is common for someone to have both Alzheimer's disease and vascular dementia together. *Vascular d.* dementia occurring when the oxygen supply to the brain is reduced because of narrowing or blockage of blood vessels, resulting in some brain cells becoming damaged or dying.

demography (də'mogrəfee) the statistical science dealing with populations, including matters of health, disease, births and mortality.

De Morgan's spots (də morgənz spotz) red or purplish raised spots in the skin consisting of a cluster of minute blood vessels. Found in middle-aged and older people, the spots becoming more numerous with increasing age. The spots may bleed if damaged, but treatment is unnecessary. *See* AGE SPOTS.

demulcent (də'mulsənt) an agent that soothes and allays irritation, especially of sensitive mucous membranes.

demyelination (dee'mieələ'nayshən) destruction of the medullary or myelin sheaths of nerve fibres, such as occurs in disseminated and multiple SCLEROSIS. Demyelinisation.

dendrite ('dendriet) one of the protoplasmic filaments of a nerve cell by which impulses are transmitted from one neurone to another. Dendron.

dendritic (den'dritik) 1. appertaining to a dendrite. 2. branching. *D. ulcer* a corneal ulcer caused by the herpes simplex virus. The ulcer has a branching appearance as it spreads.

denervation (ˌdeenər'vayshən) severance or removal of the nerve supply to a part.

dengue ('deng·gee) a painful viral haemorrhagic fever spread by mosquitoes that occurs in tropical countries throughout the world. The dengue flavivirus that causes the disease, one of four types of a group B ARBOVIRUS, is carried by *Aedes* mosquitoes that breed in stagnant water. No existing antivirals are effective. Prevention is based on public health measures to eliminate the breeding grounds of the *Aedes* mosquitoes until a vaccine is developed. Because of the intense pain in the bones, dengue is also known as breakbone fever.

denial (də'nieəl) a defence mechanism in which the existence of intolerable actions, ideas, changed circumstances, terminal illness, etc. are unconsciously denied.

dental ('dentəl) relating to dentistry or the teeth. *D. hygienist* a trained person carrying out dental procedures such as scaling of the teeth and oral cleansing, who works with the assistance of the dentist in providing preventative dental healthcare. *D. implant* a metal fixture that is inserted into the jawbone to provide permanent support for a crown, a fixed bridge or a denture. *D. nurse* a member of the dental health team who assists the dentist at the patient's side in passing instruments, preparing materials and generally assisting the dentist. *D. plaque* a sticky rough coating on the teeth formed by food deposits, bacteria and dead cells. It is the chief cause of dental decay if not removed regularly by good dental hygiene. *D. pulp* the tissue within the dental cavity containing nerves, blood and lymph vessels.

dentine (ˈdenteen) the calcified substance forming the bulk of a tooth between the pulp and the enamel.

dentist (ˈdentist) a person qualified to practise dentistry.

dentistry (ˈdentəˌstree) the art and science of the teeth, mouth and associated tissues and bone. Dentistry also includes preventative dental care and education concerned with preserving the health of the teeth and gums as well as the supplying and fitting of dentures.

dentition (denˈtishən) the process of teething. *Primary d.* deciduous dentition; cutting of the temporary or milk teeth, beginning at the age of 6 or 7 months and continuing until the end of the second year. A full set consists of 8 incisors, 4 canines and 8 premolars: 20 in all. *Secondary d.* permanent dentition; cutting of the permanent teeth, beginning in the 6th or 7th year, and being complete by the 12th to 15th year except for the posterior molars or 'wisdom teeth'. There are 32 permanent teeth: 8 incisors, 4 canines, 8 premolars or bicuspids and 12 molars. Permanent dentition. (*See* figure, p. 132.)

dentoid (ˈdentoyd) tooth-like.

denture (ˈdenchə) a removable dental prosthesis, which may contain one, several or a full set of artificial teeth.

deodorant (deeˈohdə·rənt) a substance that destroys or masks an offensive odour.

deoxycortone (deeˌokseeˈkawtohn) a naturally occurring adrenal steroid. Also known as 21-hydroxyprogesterone or desoxycortone.

deoxygenated (deeˈoksəjəˌnaytəd) deprived of oxygen. *D. blood* that which has lost much of its oxygen in the tissues and is returning to the lungs for a fresh supply.

deoxyribonucleic acid (DNA) (deeˌokseeˌriebohnyooˈklee·ik, -ˈklay-ˈasəd) a nucleic acid of complex molecular structure occurring in cell nuclei as the basic structure of the genes. It is responsible for the control and passing on of hereditary characteristics, and is present in all body cells of every species, including unicellular organisms and DNA viruses. DNA molecules are linear polymers of small molecules called nucleotides, each of which consists of one molecule of the five carbon sugar deoxyribose, bonded to a phosphate group and to one of the four bases twisted into a double helix. The four bases are two purines, adenine (A) and guanine (G), and two pyrimidines, cytosine (C) and thymine (T). The structure of DNA was described in 1953 by J.D. Watson and F.H.C. Crick.

Department of Health (deeˈpahtmənt ov helth) a department of the Australian Government that aims to provide better health and healthier ageing for all Australians by supporting universal and affordable access to medical, pharmaceutical and hospital services. This is achieved by developing evidence-based policy, providing advice, supporting research and developing partnerships with other government agencies, consumers and stakeholders. Each state and territory has a similar department.

dependence (dəˈpendəns) 1. addiction; the total psychophysical state of a user in which the usual

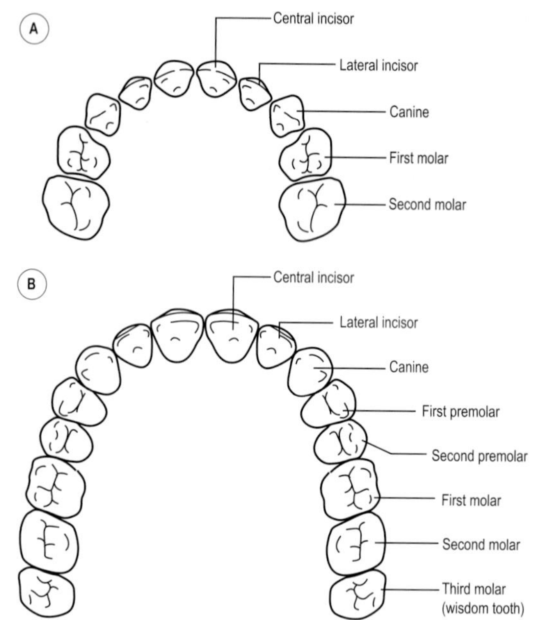

(A) Primary dentition, (B) Secondary dentition.

or increasing quantities of the drug or activity (internet, games or gambling) are required to prevent the onset of withdrawal symptoms (*see* WITHDRAWAL SYMPTOMS). 2. the level of reliance a person has on others for carrying out the activities of daily living. *See* DEPENDENCY STUDIES.

dependency (dəˈpendənsee) a state of relying on another for love, affection, mothering, comfort, security, food, warmth, shelter, protection, etc. *D. studies* the measurement of the need for care required by a patient based on the ability to carry out self-care. The main self-care activities measured are the ability to feed, the ability to carry out toilet requirements and the level of mobility, including dressing. *D. studies for staffing ratios* studies undertaken to determine the number of staff required to provide the appropriate skills to care for specific types and numbers of patients.

depersonalisation (dee,pərsənəlie'-zayshən) a condition in which the patient feels that their personality has changed so that they have become an onlooker observing their own actions. It may occur in almost any mental illness.

depilatory (də'pilətree) an agent that removes hair. Preoperative depilation reduces the risk of wound infection and, unlike shaving of the skin, is non-abrasive.

depressant (də'presənt) a drug that reduces functional activity of an organ. Anaesthetics, sedatives, tranquillisers and alcohol are all depressants.

depression (də'preshən) 1. a hollow or depressed area. 2. a lowering or decrease of functional activity. 3. in psychiatry, a morbid sadness, dejection or melancholy, distinguished from grief, which is realistic and proportionate to a personal loss. Profound depression may be symptomatic of a mental health disorder when feelings of sadness, hopelessness, helplessness, combined with a loss of interest in the social activities of life, are experienced on most days for at least 2 weeks or more. Symptoms vary with the severity of the depression, but commonly include loss of appetite or overeating, sleep disturbances, poor concentration with an overall low mood and poor self-esteem. Clinical depression may or may not be associated with stressful events or trauma. Risk factors include genetic and social issues, e.g. poverty, social isolation, substance abuse and previous history. The severely depressed may also have suicidal thoughts. Treatment is with the use of medication and/or cognitive behavioural therapy and/or psychotherapy. Seasonal affective disorder is a category of depression that occurs when the person's mood changes according to the season: for example diminished sunlight in autumn and winter. Sufferers feel low in winter and better in spring. *Endogenous d.* occurs sometimes without obvious cause as, for example, in the course of bipolar disorder psychosis. The mood change is associated with slowing of thought and action, and feelings of guilt. *Recessive d.* occurs as a result of some event, such as illness, loss of money or bereavement.

deprivation (,deprə'vayshən) loss or absence of parts, organs, powers or things that are needed. *Emotional d.* deprivation of adequate and appropriate interpersonal or environmental experience in the early developmental years. *Maternal d. syndrome* a group of symptoms, including stunted emotional and physical development, arising in infants who have been deprived of care and love provided by a mother or mothering figure. Deprivation of maternal care during the first 3 years of life is thought to be particularly critical as this is the optimal period for the forming of social attachments. *Sensory d.* deprivation of the usual external stimuli and the opportunity for perception.

Derbyshire neck ('dahbeeshə nek) *see* GOITRE.

derealisation (,dee,riəlie'zayshən) loss of a sense of reality. Surroundings and events seem unreal.

dereism ('deeri·,izəm) mental activity in which fantasy runs unhampered by logic and experience; describes autistic thinking.

dermabrasion (ˌdərmə'brayzhən) treatment to remove scars on the skin using wire brushes or sandpaper.

dermal filler (ˌdərməl 'filə) agents used to smooth out superficial contours or irregularities in the skin, such as wrinkles, scars and creases. Also called facial implants or soft tissue augmentation.

dermatitis (ˌdərma'tietəs) inflammation of the skin. *Contact d.* that arising from touching a substance to which the person is sensitive. *Exfoliative d.* widespread scaling and itching of the skin, sometimes occurring as a reaction to treatment with certain drugs. *Industrial d., occupational d.* that caused by exposure to chemicals or other substances met with at work. *Sensitisation d.* dermatitis due to an allergic reaction. *Traumatic d.* inflammation due to injury. *Varicose d.* dermatitis, usually of the lower portion of the leg, due to varicosities of the smaller veins. *X-ray d.* radiodermatitis; inflammatory reaction of the skin to radiotherapy.

dermatoglyphics (ˌdərmətoh'glifiks) study of the patterns of ridges of the skin of the fingers, palms, toes and soles. Of interest in anthropology and law enforcement as a means of establishing identity, and in medicine, both clinically and as a genetic indicator, particularly of chromosomal abnormalities.

dermatographia (ˌdərmətoh'grafi·ə) a condition in which urticarial wheals occur on the skin if a blunt instrument or fingernail is lightly drawn over it.

dermatology (ˌdərmə'toləjee) the science of skin diseases.

dermatomycosis (ˌdərmətohmie'kohsəs) a fungal infection of the skin.

dermatomyositis (ˌdərmətohˌmieoh'sietəs) a collagen disease producing inflammation of the voluntary muscles with necrosis of the muscle fibres.

dermatosis (ˌdərmə'tohsəs) any skin disease, especially one that does not produce inflammation.

dermis ('dərməs) the layer of skin just below the epidermis.

dermoid ('dərmoyd) pertaining to the skin. *D. cyst see* CYST.

descriptive/exploratory survey (də'skriptiv əks'plo·rətawree 'sərˌ-vay) a type of non-experimental research design that collects descriptions of existing phenomena for the purpose of using the data to justify or assess current conditions or to make plans for improvement of conditions.

desensitisation (deeˌsensətie'zayshən) 1. the prevention or reduction of immediate hypersensitivity reactions by the administration of graded doses of allergen; hyposensitisation. *See also* IMMUNOTHERAPY. 2. in behaviour therapy, the treatment of phobias and related disorders by intentionally exposing the patient, in imagination or in real life, to emotionally distressing stimuli.

designer drugs (də'zienə drugz) used to describe synthetic variants (drug analogues) of potent controlled drugs (including narcotics and stimulants), which are not themselves controlled. These substances currently circumvent existing drug legislation and many are relatively easy to synthesise from common industrial chemicals. Many designer drugs are extremely potent (some synthetic analogues of heroin are

1000 times as potent as heroin) and are consequently extremely dangerous.

desquamation (ˌdeskwəˈmayshən) peeling of the superficial layer of the skin, either in flakes or in powdery form.

detachment (dəˈtachmənt) separation from or state of indifference to other people, one's surroundings or environment leading to social isolation. *D. of the retina* separation of the retina, or a part of it, from the CHOROID.

detergent (dəˈtərjənt) a cleansing and antiseptic agent.

deterioration (dəˌtiə·ri·əˈrayshən) progressive impairment of function; worsening.

detoxification (deeˌtoksəfəˈkayshən) the process of neutralising toxic substances; detoxication.

detritus (dəˈtrietəs) debris; material that has disintegrated.

detrusor (deeˈtroozə) muscle of the urinary bladder, the action of which is to push down.

detumescence (ˌdeetyuhˈmesəns) 1. the subsidence of a swelling. 2. the subsidence of an erect penis after ejaculation.

development (dəˈveləpmənt) the process of growth and differentiation. *Cognitive d.* the development of intelligence, conscious thought and problem-solving ability that begins in infancy. *Psychosexual d.* the development of the psychological aspects of sexuality from birth to maturity. *Psychosocial d.* the development of the personality, including the acquisition of social attitudes and skills, from infancy through to maturity.

developmental (dəˌveləpˈment'l) pertaining to development. *D. anomaly* absence, deformity or excess of body parts as the result of faulty development of the embryo. *D. milestones* significant behaviours used to mark the process of development (*see* ACHIEVEMENT AGE). Walking is a developmental milestone in locomotor development, conversation in cognitive development.

deviance (ˈdeevi·əns) generally any pattern of behaviour that violates prevailing standards of morality or behaviour within a society. The term is usually qualified to indicate specific forms of deviance.

deviation (ˌdeeveeˈayshən) variation from the normal. In ophthalmology, lack of coordination of the two eyes. *Standard d.* in research, a method of grouping data on either side of the mean of a graph. In a normal distribution curve, 68% of the data will be covered in one standard deviation above and below the mean. A measure of dispersion of scores around the mean value. It is the square root of variance. In statistics, the 68-95-99.7 rule, or empirical rule, is a quick estimate of the spread of data in a normal distribution with a width of two, four and six standard deviations, respectively; more accurately, 68.27%, 95.45% and 99.73% of the values lie within one, two and three standard deviations of the mean, respectively. Also known as the three sigma rule.

devitalised (deeˈvietəˌliezd) devoid of vitality or life; dead.

DEXT scan *see* BONE DENSITY TESTING.

dextran (ˈdekstrən) a plasma volume expander, formed of large glucose molecules, which, given intravenously, increases the osmotic pressure of blood.

dextrin (ˈdekstrin) a soluble carbohydrate that is the first product in the breakdown of starch and glycogen to sugar.

dextrocardia (ˌdekstrohˈkahdi·ə) location of the heart in the right side of the thorax.

dextrose (ˈdekstrohz, -trohs) an old chemical name for D-glucose, an important energy source for all tissues and the sole energy source for the brain. Commonly used in intravenous infusion solutions and may also be used orally in rehydration solutions to replace electrolytes and fluids.

diabetes (ˌdieəˈbeeteez) a disease characterised by excessive excretion of urine. *See* POLYURIA. When used alone, the term refers to diabetes mellitus. *Bronze d.* haemochromatosis. *D. insipidus* diabetes marked by an increased flow of urine of low osmolality, accompanied by great thirst. Caused by deficient production or secretion of the antidiuretic hormone (ADH) or inability of the kidney tubules to respond to ADH. *D. mellitus* a complex disorder of carbohydrate, fat and protein metabolism that is primarily a result of a deficiency or complete lack of INSULIN secretion by the beta cells of the pancreas or resistance to insulin. It is characterised by chronic HYPERGLYCAEMIA and may present with characteristic symptoms such as thirst, polyuria, glycosuria, blurring of vision and weight loss. In its most severe forms, ketoacidosis or a non-ketotic hyperosmolar state may develop and lead to stupor, coma and, in the absence of effective treatment, death. (*See* DIABETIC COMPLICATIONS.) The diagnosis is confirmed by fasting plasma glucose and history. The various forms of diabetes have been organised into categories developed by the American Diabetes Association and the World Health Organisation. *Type 1 diabetes mellitus* includes people with diabetes caused by cellular-mediated autoimmune destruction of pancreatic beta cells resulting in lack of insulin. The onset of type 1 diabetes mellitus in children is sudden. Generally, individuals develop type 1 diabetes before 30 years of age, although it may occur up to the 10th decade. Individuals are prone to ketoacidosis because little or no endogenous insulin is being secreted. Type 1 diabetes mellitus is controlled by insulin, diet and exercise, and the goal is to maintain insulin–glucose homeostasis and to prevent DIABETIC COMPLICATIONS including HYPOGLYCAEMIA. Type 1 diabetes is always treated with insulin to prevent ketosis. This group was previously called insulin-dependent diabetes mellitus (IDDM), juvenile-onset diabetes, brittle diabetes or ketosis-prone diabetes. *Type 2 diabetes mellitus* is the most common form of diabetes and includes people with insulin resistance or with inadequate insulin secretion. Generally, it occurs in individuals older than 40 years of age who have central obesity and a strong genetic predisposition, but it may occur in overweight teenagers and children with a family history of diabetes. This type of diabetes may be triggered by aspects of lifestyle such as overweight and inactivity. It is frequently associated with hypertension and dyslipidaemia. The onset usually begins insidiously. Individuals are not ketosis prone. Type 2 diabetes mellitus is controlled by diet, exercise and one or more oral hypoglycaemic agents, or insulin in combination with oral agents. This group was previously called non-insulin-dependent diabetes mellitus (NIDDM), maturity-onset diabetes, adult-onset diabetes, ketosis-resistant diabetes or stable diabetes. *Gestational diabetes mellitus* occurs in women who develop glucose intolerance during pregnancy, resulting in hyperglycaemia of variable severity. Other types of diabetes are associated with pancreatic disease, hormonal changes, adverse effects of drugs, or genetic or other anomalies. A fifth subclass, the impaired glucose tolerance (IGT) group, includes persons whose blood glucose levels are abnormal, although not sufficiently beyond the normal range to be diagnosed as diabetic.

diabetic (ˌdiəˈbetik) relating to diabetes mellitus. *D. complications* include both long-term and short-term complications of diabetes mellitus. The eyes, kidneys, nervous system, skin and circulatory system may be affected by the long-term complications of either type of diabetes; infections are common, and atherosclerosis often develops. Tight control of blood glucose levels (i.e. frequent monitoring and maintenance at a level as close as possible to that of non-diabetics) significantly reduces complications such as eye disease, kidney disease and nerve damage. *See* CATARACT, GANGRENE, MICROALBUMINURIA, NEUROPATHY, RENAL FAILURE, RETINOPATHY. Although diabetes may cause complications over time, short-term complications may arise daily due to fluctuations in blood glucose levels and may be serious if untreated. *See* table below and HYPOGLYCAEMIA, HYPERGLYCAEMIA, KETOACIDOSIS. *D. diet* a diet prescribed in the treatment of diabetes mellitus, designed to prevent wide fluctuation in the amount of glucose in the blood. *See* GLYCAEMIC INDEX FACTOR. *D. ketoacidosis* (DKA) *see* KETOACIDOSIS.

Common Signs and Symptoms of Hypoglycaemia and Hyperglycaemia in Patients with Diabetes Mellitus.

Hypoglycaemia	*Hyperglycaemia*
• Heart palpitations • Fatigue • Pale skin • Shakiness • Anxiety • Sweating • Hunger • Irritability • Tingling sensation around the mouth • Crying out during sleep • Confusion, abnormal behaviour or both, such as the inability to complete routine tasks • Visual disturbances, such as blurred vision • Seizures • Loss of consciousness	• Increased thirst • Headaches • Trouble concentrating • Blurred vision • Frequent urination • Fatigue (weak, tired feeling) • Weight loss • Vaginal and skin infections • Slow-healing cuts and sores • Worse vision • Nerve damage causing painful cold or insensitive feet, loss of hair on the lower extremities or erectile dysfunction • Stomach and intestinal problems, such as chronic constipation or diarrhoea • Damage to eyes, blood vessels or kidneys

diabetogenic (ˌdieəˌbetəˈjenik) inducing diabetes. Some drugs or physical conditions, such as pregnancy or disease, precipitate the symptoms of diabetes in those prone to the disease.

diagnosis (ˌdieəgˈnohsəs) determination of the nature of a disease. *Clinical d.* diagnosis made by the study of signs and symptoms. *Differential d.* the recognition of one disease among several presenting similar symptoms. *Nursing d.* a statement of a healthcare problem or the potential for one in the health status of the patient/client for which a nurse is competent to intervene in and treat.

diagnostic-related group (DRG) (ˌdieəgˈnostik reˈlayted groop) a system for administrative purposes. *Australian refined DRG (AR-DRG)* an Australian admitted patient classification system that provides a clinically meaningful way of relating the number and type of patients treated in a hospital (i.e. its casemix) to the resources required by the hospital.

dialysate (dieˈaləˌsayt) the material passing through the membrane in dialysis.

dialyser (ˈdieəˌliezə) 1. the membrane used in dialysis. 2. the machine or 'artificial kidney' used to remove waste products from the blood in cases of renal failure.

dialysis (dieˈaləsəs) the process by which crystalline substances will pass through a semipermeable membrane, whereas colloids will not. In medicine this process is employed to remove waste and toxic products from the blood in cases of renal insufficiency. *Peritoneal d.* use of the peritoneum as the semipermeable membrane. A dialysing solution is infused into the abdominal cavity and allowed to run out again when sufficient time has elapsed for dialysis to have occurred. Waste products are thus removed from the blood. *See* HAEMODIALYSIS.

diameter (dieˈamətə) a straight line passing through the centre of a circle to opposite points on the circumference. *Cranial d.s* measurement of the fetal head at term. If these are abnormal, delivery through the vagina may not be possible. *Pelvic d.s* measurements between the bones and joints of the pelvis made in women to determine whether the fetus can pass through at the time of childbirth.

diapedesis (ˌdieəpəˈdeesəs) the passage of white blood cells through the walls of blood capillaries into the surrounding tissues.

diaphoresis (ˌdieəfəˈreesəs) perspiration; particularly profuse perspiration.

diaphragm (ˈdieəˌfram) 1. the muscular dome-shaped partition separating the thorax from the abdomen. 2. any separating membrane or structure. *Contraceptive d.* a rubber cap which occludes the cervix.

diaphragmatic breathing (ˌdieəfragˈmatik ˈbreething) a pattern of exhalation and inhalation in which most ventilator work is done by the diaphragm. It is done by contracting the diaphragm and expanding the belly during inhalation. This allows air to enter the lungs with little or no chest movement. The technique is taught to facilitate respiration, in meditation and as a relaxation technique.

diaphragmatic hernia (ˌdieəfrag-ˈmatik ˈhərni·ə) a protrusion of any part of an abdominal organ through the diaphragm into the thoracic cavity.

diaphysis (dieˈafəsəs) the shaft of a long bone.

diarrhoea (ˌdieəˈreeə) rapid movement of faecal matter through the intestine, resulting in poor absorption of water, nutritive elements and electrolytes. The most common causes of diarrhoea include bacterial or viral infections, food sensitivity, laxatives, the use of antibiotics and dietary indiscretion. Other causes include irritable bowel syndrome and systemic diseases. Diarrhoea that persists for more than a week or is recurring requires medical investigation. *Tropical d.* SPRUE.

diarthrosis (ˌdieahˈthrohsəs) a freely moving articulation, e.g. ball and socket joint. A synovial joint.

diastole (dieˈastəlee) the phase of the cardiac cycle in which the heart relaxes between contractions; specifically, the period when the two ventricles are dilated by the blood flowing into them. *See* SYSTOLE.

diathermy (ˈdieəˌthərmee) production of heat in a body tissue by a high-frequency electric current. *Medical d.* sufficient heat is used to warm the tissues but not to harm them. *Shortwave d.* used in physiotherapy to relieve pain or treat infection. *Surgical d.* of very high frequency; used to coagulate blood vessels or to dissect tissues. CAUTERY.

DIC *see* DISSEMINATED INTRAVASCULAR COAGULATION.

dichromatic (ˌdiekrohˈmatik) pertaining to colour blindness when there is ability to see only two of the three primary colours. *See* COLOUR VISION DEFICIENCY.

dicrotic (dieˈkrotik) having a double beat. *D. pulse* a small wave of distension following the normal pulse beat; occurring at the closure of the aortic valve.

didymitis (ˌdidiˈmietəs) orchitis; inflammation of a testicle.

diet (ˈdieət) 1. the customary amount and kind of food and drink taken by a person from day to day. 2. a diet planned to meet the specific requirements of the individual, including or excluding certain foods. *Bland d.* one that is free from any irritating or stimulating foods. *Elimination d.* one for diagnosis of food allergy, based on omission of foods that might cause symptoms in the patient. *High calorie d.* one that furnishes more calories than needed to maintain weight, often more than 3500–4000 kcal/day. *High fibre d.* one relatively high in dietary fibre, which decreases bowel transit time and relieves constipation. *High protein d.* one containing large amounts of protein, consisting largely of meats, fish, milk, peas, beans and nuts. *Hospital d.* a routine diet plan, provided in a hospital, which includes general, soft and liquid diets, and modifications of them, to suit the needs of specific patients. *Liquid d.* a diet limited to liquids or to foods that can be changed to a liquid state (*see also* LIQUID DIET). *Low calorie d.* one containing fewer calories than needed to maintain weight. *Low fat d.* one containing limited amounts of fat. *Low residue d.* one with a minimum of cellulose and fibre and restriction of the connective tissue found in certain cuts of meat. It is prescribed for irritations of the intestinal tract, after surgery of the large intestine, in partial intestinal obstruction, or when limited bowel movements are desirable, as in colostomy patients. Also called low fibre diet.

dietary chaos syndrome (ˈdieətəree kayˈos ˈsinˌdrohm) a syndrome in which patients believe that control of eating and body weight is the key to good health and wellbeing. A variety of approaches are used which include bulimia and periods of abstinence from food, the use of laxatives or prolonged chewing of food without swallowing. *See* ANOREXIA and BULIMIA.

dietetics (ˌdieəˈtetiks) the science of applying the principles of nutrition to the feeding of individuals or groups.

dietitian (ˌdieəˈtishən) a person who is qualified in the principles of nutrition and applies these to the feeding of an individual or of a group of people usually in a shared setting, e.g. hospitals or residential homes. May also work in the commercial sector, e.g. food processing industry.

differential (ˌdifəˈrenshəl) making a difference. *D. blood count see* BLOOD COUNT. *D. diagnosis see* DIAGNOSIS.

differentiation (ˌdifəˌrenshiˈayshən) 1. the distinguishing of one thing from another. 2. the act or process of acquiring completely individual characteristics, such as occurs in the progressive diversification of cells and tissues in the embryo. 3. increase in morphological or chemical heterogeneity.

diffuse (dəˈfyoos, -ˈfyooz) scattered or widespread, as opposed to localised.

diffusion (dəˈfyoozhən) 1. a process in which molecules of liquid or gas disperse, moving from regions of higher density to regions of lower density so that they become equally distributed. 2. dialysis.

digestion (dieˈjeschən, di-) 1. the act or process of converting food into chemical substances that may be absorbed into the blood and utilised by the body tissues. 2. the subjection of a substance to prolonged heat and moisture, so as to disintegrate and soften it.

digit (ˈdijət) a finger or toe. *Accessory d., supernumerary d.* an additional digit occurring as a congenital abnormality.

digital (ˈdijəˈtəl) coded in simple 'on–off' binary units such as in computers and the traditional view of the activation of neurones.

digitalisation (ˌdijətəlieˈzayshən) the administration of digitalis (digoxin) in a dosage schedule designed to produce and then maintain optimal therapeutic concentrations of its cardiotonic glycosides.

dilatation, dilation (ˌdieləˈtayshən; dieˈlayshən) 1. the act of dilating or stretching. 2. the condition, as of an orifice or tubular structure, of being dilated or stretched beyond normal dimensions. *D. and curettage* expanding of the opening of the womb to permit scraping of the walls of the uterus; also called D&C. *D. of the heart* compensatory enlargement of the cavities of the heart, with thinning of the walls.

dilator (dieˈlaytə) 1. an instrument used for enlarging an opening or cavity such as the rectum, the male urethra or the cervix. 2. a muscle that causes dilatation. 3. a drug that causes dilatation, e.g. a vasodilator. *Hegar's d.s* a series of dilators used to widen the cervical canal before examination of the uterus under anaesthesia.

diluent (ˈdilyooənt) 1. diluting. 2. an agent that dilutes or renders less potent or irritant.

Diogenes syndrome (dieˈojəˌneez ˈsinˌdrohm) a disorder characterised by gross self-neglect, domestic squalor, social withdrawal, apathy and lack of shame.

dioptre (dieˈoptə) *symbol* D. The unit used in measuring lenses for spectacles. When parallel light enters a lens and focuses at a distance of 1 metre, the refractive power of the lens is one dioptre, and from this basis abnormalities are calculated.

diphtheria (difˈthieə·ri·ə, dip-) a severe, notifiable, infectious disease characterised by the formation of membranes in the throat and nose and rarely the skin (in an open wound), and toxic neurological and cardiac complications; caused by the bacillus *Corynebacterium diphtheriae*. Primary prevention is provided by the routine immunisation of the population in childhood (*see* Appendix 7).

Diphyllobothrium (dieˌfilohˈbothri·əm) a genus of large tapeworm. *D. latum* the broad or fish tapeworm, grows up to 10 metres long and may infest humans after the consumption of uncooked infected fish.

diplegia (dieˈpleeji·ə) paralysis of similar parts on either side of the body.

diplococcus (ˌdipləˈkokəs) 1. any of the spherical, lanceolate or coffee-bean-shaped bacteria occurring, usually in pairs, as a result of incomplete separation after cell division in a single plane. 2. any organism of the genus *Diplococcus*.

diploid (ˈdiployd) 1. having a pair of each chromosome characteristic of a species (in humans, 46). 2. a diploid individual or cell.

Diploma in Nursing (dəplohmə in nərsing) a three- or four-semester nationally recognised program of study at TAFE or related health facility leading to registration as an enrolled nurse (Division 2 nursing).

diplopia (diˈplohpi·ə) double vision, in which two images are seen in place of one, due to lack of coordination of the external muscles of the eye.

dipsomania (ˌdipsohˈmayni·ə) a morbid craving for alcohol which occurs in bouts.

disability (ˌdisəˈbilətee) any restriction or lack (resulting from an impairment) of ability to perform an activity in the manner or within the range considered normal for a human being. *Developmental d.* a group of conditions due to an impairment in one or more domains, such as motor performance, cognition, language or behaviour, that may impact on day-to-day functioning. The condition is of indefinite duration, with onset before the age of 18 years. Some common developmental disabilities include autism spectrum disorder, cerebral palsy, epilepsy or muscular dystrophy.

disaccharide (dieˈsakəˌried) any of a class of sugars, e.g. maltose, lactose, each molecule of which yields two molecules of monosaccharide on hydrolysis. *D. intolerance* the inability to absorb disaccharides owing to an enzyme deficiency.

disarticulation (ˌdisahˌtikyəˈlayshən) separation; amputation at a joint.

disc (disk) a flattened circular structure. *Intervertebral d.* a fibrocartilaginous pad that separates the bodies of two adjacent vertebrae. *Optic d.* a white spot in the retina. It is the point of entrance of the optic nerve.

discharge (ˈdischahj) 1. a setting free, or liberation; used to describe the release of a patient from hospital, clinic or therapy program. 2. material or force set free. 3. an excretion or substance evacuated. *D. planning* the preparation required for the return of a patient/client to their usual life at home.

disciplinary action (ˈdisˌiˌplinəree ˈakshən) action taken by the employer when a member of staff has made a serious error, acted unprofessionally or negligently or has been convicted of a criminal offence. The process follows an agreed disciplinary procedure.

disciplinary process (ˈdisˌiˌplinəree prohses) in Australia, a written complaint must be received before the disciplinary process is initiated. In all jurisdictions, certain written complaints about health professionals are simultaneously referred to the relevant state or territory complaints unit or commissions. These bodies will attempt to resolve complaints through conciliation and mediation.

disclosing solution (disˈklohzing səˈlooshən) a topically applied preparation which reveals plaque and other deposits on teeth by staining them. May also be given as a tablet to be chewed; any plaque is stained red.

discography (disˈkogrəfee) radiographic examination after the injection of a radio-opaque contrast medium into an intervertebral disc.

discrete (dəˌskreet) composed of separate parts that do not become blended.

discrimination (disˈkrimˈenˈayshən) the unjust treatment of a person based on attributes such as race, religion, gender, disability or other grounds specified in anti-discrimination legislation such as the *Disability Discrimination Act (1992)* and *Age Discrimination Act (2004)*.

disease (diˈzeez) a definite pathological process having a characteristic set of signs and symptoms. It may affect the whole body or any of its parts, and its aetiology, pathology and prognosis may be known or unknown. (For separate diseases, *see* under individual names.)

disengagement (ˌdisənˈgayjmənt) the process by which an individual gradually withdraws from the community and obligations towards friends and family. The effect of this process is to lead to social isolation for the individual with alienation and disregard from the community. This situation may be compounded by physiological deficits and disabilities. *D. theory* a psychosocial theory of ageing by which both society and the individual prepare for death by gradually reducing all social contacts, which leads to poor relationships, egocentricity and sometimes depression.

disimpaction (ˌdisimˈpakshən) reduction of an impacted fracture.

disinfect (ˌdisənˈfekt) to destroy microorganisms, but not usually bacterial spores, reducing the number of microorganisms to a level which is not harmful to health.

disinfectant (ˌdisənˈfektənt) an agent that destroys infection-producing organisms. Heat and certain other physical agents, such as steam, can be disinfectants, but in common usage the term is reserved for chemical substances such as glutaraldehyde, sodium hypochlorite or phenol.

Disinfectants are usually applied to inanimate objects because they are too strong to be used on living tissues. Chemical disinfectants are not always effective against spore-forming bacteria.

disinfection (disən'fekshən) the act of disinfecting. *Terminal d.* disinfection of a sick room and its contents at the termination of a disease.

disinfestation (ˌdisinfe'stayshən) destruction of insects, rodents or pests present on the person or the clothes or in the surroundings, and which may transmit disease.

dislocation (ˌdislə'kayshən) the displacement of a bone from its natural position upon another at a joint; luxation.

dismemberment (dis'membəmənt) the amputation of a limb or a part of it.

disorientation (disˌawreeənt'tayshən) the loss of proper bearings, or a state of mental confusion as to time, place or identity.

dispensary (də'spensə·ree) any place where drugs or medicines are actually dispensed.

displacement (dəs'playsmənt) removal to an abnormal location or position. *D. activity* in psychology, unconscious transference of an emotion from its original object onto a more acceptable substitute.

disposition (ˌdispə'zishən) a tendency to suffer from certain diseases.

dissect (die'sekt, di-) 1. to cut carefully in the study of anatomy. 2. during operation, to separate according to natural lines of structure.

disseminated (də'semiˌnaytəd) widely scattered or dispersed. *D. intravascular coagulation (DIC)* widespread formation of microthromboses in the capillaries, leading to the consumption of clotting factors and thus resulting in the failure of the clotting mechanism at a site of bleeding. The result is a bleeding tendency, which may be catastrophic and difficult to control. It is a secondary complication of a diverse group of obstetric, surgical, haemolytic and neoplastic disorders.

dissociation (dəˌsohsee'ayshən, -'sohshee-) separation. 1. the splitting up of molecules of matter into their component parts, e.g. by heat or electrolysis. 2. in psychology, the separation of ideas, emotions or experiences from the rest of the mind, giving rise to a lack of unity of which the patient is unaware.

distal ('dist'l) situated away from the centre of the body or point of origin. The opposite of proximal.

distension (dis'tenshən) enlargement. *Abdominal d.* enlargement of the abdomen by gas in the intestines or fluid in the abdominal cavity.

distractibility (ˌdə'straktəˌbilətee) inability to focus or maintain attention on any one subject.

distraction (ˌdə'strakshən) 1. anything that diverts a person's attention. 2. the location of joint surfaces caused by extension but without injury to the parts involved. 3. mental or emotional distress, anguish or confusion. *D. therapy* diverting the focus of attention on one activity, object or person to another. Used in the management of pain.

distribution (ˌdəs'trəbyooshən) 1. the sharing out or spreading of an agent, object or population within an area. 2. in research, the relative frequencies with which scores of a different size occur.

diuresis (ˌdieyə'reesəs) increased excretion of urine.

diuretic (ˌdieyəˈretik) 1. increasing urine excretion or the amount of urine. 2. an agent that promotes urine secretion. Diuretic drugs are classified by chemical structure and pharmacological action, although a diuretic medication may contain drugs from one or more groups, e.g. loop diuretics, osmotic and potassium sparing diuretics and thiazides.

diurnal (dieˈərnəl) occurring during daytime or period of light. Diurnal animals have one period of rest and one of activity in 24 hours.

diverticulitis (ˌdievəˈtikyəˈlietəs) inflammation of a diverticulum. It is most common in the colon; lower abdominal pain with colic and constipation may occur. Intestinal obstruction or abscesses may develop as a result of collections of bacteria and irritating agents being trapped in small blind pouches formed in the intestinal walls.

diverticulosis (ˌdievəˌtikyəˈlohsəs) the presence of diverticula in the colon without inflammation.

diverticulum (dievəˈtikyələm) a pouch or pocket in the lining of a hollow organ, as in the bladder, oesophagus or large intestine. *Meckel's d.* a small sac occurring in the ileum as a congenital abnormality.

diving reflex (ˈdievˌing ˈreefleks) decrease in the heart rate that occurs when the face is immersed in cold water.

dizygotic, dizygous (ˌdiezieˈgotik; dieˈziegəs) pertaining to or derived from two separate zygotes (fertilised ova); said of non-identical twins.

dizziness (ˈdizeenəs) a feeling of unsteadiness or haziness, accompanied by anxiety. *See* VERTIGO.

DKA diabetic ketoacidosis. *See* KETOACIDOSIS.

DNA *see* DEOXYRIBONUCLEIC ACID.

Döderlein's bacillus (ˈdərdəˌlienz bəˈsiləs) *Albert Döderlein, German obstetrician and gynaecologist, 1860–1941.* A lactobacillus occurring normally in vaginal secretions.

dolor (ˈdolə, ˈdohlə) [L.] pain.

dominant (ˈdomənənt) in genetics, capable of expression when carried by only one of a pair of homologous chromosomes. The opposite to recessive. *D. gene* one which will produce its characteristics when it is present in either a heterozygous or a homozygous state, i.e. it may be inherited from one parent only.

donor (ˈdohnə) 1. an organism that supplies living tissue to be used in another body, as a person who furnishes blood for transfusion or an organ for transplantation. 2. a substance or compound that contributes part of itself to another substance (acceptor). *D. register* a register for people to record their decision about becoming an organ and tissue donor for transplantation after death. In Australia, family consent is always sought before donation can proceed. It is important that family members know of decisions relating to the donor's wishes. *Universal d.* a person with group O blood; such blood is sometimes used in emergency transfusion. Transfusion of blood cells rather than whole blood is preferred.

dopa (ˈdohpə) the precursor of dopamine and an intermediate product in the biosynthesis of noradrenaline and adrenaline. It is used in PARKINSON'S DISEASE and manganese poisoning. Also called L-dopa and levodopa.

dopamine (ˈdohpəˌmeen) a substance allied to noradrenaline and used in the treatment of cardiogenic shock. Also occurs naturally in the adrenal medulla and the brain, where it functions as a transmitter of nervous impulses.

Doppler effect (ˈdopləˌ eˈfekt) the relationship of the apparent frequency of waves, as of sound, light and radio waves, to the relative motion of the source of the waves and the observer.

Doppler ultrasound flowmeter (doplə ˈultrəsownd ˈflohˌmeetə) a device for measuring blood flow that transmits sound at a frequency of several megahertz along a blood vessel. Rapid pulsatile changes in flow as well as steady flow can be recorded; hence, it is helpful in assessing intermittent claudication, thrombus obstruction of deep veins and other abnormalities of blood flow in the major arteries and veins.

dorsal (ˈdawsəl) relating to the back or posterior part of an organ.

dorsalis pedis pulse (ˌdawˈsahlis pedis puls) the pulse of the dorsalis pedis artery, palpable between the first and second metatarsal bones of the top of the foot.

dorsiflexion (ˌdawsəˈflekshən) bending backwards of the fingers or toes, i.e. upwards.

dorsum (ˈdawsəm) 1. the back. 2. the upper or posterior surface.

dose (dohs) the amount of a drug taken at a given time or the amount of irradiation given to a patient. Drug dose can be expressed in terms of the weight of its active ingredient, the volume of liquid to be drunk or its effects on the body tissues. The amount of radiation absorbed during a session of radiotherapy is expressed in units called millisieverts. *See* RADIATION.

dosimeter (dohˈsimətə) one of various devices used to detect and measure exposure to radiation; worn by personnel near to radiation sources.

double-blind trial (dubəl bliend ˈtrie·əl) a test for the real effect of a new drug or treatment in clinical practice. Neither the patient nor the staff administering the treatment know which of two apparently identical treatments is the new one being tested.

douche (doosh) a stream of fluid directed to flush out a cavity of the body.

download (ˈdownˌlohd) an action that is designed to transfer a file from a computer on the internet to a personal computer by means of a modem and telephone line or wireless connection to the internet.

Down syndrome (down ˈsindrohm) *John Langdon Down, British physician, 1828–1896.* A chromosomal abnormality, the most common type having 47 instead of 46 chromosomes. The extra one is attached to the 21st pair, so the condition is also called trisomy 21. This condition is associated with increasing maternal age. In the other form of Down syndrome, a translocation occurs, usually between chromosomes 14 and 21, as a structural rearrangement originating in the child, although the parents have normal chromosomes. Alternatively, the translocations may occur as a result of a similar translocated chromosome in the parents; this increases the risk of the condition recurring in further pregnancies by 10%. The child exhibits certain features which include slanting eyes with specked iris, broad hands with a single palmar crease, short neck with loose skin and hypotonia. Other abnormalities may also occur, e.g. congenital heart disease. Learning difficulties are also present but the range of ability is wide.

dracontiasis (ˌdrakonˈtieəsəs) a tropical disease caused by infestation with the GUINEA-WORM; acquired by drinking contaminated water.

Dracunculus (drəˈkungkyələs) a genus of roundworms; includes the GUINEA-WORM.

drain (drayn) 1. to withdraw liquid generally. 2. any device by which a channel or open area is established for exit of fluids or purulent material from a cavity, wound or infected area.

drama-therapy (drahmə therəpee) the therapeutic use of drama, in which clients are encouraged to act out their feelings in order to overcome problems.

drawsheet (ˈdrawˌsheet) a narrow sheet placed across the bed under a patient to prevent soiling of the main sheet. The sheet is twice the width of the bed to enable a clean piece to be drawn under the patient without the whole sheet being changed.

dream (dreem) mental activity that occurs during deep (*see* REM) sleep, usually in the form of vivid images, emotions and imagined events. Often rapidly forgotten on waking.

dreaming (dreeming) the activity of engaging in fantasies or speculation during quiescent waking periods. Also called daydreaming. Some research suggests that this activity helps to promote positive mental health for the individual concerned.

dressing (dresing) material applied to cover a wound or a diseased surface of the body. *See* WOUND DRESSING.

DRG *see* DIAGNOSTIC-RELATED GROUP.

drip (drip) a colloquial term used to denote intravenous infusion of fluid (blood, saline, glucose) into the body.

drive (driev) in psychology, an urge or motivating force.

droplet infection (ˈdroplət inˈfekshən) infection due to inhalation of respiratory pathogens suspended in liquid particles exhaled from someone already infected.

dropsy (ˈdropsee) an old-fashioned term used to describe excess fluid in the tissues (oedema).

drowning (ˈdrowning) asphyxiation due to immersion in a liquid medium.

drug (drug) 1. any medicinal substance. 2. a narcotic. 3. to administer a drug. *D. abuse* the overuse of a drug for a non-therapeutic effect. The major groups of drugs most commonly abused are stimulants ('uppers'), depressants ('downers'), psychedelics and narcotics. Also known as substance abuse. *D. addiction* a state of periodic or chronic intoxication produced by the repeated consumption of a drug, characterised by: (a) an overwhelming desire or need (compulsion) to continue use of the drug and to obtain it by any means; (b) a tendency to increase the dosage; (c) a psychological and usually a physical dependence on its effects; and (d) a detrimental effect on the individual and on society. *D. idiosyncrasy* an individual response to a drug that is unique to that person and quite different from what is expected. *D. interaction* modification of the potency of one drug by another (or others) taken concurrently or sequentially. Some drug interactions are harmful and some may have therapeutic benefits. Present knowledge of these interactions is limited. Drugs may also interact with various foods. In general, these interactions fall into three categories: (a) food malabsorption; (b) nutritional status; and (c) alteration of drug response by nutrients. In teaching patients self-care in the taking of prescribed medications, the need to follow directions should be emphasised, especially with respect to the intake of food and drink while the medication regimen is being followed. *D. misuse* the use of drugs for purposes other than those for which they are prescribed or recommended. Most often refers to prescription medications, e.g. taking an extra medication, taking a medication not prescribed for you or taking a medication for a reason other than the one for which it was originally prescribed. *D. tolerance* a progressive reduction in the effect of a drug following repeated use. To achieve the desired effect, increasingly larger doses of the medication are needed. *D. trial* the testing undertaken of any new drug before it becomes available for medical use.

dry eye syndrome (drie ie ˈsin͵drohm) a common condition in which the eyes do not make sufficient tears. Also known as keratoconjunctivitis sicca or dry eyes.

dry socket (drie sokət) infection of the soft tissues of a tooth socket, occurring 2 or 3 days after tooth extraction, often a lower molar. It is a painful condition requiring dental treatment with socket irrigation and local and/or systemic antibiotics.

DSM (Diagnostic and Statistical Manual of Mental Disorders) a publication of the American Psychiatric Association. It contains sets of diagnostic criteria grouped into categories (disorders) to assist clinicians with effective diagnoses and care of people with mental health disorders.

dual-energy X-ray absorptiometry (DXA) (dyooˈl enərjee ˈeks͵ray əbˈsawptiometree) an imaging technique for quantifying bone mineral density. It is used in the diagnosis and management of osteoporosis.

Dubowitz score (dooˈboh͵wits skor) *Victor Dubowitz, South African-English paediatrician, b. 1931.* A method used to assess gestational age in a low-birth-weight infant.

Duchenne dystrophy (doo͵shen ˈdistrəfee) *Guillaume Duchenne, French neurologist, 1806–1875.* Progressive muscular dystrophy occurring in childhood. *See* DYSTROPHY.

duct (dukt) a tube or channel for the passage of fluid, particularly one conveying the secretion of a gland.

ductless (ˈduktləs) without an excretory duct. *D. glands* ENDOCRINE GLANDS.

ductus (ˈduktəs) a duct. *D. arteriosus* a passage connecting the pulmonary artery and aorta in intrauterine life, which normally closes at birth. When it remains open, it is called persistent ductus arteriosus. *See also* PATENT DUCTUS ARTERIOSUS. *D. (vas) deferens see* VAS.

dumping (ˈdumping) the rapid evacuation of the contents of an organ. *D. syndrome* a feeling of fullness, weakness, sweating and dizziness which may occur after meals following a partial gastrectomy.

duodenal (͵dyooəˈdeenəl) pertaining to the duodenum. *D. intubation* the use of a special tube which is passed via the mouth and stomach into the duodenum. Used for withdrawal of duodenal contents for pathological examination. *D. ulcer* a peptic ulcer occurring in the duodenum near the pylorus.

duodenostomy (ˌdyooədəˈnostəmee) the formation of an artificial opening into the duodenum, through the abdominal wall, for the purposes of feeding in cases of gastric disease.

duodenum (ˌdyooəˈdeenəm) the first 20–25 cm of the small intestine, from the pyloric opening of the stomach to the JEJUNUM. The pancreatic and common bile ducts open into it.

Dupuytren's contraction or contracture (ˌduhpwiˈtrenz kənˌtrakshən or kənˈtrakchə) *Baron Guillaume Dupuytren, French surgeon, 1777–1835.* Contracture of the palmar fascia, causing permanent bending and fixation of one or more fingers (*see* figure below).

dura mater (ˈdyoorə mahtə, -maytə) a strong fibrous membrane forming the outer covering of the brain and spinal cord.

duty of care (dyootee ov kair) 1. the legal responsibility in the law of negligence that a person must take reasonable care to avoid causing harm. 2. a nurse, midwife, allied health or medical practitioner has an accepted duty to a patient or client irrespective of any contractual agreement existing between the parties. The law has developed a set of rules on the expected standard of care to assist in determining whether or not a professional has neglected their duty of care, based on the standards prevailing at the time of any case questioning the issue.

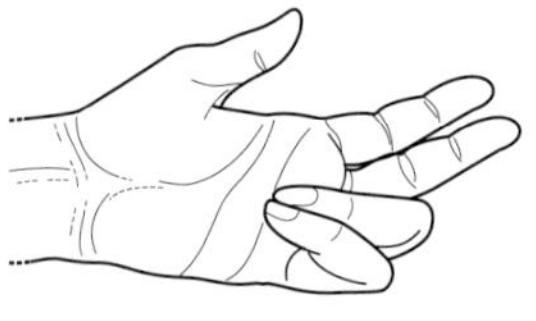

Dupuytren's contracture.

DVT *see* DEEP VENOUS THROMBOSIS.

dwarfism (ˈdwawfizəm) the state of being short in stature. Arrest of growth and development, e.g. due to renal rickets, cretinism or deficient pituitary function.

DXA *see* DUAL-ENERGY X-RAY ABSORPTIOMETRY.

dysarthrosis (ˌdisahˈthrohsəs) a deformed, dislocated or false joint.

dyschondroplasia (ˌdiskondroh-ˈplayzi·ə) a condition in which cartilage is deposited in the shaft of some bones. The affected bones become shortened and deformed.

dyscrasia (disˈkrayzi·ə) a morbid condition, usually referring to an imbalance of component elements. *See* BLOOD DYSCRASIA.

dysdiadochokinesis (ˌdisdieˌadəkoh-kəˈneesəs) a sign of cerebellar disease in which the ability to perform rapid alternating movements, such as rotating the hands, is lost.

dysentery (ˈdisəntree) inflammation of the intestine, especially of the colon, with abdominal pain, tenesmus and frequent stools, often containing blood and mucus. The causative agent may be chemical irritants, bacteria, protozoa, viruses or parasitic worms. *Amoebic d.* common in tropical countries; caused by the protozoon *Entamoeba histolytica*. Also called amoebiasis. *Bacillary d.* the most common and acute form of the disease, caused by bacteria of the genus *Shigella*.

dysfunction (dis'fungkshən) impairment of function.

dysgammaglobulinaemia (dis,gamə,globyələ'neemi·ə) an immunological deficiency state marked by selective deficiencies of one or more, but not all, classes of immunoglobulin, resulting in heightened susceptibility to infectious diseases.

dysgerminoma (,disjərmə'nohmə) a malignant tumour derived from germinal cells that have not been differentiated to either sex, occurring in either the ovary or the testicle.

dyshidrosis (dis·hie'drohsəs) a disturbance of the sweat mechanism in which an itching vesicular rash may be present.

dyskinesia (,diskə'neezi·ə) impairment of voluntary movement.

dyslalia (dis'layli·ə) impairment of speech, caused by a physical disorder.

dyslexia (dis'leksi·ə) difficulty in reading or learning to read; accompanied by difficulty in writing and spelling correctly.

dysmaturity (,dismə'tyoorətee) the condition of being small or immature for gestational age; said of fetuses that are the product of a pregnancy involving placental insufficiency or dysfunction. Also called small for dates or light for gestational age.

dysmenorrhoea (dis,menə'reeə) painful menstruation. *Primary (spasmodic) d.* painful menstruation occurring without apparent cause. The onset is usually shortly after puberty and occurs with each subsequent period. May be helped by hormonal therapy. *Secondary (congestive) d.* painful menstruation occurring in a woman who has previously had normal periods for some years. Often due to ENDOMETRITIS. The condition tends to worsen as the local congestion increases.

dysostosis (,diso'stohsəs) abnormal development of bone.

dyspareunia ('dispə'rooni·ə) painful or difficult coitus in women.

dyspepsia (dis'pepsi·ə) indigestion. There may be abdominal discomfort, flatulence, nausea and sometimes vomiting. *Nervous d.* dyspepsia in which anxiety and tension aggravate the symptoms.

dysphagia (dis'fayji·ə) difficulty in swallowing.

dysphasia (dis'fayzi·ə) difficulty in speaking as a result of a brain lesion. There is a lack of coordination and an inability to arrange words in their correct order.

dysplasia (dis'playzi·ə) abnormal development of tissue.

dyspnoea (disp'neeə) difficult or laboured breathing. *Expiratory d.* difficulty in expelling air. *Inspiratory d.* difficulty in taking in air.

dyspraxia (dis'praksi·ə) partial loss of ability to perform coordinated movements. Also known as developmental coordination disorder (DCD).

dysrhythmia (dis'rithmi·ə) disturbance of a regularly occurring pattern. Often applied to an abnormality of rhythm of the brain waves, as shown in an electroencephalogram.

dystaxia (dis'taksi·ə) difficulty in controlling voluntary movements.

dystonia (dis'tohni·ə) a lack of tonicity in a tissue, often referring to the muscles.

dystrophia (dis'trohfi·ə) DYSTROPHY. *D. myotonica* a rare hereditary disease of early adult life in which there is progressive muscle wasting and gonadal atrophy.

dystrophy (ˈdistrəfee) a disorder of an organ or tissue caused by faulty nutrition of the affected part; DYSTROPHIA. *Muscular d.* a group of hereditary diseases in which there is progressive muscular weakness and wasting.

dysuria (disˈyoori·ə) difficult or painful micturition.

Ee

ear (iə) the organ of hearing and of equilibrium. It consists of three parts: (a) the *external e.*, made up of the expanded portion or pinna, and the auditory canal, separated from the middle ear by the drum, or tympanum; (b) the *middle e.*, an irregular cavity containing three small bones (incus, malleus and stapes) that link the tympanic membrane to the internal ear (it also communicates with the pharyngotympanic tube and the mastoid cells); (c) the *internal e.*, which consists of a bony and a membranous labyrinth (the cochlea and semicircular canals).

eating disorders (ˈeeting disawdəz) a general term for disturbed behaviour involving food, eating and body weight. *See* ANOREXIA, BULIMIA and DIETARY CHAOS SYNDROME.

EBM expressed breast milk.

Ebola virus disease (EVD) (ˌeˈbowlə vierəs diˈzeez) a severe and acute, often fatal, haemorrhagic viral disease, principally seen in central African countries and caused by the Ebola virus, of the family *Filoviridae*. The incubation period ranges from 2 to 21 days and the patient presents with abrupt onset of high fever, weakness, muscle pain, headache and sore throat. This is quickly followed by more severe symptoms, including vomiting, diarrhoea, rash, decreased kidney and liver functioning, and, in some cases, both internal and external bleeding. Fatality rate is approximately 50% of cases. Ebola virus can be transmitted in several ways, the most significant being person-to-person through direct contact with body fluids (e.g. blood, semen, vaginal fluid) of an infected person. Formerly know as Ebola haemorrhagic fever. *See also* MARBURG VIRUS DISEASE.

EBP *see* EVIDENCE-BASED PRACTICE.

ecchymosis (ˌekiˈmohsəs) a bruise; an effusion of blood under the skin causing discolouration.

eccrine (ˈekrien, -rin) secreting externally. Applied particularly to the sweat glands, which are generally distributed over the body. *See* APOCRINE.

ECG *see* ELECTROCARDIOGRAM.

Echinococcus (eˌkienəˈkokəs) a genus of tapeworm. *E. granulosus* infests dogs and may also infect humans. The larval form develops into cysts (hydatids), which occur in the liver, lung, brain and other organs.

echocardiography (ˌekohˌkahdee-ˈogrəfee) a method of studying the movements of the heart by the use of ultrasound.

echoencephalography (ˌekoh·enˌ-kefəˈlogrəfee, -ˌsef-) a method of brain investigation by ultrasonic echoes.

echolalia (ˌekohˈlayli·ə) the pathological involuntary repetition of phrases or words spoken by another person.

echopraxia (ˌekohˈpraksi·ə) the automatic repetition of the movements of others.

echovirus ('ekoh,vierəs) a group of viruses (enteroviruses), the name of which was derived from the first letters of the description 'enteric cytopathogenic human orphan'. At the time of the isolation of the viruses, the diseases they caused were not known, hence the term 'orphan'. It is now known that these viruses produce many types of human disease, especially aseptic meningitis, diarrhoea and respiratory diseases.

eclampsia (ə'klampsi·ə) a severe condition of pregnancy-induced hypertension in which convulsions may occur as a result of an acute toxaemia of pregnancy.

ecology (ee'koləjee) the study of the relationship between living organisms and the environment.

economy (ee'konəmee) the management of money or domestic affairs. *E. class syndrome see* DEEP VENOUS THROMBOSIS. *Token e.* in behaviour therapy, a program of treatment in which the patient earns tokens, exchangeable for tangible rewards, by engaging in appropriate personal and social behaviour, and loses tokens for antisocial behaviour.

ecstasy ('ekstəsee) 1. a feeling of exaltation. It may be accompanied by sensory impairment and lack of activity, but with an expression of rapture. 2. an illegal drug. It is widely used as an accompaniment to modern dance music and has resulted in several fatalities in young people. Causes intense thirst, leading to the drinking of large quantities of water, resulting in fatal damage of the body's fluid balance, kidney failure and coma. Also known as MDMA, 'E' or 'ecky'.

ECT *see* ELECTROCONVULSIVE THERAPY.

ectoderm ('ektə,dərm) the outer germinal layer of the developing embryo from which the skin and nervous system are derived.

ectogenous (ek'tojənəs) produced outside an organism. *See* ENDOGENOUS.

ectoparasite (,ektoh'parə,siet) a parasite that spends all or part of its life on the external surface of its host, e.g. a louse.

ectopia (ek'tohpi·ə) displacement or abnormal position of any part. *E. cordis* congenital malposition of the heart outside the thoracic cavity. *E. vesicae* a defect of the abdominal wall in which the bladder is exposed.

ectopic (ek'topik) 1. pertaining to or characterised by ECTOPY. 2. located away from the normal position. 3. arising or produced at an abnormal site or in a tissue where it is not normally found. *E. beat* an impulse that originates at a site in the heart other than the sinoatrial node. *E. pregnancy* pregnancy in which the fertilised ovum becomes implanted outside the uterus instead of in the wall of the uterus. Also called extrauterine pregnancy.

ectopy ('ektəpee) displacement or malposition, especially if congenital.

ectropion (ek'trohpi·ən) eversion of an eyelid, often due to contraction of the skin or to paralysis. It causes a persistent overflow of tears and hypertrophy of exposed conjunctiva.

eczema ('eksimə, 'eksmə) a general term for any superficial inflammatory process involving primarily the epidermis, marked early by redness, itching, minute papules and vesicles, weeping, oozing and crusting, and later by scaling, lichenification and often pigmentation. Eczema is a common allergic reaction in children, but also occurs in adults. Childhood eczema often begins in infancy, the rash appearing on the face, neck and folds of elbows and knees. It may disappear by itself when an offending food is removed from the diet, or it may become more extensive and, in some instances, cover the entire surface of the body. Severe eczema can be complicated by skin infections. The cause of eczema may be either exogenous (due to external or traumatic factors) or endogenous (due to internal or constitutional factors). Also called atopic dermatitis. *Discoid e.* a chronic skin condition that causes coin-shaped spots to develop on the skin. These spots are itchy, reddened and swollen and can crack. Also known as nummular or discoid dermatitis.

edentulous (ee'dentyələs, -'dench-) without natural teeth.

Edwards' syndrome (Ehd'werds' sin͵drohm) a serious and rare genetic condition caused by an additional copy of chromosome 18. Babies born with Edwards' syndrome tend to be very small and will have serious complications. They will rarely live for more than a few weeks and if they survive are likely to have severe physical and learning disabilities. Also known as trisomy 18.

EEG *see* ELECTROENCEPHALOGRAM.

EEN endorsed enrolled nurse. *See* NURSE.

effacement (ə'faysmənt) taking up of the cervix. The process during labour by which the internal os dilates, thus opening out the cervical canal and leaving only a circular orifice, the external os. In a PRIMIGRAVIDA, this process precedes cervical dilatation, whereas in a MULTIGRAVIDA the two processes occur simultaneously.

effective (͵e'fektiv) 1. the extent to which something succeeds. 2. a result produced by an agent, action or force, e.g. resources to achieve desired outcomes. Cost effectiveness. *E. dose* the amount of a drug given to a patient to achieve the required treatment result.

effector (ə'fektə) a motor or sensory nerve ending in a muscle, gland or organ.

efferent ('efə·rənt) conveying from the centre to the periphery. *E. nerves* nerves coming from the brain to supply the muscles and glands. *See also* AFFERENT.

effleurage (͵eflə'rahzh) [Fr.] stroking movement in massage. In NATURAL CHILDBIRTH, a light circular stroke of the lower abdomen, performed in rhythm to control breathing, aid in relaxation of the abdominal muscles and increase concentration during a uterine contraction. The stroking is accomplished by moving the wrist only.

effort syndrome ('efət 'sindrohm) a condition characterised by breathlessness, palpitations, chest pain and fatigue, associated with abnormal anxiety for which no pathological explanation has been found.

effusion (ə'fyoozhən) the escape of blood, serum or other fluid into surrounding tissues or cavities.

ego ('eegoh) in psychoanalytical theory, that part of the mind which the individual experiences as 'self'. The ego is concerned with satisfying the unconscious primitive demands of the 'id' in a socially acceptable form.

egocentrism (͵eegoh'sentrəsm) a type of thinking in which a person has difficulty in seeing another's point of view. This self-centring is normal in young children, but in adults may indicate delayed cognitive development.

Ehlers-Danlos syndrome (EDS) (el'lez dan'loss 'sin͵drohm) *'Edvard' Ehlers, Danish dermatologist, 1863–1937; Henri-Alexandre Danlos, French dermatologist, 1844–1912.* A group of rare inherited disorders that weaken the body's connective tissues in areas such as joints and skin and the walls of blood vessels. There are several types of EDS, with some people displaying mild symptoms while other people may have life-threatening ones.

eidetic (ie'detik) having the ability to visualise exactly objects or events that have previously been seen. Having a photographic memory.

ejaculation (ee͵jakyə'layshən) the act of ejecting semen, a reflex action that occurs as the result of sexual stimulation. 2. a sudden utterance or exclamation, which may be out of context.

elastic (ə'lastik) capable of stretching. *E. bandage* one that will stretch and exert continuous pressure on the part bandaged. *E. stocking* a woven elastic stocking worn to prevent deep vein thrombosis. *E. tissue* connective tissue containing yellow elastic fibres.

elation (ə'layshən) in psychiatry, a feeling of wellbeing or a state of excitement. It occurs to a marked degree in hypomania and to an intense degree in mania. *See* EUPHORIA.

elbow ('elboh) the joint between the upper arm and the forearm. It is formed by the humerus above, and the radius and ulna below.

elder abuse (eldə 'ə'byoos) can be unintentional or deliberate and relates to any act which causes harm to an older person and is carried out by someone they know and trust. Harm includes all forms of physical assault, along with the use of restraint by physical or chemical methods, as well as emotional and financial loss incorporating the loss of a home and belongings. Compulsory reporting of abuse in aged care was introduced by the Australian Government in the *Aged Care Act (2007)*, and refers to both unlawful sexual contact with a resident of an aged care home and the unreasonable use of force on a resident in an aged care setting.

elective (ə'lektiv) usually pertaining to a surgical procedure that is performed by choice, as opposed to an emergency life-saving procedure. Timing of the procedure may also be arranged to be mutually convenient for the patient and the surgeon.

Electra complex (ə'lektrə 'kompleks) libidinous fixation of a daughter towards her father. The female version of the Oedipus complex.

electrocardiogram (ECG) (ə'lek-troh'kahdiə͵gram) a tracing made of the various phases of the heart's action by means of an electrocardiograph. The normal electrocardiogram (*see* figure, p. 155) is composed of a P wave, Q, R and S waves (known as the QRS COMPLEX, or QRS wave), and a T wave. The P wave occurs at the beginning of each contraction of the atria. The QRS wave occurs at the beginning of each contraction of the ventricles. The T wave seen in a normal electrocardiogram occurs as the ventricles recover electrically and prepare for the next contraction. There is a refractory period between these waves.

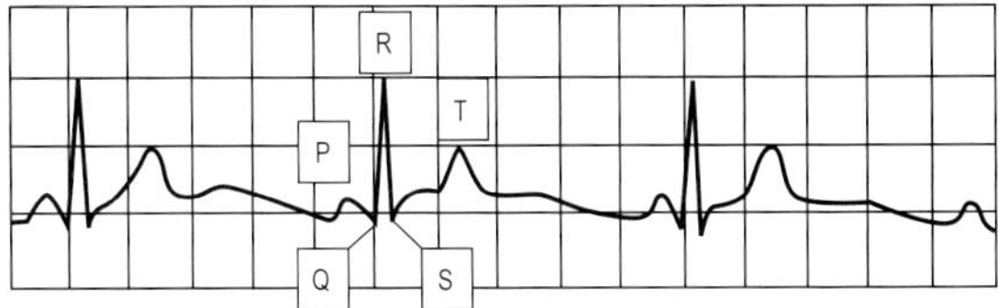

Electrocardiogram.

electrocardiograph (əˌlektroh-ˈkahdeeəˌgrahf, -ˌgraf) an instrument that records the electrical potential of the heart from electrodes on the chest and limbs.

electrocautery (əˈlektrohˈkawtə·ree) an instrument for the destruction of tissue by means of an electrically heated needle or wire loop.

electrocoagulation (əˌlektrohkoh-ˌagyəˈlayshən) a method of coagulation using a high-frequency current. A form of surgical diathermy.

electroconvulsive therapy (ECT) (əˌlektrohkənˈvulsiv ˈtherəpee) the passage of an electric current through specific areas of the brain, which causes a convulsion. It is used in the treatment of severe depression. A general anaesthetic and muscle relaxant are given before treatment.

electrocorticography (əˌlek-trohˌkawtəˈkogrəfee) electro-encephalography with the electrodes applied directly to the cortex of the brain during surgery to locate a small lesion, e.g. a scar.

electrode (əˈlektrohd) the terminal of a conducting system or cell of a battery, through which electricity enters or leaves the body; may be in the form of a plate or pad.

electroencephalogram (EEG) (əˌlektroh·enˈkefələˌgram) a tracing of the electrical activity of the brain. Abnormal rhythm is an aid to diagnosis in epilepsy and cerebral tumour.

electroencephalograph (əˌlektroh·enˈkefələˌgrahf) an instrument for recording the electrical activity of the cortex of the brain. The electrodes are applied to the scalp.

electrolysis (əˌlekˈtroləsəs) 1. chemical decomposition by means of electricity, e.g. an electric current passed through water decomposes it into oxygen and hydrogen. 2. the destruction of tissue by means of electricity, e.g. the removal of surplus hair.

electrolyte (əˈlektrəˌliet) a compound which, when dissolved in a solution, will dissociate into ions. These ions are electrically charged particles and will therefore conduct electricity. *E. balance* the maintenance of the correct balance between the different elements in the body tissues and fluids.

electron (əˈlektron) a negatively charged particle revolving round the nucleus of an atom. *See* ATOM. *E. microscope* a type of microscope employing a beam of electrons rather than a beam of light, which allows very small particles (such as viruses) to be identified.

electronic health record (EHR) (ˈeləktronik helth rekawd) longitudinal record of a patient's health and healthcare which combines information from primary healthcare with periodic care from other institutions.

electronic patient record (EPR) (ˈeləktronik ˈpayˌshənt rekawd) a computerised record of the care provided for a patient in both primary and secondary healthcare settings.

electrophoresis (əˌlektrohfəˈreesəs) a method of analysing the different proteins in blood serum by passing an electric current through the serum to separate the electrically charged particles. The particles gradually separate into bands as a result of the difference in rate of movement according to the electrical charge on the particles.

electroretinography (əˈlektrohˌretə-ˌnogrəfee) a method of examining the retina of the eye by means of electrodes and light stimulation for assessment of retinal damage.

element (ˈeləmənt) 1. any of the primary parts or constituents of a compound. 2. in chemistry, a simple substance that cannot be decomposed by ordinary chemical means; the basic 'stuff' of which all matter is composed.

elephantiasis (ˌeləfənˈtieəsəs) a chronic disease of the lymphatics producing excessive thickening of the skin and swelling of the parts affected, usually the lower limbs. It may be due to FILARIASIS in tropical and subtropical climates.

elimination (əˌliməˈnayshən) the removal of waste matter, particularly from the body. Excretion.

ELISA (əˈliezə) *see* ENZYME-LINKED IMMUNOSORBENT ASSAY (also called enzyme immunoassay—EIA), a laboratory technique to identify the presence of an antibody or an antigen in a sample, such as blood or saliva. It is the principal technique used in testing for human immunodeficiency virus (HIV) infection. It is a highly accurate test, but positive results are always confirmed by additional testing.

elixir (əˈliksə) a sweetened spirituous liquid, used largely as a flavouring agent to hide the unpleasant taste of some drugs.

emaciation (əˌmayseeˈayshən) excessive wasting of body tissues. Extreme thinness.

email (ˈeemayl) an electronic method of exchanging digital messages between healthcare professionals using digital devices such as computers, mobile phones or other electronic devices. Email operates primarily across the internet. *E. address* a series of characters that precisely identifies the location of an individual electronic mailbox.

emasculation (əˌmaskyəˈlayshən) the removal of the penis or testicles; castration.

embolectomy (ˌembəˈlektəmee) surgical removal of an EMBOLUS, frequently arterial emboli that are cutting off the blood supply to the limbs.

embolism (ˈembəˌlizəm) obstruction of a blood vessel by a travelling blood clot or particle of matter. *Air e.* the presence of gas or air bubbles, usually sucked into the large veins from a wound in the neck or chest. *Cerebral e.* obstruction of a vessel in the brain. *Coronary e.* the blockage of a coronary vessel with a clot. *Fat e.* globules of fat released into the blood from a fractured long bone. *Infective e.* detached particles of infected blood clot from an area of inflammation which, by obstructing small vessels, results in pus or abscess formation. Also known as septic or pyaemic embolism. *Pulmonary e.* blocking of the pulmonary artery or one of its branches by a detached clot, usually due to thrombosis in the femoral or iliac veins. *Retinal e.* blockage, due to air or a blood clot, of the central retinal artery, resulting in loss of vision.

embolus (ˈembələs) a substance carried by the bloodstream until it causes obstruction by blocking a blood vessel. *See* EMBOLISM.

embrocation (ˌembrohˈkayshən) a liquid applied to the body by rubbing to treat strains. A liniment.

embryo (ˈembreeˌoh) the fertilised ovum in its earliest stages, i.e. until it shows human characteristics during the second month. After this, it is termed a FETUS.

embryology (ˌembreeˈoləjee) the study of the growth and development of the embryo from the unicellular stage until birth.

emergency (əˈmərjənsee) a sudden crisis requiring urgent intervention. *E. planning* creating a plan outlining how to manage a serious incident, such as a major road or rail accident, bomb, terrorist incident, outbreak of an infectious disease or chemical spill. Each level and part of a health service has an emergency plan, which must relate to the emergency plans of other agencies such as local authorities, police and fire services. *E. protection order* a court order whereby a child is removed from the care of the parents in the interests of the child's safety.

emesis (ˈeməsəs) vomiting.

emetic (əˈmetik) an agent that can induce vomiting.

emic (ˈeemik) perspectives that are shared and understood by members of a group, community or culture, i.e. the 'insiders'. These views may contrast to those of 'outsiders' (*see* ETIC). Used in ethnographic and qualitative research.

eminence (emənəns) a projection, usually rounded, from a surface, e.g. of a bone.

emission (əˈmishən) involuntary ejection (of semen). *Positron e. tomography* (PET) *see* POSITRON EMISSION TOMOGRAPHY.

emollient (əˈmoli·ənt, -ˈmoh-) any substance used to soothe or soften the skin.

emotion (əˈmohshən) feeling or affect; a state of arousal characterised by alteration of feeling tone and by physiological behavioural changes. The physical form of emotion may be outward and evident to others, as in crying, laughing, blushing or a variety of facial expressions. However, emotion is not always reflected in the appearance and actions even though psychic changes are taking place. Joy, grief, fear and anger are examples of emotions.

emotional (ˈəmohshənəl) 1. relating to the emotions. 2. arousing emotions or readily showing the emotions. *E. bias* situation in which emotional attitudes affect logical judgement; an emotional reaction. *E. deprivation* a lack of loving attention during a child's early years when there has been a failure to achieve a psychological and emotional tie between parent and child. This may lead to impulsive behaviour and an inability to sustain trusting relationships in later life. *See* BONDING. *E. intelligence* the ability to recognise your own and others' emotions to guide thinking and behaviour. Generally speaking this means that the person has the skills of being: emotionally aware; able to harness emotions and apply them to tasks such as thinking and problem solving; and able to manage both one's own and others' emotions, especially when under pressure. *E. lability* characterised by exaggerated swings in mood, ranging from extreme excitement to one of depression. *E. maturity* the achievement of maximum emotional control.

empathy (ˈempəthee) the capacity to understand the problems and feelings of another person by placing oneself within the other person's frame of reference.

emphysema (ˌemfəˈseemə, -fie-) the abnormal presence of air in tissues or cavities of the body. *Pulmonary e.* a chronic disease of the lungs. Distension of alveoli causes intervening walls to be broken down and bullae to form on the lung surface. It also causes distension of the bronchioles and eventual loss of elasticity so that inspired air cannot be expired, making breathing difficult. *Surgical e.* the presence of air or any other gas in the subcutaneous tissues, introduced through a wound and evidenced by crepitation on pressure. Also known as tissue emphysema.

empirical (emˈpirikəl) based on observation and experiment, rather than theory; the obtaining of evidence or scientific data.

empowerment (emˈpowəmənt) the capacity to empower, to give power or authority, e.g. to a person to take control over their own care and to work in partnership with care providers.

empyema (ˌempieˈeemə) a collection of pus in a cavity, most commonly referring to the pleural cavity.

emulsion (əˈmulshən) a mixture in which an oil is suspended in water by the addition of an emulsifying agent.

EN enrolled nurse. *See* NURSE.

enamel (əˈnaməl) the hard outer covering of the crown of a tooth.

enarthrosis (ˌenahˈthrohsəs) a freely moving joint, e.g. a ball-and-socket joint.

encanthis (enˈkanthəs) a small, fleshy growth at the inner canthus of the eye, which may form an abscess.

encapsulated (enˈkapsyəˌlaytəd) enclosed in a capsule.

encephalin (enˈkefələn, -ˈsef-) an opiate-like substance produced by the pituitary gland which has analgesic effects. This substance may also be produced synthetically. *See* ENDORPHIN. Also spelt enkephalin.

encephalitis (enˈkefəˈlietəs, -ˈsef-) inflammation of the brain. There are many causes of encephalitis, most usually viral but may be bacterial. At first, the symptoms may be mild, with headache, general malaise and muscle ache similar to that associated with influenza. The more acute and serious symptoms may include fever, delirium, convulsions and coma, and in a significant number of patients may result in death.

encephalocele (enˈkefəlohˌseel, -ˈsef-) herniation of the brain through the skull.

encephalography (enˌkefəˈlogrəfee, -ˌsef-) radiographic examination of the ventricles of the brain after the insertion of air or a gas through a lumbar or cisternal puncture.

encephalomalacia (enˌkefəlohməˈlayshi·ə, -ˌsef-) softening of the brain.

encephalomyelitis (en,kefəloh,-mieə'lietəs, -,sef-) inflammation of the brain and spinal cord.

encephalomyelopathy (en,kefə-loh,mieə'lopəthee, -,sef-) any disease condition of the brain and spinal cord.

encephalopathy (en,kefə'lopəthee, -,sef-) cerebral dysfunction with diffuse disease or damage of the brain. Especially chronic degenerative conditions of toxic, nutritional or metabolic aetiology.

encephalotrigeminal (en,kefə'-lopəthee-trie'jeminəl) angiomatosis *see* STURGE-WEBER SYNDROME.

encopresis (,enkə'preesəs) incontinence of faeces not due to organic defect or illness.

endarterectomy (,endahtə'rektə-mee) the surgical removal of the lining of an artery, usually because of narrowing of the vessel by atheromatous plaques. *Thrombo e.* removal of a clot with the lining.

endarteritis (,endahtə'rietəs) inflammation of the innermost coat of an artery. *E. obliterans* a type that causes collapse and obstruction in small arteries.

endemic (en'demik) pertaining to a disease prevalent in a particular locality. *See* EPIDEMIC.

endemiology (en,deemeeoləgee) the study of all the factors pertaining to endemic disease.

endocarditis (,endohkah'dietəs) inflammation of the endocardium characterised by vegetations on the endocardium and heart valves. Due to infection by microorganisms, fungi or *Rickettsia*, or to rheumatic fever. Can affect all ages.

endocardium (,endoh'kahdi·əm) the membrane lining the heart.

endocervicitis (,endoh,sərvə'sietəs) inflammation of the membrane lining the uterine cervix.

endocrine ('endə,krin, -,krien) secreting within. Applied to those glands whose secretions (hormones) flow directly into the blood and not outwards through a duct. The chief endocrine glands are the thyroid, parathyroids, suprarenals and pituitary. The pancreas, stomach, liver, ovaries and testes also produce internal secretions. *See* EXOCRINE.

endocrinology (,endəkrə'noləjee) the science of the endocrine glands and their secretions.

endoderm ('endoh,dərm) *see* ENTODERM.

end of life care (,end ov lief 'kair) covers care provided for the person who is likely to die within the next 12 months. This also includes people whose death is imminent (expected within a few hours or days) and those with advanced progressive and incurable conditions. Care is provided by a multidisciplinary team with the support of families and carers.

endogenous (en'dojənəs) produced within the organism. *See* EXOGENOUS. *E. depression* one in which the disease derives from internal causes.

endolymph ('endoh,limf) the fluid inside the membranous labyrinth of the ear.

endometriosis (,endoh,meetree-'ohsəs) the presence of endometrium in an abnormal situation, e.g. in the ovaries, the intestines or the urinary bladder. The ectopic tissue undergoes the same hormonal changes as normal endometrium (*see* figure, p. 160). As there is no outlet for bleeding when menstruation occurs, the woman suffers considerable pain.

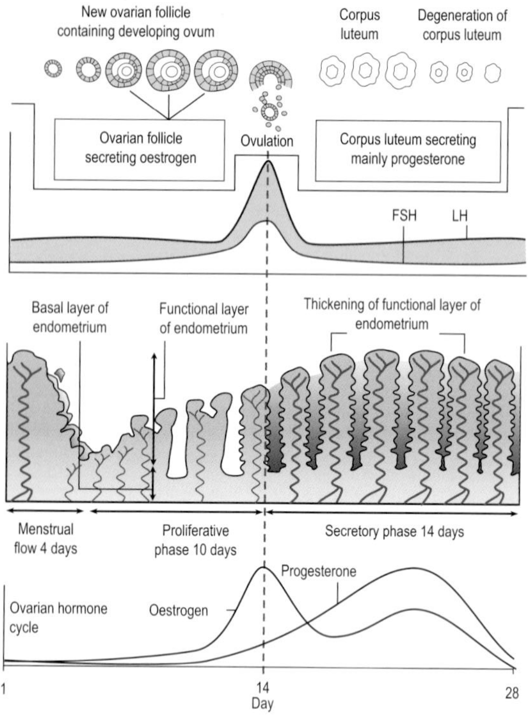

Endometrial and follicular changes during the menstrual cycle.

endometritis (ˌendohmə'trietəs) inflammation of the endometrium.

endometrium (ˌendoh'meetri·əm) the mucous membrane lining the uterus.

endomyocarditis (ˌendohˌmieoh-kah'dietəs) inflammation of the lining membrane and muscles of the heart.

endoparasite (ˌendoh'parəˌsiet) a parasite that lives within the body of its host.

endophthalmitis (ˌendof'thal'mie-təs) inflammation of the ocular cavity and adjacent structures.

endorphin (en'dawfən) one of a group of opiate-like peptides produced naturally by the body at neural synapses at various points in the central nervous system, where they modulate the transmission of pain perceptions. Endorphins raise the pain threshold and produce sedation and euphoria; the effects are blocked by naloxone, a narcotic antagonist. Also known as encephalins.

endoscope (ˈendəˌskohp) fibre-optic endoscopes are in general use for visualisation of tubular structures and cavities within the body. Light is carried by very fine glass fibres along a flexible tube that can 'see' around corners. This allows for examination, photography, biopsy and treatment of body cavities or organs in a conscious, relaxed (sometimes sedated) patient. Older style endoscopes are rigid and made of metal.

endosteoma (enˌdosteeˈohmə) a neoplasm in the medullary cavity of a bone.

endosteum (enˈdostee·əm) the lining membrane of bone cavities.

endothelioma (ˌendohˌtheelee-ˈohmə) a malignant growth originating in the endothelium.

endothelium (ˌendohˈtheelee·əm) the membranous lining of serous, synovial and other internal surfaces.

endotoxin (ˌendohˈtoksən) a poison produced by, and retained within, a bacterium, e.g. *Salmonella typhi*, which is released only after the destruction of the bacterial cell. *See* EXOTOXIN.

endotracheal (ˌendohˈtrayˌkeeəl) within the trachea. *E. tube* an airway catheter which is inserted into the trachea when a patient requires ventilatory support. It also allows for the removal of secretions by suction.

end-stage disease (end stayj diˈzeez) a disease condition that is essentially terminal. Kidney or renal end-stage disease is defined as a point at which the kidneys are so badly damaged or scarred that dialysis or transplantation is required for patient survival.

enema (ˈenəmə) 1. introduction of fluid into the rectum. 2. a solution introduced into the rectum to promote evacuation of faeces or as a means of administering nutrient or medicinal substances. 3. introduction of a radio-opaque material in a radiological examination of the colon (*barium e.*), or via a tube inserted into the JEJUNUM in a radiological examination of the small bowel (*small bowel e.*).

energy (ˈenəjee) the ability to do work or effect a physical change in status. Energy has many forms, including light, heat and sound. Food, through its breakdown within the body, provides energy for human activity, strength, growth and vitality, and is measured in calories or joules. Carbohydrates provide 4 kcal/g and fats provide 9 kcal/g. *E. conservation* an occupational therapy technique that seeks to assist patients/clients in minimising muscle fatigue, joint stress and pain. By using the body effectively, energy can be conserved and the person can remain independent for as long as possible. This approach is used by nurses and other healthcare workers working with older people and the physically disabled in the community. *E. requirements* the amount of energy required by a person for cell metabolism, growth and activity. This is influenced by age, gender, activity and health. *See* METABOLISM. A woman requires approximately 2000 cal (8372 kJ) per day. A man requires 2500 cal

(10 465 kJ) per day. Excess energy foods are stored as fat. This fat provides a supplementary source of energy if the diet is inadequate.

enervation (ˌenəˈvayshən) 1. general weakness and loss of strength. 2. removal of a nerve.

en face (ˌonh ˈfahs) [Fr.] a position in which the mother's face and that of her infant are on the same plane and approximately 20 cm apart; a position usually held during breastfeeding.

engagement (ənˈgayjmənt) the entry of the presenting part of the fetus, normally the head, into the true pelvis. Occurs in the last stage of pregnancy.

engorgement (enˈgawjmənt) distension or vascular congestion of body tissues, such as the swelling of breast tissue caused by an increased flow of blood and lymph before true lactation.

enkephalin (enˈkefələn, -ˈsef-) *see* ENCEPHALIN.

enophthalmos (ˌenofˈthalməs) a condition in which the eyeball is abnormally sunken into its socket.

ensiform (ˈensəˌfawm) xiphoid; sword shaped. *E. cartilage* the lowest portion of the sternum.

Entamoeba (ˌentəˈmeebə) a genus of protozoa, some of which are parasitic in humans. *E. histolytica* the cause of amoebic dysentery.

enteral (ˈentə·rəl) within the gastrointestinal tract. *E. diets* or *e. nutrition* a technique for providing nutrition to patients who are unable to ingest sufficient nutrients orally, but who are able to utilise them in the body to provide for energy requirements and for healing. Nutrition may be delivered through nasogastric, gastrostomy or jejunostomy tubes by bolus, gravity or pump assisted. *See* PARENTERAL FEEDING.

enteric (enˈterik) pertaining to the intestine. *E.-coated* refers to a special coating applied to tablets or capsules which prevents release and absorption of their contents until they reach the intestine.

enteritis (ˌentəˈrietəs) inflammation of the small intestine.

Enterobacteriaceae (ˌentə·roh-baktiə·reeˈaysee·ie) a family of Gram-negative, rod-shaped bacteria, many of which are normally found in the human intestine.

enterobiasis (ˌentə·rohˈbieəsəs) infestation by threadworms.

Enterobius (ˌentəˈrohbi·əs) a genus of nematode worms. *E. vermicularis* the threadworm or pinworm, a small white worm parasitic in the upper part of the large intestine. Gravid females migrate to the anal region to deposit their eggs, sometimes causing severe itching. Infection and re-infection is frequent in children.

enterococcus (ˌentə·rohˈkokəs) any streptococcus of the human intestine. An example is *Streptococcus faecalis*, only harmful out of its normal habitat, when it may cause a urinary infection or endocarditis.

enterocolitis (ˌentə·rohkəˈlietəs, -koh-) inflammation of both the large and the small intestine.

enterokinase (ˌentə·rohˈkinayz) an intestinal enzyme that converts trypsinogen into trypsin; enteropeptidase.

enterostomy (ˌentəˈrostəmee) the formation of an external opening into the small intestine. It may be: (a) temporary, to relieve obstruction; or (b) permanent, in the form of an ileostomy in cases of total COLECTOMY.

enterotomy (ˌentəˈrotəmee) any incision of the intestine.

enterotoxin (ˌentə·rohˈtoksən) a toxin that is produced by one of the many organisms that cause food poisoning. Such toxins frequently prove more resistant to destruction than the bacteria themselves.

enterovirus (ˌentə·rohˈvierəs) a virus that infects the gastrointestinal tract and then attacks the central nervous system. This subgroup includes Coxsackie, polio and echoviruses, which are now known, together with rhinoviruses, as PICORNAVIRUSES.

entoderm (ˈentohˌdərm) the innermost of the three germ layers of the embryo. It gives rise to the lining of most of the respiratory tract and to the intestinal tract and its glands. Also called endoderm.

entropion (enˈtrohpi·ən) inversion of an eyelid, so that the lashes rub against the eyeball.

enucleation (əˌnyookleeˈayshən) removal of an organ or other mass intact from its supporting tissues, as of the eyeball from the orbit.

enuresis (ˌenyəˈreesəs) involuntary passing of urine, usually during sleep at night (bed-wetting).

environment (enˈvierənmənt) the surroundings of an organism which influence its development and behaviour.

environmental health (ˌənˈvierən-məntəl helth) the concept that an individual's living and working environment has an impact on health and wellbeing. Factors that may influence health include housing, food hygiene, refuse collection, infestation, air and noise pollution and so on.

enzyme (ˈenziem) a protein that will catalyse a biological reaction. *See* CATALYST.

enzyme-linked immunosorbent assay (ˈenziem linkt ˌimyənohˈsawbənt asay) *see* ELISA.

eosin (ˈeeohsən) a red dye used to stain biological specimens. A derivative of bromine and fluorescein.

eosinophil (eeəˈsinəfil) a cell having an affinity for eosin. A type of white blood cell containing eosin-staining granules.

eosinophilia (ˌeeəˌsinəˈfili·ə) excessive numbers of eosinophils present in the blood.

ependyma (eˈpendəmə) the membrane lining the cerebral ventricles and the central canal of the spinal cord.

ependymoma (eˌpendəˈmohmə) a neoplasm arising from the lining cells of the ventricles or central canal of the spinal cord. It gives rise to signs of HYDROCEPHALUS and is treated by surgery and radiotherapy.

ephidrosis (ˌefəˈdrohsəs) profuse sweating; hyperhidrosis.

epiblepharon (ˌepeeˈblefə·ron) a congenital condition in which an excess of skin of the eyelid folds over the lid margin so that the eyelashes are pressed against the eyeball.

epicanthus (ˌepeeˈkanthəs) a vertical fold of skin on either side of the nose, sometimes covering the inner canthus; a normal characteristic in persons of certain races, but anomalous in others.

epicardium (ˌepeeˈkahdi·əm) the visceral layer of the pericardium.

epicondyle (ˌepeeˈkondiel) a protuberance on a long bone above its condyle.

epicondylitis (ˌepeeˈkondiˈlietəs) caused by strenuous overuse of the muscles and tendons of the forearm. Also known as tennis or golfer's elbow.

epicritic (ˌepeeˈkritik) pertaining to sensory nerve fibres in the skin which give the appreciation of touch and temperature.

epidemic (ˌepəˈdemik) the presence in a population of disease or infection in excess of that usually expected.

epidemiology (ˌepəˈdeemeeˈoləjee) the study of the distribution of diseases in populations. It includes the attack rate (incidence), risk factors, other influences and the numbers affected at any one time (prevalence).

epidermis (ˌepeeˈdərməs) the non-vascular outer layer or cuticle of the skin. It consists of layers of cells which protect the dermis.

epidermoid (ˌepeeˈdərmoyd) pertaining to certain tumours which have the appearance of epidermal tissue.

Epidermophyton (epeeˌdərməˈfietən) a genus of fungi that attacks skin and nails, but not hair. The cause of ringworm and athlete's foot.

epididymis (ˌepeeˈdidəməs) [Gr.] an elongated, cord-like structure along the posterior border of the testis; its coiled duct provides for the storage, transport and maturation of spermatozoa.

epididymitis (ˌepeeˌdidəˈmietəs) inflammation of the epididymis.

epididymo-orchitis (ˌepeeˌdidəmoh·awˈkietəs) inflammation of the epididymis and the testis.

epidural (ˌepeeˈdyoorəl) outside the DURA MATER. *E. analgesia* also known as extradural or peridural anaesthesia. A form of pain relief for labour and chronic pain, obtained by a single injection of a local analgesic or intermittently via a catheter into the epidural space in order to block the spinal nerves. It may be approached by two routes: (a) caudal, through the sacrococcygeal membrane covering the sacral hiatus; or (b) lumbar, through the intervertebral space and ligamentum flavum.

epigastrium (ˌepeeˈgastri·əm) that region of the abdomen situated over the stomach.

epiglottis (ˌepeeˈglotəs) a cartilaginous structure which covers the opening from the pharynx into the larynx during swallowing and prevents food from passing into the trachea.

epilation (ˌepəˈlayshən) removal of hairs with their roots. It may be effected by pulling out the hairs by electrolysis or the application of an epilatory cream/ointment.

epilatory (eˈpilətə·ree) an agent that produces epilation.

epilepsy (ˈepəˈlepsee) a group of neurological disorders characterised by recurring convulsive or non-convulsive seizures. Approximately 10% of the population are at risk of experiencing a seizure during their lifetime, while only 3–4% will go on to be diagnosed with epilepsy. A seizure is caused by an episode of disrupted electrical activity in the brain and can vary greatly depending on the part of the brain involved. There are three main seizure types: focal onset, generalised and unknown. Most people will only have one or two seizure types. Sometimes a person with more complex or severe epilepsy may experience a number of different seizure types. Generalised tonic-clonic seizures are one of the best recognised and they begin with a sudden loss of consciousness, the body then becomes stiff, followed by jerking of the muscles. Turning red or blue, tongue-biting and loss of bladder control are common. Confusion, drowsiness, memory loss, headache and agitation can occur on regaining consciousness. Previously known as grand mal seizures. *Focal* or *Jacksonian e.* a symptom of a cerebral lesion. The convulsive movements are often localised and close observation of the onset and course of the attack may greatly assist diagnosis. *Temporal lobe e.* characterised by hallucinations of sight, hearing, taste and smell, paroxysmal disorders of memory, and automatism. Caused by temporal or parietal lobe disease.

epileptiform (ˌepee'leptəˌfawm) resembling an epileptic fit.

epiloia (ˌepee'loyə) tuberous SCLEROSIS. A congenital disorder with areas of hardening in the brain, skin and other organs.

epinephrine (ˌepee'nefrən) adrenaline.

epineurium (ˌepee'nyoori·əm) the sheath of tissue surrounding a nerve.

epiphora (ə'pifərə) persistent overflow of tears, often due to obstruction in the lacrimal passages or to ectropion.

epiphysis (ə'pifəsəs) the end of a long bone, developed separately from, but attached by cartilage to, the diaphysis (the shaft), with which it eventually unites. Growth in length takes place from the line of junction.

episcleritis (ˌepee·sklə'rietəs) inflammation of the outer coat of the eyeball. It is seen as a slightly raised bluish nodule under the CONJUNCTIVA.

episiotomy (əˌpeezee'otəmee) an incision made in the perineum when it will not stretch sufficiently during the second stage of labour.

epispadias (ˌepee'spaydi·əs) a malformation in which there is an abnormal opening of the urethra on the dorsal surface of the penis. *See* HYPOSPADIAS.

epistaxis (ˌepee'staksəs) bleeding from the nose.

epithelioma (ˌepee'theeleeˌohmə) any tumour originating in the epithelium.

epithelisation (ˌepeeˌtheelie'zayshən) development of epithelium. The final stage in the healing of a surface wound. Epithelialisation.

epithelium (ˌepee'theeli·əm) the surface layer of cells of the skin or lining tissues.

Epstein-Barr virus (ˌepstien'bah vierəs) *Michael Epstein, British pathologist, b. 1921*; *Yvonne Barr, English virologist, 1932–2016*. A herpes virus that causes INFECTIOUS MONONUCLEOSIS. It has been isolated from cells cultured from Burkitt's lymphoma, and has been found in certain cases of nasopharyngeal cancer. Also called EB virus.

Erb's palsy (airbs 'pawlzee) *Wilhelm Erb, German physician, 1840–1921*. Paralysis of the arm, often due to birth injury causing pressure on the brachial plexus or lower cervical nerve roots.

erectile (ə'rektiel) having the power of becoming erect. *E. tissue* vascular tissue which, under stimulus, becomes congested and swollen, causing erection of that part. The penis consists largely of erectile tissue.

erection (ə'rekshən) the enlarged and rigid state of the sexually aroused penis. Erection can also occur in the clitoris and the nipples of the female.

erepsin (ə'repsən) the enzyme of succus entericus, secreted by the intestinal glands, which splits peptones into amino acids.

ergonomics (ˌergəˈnomiks) the scientific study of human beings in relation to their work and the effective use of human energy.

ergosterol (ərˈgostəˌrol) a sterol occurring in animal and plant tissues which, on ultraviolet irradiation, becomes a potent antirachitic substance, vitamin D_2 (ergocalciferol).

erogenous (əˈrojənəs) arousing erotic feelings. *E. zones* areas of the body, stimulation of which produces erotic desire, e.g. the genitalia, oral and anal orifices, and the nipples.

erosion (əˈrohzhən) the breaking down of tissue, usually by ulceration. *Cervical e.* a covering of columnar epithelium on the vaginal part of the uterine cervix, arising from erosion of the squamous epithelium, which normally covers it.

erotic (əˈrotik) pertaining to sexual love or lust.

eroticism, erotism (əˈrotəˌsizəm; ˈerəˌtizəm) a sexual instinct or desire; the expression of one's instinctual energy or drive, especially the sex drive.

eructation (ˌərukˈtayshən) belching; the escape of gas from the stomach through the mouth.

eruption (əˈrupshən) a breaking out (e.g. of a skin lesion) or the cutting of teeth.

erysipelas (ˌerəˈsipələs) a febrile disease characterised by inflammation and redness of the skin and subcutaneous tissues, and caused by group A haemolytic streptococci.

erysipeloid (ˌerəˈsipəˌloyd) an infective dermatitis or cellulitis due to infection with *Erysipelothrix insidiosa*. It usually begins in a wound (often the result of a prick by a fish bone) and remains localised, rarely becoming generalised and septicaemic.

erythema (ˌerəˈtheemə) redness of the skin caused by congestion of the capillaries in its lower layers. It occurs with any skin injury, infection or inflammation. *E. induratum* a manifestation of VASCULITIS. *E. multiforme* an acute eruption of the skin and sometimes the mucous membrane, which may be due to an allergy or to drug sensitivity. *E. nodosum* a painful disease in which bright red, tender nodes occur below the knee or on the forearm; it may be associated with tuberculosis.

erythematous (ˌerəˈtheemətəs) characterised by erythema.

erythrasma (ˌerəˈthrazmə) a skin disease due to infection by *Corynebacterium minutissimum* attacking the armpits or groin. It causes no irritation but is contagious.

erythroblast (əˈrithrohˌblast) originally any nucleated erythrocyte, but now more generally used to designate the nucleated precursor from which an erythrocyte develops.

erythroblastosis (əˈrithrohblasˈtohsəs) the presence of erythroblasts in the blood. *E. fetalis* a severe haemolytic anaemia with an excess of erythroblasts in the newly born. Due to incompatibility of Rh antibodies in the child's and the mother's blood.

erythrocyte (əˈrithrəˌsiet) a mature red blood cell. The cells contain haemoglobin and serve to transport oxygen. They are developed in the red bone marrow found in the cancellous tissue of all bones (*see* figure, p. 167). The haematopoietic factor vitamin B_{12} is essential for the change from proerythroblast to normoblast, and iron, thyroxine and

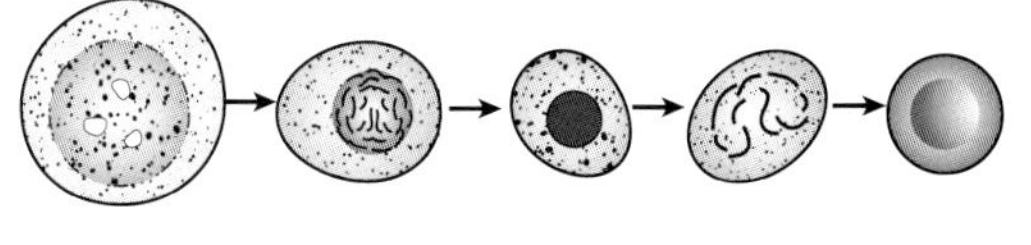

Erythrocyte development in bone marrow.

vitamin C are also necessary for its perfect structure. *E. sedimentation rate (ESR)* the rate at which the cells of citrated blood form a deposit in a graduated 200 mm tube (Westergren method). The normal rate is less than 10 mm of clear plasma in 1 hour. This is much increased in severe infection and acute rheumatism.

erythrocythaemia (əˌrithrohsieˈthee-mi·ə) increase in numbers of red blood cells due to overactivity of the bone marrow; Vaquez' disease; polycythaemia vera.

erythrocytopenia (əˌrithrohˌsietoh-ˈpeeni·ə) erythropenia; deficiency in the number of red blood cells.

erythrocytosis (əˈrithrohsieˈtohsəs) ERYTHROCYTHAEMIA.

erythroderma (əˌrithrəˈdərmə) abnormal redness of the skin, usually over a large area.

erythropoiesis (əˌrithrohpoyˈeesəs) the manufacture of red blood corpuscles.

erythropoietin (əˌrithrohˈpoyətən, -poyˈee-) a hormone produced by the kidney which stimulates the production of red blood cells in the bone marrow. *E. therapy* the use of erythropoietin to promote new blood formation in the treatment of anaemia.

erythropsia (ˌeriˈthropsi·ə) a defect of vision in which all objects appear red. May occur after a cataract operation.

eschar (ˈeskar) a slough or scab which forms after the destruction of living tissue by gangrene, infection or burning.

Escherichia (ˌesh·əˈriki·ə) a genus of *Enterobacteriaceae*. *E. coli* an organism normally present in the intestines of humans and other vertebrates. Although not generally pathogenic, it may cause infections of the gallbladder, bile ducts and urinary and intestinal tracts. It was formerly called *Bacillus coli*. Strain O157, normally found in the gut of cattle, has occasionally been responsible for serious outbreaks of food poisoning in humans.

esophoria (ˌeesəˈfaw·ri·ə) latent convergent STRABISMUS. The eyes turn inwards only when one is covered up.

esotropia (ˌeesohˈtrohpi·ə) convergent STRABISMUS. One or other eye turns inwards, resulting in double vision.

ESP *see* EXTRASENSORY PERCEPTION.

ESR *see* ERYTHROCYTE SEDIMENTATION RATE.

ESRD end-stage renal disease. *See* RENAL.

essence (ˈesəns) 1. an indispensable part of anything. 2. a volatile oil dissolved in alcohol.

essential (əˈsenshəl) indispensable. *E. amino acids* those amino acids that must be obtained in the diet and are necessary for the maintenance of tissue growth and repair. *See* AMINO

ACID. *E. fatty acids* unsaturated fatty acids that are necessary for body growth. *E. oils* specially prepared aromatic oils which are obtained from the different parts of plants including flowers, leaves, seeds, wood, roots and bark. Used in aromatherapy.

ester (ˈestə) a compound formed by the combination of an acid and an alcohol, with the elimination of water.

esterase (ˈestəˌrayz) an enzyme that causes the hydrolysis of esters into acids and alcohol.

estimated date of delivery (EDD) (ˈestəmayˌted ˌdayt ov dəˈlivə·ree) used in midwifery and obstetrics to calculate the date of delivery of a baby. This is calculated by counting forwards 9 months and adding 7 days (or counting back 3 months and adding 7 days) from the first day of the last normal menstrual period.

ethanol (ˈethəˌnol, ˈeethə-) alcohol.

ethanolamine (ˌethəˈnoləˌmeen) an intravenous sclerosing agent used in the treatment of varicose veins and oesophageal varices.

ether (ˈeethə) a volatile inflammable liquid formerly used as a general anaesthetic agent.

ethics (ˈethiks) a code of moral principles. Each practitioner, upon entering a profession, is invested with the responsibility to adhere to the standards of ethical practice and conduct set by that profession. The Code of ethics and Code of conduct for nurses and Code of conduct for midwives in Australia provide guidance and advice for standards of practice and conduct that are essential for the ethical discharge of the practitioner's responsibility. (*See* Appendix 8.) *E. committee* a group of lay people with professional healthcare practitioners, nurses, doctors and other experts, who consider and discuss ethical issues and monitor the integrity of research projects, to ensure the safety, integrity and human rights of study participants.

ethmoid (ˈethmoyd) a sieve-like bone separating the cavity of the nose from the cranium. The olfactory nerves pass through its perforations.

ethnic (ˈethnik) pertaining to a social group, members of which share cultural bonds or physical (racial) characteristics. *E. minority* a social grouping of people who share cultural or racial factors but who constitute a minority within the greater culture or society.

ethnocentrism (ˌethnohˈsentriz'm) the belief that one's own group, community, society or way of doing things is superior to those of others, leading to mistrust or doubt about others' values and beliefs.

ethnography (ethˈnogrəfee) a qualitative research approach developed by anthropologists with the purpose of describing an aspect of a culture, but also aimed at learning about the culture or factor being studied.

ethnology (ethˈnoləjee) the science dealing with the human races, their descent, relationships, etc.

ethnomethodology (ˈethnohˌmethə-doləjee) a sociological theory which concentrates on the case study using participant or non-participant observation.

ethyl chloride (ˌethəlˈklor·ied) a volatile liquid used as a local anaesthetic. When sprayed on intact skin, it causes local insensitivity through freezing.

ethylene oxide (ˈethəleen oksied) a gas that is sporicidal and virucidal and capable of penetrating relatively inaccessible parts of an apparatus during sterilisation. It is used for equipment which is too delicate to be sterilised by other methods.

etic (ˈetik) the perspectives of a group community or culture held by observers who are 'outsiders' or non-participants. *See* EMIC.

etiolation (ˌeetee·əˈlayshən) paleness of the skin due to lack of exposure to sunlight.

etiology (ˌeeteeˈoləjee) *see* AETIOLOGY.

eucalyptus oil (ˌyookəˈliptəs oyl) an oil derived from the leaves of the eucalyptus tree; it has mild antiseptic properties and is used in the treatment of nasal catarrh.

eugenics (yooˈjeniks) the study of measures that may be taken to improve future generations, both physically and mentally.

eukaryote (yooˈkareeˌoht) a cell with a true nucleus. Also eucaryote.

eugeria (yooˈger·ri·ə) the state of a high quality of life in old age. Eugeria should be the normal state for older people but may be affected by physical or mental illness.

eunuch (ˈyoonək) a castrated male.

euphoria (yooˈfor·ri·ə) an exaggerated feeling of wellbeing, often not justified by circumstances. Less extreme than ELATION.

eurhythmics (yooˈrithmiks) gentle body exercises performed to music.

eustachian tube (yooˈstayshən) *Bartolomeo Eustachi, Italian anatomist, 1520–1574.* The PHARYNGOTYMPANIC TUBE.

eustachitis (yooˈstayˈkietəs) inflammation of the eustachian tube.

euthanasia (ˌyoothəˈnayzi·ə, -zhə) 1. an easy or good death. 2. the deliberate ending of the life of a person suffering from an incurable disease painlessly in order to relieve suffering. Euthanasia is illegal in Australia.

euthyroid (yooˈthieroyd) normally functioning thyroid gland.

evacuant (eeˈvakyooənt) 1. promoting evacuation. 2. an agent that promotes evacuation.

evacuation (eeˌvakyooˈayshən) 1. an emptying or removal, especially the removal of any material from the body by discharge through a natural or artificial passage. 2. material discharged from the body, especially the discharge from the bowels.

evacuator (eeˈvakyooˌaytə) an instrument that produces evacuation, e.g. one designed to wash out small particles of stone from the bladder after lithotripsy.

evaluation (eeˌvalyooˈayshən) a critical appraisal or assessment; a judgement of the value, worth, character or effectiveness of that which is being assessed. In the healthcare field, this includes assessment of the patient's position on the health–illness continuum, and evaluation of the effectiveness of patient care activities in bringing about a change in the patient's position. Accepted as the last phase of the nursing process.

eventration (ˌeevənˈtrayshən) 1. the protrusion of the intestines through the abdominal wall. 2. removal of abdominal viscera.

eversion (eeˈvərzhən) turning outwards. *E. of the eyelid* ECTROPION. The upper eyelid may be everted for examination of the eye or for the removal of a foreign body.

evidence-based practice (EBP) (ˈevədəns bayst ˈpraktis) systematically appraising clinical situations and then using up-to-date research findings as a basis for decisions by the nursing or other health-related professions. An approach to clinical practice first developed at McMasters University (Canada) which is based on the following four principles: (a) clinical and other healthcare decisions should be based on the best evidence available from patients and populations as well as from the laboratory; (b) the patient's problem determines the nature and source of evidence to be sought, rather than habit, protocol or tradition; (c) identifying the best evidence calls for the integration of epidemiological and biostatistical ways of thinking with those derived from pathophysiology and clinical experience; and (d) the conclusions of this search and critical appraisal of evidence are worthwhile only if they are translated into actions that affect patients.

evisceration (ee͵visəˈrayshən) removal of internal organs. *E. of the eye* removal of the contents of the eyeball, but not the SCLERA.

evolution (͵eevəˈlooshən) the development of living organisms whose characteristics change during succeeding generations.

evulsion (eeˈvulshən) extraction by force.

Ewing's tumour (ˈyooingz ˈtyoomə) *James Ewing, American pathologist, 1866–1943*. A form of sarcoma usually affecting the shaft of a long bone in young adults.

exacerbation (ekˈsasəˈbayshən, ig͵zasə-) an increase in the severity of the symptoms of a disease.

exanthem (egˈzanthəm, ekˈs-) an infectious disease characterised by a skin rash.

exanthematous (͵egzanˈthemətəs, eks-) pertaining to any disease associated with a skin eruption.

excavation (͵ekskəˈvayshən) scooping out. *Dental e.* the removal of decay from a tooth before inserting a filling.

excision (ekˈsizhən) the cutting out of a part.

excitation (͵eksieˈtayshən) the act of stimulating.

excitement (əkˈsietmənt) a physiological and emotional response to a stimulus.

excoriation (ek͵skor·reeˈayshən) an abrasion of the skin.

excrement (ˈekskrəmənt) faecal matter; waste matter from the body.

excrescence (ekˈskresəns) abnormal outgrowth of tissue, e.g. a wart.

excreta (ekˈskreetə) the natural discharges of the excretory system: faeces, urine and sweat.

excretion (ekˈskreeshən) the discharge of waste from the body.

exercise (ˈeksə͵siez) performance of physical exertion for improvement of health or correction of physical deformity. *Active e.* motion imparted to a part by voluntary contraction and relaxation of its controlling muscles. *Isometric e.* active exercise performed against stable resistance, without change in the length of the muscle. No movement occurs at any joints over which the muscle passes. *Passive e.* motion imparted to a segment of the body by another individual, machine or other outside force, or produced by voluntary effort of another segment of the patient's own body. *Range of movement (ROM) e.* Refers to exercises that move each joint through its full range of movement, that is, to the highest degree of movement of which each joint is normally capable.

exfoliation (eks͵fohleeˈayshən) the splitting off from the surface of dead tissue in thin flaky layers.

exhalation (ˌeks·həˈlayshən) 1. the giving off of a vapour. 2. the act of breathing out.

exhibitionism (ˌeksəˈbishəˌnizəm) 1. showing off; a desire to attract attention. 2. exposing the genitals to persons of the opposite sex in socially unacceptable circumstances.

exocrine (ˈeksəˈkrin, -ˌkrien) pertaining to those glands that discharge their secretion by means of a duct, e.g. salivary glands. *See* ENDOCRINE.

exogenous (ekˈsojənəs) of external origin.

exomphalos (ekˈsomfələs) 1. hernia of the abdominal viscera into the umbilical cord. 2. congenital umbilical hernia.

exophthalmometer (ˌeksof·thal-ˈmomətə) an instrument for measuring the extent of protrusion of the eyeball.

exophthalmos (ˌeksofˈthalməs) abnormal protrusion of the eyeball which results in a marked stare. May be due to injury or disease and is often associated with THYROTOXICOSIS.

exostosis (ˌeksoˈstohsəs) a bony outgrowth from the surface of a bone.

exotoxin (ˌeksohˈtoksən) a poison produced by a bacterial cell and released into the tissues surrounding it. *See* ENDOTOXIN.

exotropia (ˌeksohˈtrohpi·ə) divergent strabismus; the eyes turn outwards.

expanded role (ˌekˈspandəd rohl) the opportunity for nurses and midwives to undertake an expanded role in relation to patient care beyond that traditionally recognised. The professional framework for nurses and midwives in relation to the expanded role is contained within separate codes: the Code of conduct for nurses and the Code of conduct for midwives (*see* Appendix 8).

expected outcome (ˈekspektəd ˈowtˌkum) in a nursing care plan, the rationale for a statement regarding a nursing intervention and what it is expected to achieve.

expectorant (əkˈspektə·rənt) a remedy that promotes and facilitates expectoration.

expectoration (əkˌspektəˈrayshən) sputum; secretions coughed up from the air passages. Its characteristics are a valuable aid in diagnosis and note should be taken of the quantity ejected, its colour and the amount of effort required. Frothiness denotes that it comes from an air-containing cavity; fluidity indicates oedema of the lung.

experiential learning (ˈekspə-reeˌənshəl lərning) learning from experiencing a situation. May also be facilitated with the use of role play or of a simulated situation and reflecting on the experience.

experiment (əksˈperəmənt) a scientific investigation in which observations are made and data collected by means of the characteristics of control, randomisation and manipulation.

experimental group (əksˌperəˈ-mentˈl groop) the group in an experimental investigation which receives an intervention or treatment.

expertise (ekˈspəteez) special skills or knowledge acquired by a person through education, training or experience.

expiration (ˌekspəˈrayshən) 1. the act of breathing out. 2. termination or death.

exploration (ˌeksplәˈrayshən) the operation of surgically investigating any part of the body.

expression (ək'spreshən) 1. the aspect or appearance of the face as determined by the physical or emotional state. 2. the act of squeezing out or evacuating by pressure, e.g. the removal of breast milk by hand or breast pump. 3. the manifestation of a heritable trait in an individual carrying the gene or genes that determine it.

exsanguination (ək,sang·gwə'-nayshən) extensive blood loss due to internal or external haemorrhage.

extended family (ek'stendəd faməlee) one that includes aunts, uncles, cousins and grandparents. *See* FAMILY.

extension (ək'stenshən) 1. the straightening out of a flexed joint, such as the knee or elbow. 2. the application of traction to a fractured or dislocated limb by means of a weight.

extensor (ek'stensə, -saw, ək-) a muscle that extends or straightens a limb.

exterior (ek'stiə·ri·ə, ək-) on the outside.

exteriorise (ek'stiə·ri·ə,riez, ək-) 1. to bring an organ or part of one to the outside of the body by surgery. 2. in psychiatry, to turn one's interests outwards.

extra (ekstrə) prefix denoting outside, additional or beyond.

extracapsular (,ekstrə'kapsyələ) outside the capsule. May refer to a fracture occurring at the end of the bone, but outside the joint capsule, or to cataract extraction.

extracellular (,ekstrə'selyələ) outside the cell. *E. fluid* tissue fluid that surrounds the cells.

extracorporeal membrane oxygenation (ECMO) (,ekstrə-caw'pawreeəl 'mem,brayn ,oksəjə'nayshən) a life support procedure using an extracorporeal technique providing both cardiac and respiratory oxygen to patients whose heart and lungs are severely diseased or damaged. Blood is taken from the patient, directed through a machine (artificial kidney or 'heart-lung') for removal of carbon dioxide and water and oxygenation, and is then returned to the general circulation.

extract ('ekstrakt) a concentrated preparation of a drug made by extracting its soluble principles by steeping in water or alcohol and then evaporating the fluid.

extraction (ek'strakshən, ək-) 1. the process or act of pulling or drawing out. 2. the preparation of an extract. *Breech e.* extraction of an infant from the uterus in cases of breech presentation. *Vacuum e.* removal of the uterine contents by application of a vacuum. An alternative to the forceps method of delivering a baby.

extrapyramidal (,ekstrəpə'ramәd'l) outside the pyramidal (cerebrospinal) tract. *E. system* the nerve tracts and pathways which are not within the pyramidal tracts.

extrasensory (,ekstrə'sensə·ree) outside or beyond any of the known senses. *E. perception (ESP)* appreciation of the thoughts of others or of current or future events without any normal means of communication.

extrasystole (,ekstrə'sistəlee) premature contraction of the atria or ventricles. *See* SYSTOLE.

extrauterine (,ekstrə'yootə,rien) occurring outside the uterus. *E. pregnancy* ectopic gestation; development of a fetus outside the uterus.

extravasation (ək,stravə'sayshən) effusion or escape of fluid from its normal course into surrounding tissues. *E. of blood* a bruise.

extremity (ək'streməteе) distal part; a hand or foot.

extrinsic (ək'strinsik, -zik) originating externally. *E. factor* a substance present in meat and other foodstuffs. Also called CYANOCOBALAMIN (vitamin B_{12}), it is necessary for the manufacture of red blood cells. The intrinsic factor produced in the stomach is necessary for the absorption of vitamin B_{12}. *E. muscle* a muscle originating away from the part that it controls, such as those controlling the movements of the eye.

extroversion (ˌekstrə'vərzhən) turning inside out, e.g. of the uterus, as sometimes occurs after labour, or in psychology the turning of thoughts to the external environment.

extrovert ('ekstrəˌvərt) a person who is sociable, a good mixer, outgoing and interested in what is going on in the social environment. A personality type first described by Jung. *See* INTROVERT.

extubation (ˌekstyoo'bayshən) removal of a tube used in intubation.

exudation (ˌeksyoo'dayshən) the slow discharge of serous fluid through the walls of the blood cells and its deposition in or on the tissues.

eye (ie) the organ of sight. A globular structure with three coats. The nerve tissue of the retina receives impressions of images via the pupil and lens. From this, the optic nerve conveys the impressions to the visual area of the cerebrum. *E. contact* two people making direct contact in the vicinity of the other's eyes. Also called mutual gaze. Forms an important component of non-verbal communication in many cultures between people, although the healthcare professional will need to be sensitive to the cultural background of the person, as some cultures consider direct eye contact inappropriate. *E. strain* fatigue of the eye(s) from overuse and tiredness, often associated with headaches. May be due to poor lighting or an uncorrected defect in focusing.

eyelid ('ieˌlid) a protective covering of the eye, composed of muscle and dense connective tissue covered with skin, lined with conjunctiva, and fringed with eyelashes. Eyelids contain the Meibomian glands.

eyetooth (ie'tooth) an upper canine tooth.

Ff

F symbol for *Fahrenheit* and *fluorine*.

f waves (ef wayvz) waves that represent fibrillation or flutter on an ECG.

face (fays) the front of the head from the forehead to the chin. *F. lift* a surgical procedure to remove excess skin and reduce signs of ageing in the face and neck. Facial muscles may also be tightened to enhance tone. Also known as meloplasty or rhytidectomy. *F. presentation* the appearance of the face of the fetus first at the cervix during labour.

facet (ˈfasət) a small flat area on the surface of a bone. *F. syndrome* a slight dislocation of the small facet joints of the vertebrae giving rise to pain and muscle spasm.

facial (ˈfayshəl) pertaining to the face or lower anterior portion of the head. *F. nerve* the seventh cranial nerve, which supplies the salivary glands and superficial face muscles. *F. paralysis see* PARALYSIS.

facies (ˈfayseeˌeez, ˈfayshee-) facial expression; it often gives some indication of the person's condition. *Adenoid f.* the open mouth and vacant expression associated with mouth breathing and nasal obstruction. *Parkinson f.* fixed expression, due to paucity of movement of facial muscles, characteristic of parkinsonism. *F. factor V Leiden see* THROMBOPHILIA.

factor analysis (ˈfaktə əˈnaləsəs) a type of validity that uses a statistical procedure for determining the underlying dimensions or components of a variable.

fadoobadas (fadˈuhbahˌdahs) colloquial term for flabby fatty skin which hangs down from the underside of the upper arms over the triceps. Loss of skin elasticity and ageing are contributing factors. Also know as bat wings or flabby triceps.

faeces (ˈfeeseez) waste matter excreted by the bowel, consisting of indigestible cellulose, food which has escaped digestion, bacteria (living and dead) and water.

Fahrenheit scale (ˈfarənˌhiet ˌskayl) *Gabriel Fahrenheit, German physicist, 1686–1736.* A scale of heat measurement. It registers the freezing point of water at 32°, the normal heat of the human body at 98.4°, and the boiling point of water at 212°. *Symbol* F. *See* CELSIUS.

failure (ˈfaylyə) inability to perform or to function properly. *Heart f.* inability of the heart to maintain a circulation sufficient to meet the body's needs. *Kidney f., renal f.* inability of the kidney to excrete metabolites at normal plasma levels under normal loading, or inability to retain electrolytes when intake is normal; in the acute form, marked by uraemia and usually by oliguria, with hyperkalaemia and pulmonary oedema. *Respiratory f., ventilatory f.* a life-threatening condition in which respiratory function is inadequate to maintain the body's needs for oxygen supply and carbon dioxide removal while at rest.

fainting (ˈfaynting) *see* SYNCOPE.

faith healing (fayth heeling) an attempt to cure disease or disability with the use of spiritual powers or by the influence of the personality of the healer.

falciform (ˈfalsə͵fawm) sickle-shaped. *F. ligament* a fold of peritoneum which separates the two main lobes of the liver and connects it with the anterior abdominal wall and the diaphragm.

fall (fawl) moving downwards quickly and without control. The tendency to fall to the ground increases with age when reflex actions are slower. Various conditions of older people, such as poor sight or walking disorders, increase the risk of falls, as does the taking of certain medications to induce sleep or for the treatment of anxiety and tension. Bone fractures are a common complication; this occurs most usually in women, who are more prone to osteoporosis. A fall or the fear of falling can have an adverse psychological effect on an older person, who may become reluctant to leave home. Community care staff can provide practical advice and support to prevent or minimise further falls, e.g. ensuring that floor coverings and electrical cords are made safe, suitable footwear is worn, good lighting is available and hand rails are safe and secure.

fallopian tube (fəˈlohpee ən tyoob) *Gabriele Fallopius, Italian anatomist, 1523–1563.* Uterine tube. One of a pair of tubes, about 10–14 cm long, arising out of the upper part of the uterus. The distal end of each tube is fimbriated and lies near an ovary. The tubes' function is to conduct the ova from the ovaries to the interior of the uterus. An oviduct.

falx (falks) a sickle-shaped structure. *F. cerebri* the fold of DURA MATER that separates the two cerebral hemispheres.

familial (fəˈmilee əl) occurring in or affecting members of a family more than would be expected by chance.

family (ˈfaməlee) 1. a group of people who reside together and who may be related by blood or marriage (registered or de facto), typically consisting of one or two parents and their children. 2. a taxonomic category below an order and above a genus. *Blended f.* a family unit composed of a couple and the children they had together and their children from previous relationship(s). *Extended f.* a nuclear family and their close relatives, such as the children's grandparents, aunts and uncles. *Extended nuclear f.* a nuclear family who make frequent social contact with the extended family group despite geographical distance. *F. centred care* a nursing approach to care and treatment of children which recognises the needs of the family and their circumstances in the planning and delivery of services being provided for the child. *F. planning* the arrangement, spacing and limitation of the children in a family, depending on the wishes and social circumstances of the parents. *F. therapy* a therapeutic process whereby the psychotherapist uses family group therapy to resolve problems for one member of the family. *Nuclear f.* a couple and their children, by birth or adoption, who are living together and are more or less isolated from their extended family. *Single parent f.* a lone parent and offspring living together as a family unit.

Fanconi's syndrome (fanˈkohneez ˈsin͵drohm) *Guido Fanconi, Swiss paediatrician, 1892–1979.* A rare inherited disorder of metabolism in which reabsorption of phosphate, amino acids and sugar by the renal tubules is impaired. The kidneys fail to produce acid urine, and the resulting features are thirst, POLYURIA and rickets, leading to chronic renal failure.

fang (fang) the root of a tooth.

fantasy (ˈfantəsee) an imagined sequence of events or mental images that serves to satisfy unconscious wishes or to express unconscious conflicts.

farmer's lung (ˈfahməz lung) extrinsic allergic alveolitis, a disease occurring in those in contact with mouldy hay. Due to a hypersensitivity, with widespread reaction in the lung tissue. It causes excessive breathlessness. Also known as hypersensitivity pneumonitis.

FAS *see* FETAL ALCOHOL SYNDROME.

fascia (ˈfashi·ə) a sheath of connective tissue enclosing muscles or other organs.

fasciculation (fəˌsikyəˈlayshən) isolated fine muscle twitching which gives a flickering appearance.

fasciculus (fəˈsikyələs) a small bundle of nerve or muscle fibres; a fascicle.

fasciotomy (ˌfasheeˈotəmee) a surgical incision into the fascia.

fast (fahst) 1. resisting change. 2. to abstain from food. 3. moving or capable of moving at high speed.

FAST (fahst) acronym used to easily remember and detect the early signs of a stroke. Getting the person to hospital quickly is more likely to lead to better health outcomes and fewer hospital days. *See table* below and STROKE.

fat (fat) 1. the adipose or fatty tissue of the body. 2. neutral fat; a triglyceride which is an ester of fatty acids and glycerol. *F. soluble vitamins* those vitamins that are soluble in fat, i.e. vitamins A, D, E and K. *Wool-f.* lanolin. *See also* BROWN FAT.

fatigue (fəˈteeg) a state of weariness which may range from mental disinclination for effort to profound exhaustion after great physical and mental effort. *Muscle f.* may occur during prolonged effort, owing to lack of oxygen and to accumulation of waste products.

fatty (ˈfatee) containing or similar to fat. *F. acid see* ESSENTIAL FATTY ACIDS. *F. degeneration* a degenerative change in tissue cells due to the invasion of fat and consequent weakening of the organ. The change occurs as a result of incorrect diet, shortage of oxygen in the tissues or excessive consumption of alcohol. *F. liver disease* a build-up of fat in the liver which can cause serious complications such as cirrhosis. *Non-alcoholic f. liver disease (NAFLD)* a common disease in Australia and risk factors are increasing age, obesity and diabetes.

Use FAST to remember the warning signs of a stroke		
F	Facial drooping	One side or section of the face droops.
A	Arm weakness	Difficulty or inability to raise one arm.
S	Speech difficulties	Speech is slurred or difficult to understand.
T	Time to call emergency services	Time is important. If you observe any of these signs in a person, call 000 (in Australia, or the emergency number for your particular country) or take the person to the nearest hospital immediately.

fauces (ˈfawseez) the opening from the mouth into the pharynx. *Pillars of the f.* the two folds of muscle covered with mucous membrane that pass from the soft palate on either side of the fauces. One fold passes into the tongue, the other into the pharynx, and between them is situated the tonsil.

favism (ˈfayvizəm) an acute haemolytic anaemia caused by ingestion of fava beans or inhalation of the pollen of the plant, usually occurring in certain individuals as a result of a genetic abnormality with a deficiency in an enzyme, glucose-6-phosphate dehydrogenase, in the erythrocytes. Also called fabism.

favus (ˈfayvəs) a type of ringworm infection, with formation of scabs, in appearance like a honeycomb. It usually affects the scalp and is due to a fungus infection (*Trichophyton schoenleinii*).

Fe symbol for *iron* [L. *ferrum*].

fear (fiə) a normal emotional response, in contrast to anxiety and phobia, to consciously recognised external sources of danger; it is manifested by alarm, apprehension or disquiet. *Obsessional f.* a recurring irrational fear that is not amenable to ordinary reassurance; a phobia.

febrile (ˈfeebriel, ˈfeb-) characterised by, or relating to, fever. *F. convulsion* a convulsion which occurs in childhood, between the ages of six months and six years and is associated with FEVER.

fecundation (ˌfekənˈdayshən, fee-) fertilisation.

fecundity (fəˈkundətee) the ability to produce offspring frequently. In demography, the physiological ability to reproduce, as opposed to fertility.

feedback (ˈfeedˌbak) a method of homeostatic control where some of the output is returned as input for monitoring purposes. Feedback mechanisms are important in the regulation of such physiological processes as hormone and enzyme reactions. *F. treatment* see BIOFEEDBACK. *Negative f.* a rise in the output of a substance is detected and further output is thus inhibited. *Positive f.* a rise in output causes either a direct or an indirect rise in the output of another substance.

Felty's syndrome (ˈfelteez ˈsinˌdrohm) *Augustus Felty, American physician, 1895–1963.* The triad of rheumatoid arthritis, SPLENOMEGALY and LEUCOPENIA. Often associated with anaemia, LYMPHADENOPATHY and vasculitic cutaneous ulceration.

female (ˈfeeˈmael) a person with two X chromosomes and normally having a vagina and uterus and the ability to reproduce after puberty. *F. genital mutilation* is the intentional, non-therapeutic, physical modification of female genitalia by either partial or total removal of the external female genitalia or other injury to the female genital organs in young girls before puberty. Still performed ritualistically in certain countries, the extent of the injury varying from one culture to another. Long-term complications from the procedure include excessive scar tissue formation, sexual dysfunction and chronic genital, reproductive and urinary problems. Psychological consequences may also occur, such as post-traumatic stress disorder. During pregnancy special care will be required throughout the antenatal period, and during labour, birth and the immediate postnatal period. Alternatively a caesarean section may be considered. Female genital mutilation is illegal in most countries, including all Australian states and territories. Also known as female circumcision.

feminisation (ˈfemənieˈzayshən) 1. the normal induction or development of female sexual characteristics. 2. the induction or development of female secondary sexual characteristics in the male. *Testicular f. syndrome* now called COMPLETE ANDROGEN INSENSITIVITY SYNDROME is a condition in which the subject is phenotypically female, but lacks nuclear sex chromatin and is of XY chromosomal sex.

feminist theory (femənəst thiəree) theory based on general theories about the origins of inequality and social construction of gender roles in various disciplines. It offers both a philosophical approach to the conduct of therapy and a specific type of theory. The focus of both types is on consciousness raising that highlights the presence of sexism and gender-role stereotyping in society.

femoral (ˈfemərəl) pertaining to the femur. *F. artery* that of the thigh from groin to knee. *F. canal* the opening below the inguinal ligament through which the femoral artery passes from the abdomen to the thigh.

femur (ˈfeemə) the thigh bone.

fenestra (fəˈnestrə) a window-like opening. *F. ovalis* the oval opening between the middle and the internal ear.

ferritin (ˈferətən) a complex formed of an iron and protein molecule; one of the forms in which iron is stored in the body.

ferrous (ˈferəs) containing iron. *F. fumarate*, *f. gluconate*, *f. succinate* and *f. sulphate* are iron salts which are given orally to treat iron-deficiency anaemia.

ferrule (ˈferool, -rəl) a rubber cap used on the end of walking sticks, frames and crutches to prevent slipping.

fertilisation (ˌfərtəlieˈzayshən) the impregnation of the female sex cell, the ovum, by a male sex cell, a spermatozoon. *In vitro f.* artificial fertilisation of the ovum in laboratory conditions. The timing and conditions for implantation into a uterus have to be perfect if successful pregnancy is to ensue.

fester (ˈfestə) to become superficially inflamed and to suppurate.

festination (ˌfestəˈnayshən) an involuntary tendency to take short accelerating steps in walking; seen in conditions such as PARKINSON'S DISEASE.

fetal (ˈfeet'l) pertaining to the fetus. *F. alcohol syndrome (FAS)* physical and mental abnormalities due to excessive maternal alcohol intake during pregnancy. Abnormalities may include MICROCEPHALY, poor growth, learning difficulties, hyperactivity, heart murmurs and skeletal malformation. The exact amount of alcohol consumption that will produce fetal damage is unknown, but the periods of gestation during which the alcohol is most likely to result in fetal damage are 3–4.5 months after conception and during the last trimester. *F. assessment* determination of the wellbeing of the fetus. Assessment techniques and procedures include: (a) medical and family histories and physical examination of the mother; (b) ULTRASONOGRAPHY; (c) assessment of fetal activity, with the mother recording fetal movements over a given period of time (usually used in conjunction with other fetal wellbeing tests); (d) chemical assessment of placental function; (e) assays of amniotic fluid obtained by AMNIOCENTESIS; and (f) electronic and ultrasonic fetal heart rate monitoring. *F. distress* the clinical manifestation of fetal hypoxia which may be due to maternal or fetal causes. *F. position* a position resembling that of the fetus in the womb, sometimes adopted by a child or adult in a state of distress or depression.

fetishism (ˈfetiˌshizəm) a state in which an object is regarded with an irrational fear, or an erotic attraction which may be so strong that the object is necessary for achieving sexual excitement.

fetor (ˈfeetə, -taw) an offensive smell.

fetoscope (ˈfeetəˌskohp) 1. an endoscope for viewing the fetus in utero. 2. a type of stethoscope designed for listening to the fetal heartbeat.

fetus, foetus (ˈfeetəs) the developing baby between the eighth week and the end of pregnancy.

fever (ˈfeevə) 1. an abnormally high body temperature; PYREXIA. 2. any disease characterised by marked increase of body temperature.

fibre (ˈfiebə) a thread-like structure.

fibre optics (ˌfiebəˈroptiks) the transmission of light rays along flexible tubes by means of very fine glass or plastic fibres. Use is made of this in endoscopic instruments such as the gastroscope.

fibrescope (ˈfiebəˌskohp) an endoscope in which fibre optics are used.

fibrillation (ˌfibrəˈlayshən) a quivering, vibratory movement of muscle fibres. *Atrial f.* rapid contractions of the atrium causing irregular contraction of the ventricles in both rhythm and force. *Ventricular f.* fine rapid twitchings of the ventricles leading to circulatory arrest. Rapidly fatal unless it may be controlled.

fibrin (ˈfiebrən) an insoluble protein that is essential to CLOTTING of blood, formed from fibrinogen by the action of THROMBIN.

fibrinogen (fieˈbrinəjən) a soluble protein which is present in blood plasma and is converted into fibrin by the action of thrombin when the blood clots.

fibrinolysin (ˌfiebriˈnoləsən) a proteolytic enzyme that dissolves fibrin.

fibrinolysis (ˌfiebrəˈnoləsəs) the dissolution of fibrin by the action of fibrinolysin. The process by which clots are removed from the circulation after healing has taken place.

fibrinopenia (ˌfiebrənohˈpeeni·ə) a deficiency of fibrinogen in the blood. There is a tendency to bleed because the coagulation time is increased.

fibroadenoma (ˌfiebrohˌadəˈnohmə) a benign tumour of glandular and fibrous tissue. *See* ADENOMA.

fibroangioma (ˌfiebrohˌanjeeˈohmə) a benign tumour containing both fibrous and vascular tissue.

fibroblast (ˈfiebrohˌblast) a connective tissue cell.

fibrocartilage (ˌfiebrohˈkahtəlij) cartilage with fibrous tissue in it.

fibrochondritis (ˌfiebrohkonˈdrietəs) inflammation of fibrocartilage.

fibrocystic (ˌfiebrohˈsistik) fibrous and cystic. *F. disease of the pancreas* an inherited disease affecting the mucus-secreting glands, the sweat glands and the pancreas. It is characterised by fatty stools and repeated lung infections. MUCOVISCIDOSIS; *see* CYSTIC FIBROSIS.

fibroid (ˈfiebroyd) 1. having a fibrous structure. 2. a FIBROMA or a FIBROMYOMA, usually one occurring in the uterus.

fibroma (fie'brohmə) a benign tumour of connective tissue.

fibromyoma (ˌfiebrohmie'ohmə) a tumour consisting of fibrous and muscle tissue; frequently found in or on the uterus.

fibroplasia (ˌfiebroh'playzi·ə) the formation of fibrous tissue when a wound heals. *Retrolental f. see* RETINOPATHY OF PREMATURITY.

fibrosarcoma (ˌfiebrohsah'kohmə) a malignant tumour arising in fibrous tissue.

fibrosis (fie'brohsəs) fibrous tissue formation, such as occurs in scar tissue or as the result of inflammation. It is the cause of adhesions of the peritoneum or other serous membranes. *F. of the lung* condition that may precede BRONCHIECTASIS and EMPHYSEMA.

fibrositis (ˌfiebrə'sietəs) inflammation of fibrous tissue. The term is loosely applied to pain and stiffness, particularly of the back muscles, for which no other cause can be found.

fibula ('fibyələ) the slender bone from knee to ankle, on the outer side of the leg.

field of vision (ˌfeeld ov 'vizhən) the area within view, as for the fixed eye, a camera or in an operation.

fifth disease ('fif·th 'di'zeez) a mild but contagious childhood infection caused by the human parvovirus B19 virus which produces a bright red rash on the cheeks that normally clears up without treatment. Also known as slapped cheek syndrome or erythema infectiosum.

fight or flight response (fiet aw fliet rə'spons) activation of the sympathetic nervous system in response to danger or stress.

filament ('filəmənt) a small thread-like structure.

filaria (fi'lair ri·ə) a genus of nematode worms which may be found in the connective tissues and lymphatics, having been transmitted to humans by mosquitoes. Found mainly in the tropics and subtropics.

filariasis (ˌfilə'rieəsəs) an infection by filaria, particularly by *Wuchereria bancrofti*, resulting in blockage of the lymphatics, which causes swelling of the surrounding tissues. ELEPHANTIASIS may occur.

filiform ('filəˌfawm, 'fie-) thread-like. *F. papillae* the fine thread-like processes that cover the anterior two-thirds of the tongue.

filter ('filtə) a device for eliminating certain elements, such as: (a) particles of a certain size from a solution; or (b) rays of a certain wavelength from a stream of radiant energy.

filtrate ('filtrayt) the fluid that passes through a filter.

filtration (fil'trayshən) 1. the removal of precipitate from a liquid by means of a filter. 2. the removal of rays of a certain wavelength from an electromagnetic beam. *F. angle* the angle of the anterior chamber of the eye through which the aqueous humour drains; blockage of this channel gives rise to glaucoma.

fimbria ('fimbri·ə) a fringe. *F. of the uterine tube* the thread-like projections that surround the pelvic opening of the uterine tube.

finger ('fing·gə) a digit of the hand. *Clubbed f.* one with enlargement of the terminal phalanx with constant osseous changes; occurs in many heart and lung diseases. *F. spelling see* SIGN LANGUAGE. *Hammer f., mallet f.* permanent flexion of the distal phalanx of a finger due to avulsion of the extensor tendon. *Trigger f.* temporary flexion of a finger which is overcome in a sudden jerk by active or passive extension of the finger. It is caused by thickening of the flexor tendon in a narrowed tendon sheath. *Webbed f.s* fingers more or less united by strands of tissue; syndactyly.

fingerprint (ˈfingəprint) the impression left on a surface of the ridged pattern of the skin of the fingertips. Loops, whorls, arches and combinations of these form distinct patterns for each human individual—not even identical twins have the same fingerprint pattern.

first aid (ˌfərst ˈayd) emergency care and treatment of an injured person before complete medical and surgical treatment can be secured.

fission (ˈfishən) a form of asexual reproduction by dividing into two equal parts, as in bacteria. *Binary f.* the splitting in two of the nucleus and the protoplasm of a cell, as in protozoa. *Nuclear f.* the splitting of the nucleus of an atom, with the release of a great quantity of energy.

fissure (ˈfishə) a narrow slit or cleft. *Anal f.* a painful crack in the mucous membrane of the anus. *F. of Rolando* a furrow in the cortex of each cerebral hemisphere, dividing the sensory from the motor area; the central sulcus.

fistula (ˈfistyələ) an abnormal passage between two epithelial surfaces, usually connecting the cavity of one organ with another or a cavity with the surface of the body. *Anal f.* the result of an ischiorectal abscess where the channel is from the anus to the skin. *Arteriovenus (AV) f.* an abnormal connection between an artery and vein allowing increased bloodflow through the vein. It may be congenital or acquired due to trauma or erosion of an arterial aneurysm. AV fistulas can also be surgically created for use in haemodialysis in people with severe kidney disease. The fistula is usually formed in the arm (wrist, forearm or upper arm) and will take about 6 weeks to grow and mature. Recently, non-surgical, percutaneous procedures have been trialled to create AV fistulas for dialysis access. *Biliary f.* a leakage of bile to the exterior, following an operation on the gallbladder or ducts. *Blind f.* one which is open at only one end. *Faecal f.* one in which the channel is from the intestine through the wound caused by an operation on the intestines when sepsis is present. *Rectovaginal f.* fistula from the rectum to the vagina, which may result from a severe perineal tear during childbirth. *Tracheo-oesophageal f.* an opening from the trachea into the oesophagus; a congenital deformity. *Vesicovaginal f.* an opening from the bladder to the vagina, either from error during operation or from ulceration, as may occur in carcinoma of the cervix.

fit (fit) a commonly used term for paroxysmal motor discharges leading to sudden convulsive movements, as in epilepsy, ECLAMPSIA and hysteria.

fitness (fitnəs) associated with a sense of wellbeing, and the ability to undertake sustained physical exertion without undue breathlessness. Fitness needs to be maintained on a regular basis by the person engaging in physical exertion or exercise.

fixation (fikˈsayshən) 1. the process of rendering something immovable, such as a joint or a fractured bone. 2. in psychology, a term used to describe a failure to progress wholly or in part through the normal stages of psychological development to a fully developed personality. 3. in ophthalmology, directing the sight straight at an object.

flaccid (ˈflaksəd, ˈflasəd) soft, flabby. *F. paralysis see* PARALYSIS.

flail (flayl) exhibiting abnormal or pathological mobility. *F. chest* a loss of stability of the chest wall due to multiple rib fractures or detachment of the sternum from the ribs as a result of a severe crushing chest injury. The loose chest segment moves in a direction that is the reverse of normal. *F. joint* an unusually movable joint.

flap (flap) a mass of tissue, used for grafting in plastic surgery, which is left attached to its blood supply and used to repair defects either adjacent to it or at some distance from it.

flare (flair) the response of the skin to an allergic or hypersensitivity reaction. Reddening of the skin that spreads outwards.

flatfoot (ˈflatˌfuht) a condition due to absence or sinking of the medial longitudinal arch of the foot, caused by weakening of the ligaments and tendons.

flatulence (ˈflatyələns) excessive formation of gases in the stomach or intestine.

flatulent (ˈflatyələnt) suffering from flatulence. *F. distension* swelling due to gas in the stomach or intestines. It is a common complication after abdominal operations and is caused by intestinal stasis.

flatus (ˈflaytəs) gas in the stomach or intestine.

flea (flee) a small, wingless, blood-sucking insect parasite. The common human flea, *Pulex irritans*, rarely transmits disease. Cat and dog fleas, *Ctenocephalides*, are also relatively harmless. The rat fleas *Xenopsylla* and *Nosopsyllus* are the vectors of bubonic plague.

flexion (ˈflekshən) bending; moving a joint so that the two or more bones forming it draw towards each other. *Plantar f.* bending the fingers or toes downwards.

Flexner's bacillus (ˈfleksnəz bəˈsiləs) *Simon Flexner, American bacteriologist, 1863–1946.* One of the group of pathogenic bacteria which cause bacillary dysentery; *Shigella flexneri*.

flexor (ˈfleksə) any muscle causing flexion of a limb or other part of the body.

flexure (ˈflekshə) a bend or curve.

flight of ideas (fliet ov ieˈdiəz) the rapid movement of ideas and speech from one fragmentary topic to another that occurs in mania.

floaters (ˈflohtəz) wisps or strands within the eye that are visible to the person. Usually caused by detachment and collapse of the vitreous humour and the normal ageing process.

flooding (ˈfluding) 1. excessive loss of blood from the uterus often associated with childbirth or severe cases of menorrhagia. 2. a technique used in behaviour therapy for the reduction of anxiety related to phobias and other related disorders. The patient is repeatedly exposed, in imagination or in real life, to emotionally distressing aversive stimuli of high intensity. Also called EXPOSURE THERAPY.

florid (ˈflo·rid) having a flushed facial appearance.

flowmeter (ˈflohˌmeetə) an instrument used to measure the flow of liquids or gases.

fluctuation (ˌfluktyooˈayshən, -chyoo-) a wave-like motion felt on palpation of the abdomen.

fluid (ˈflooəd) 1. a liquid or gas; any liquid of the body. 2. composed of molecules which freely change their relative positions without separation of the mass. *Amniotic f.* the fluid within the amnion that bathes the developing fetus and protects it from mechanical injury. *Body f.s* any fluid in the body, such as blood, cerebrospinal fluid, urine, saliva, sputum, tears, semen, breast milk or vaginal secretions. *Total body f.s* the fluids within the body, composed of water, electrolytes and non-electrolytes. The volume and distribution of body fluids vary with age, gender and amount of adipose tissue. For the average adult, approximately 60% of the total body weight is water—40% of total body water is held within cells as intracellular fluid; the remaining 20% is within the extracellular space as the extracellular fluid. *Cerebrospinal f.* the fluid contained within the ventricles of the brain, the subarachnoid space and the central canal of the spinal cord. *Extracellular f.* fluid outside the cell, constituting one-third of the total body fluid. *F. chart* a chart used to record the daily intake and output of fluids for a patient. The amount of intake and output is usually totalled every 24 hours. The chart provides a crude indicator for the patient's fluid balance status. *F. overload* an excessive accumulation of fluid in the body caused by too much parenteral infusion or deficiencies in cardiovascular or renal fluid volume regulation. *Interstitial f.* the extracellular fluid bathing most tissues, excluding the fluid within the lymph and blood vessels. *Intracellular f.* fluid within the cell, constituting two-thirds of the total body fluid.

fluid balance (flooəd baləns) a state in which the volume of body water and its solutes (electrolytes and non-electrolytes) is within normal limits and there is normal distribution of fluids within the intracellular and extracellular compartments. The total volume of body fluids should be about 60% of the body weight.

fluke (flook) one of a group of parasitic flatworms (*Trematoda*). Different varieties may affect the blood, the intestines, the liver or the lungs.

fluorescein (ˌflooˈrəsee·ən) a dye used to detect corneal ulceration. When it is dropped on the eye, the ulcer stains green.

fluorescence (ˌflooˈresəns) the property of reflecting back light waves, usually of a lower frequency than that absorbed, so that invisible light (e.g. ultraviolet) may become visible.

fluorescent (ˌflooˈresənt) capable of producing fluorescence. *F. screen* a screen that becomes fluorescent when exposed to X-rays. *F. treponemal antibody test* a serological test for syphilis; the first to become positive after infection.

fluoridation (ˌflooraˈdayshən) the adding of fluoride compounds to water, in those areas where it is lacking, in order to reduce the incidence of dental caries. Fluoride compounds may also be added to tooth paste as a caries preventative.

fluoride (ˈflooried) *symbol* F. Any binary compound of fluorine. *F. dental treatment* the delivery of fluoride compounds topically to the teeth to reduce the incidence of dental caries.

fluoroscope (ˈflooraˌskohp) an instrument for the study of moving internal organs and contrast medium using X-rays.

flush (flush) a redness of the face and neck. *Hectic f.* one occurring in conditions such as septic poisoning and pulmonary tuberculosis. *Hot f.* one occurring during the menopause, accompanied by a feeling of heat.

flutter (ˈflutə) an irregularity of the heartbeat.

focus (ˈfohkəs) 1. the point of convergence of light or sound waves. 2. the local seat of a disease. *F. group* small group led by a facilitator, with the aim of generating data on a designated topic through discussion and interaction. A research technique.

focusing (ˈfohkəsing) the ability of the eye to alter its lens power to focus correctly at different distances.

foetus (ˈfeetəs) *see* FETUS.

Foley catheter (ˈfohlee ˈkathətə) *Frederick Foley, American physician, 1891–1966.* Rubber catheter with a balloon tip that is filled with sterile water after it is placed in the bladder. Used for continuous drainage of the bladder.

folic acid (ˈfohlik ˈasəd) one of the VITAMINS of the B complex. Folic acid is involved in the synthesis of amino acids and DNA; its deficiency causes megaloblastic anaemia. Green vegetables, liver and yeast are major sources. *F. a. antagonist* any antimetabolite cytotoxic drug that inhibits the action of the folic acid enzyme.

folie à deux (foˈlee ə ˌdər) [Fr.] the occurrence of identical psychoses simultaneously in two closely associated persons.

follicle (ˈfolikəl) a very small sac or gland. *Graafian f.* a vesicular ovarian follicle. *See* GRAAFIAN FOLLICLE. *Hair f.* the sheath in which a hair grows. *F. stimulating hormone (FSH)* a hormone, produced by the anterior pituitary gland, which controls the maturation of the Graafian follicles in the ovary.

follicular (fəˈlikyələ) pertaining to a follicle. *F. conjunctivitis* inflammation occurring in the lower conjunctival fornix. *F. tonsillitis* tonsillitis arising from infection of the tonsillar follicles.

folliculosis (fəˌlikyəˈlohsəs) an abnormal increase in the number of lymph follicles. *Conjunctival f.* a benign non-inflammatory overgrowth of follicles of the conjunctiva of the eyelids.

fomentation (ˌfohmenˈtayshən) treatment by warm, moist applications; also, the substance thus applied.

fomes (ˈfohmeez) *see* FOMITES.

fomites (fəˈmieteez, ˈfohmə-) inanimate objects or material on which disease-producing agents may be conveyed.

fontanel (ˌfontəˈnel) a soft membranous space between the cranial bones of an infant (*see* figure, p. 185). *Anterior f.* that between the parietal and frontal bones, which closes at about the age of 18 months. Rickets causes delay in this process. *Posterior f.* the junction of the occipital and parietal bones, at the sagittal suture, which closes within 3 months of birth.

food (food) anything which, when taken into the body, serves to nourish or build up the tissues or to supply body heat. *F. additives see* ADDITIVES. *F. allergy* sensitivity to one or more of the components of a normal diet, e.g. peanuts, cow's milk or eggs. The reaction to the allergen usually occurs within a short period of ingesting the trigger food and includes lip swelling, vomiting, abdominal distension and diarrhoea. Serious allergies can cause anaphylactic shock requiring an injection of adrenaline. The only effective treatment is total avoidance of the offending food. *See* ANAPHYLAXIS. *F. intolerance* an adverse reaction to a food or to a specific food ingredient that

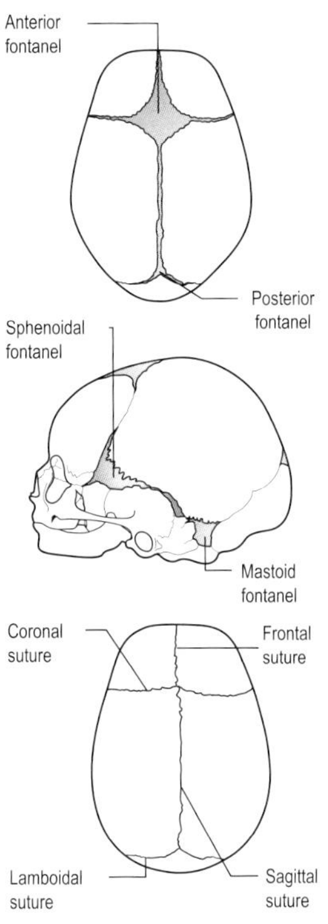

The fontanels.

occurs each time the substance is ingested that is not due to food poisoning or involves the immune system. The specific cause of food intolerance may be difficult to trace, others more recognisable, e.g. lactose intolerance is due to a genetic deficiency of the enzyme lactase needed for the digestion of lactose in milk. *F. poisoning* a group of notifiable acute illnesses caused by ingestion of contaminated food. It may result from toxaemia from foods, such as those inherently poisonous or those contaminated by poisons, foods containing poisons formed by bacteria or food-borne infections. Food poisoning usually causes inflammation of the gastrointestinal tract (gastroenteritis). This may occur quite suddenly, soon after the food has been eaten. The symptoms are acute, and include tenderness, pain or cramps in the abdomen, nausea, vomiting, diarrhoea, weakness and dizziness. *See* BOTULISM.

Food Standards Code (food standərdz kohd) a code that sets legal requirements to ensure food in Australia and New Zealand is safe and suitable for consumers to eat. It includes standards for food additives, food safety, labelling and foods that need pre-approval, such as genetically modified foods.

foot (fuht) the terminal part of the lower limb. *Athlete's f.* ringworm of the foot; tinea pedis. *F. drop* inability to keep the foot at the correct angle owing to paralysis of the flexors of the ankle. *F. presentation* the presentation of one or both legs instead of the head during labour.

foramen (fə'raymən) an opening or hole, especially in a bone. *F. magnum* the hole in the occipital bone through which the spinal cord passes. *F. ovale* the hole between the left and right atria in the fetus. *Obturator f.* the large hole in the innominate bone. *Optic f.* the opening in the posterior part of the orbit through which the optic nerve and the ophthalmic artery pass.

forceps (ˈfawseps) surgical instruments with two opposing blades used for lifting or compressing an object. *Artery f.* (*Spencer Wells f.*) compress bleeding points during an operation. *Cheatle f.* long forceps for lifting utensils. *Obstetric f.* used in difficult labour to assist delivery of the fetal head. *Vulsellum f.* have claw-like ends for exerting traction.

foreign body (forən bodee) any object or substance found in an organ or tissue in which it does not belong under normal circumstances, e.g. dust or a small piece of metal in the eye.

forensic (fəˈrenzik, -sik) pertaining to or applied in legal proceedings. *F. medicine* the branch that is concerned with the law and has a bearing on legal problems. It includes the investigation of unexplained death or injury. *F. psychiatry* the consideration of current mental health laws and their relationship to mental healthcare and the consideration of issues such as diminished responsibility and fitness to stand trial. Mental health nurses work closely with the justice system and courts for offenders with mental health problems.

foreskin (ˈfawˌskin) a loose fold of skin that covers the end of the penis or clitoris. Its removal constitutes circumcision. Also called PREPUCE.

forgetfulness (ˌfawˈgetfəlnəs) the inability to remember or recall events, appointments, objects, etc. that make for daily life. Failure to retrieve memories may occur as a normal result of inattention, although it is a common difficulty that develops with increasing age. In the older person, worsening forgetfulness may be associated with the development of dementia.

formaldehyde (fawˈmaldəˌhied) a gaseous compound with strongly disinfectant properties. It is used in solution (formol) for disinfection of excreta and utensils and also in the preparation of toxoids from toxins.

formula (ˈfawmyələ) [L.] 1. an expression, using numbers or symbols, of the composition of a compound; an expression of directions for preparing such a compound, such as a medicine; an expression of the procedure to follow to obtain a desired result; or an expression of a single concept. 2. a mixture for feeding an infant, composed of milk and/or other ingredients.

formulary (ˈfawmyələ·ree) a prescriber's handbook of drugs. *Prescribing f. for midwives* The Nursing and Midwifery Board of Australia (NMBA) has the power to endorse the registration of suitably qualified midwives to prescribe and/or supply NMBA approved schedule 2, 3, 4 and 8 medicines for the management of women and their infants in the antenatal, intrapartum and postnatal stages of pregnancy and birth.

fornix (ˈfawniks) an arch. *Conjunctival f.* the reflection of the conjunctiva from the eyelids onto the eyeball. *F. cerebri* an arched structure at the back and base of the brain. *F. of the vagina* the recesses at the top of the vagina in front (*anterior f.*), back (*posterior f.*) and sides (*lateral f.*) of the cervix uteri.

fossa (ˈfosə) a small depression or pit. Usually applied to fossae in bones. *Cubital f.* the triangular depression at the front of the elbow. *Iliac f.* the depression on the inner surface of the iliac bone. *Pituitary f.* the depression in the sphenoid bone. *See* SELLA TURCICA.

Fothergill's operation (ˈfothəˌgilz ˌopəˈrayshən) *William Fothergill,*

British gynaecologist, 1865–1926. A technique used in gynaecological surgery for prolapse of the uterus by fixation of the cardinal ligaments and shortening the cervix. The aim is to reduce the cystourethrocele and to reposition the uterus within the pelvis. Also known as Manchester repair or operation.

fourchette (faw'shet) [Fr.] the fold of membrane at the perineal end of the vulva.

fovea ('fohvi·ə) a fossa; a small depression. *F. centralis* an area at the centre of the retina which contains a large number of cones, giving form and colour to vision; the area of most accurate vision.

Fowler's position ('fowləz pə'zishən) *George Fowler, American surgeon, 1848–1906.* The position of a patient lying face up with the head of the bed elevated 45° to 60° and with the knees slightly elevated.

fracture ('frakchə) 1. to break apart, especially a bone. 2. a break in the continuity of bone. The signs and symptoms are pain, swelling, deformity, shortening of the limb, loss of power, abnormal mobility and CREPITUS. Fractures are generally caused by trauma, by either a direct or an indirect force on the bone. Fractures may also be caused by muscle spasm or by disease that results in decalcification of the bone. The different types and classification of fractures are shown in the figure on p. 188. *March f.* a hairline crack in the long bone of the foot caused by repeated trauma associated with long marches and with jogging. Also known as fatigue or stress fracture. *Pathological f.* one due to weakening of the bone structure by pathological processes, such as NEOPLASIA, OSTEOMALACIA or OSTEOMYELITIS. *Pott's f.* a fracture dislocation of the ankle involving the lower end of the fibula and sometimes the internal malleolus of the tibia. *Spontaneous f.* one that occurs as a result of little or no violence, usually of a bone weakened by disease.

frailty (fray'əltee) associated with age-related decline and characterised by a combination of fatigue, weakness, malnutrition and greater vulnerability to stressors. It is also an indicator of poorer health outcomes in older adults. *Clinical F. Scales* assessment tools for assessing elderly patients at risk of having frailty and consider a person's physical performance, nutritional status, cognition, mental health and health assets.

frame (fraym) a rigid supporting structure or a structure for immobilising a part. *Braun f.* a metal frame used to elevate the lower limb in fractures of the tibia and fibula. *Quadriplegic standing f.* a device for supporting in the upright position a patient whose four limbs are paralysed. *Stryker f.* one consisting of canvas stretched on anterior and posterior frames, on which the patient can be rotated around the longitudinal axis. *Walking f.* a walking aid with three or four legs. *Zimmer f. see* ZIMMER.

freckle ('frekəl) a brown pigmented spot on the skin. *Hutchinson's melanotic f.* a non-invasive malignant melanoma which occurs mainly on the faces of middle-aged women.

free association (free ə,sohsee'-ayshən) in psychoanalysis, a spontaneous mental process whereby words used in a non-logical chain suggest ideas, thoughts or feelings without selection or repression.

freedom of information (freedəm ov infaw'mayshən) all jurisdictions within Australia have enacted

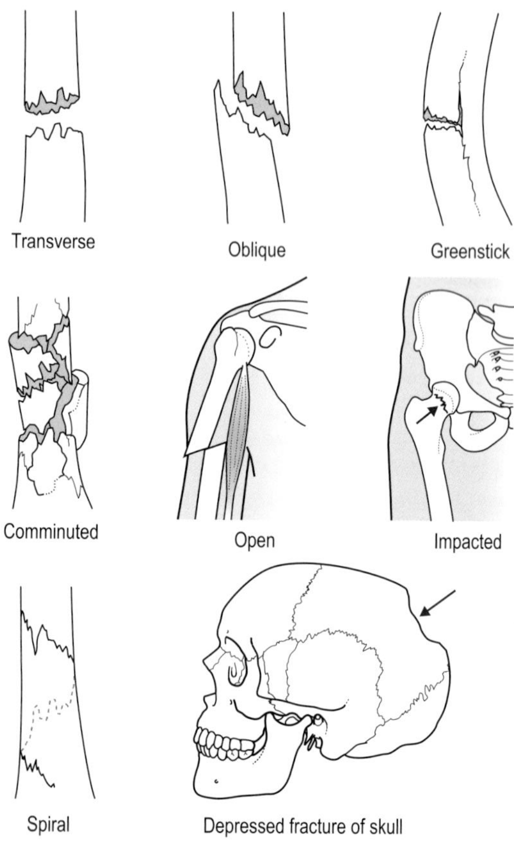

Fractures of bones.

legislation that provides individuals with accessibility to documents including health records. Access is usually governed by Acts, such as the *Freedom of Information Act 1982* (C'wlth) and the *Health Records and Information Privacy Act 2002* (NSW), which provide conditions under which access can be obtained.

Frei's test (friez ˌtest) *Wilhelm Frei, German dermatologist, 1885–1943.* An intradermal test to aid the diagnosis of LYMPHOGRANULOMA VENEREUM.

Freiberg's disease (friebərgz di'zeez) *Albert Freiberg, American surgeon, 1868–1940.* OSTEOCHONDRITIS of the second metatarsal bone, in which there is pain on walking and standing.

frenotomy (frə'notəmee) the cutting of the frenulum of the tongue to cure tongue-tie.

frenulum ('frenyələm) frenum; a fold of mucous membrane which limits the movement of an organ. *F. of the tongue* the fold under the tongue.

Freudian ('froydee·ən) *Sigmund Freud, Austrian psychiatrist, 1856–1939.* Relating to the theories of Freud, who was the originator of psychoanalysis and the psychoanalytical theory of the cause of neurosis.

friable ('frieəbəl) easily crumbled or torn.

friction ('frikshən) the act of rubbing one object against another. *F. massage* a circular or transverse pressure applied by fingertip or thumb to a localised area. Used for the relief of pain. *F. murmur* the grating sound heard in auscultation when two rough surfaces rub together, as in dry pleurisy.

Friedländer's bacillus ('freedˌlendəz bə'siləs) *Karl Friedländer, German pathologist, 1847–1887.* The cause of a rare form of pneumonia. *Klebsiella friedländeri.*

Friedreich's ataxia or disease ('freedrieks ə'taksi·ə aw di'zeez) *Nikolaus Friedreich, German physician, 1825–1882.* A rare form of hereditary ATAXIA.

frigidity (frə'jidətee) an absence of normal sexual desire; usually refers to women.

Frölich's syndrome ('frərliks 'sinˌdrohm) *Alfred Frölich, Austrian neurologist, 1871–1953.* A group of symptoms associated with disease of the pituitary body: increased adiposity, atrophy of the genital organs and development of feminine characteristics. Also known as adiposogenital dystrophy.

frontal ('frunt'l) 1. relating to the forehead. 2. relating to the front or anterior aspect of a structure.

frostbite ('frostˌbiet) impairment of circulation chiefly affecting the fingers, the toes, the nose and the ears due to exposure to severe cold. The first stage is represented by chilblains. Advanced cases show thrombosis and dry gangrene.

frottage (fro'tahzh) [Fr.] 1. a rubbing movement in massage. 2. sexual gratification by rubbing against another person's body.

frozen shoulder ('frohzən 'shohldə) inflammation between the joint capsule and the peripheral articular shoulder cartilage that causes pain whether in motion or at rest; also called adhesive capsulitis. Treatment may include stretching under anaesthesia, combined with exercises. The cause is unknown.

frozen watchfulness ('frohzən 'wochfuhlnes) the state of a young child who is unresponsive to its surroundings, but is clearly aware of them. The state of frozen watchfulness is usually a marker of child abuse.

fructose (ˈfruktohs, -tohz, ˈfruhk-) fruit sugar, a monosaccharide.

FSH *see* FOLLICLE-STIMULATING HORMONE.

fugue (fyoog) a period of altered awareness during which a person may wander for hours or days and perform purposive actions although memory for the period may be lost. It may follow an epileptic fit or occur in hysteria or schizophrenia.

fulguration (ˌfulgyəˈrayshən) the destruction of tissue by diathermy.

fulminating (ˈfuhlməˌnayting, ˈful-) sudden in onset and rapid in course.

fumigation (ˌfyooməˈgayshən) disinfection by exposure to the fumes of a vaporised germicide.

function (ˈfungkˌshən) 1. the natural action or intended purpose of a person, organ or structure. 2. to perform special work or an action.

fundus (ˈfundəs) the base of an organ or the part furthest removed from the opening. *F. of the eye* the posterior part of the inside of the eye as shown by an ophthalmoscope. *F. of the stomach* that part above the cardiac orifice. *F. of the uterus* the top of the uterus; that part furthest from the cervix.

fungal infection of the nail (ˈfungˈgul ˈinˈfekshən of the ˈnayl) an infection of the horny cutaneous plates of fingers and toes. It is difficult to treat and management is with local or systemic anti-fungal medication. Also called ONYCHOMYCOSIS or *tinea unguium*.

fungate (ˈfungˌgayt) to grow rapidly and produce fungus-like growths. Often occurs in the late stages of malignant tumours.

fungicide (ˈfunjəˌsied) a preparation that destroys fungal infection.

fungiform (ˈfunjəˌfawm) shaped like a fungus or mushroom.

fungus (ˈfungˌgəs) a low form of vegetable life which includes mushrooms and moulds. Some varieties cause disease, such as ACTINOMYCOSIS and ringworm.

funnel chest (ˈfun'l chest) a developmental deformity in which there is a depression in the sternum and an inward curvature of the ribs and costal cartilages.

funnel-web spider (funəl web spiedə) a medium to large, black venomous spider from the *Atrax* and *Hadronyche* genera. Clinical symptoms develop quickly after systemic envenomation and resemble a catecholamine storm with profuse sweating, piloerection, hypertension, tachycardia and painful muscle spasm. First aid management includes pressure and immobilisation. This must be carried out immediately. These strategies compress surface tissues and reduce muscle movement, inhibiting lymphatic flow. Deaths are uncommon. Specific antivenom is available.

furor (ˈfyooˌraw) a state of intense excitement during which violent acts may be performed. This may occur after an epileptic fit.

furuncle (ˈfyooˌrungkəl) a boil.

furunculosis (fyəˌrungkyəˈlohsəs) a staphylococcal infection represented by many, or crops of, boils.

furunculus (fyəˈrungkyələs) a furuncle. *F. orientalis* a protozoal infection, mainly of the tropics, which causes a chronic ulceration. Cutaneous LEISHMANIASIS.

fusiform (ˈfyoozəˌfawm) shaped like a spindle.

fusion (ˈfyoozhən) 1. the union between two adjacent structures. 2. the coordination of separate images of the same object in the two eyes into one image.

Gg

g symbol for *gram*.

G symbol for *guanine*.

Ga symbol for *gallium*.

gag (gag) 1. an instrument placed between the teeth to keep the mouth open. 2. the reflex action that occurs when the back of the throat is stimulated.

gait (gayt) manner of walking. *Ataxic g.* the foot is raised high, descends suddenly, and the whole sole strikes the ground. *Cerebellar g.* a staggering walk indicative of cerebellar disease. *Four-point g.* a method that may be adopted when using sticks or crutches, which allows maximum stability. *Spastic g.* stiff, shuffling walk, the legs being kept together.

galactorrhoea (ˌgaləktəˈreeə) 1. an excessive flow of milk. 2. secretion of milk after breastfeeding has ceased.

galactosaemia (gəˈlaktəˈseemi·ə) an inborn error of metabolism in which there is an inability to convert galactose to glucose. This rare genetic disorder becomes apparent soon after birth and is characterised by feeding problems, vomiting, diarrhoea, abdominal distension, enlargement of the liver and intellectual disability. Treatment consists of exclusion from the diet of milk and all foods containing galactose or lactose.

galactose (gəˈlaktohz, -ohs) a monosaccharide derived from lactose. D-galactose is found in lactose or milk sugar and cerebrosides of the brain. *G. tolerance test* a laboratory test to determine the liver's ability to convert the sugar galactose into glycogen.

gall (gawl) bile, a digestive fluid secreted by the liver and stored in the gallbladder.

gallbladder (ˈgawlˌbladə) the sac under the lower surface of the liver which acts as a reservoir for bile. *See also* GALLSTONE.

gallium (ˈgali·əm) *symbol* Ga. A radioisotope used in detecting some soft tissue disorders. *G. scan* a radioactive isotope of gallium may be administered intravenously in a total body scan to detect metastatic spread, lymphomas or a focus of infection.

gallop rhythm (ˈgaləp ˈrithəm) heart rhythm that may occur when there is ventricular overload.

gallstone (ˈgawlˌstohn) a concretion formed in the gallbladder or bile ducts. Gallstones vary in size and may be multiple and faceted. *G. colic see* BILIARY COLIC.

gamete (ˈgameet) a sex cell which combines with another to form a zygote, from which a complete organism develops; a SPERMATOZOON or an OVUM.

gamete intrafallopian transfer (GIFT) (gameet ˌintrəˈfalohpeeən transfə) a technique for assisting conception. The woman must have at least one patent fallopian tube. Oocytes and spermatozoa are mixed in the laboratory and introduced into a fallopian tube, and the fertilised egg may then become embedded in the uterus. The GIFT procedure is used less nowadays with current advances in in vitro fertilisation (IVF) techniques.

gametocyte (gə'meetoh,siet) a cell that is undergoing gametogenesis.

gametogenesis (,gameetoh'jenəsəs) the production of gametes by the gonads.

gamma ('gamə) the third letter in the Greek alphabet. *G. camera* an apparatus for depicting a part of the body into which radioactive isotopes emitting gamma rays have been introduced. *G. encephalography* a method of localising a brain tumour by using radioactive isotopes emitting gamma rays. *G. globulin* a class of plasma proteins composed almost entirely of IgG, an IMMUNOGLOBULIN protein that contains most antibody activity. *G. rays* electromagnetic rays, of shorter wavelength and with greater penetration than X-rays, which are given off by certain radioactive substances and which are used in radiotherapy. Also used in the sterilisation of articles that would be destroyed by the heat and moisture required in autoclaving.

ganglion ('gang·glee·ən) 1. a collection of nerve cells and fibres forming an independent nerve centre, as found in the sympathetic nervous system. 2. a cystic swelling on a tendon.

ganglionectomy (,gang·glee·ə'nek-təmee) excision of a ganglion.

gangrene ('gang·green) death of body tissue, generally in considerable mass, due either to loss of blood supply or to the effects of certain infections. *Dry g.* occurs gradually and results from slow reduction of blood flow in the arteries. There is no subsequent bacterial decomposition; the tissues become dry and shrivelled. It occurs only in the extremities, and can occur with ARTERIOSCLEROSIS and DIABETES MELLITUS. *Gas g.* serious wound infection resulting from wounds/lacerations infected by anaerobic bacteria, especially species of *Clostridium*, a soil microbe often found in the intestines of humans and animals. It is an acute, severe and painful condition in which muscles and subcutaneous tissues become filled with gas and a serosanguineous exudate. It is fatal without appropriate antibiotics and supportive therapy. *Moist g.* is caused by sudden stoppage of blood, resulting from burning by heat or acid, severe freezing, physical accident that destroys the tissue or a clot or other embolism. At first, tissue affected by moist gangrene has the colour of a bad bruise, is swollen and is often blistered. The gangrene is likely to spread with great speed. Toxins are formed in the affected tissues and absorbed.

Ganser's syndrome (state) ('ganzəz 'sindrohm ('stayt)) *Sigbert Ganser, German psychiatrist, 1853–1931.* Amnesia, disturbance of consciousness and hallucinations, associated with senseless answers to questions and absurd acts. Usually a transient response to a troublesome situation, e.g. prisoners on remand (prison psychosis).

gargle ('gahgəl) 1. a solution for rinsing the mouth and throat. 2. to rinse the mouth and throat by holding a solution in the open mouth and agitating it by expulsion of air from the lungs.

gargoylism ('gahgoy·lizəm) *see* HURLER'S SYNDROME.

gas (gas) molecules of a substance combined very loosely; a vapour. *G. and air analgesia* an authorised form of analgesia using nitrous oxide and air, by which the pains of labour are lessened without affecting uterine contractions. *Laughing g.* nitrous oxide. *Marsh g.* methane. *Sternutatory g.* one that causes sneezing. *Tear g.* one that is irritating to the eyes and causes excessive lacrimation.

Gasser's ganglion (ˈgasəz ˈgang·glee·ən) *Johann Gasser, Austrian anatomist, 1723–1765.* The trigeminal ganglion. The ganglion of the sensory root of the fifth cranial nerve.

gastrectomy (gaˈstrektəmee) excision of part or whole of the stomach. It is performed to remove a malignancy or to stop haemorrhage in a perforation of the stomach wall. *Sleeve g.* used to treat people with potentially life-threatening obesity. Surgery reduces the stomach size by up to 75%, resulting in a reduction in volume of the stomach, reducing satiety and causing an inability to eat large amounts of food, subsequently resulting in weight loss.

gastric (ˈgastrik) pertaining to the stomach. *G. analysis* analysis of the stomach contents by microscopy and tests to determine the amount of acid present. *G. band* a silicone band placed around the top portion of the stomach reducing the need to eat as much food to feel full. Also known as a lap band or LAGB (laparoscopic adjustable gastric band). Used in the treatment of obesity. *G. bypass* surgical creation of a small gastric pouch that empties directly into the JEJUNUM through a gastrojejunostomy, thereby causing food to bypass the duodenum; performed for the treatment of morbid OBESITY. *G. flu* a popular term for what may be any of several disorders of the stomach and intestinal tract. The symptoms are nausea, diarrhoea, abdominal cramps and fever. *G. juice* the clear fluid secreted by the glands of the stomach to assist digestion. It contains an enzyme called pepsin, which acts upon proteins in the presence of weak hydrochloric acid. *G. lavage* a treatment for some types of poisoning where the stomach contents are washed out through a stomach tube. *G. ulcer* ulceration of the gastric mucosa, associated with hyperacidity and often precipitated by *Helicobacter pylori* organisms. The condition is often aggravated by stress.

gastrin (ˈgastrin) a hormone, secreted by the walls of the stomach, which excites continued secretion of digestive juice while food is in the stomach.

gastritis (gaˈstrietəs) inflammation of the lining of the stomach.

gastro-oesophagostomy (ˌgastroh·-əˌsofəˈgostəmee) a surgical anastomosis between the stomach and the oesophagus.

gastrocnemius (ˌgastrokˈneemee·əs) the principal muscle of the calf of the leg. It flexes both the ankle and the knee.

gastrocolic (ˌgastrohˈkolik) pertaining to the stomach and colon. *G. reflex* after a meal, increased peristalsis causes the colon to empty into the rectum. This gives rise to a desire to defecate.

gastroduodenostomy (ˌgastroh-ˌdyooədeeˈnostəmee) a surgical anastomosis between the stomach and the duodenum.

gastroenteritis (ˌgastrohˌentəˈrietəs) inflammation of the stomach and intestines causing episodes of nausea, vomiting, appetite loss, fever, abdominal pain and diarrhoea.

A mild episode usually only lasts a few days but a severe one may cause dehydration, shock and collapse, especially in children and older people. The illness may be caused by any one of a number of organisms: bacteria, bacterial toxins, viruses and other organisms in food and water.

gastroenterology (ˌgastrohˌentə'roləjee) the study of diseases of the gastrointestinal tract.

gastroenterostomy (ˌgastrohˌentə'rostəmee) a surgical anastomosis between the stomach and small intestine.

gastroileac (ˌgastroh'ileeak) pertaining to the stomach and ileum. *G. reflex* food entering the stomach sets up powerful peristalsis in the ileum and opening of the ileocaecal valve.

gastrointestinal (ˌgastroh·in'testə-n'l) pertaining to the stomach and intestine. *G. tract* the alimentary tract.

gastrojejunostomy (ˌgastrohˌjejə'nostəmee) a surgical anastomosis between the stomach and the JEJUNUM.

gastro-oesophageal reflux (gastroh-ohsofəgee'l 'reefluks) a backflow of contents of the stomach into the oesophagus, which is often the result of the lower oesophageal sphincter not closing properly and stomach contents leaking back, or reflux, and therefore producing burning pain in the oesophagus. Repeated episodes of reflux may cause oesophagitis. In uncomplicated cases, treatment includes lifestyle changes and regular administration of antacid medication. Also known as GORD.

gastroparesis ('gastrəˌparee'sis) a chronic digestive condition where the stomach cannot empty solids or liquids properly; caused by damage to nerves and muscle.

gastroscope ('gastrəˌskohp) a fibre optic endoscope especially designed for passage into the stomach to permit examination of its interior.

gastrostomy (ga'strostəmee) the creation of an opening into the stomach. This surgical procedure is done to provide for the administration of food and liquids when stricture of the oesophagus or other conditions make swallowing impossible. *See* ARTIFICIAL FEEDING.

gastrotomy (ga'strotəmee) a surgical incision of the stomach.

gastrula ('gastrələ) an early stage in the development of the fertilised ovum.

gate control theory of pain (gayt ˌkən'trohl thiəree ov payn) theory proposing that a neural mechanism in the dorsal horns of the spinal cord acts like a gate that can increase or decrease the flow of nerve impulses from peripheral fibres to the central nervous system. It is the position of the gate that determines how much information is transmitted to the brain and therefore the amount of pain generated. Influences, such as anxiety and anticipation, cause the gate to open and therefore increase the level of pain experienced, whereas other factors may cause the gate to close, thereby reducing the pain.

gatekeepers ('gaytˌkeepəz) the individuals or groups in an organisation who regulate access to goods and services, e.g. a general practitioner's receptionist.

gateway drug (gaytway drug) generic name for less deleterious drugs, such as ALCOHOL, TOBACCO or CANNABIS, referring to their supposed roles as conduits leading on to the taking of harder drugs like COCAINE or amphetamines.

Gaucher's disease (gho'shayz di'zeez) *Phillipe Gaucher, French physician, 1854–1918*. A rare familial disease in which fat is deposited in the reticuloendothelial cells, causing an enlarged spleen and anaemia.

gauze (gawz) a thin, open-meshed material used for dressing wounds.

gavage ('gavahzh) [Fr.] forced feeding; the giving of fluids and nourishment by oesophageal or other type of tube directly into the stomach.

gay (gay) 1. popular term for a homosexual, usually male. 2. pertaining to homosexuality. *G. bowel syndrome* the damaging effects of male homosexual practices on the lower bowel; also includes anal fissures, anal fistulas, haemorrhoids and ulcers.

Geiger counter ('giegə 'kowntə) *Hans Geiger, German physicist, 1882–1945*. An instrument for detecting and registering radioactivity. The apparatus is sensitive to the rays emitted.

gelatin ('jelətən) an albuminoid, obtained from connective tissue or bone. Used in pharmacy for suppositories and capsules, and in bacteriology as a culture medium. It is used in surgical procedures in absorbable film and sponge forms.

gender ('jendə) the perceived differences between the two sexes that generate social differentiation, inequality, discrimination and prejudice. Gender refers to social and cultural differences rather than biological differences between men and women. *G. identity* the concept or inner feeling that a person has of being male and masculine or female and feminine. Differentiation of gender identity begins in infancy, continues through childhood and is reinforced in adolescence. This includes parental attitudes and expectations, as well as psychological and social pressures. *G. identity disorders* a term used for those disorders marked by a persistent sense of a mismatch between one's experienced gender and assigned gender. Also known as gender dysmorphia and gender dysphoria.

gene (jeen) one of the biological units of inheritance that is composed of a sequence of DNA and occupies a specific position (locus) on a particular chromosome. Genes control the characteristics that an offspring will have by transmitting information in the sequence of nucleotides on short sections of DNA. *Dominant g.* one that is capable of transmitting its characteristics, irrespective of the genes from the other parent. *G. therapy* the use of 'healthy' genes, the process being known as somatic-gene cell therapy, to cure or treat a hereditary disease. *Recessive g.* one that can pass on its characteristics only if it is present with a similar recessive gene from the other parent. *See* MENDEL'S THEORY.

general anaesthesia (jenrəl ˌanəs'theezi·ə) the practice of administering medications either by injection or by inhalation to bring about a state of controlled and temporary loss of sensation or awareness. It is carried out to permit medical and surgical procedures to be undertaken that would otherwise be unbearably painful for the patient.

general practice (jenrəl ˌpraktis) a medical specialty providing person-centred, continuing, comprehensive and coordinated whole-person healthcare to individuals and families in their communities.

general practitioner (GP) (jenrəl ˌprak'tishənə) a general practice physician whose practice consists of providing ongoing care covering a variety of medical problems in patients of all ages, often including referral to appropriate specialists. GPs play a central role in the delivery of healthcare in the Australian community.

generalised anxiety disorder (GAD) (jenrəl'iezd ˌang'zieətee ˌdə'sawdə) a type of anxiety disorder characterised by excessive and uncontrollable anxiety and worry that often impacts on everyday life.

generic (jə'nerik) 1. pertaining to a genus. 2. non-proprietary, relating to a drug name not protected by a trademark, usually descriptive of the drug's chemical structure.

genetic (jə'netik) 1. pertaining to reproduction or to birth or origin. 2. inherited. *G. code* the arrangement of genetic material stored in the DNA molecule of the chromosome. *G. counselling* supportive service for prospective parents who can receive advice as to the likelihood of their children being born with a genetically transmitted disorder. *G. engineering* the alteration of a genome of an organism to change its heritable characteristics. In practice, this technique currently is used to mass produce a variety of drugs and vaccines used in medical treatment, e.g. growth hormone and human insulin. Further development offers enormous scope for the advancement of medicine in the treatment of disease and genetic disorders. *G. screening* 1. tests used to screen individuals whose genotypes are associated with specific diseases. These individuals may develop the disease itself or pass it on to their offspring. 2. testing a specific population for the presence of a genetic disease, e.g. testing neonates for cystic fibrosis.

genetics (jə'netiks) the study of heredity and natural development.

genital herpes (ˌjen'ital 'hərpeez) caused by the herpes simplex virus (HSV types 1 or 2) and presents with painful blisters on or around the genitalia and transmitted through sexual contact.

genital warts ('jenˌit'l 'wawtz) small fleshy lumps appearing on the genitalia, caused by strains of the human papillovirus (HPV) and transmitted through sexual contact.

genitalia ('jenəˌtayliə') the male and female reproductive organs. Also called genitals.

genitourinary (ˌjenitoh'yoo·rienə·ree) referring to both the reproductive organs and the urinary tract.

genome ('jeenohm) the complete set of genes in the chromosomes, including DNA in chromosomes, as well as the DNA in mitochondria.

genotype ('jenohˌtiep, 'jeenoh-) the genetic characteristics of an individual, either over the genome as a whole or at one particular locus.

genu ('jenyoo) [L.] the knee. *G. valgum* knock-knee. *G. varum* bowleg.

genupectoral (ˌjenyoo'pektə·rəl) relating to the knee and chest. *G. position* the knee–chest position. *See* POSITION.

genus ('jeen'əs) a taxonomic rank used in biological classifications of living organisms.

geriatrics (ˌjeree'atriks) the branch of medicine covering older people and the disorders arising from it.

germ (jərm) 1. a microbe. 2. that from which something may develop; a seed.

German measles (ˈjərmən ˈmeezəlz) *see* RUBELLA.

germicide (ˈjərməˌsied) an agent capable of destroying pathogenic microorganisms.

germinoma (ˌjərməˈnohmə) a neoplasm of the testis or ovum.

gerontology (ˌjeronˈtoləjee) the study of the changes associated with older people and the ageing processes. Includes both mind and body and involves many disciplines, e.g. psychology, sociology, pharmacology, biology and social care.

gestaltism (gəˈshtaltizəm) a theory of holism in psychology which claims that ideas come as a whole and are not subdivisible.

gestation (jeˈstayshən) the period of development of the young in mammals, from the time of fertilisation of the ovum to birth. *See also* PREGNANCY. *Ectopic g.* fetal development in some part other than the uterus, usually the uterine tube. *G. period* the duration of pregnancy; in the human female about 280 days when measured from the first day of the last menstrual period. *See also* EXPECTED DATE OF DELIVERY.

gestational diabetes (jeˈstay·shənˈəl ˌdieəˈbeeteez) any degree of glucose intolerance first recognised during pregnancy. It usually resolves following birth, but women who have had the condition should be screened annually as they have a greater risk of developing type 2 diabetes.

gestational trophoblastic disease (jeˈstayshənˈəl ˈtrofəˌblastik diˈzeez) a group of pregnancy-related tumours arising from the tissue that helps form the placenta during pregnancy.

Ghon focus (gon ˈfohkəs) *Anton Ghon, Czechoslovakian pathologist, 1866–1936*. The primary lesion of pulmonary tuberculosis, as seen on chest radiograph, after it has healed by fibrosis and calcification.

giant cell arteritis (ˈjieənt ˈsel ahtəˈrietəs) a condition in which the medium and large arteries in the scalp, head and neck become inflamed. Also known as temporal arteritis.

giardiasis (ˌjiahˈdieəsəs) *Alfred Giard, French biologist, 1846–1908*. An infection with *Giardia lamblia*, a pear-shaped protozoon that causes a persistent protracted diarrhoea, often resulting in intestinal malabsorption.

gigantism (ˈjieganˌtizəm, jieˈgantizəm) abnormal condition characterised by excessive size and stature. It is most often caused by the hypersecretion of growth hormone (GH).

Gilbert's syndrome (ˈgilbərtz ˈsinˌdrohm) a relative mild condition where higher levels of bilirubin build up in the blood leading to episodes of jaundice.

Gilles de la Tourette's syndrome (disease) (ˌzheel də lah tooˈrets ˈsinˌdrohm (diˈzeez)) *Georges Gilles de la Tourette, French neurologist, 1857–1904*. Multiple tics, especially of the face and upper part of the body, and in some cases is associated with involuntary obscene utterances. The condition usually has its onset in childhood and often becomes chronic. The cause is unknown, but the disorder is likely to be passed down through families. Also called Tourette's syndrome.

gingiva (ˈjinjəvə, jinˈjievə) the gum; connective tissue surrounding the necks of the teeth.

gingivectomy (ˌjinjəˈvektəmee) the surgical removal of the gum margins to eliminate periodontal pockets and improve the shape of the gums. Performed to stop the progress of periodontal disease.

gingivitis (ˌjinjəˈvietəs) inflammation of the gums.

ginkgo (gingkoh) a herbal extract from the maidenhair tree, *Ginkgo biloba*, used by herbalists and naturopaths and claimed to be helpful in circulatory disorders, reduced circulation in the brain, senility, depression and premenstrual syndrome.

ginseng (ginseng) extract from the root of plants of genus *Panax*, used widely in Chinese medicine, reputed to have the power to cure many diseases and to have properties to improve sexual health and impotence.

gland (gland) an organ composed of cells which secrete fluid prepared from the blood, either for use in the body or for excretion as waste material. *Ductless* (endocrine) *g.* one that produces an internal secretion but has no canal (duct) to carry the secretion away, e.g. the thyroid gland. *Exocrine g.* one that discharges its secretion through a duct, e.g. the parotid gland. *Lymph g. see* LYMPH NODES. *Mucous g.* one that secretes mucus.

glanders (ˈglandəz) a disease of horses communicable to humans and caused by the bacterium *Burkholderia mallei*.

glandular (ˈglandyələ) pertaining to a gland. *G. fever see* INFECTIOUS MONONUCLEOSIS.

glans (glanz) an acorn-shaped body, such as the rounded end of the penis or the clitoris.

Glasgow Coma Scale (GCS) (ˌglazgoh kohmə skayl) a standardised system for quickly evaluating the level of consciousness in the critically ill. Measures include: eye opening according to four (4) criteria, verbal response against five (5) criteria and motor response using six (6) criteria, giving a possible total GCS of 15, which reflects a patient who is alert, aware and orientated, whereas the lowest possible GCS is 3, which indicates a deeply unconscious patient. Generally classifications are—severe: GCS score of 3–8, moderate: GCS 9–12 and mild: GCS 13–14. Any patient who has a declining or waxing and waning GCS in any setting needs to be reported to the responsible clinician immediately and further management decisions should be considered in the context of the patient's overall clinical picture.

glaucoma (glawˈkohmə) raised intraocular pressure. *Closed-angle g.* one that occurs when there is a mechanical defect in the drainage angle; may be primary or secondary. It may be acute, when there is pain and blurring of vision, or chronic, when there may be no pain, but a gradual loss of vision. *Open-angle g.* chronic primary glaucoma in which the angle remains open but drainage becomes gradually diminished; tends to run in families. *Primary g.* one that occurs without any previous disease. It is a common cause of blindness, partial or complete, in older people. *Secondary g.* one that occurs when some ocular disease is complicated by an increase in intraocular pressure.

gleet (gleet) chronic gonococcal URETHRITIS marked by a transparent mucous discharge.

glenoid (ˈgleenoyd) resembling a hollow. *G. cavity* the socket of the shoulder joint.

glia (ˈglieə) neuroglia; the connective tissue of the brain and spinal cord.

glioblastoma (ˌglieohˈblastohmə) a malignant GLIOMA arising in the cerebral hemispheres.

glioma (glieˈohmə) a malignant tumour composed of neuroglial cells affecting the brain and spinal cord; seldom metastasises.

globulins (ˈglobyələns) a protein group, forming constituents of the blood (*serum g.*) and cerebrospinal fluid.

globus (ˈglobəs) a ball or globe. *G. hystericus* a symptom of hysteria whereby a patient feels unable to swallow because there is a lump in the throat. *G. pallidus* the pale medial part of the lentiform nucleus of the brain.

glomerulitis (gloˌmeryəˈlietəs) inflammation of the glomeruli of the kidney.

glomerulonephritis (gloˌmeryəloh-nəˈfrietəs) a bilateral, non-infectious inflammation of the kidneys. The cause is unknown but the condition is associated with immunological disturbance. It may be acute, presenting rapidly but reversibly, or it may be chronic, presenting slowly and irreversibly.

glomerulosclerosis (gloˌmeryəloh-skləˈrohsəs) degenerative changes in the glomerular capillaries of the renal tubule, leading to renal failure.

glomerulus (gloˈmeryələs) the tuft of capillaries within the nephron, which filters urine from the blood.

glossal (ˈglosəl) relating to the tongue.

glossitis (gloˈsietəs) inflammation of the tongue.

glossolalia (ˌglosəˈlayli·ə) 'speaking in tongues'; unintelligible speech. The patient speaks in an imaginary language.

glossopharyngeal (ˌglosohfəˈrinji·əl, -ˌfarənˈji·əl) pertaining to the tongue and pharynx. *G. nerve* the ninth cranial nerve.

glossoplegia (ˌglosohˈpleeji·ə) paralysis of the tongue.

glottis (ˈglotəs) the space between the vocal cords. The term is sometimes used for that part of the larynx which is associated with voice production.

glucagon (ˈglookəˌgon) a polypeptide produced by the pancreas. It stimulates the conversion of glycogen to glucose in the liver and raises the blood sugar level. Glycogen secretion is stimulated by hypoglycaemia and by growth hormone in the anterior pituitary gland. A crystallised glucagon preparation is used in the treatment of severe hypoglycaemia.

glucocorticoid (ˌglookohˈkawtəˌ-koyd) any corticoid substance that raises the concentration of liver glycogen and blood sugar, i.e. cortisol (hydrocortisone), cortisone and corticosterone.

gluconeogenesis (ˌglookohˌneeoh-ˈjenəsəs) the production of glucose from the non-nitrogen portion of the amino acids after deamination. It occurs in the liver and kidneys.

glucose (ˈglookohs, -kohz) a simple sugar, a monosaccharide in certain foodstuffs, especially fruit, and in normal blood; the chief source of energy for living organisms. *See also* DEXTROSE. *G.-6-phosphate dehydrogenase* (G6PD) a red-cell enzyme. Inherited deficiency that occurs most often in males and causes a tendency to haemolytic anaemia. *See* FAVISM. *G. tolerance test* test in which a quantity of glucose is given and the concentration of glucose in the blood is estimated at intervals afterwards (*see* figure, p. 200). Used mainly when DIABETES MELLITUS is suspected.

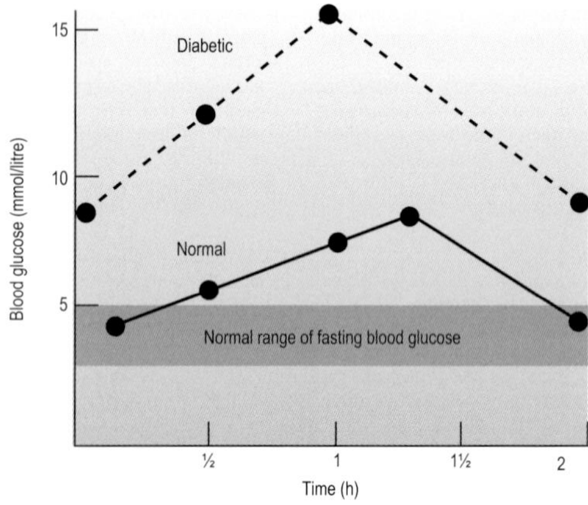

Glucose tolerance test.

glue ear (ˈgloo iə) the accumulation of sticky glue-like material in the middle ear resulting in impaired hearing; most common in young schoolchildren. Glue ear often follows repeated ear infections, and can affect hearing and lead to other problems. Also known as middle ear effusion.

glue sniffing (ˈgloo ˌsnifing) solvent abuse.

glutamic acid (glooˈtamik ˈasəd) one of the 22 amino acids formed by the digestion of dietary protein. *g. a. decarboxylase (GAD) autoantibody* an antibody found in patients with type 1 diabetes mellitus.

glutamic oxaloacetic transaminase (glooˈtamik oksəloh·əˈseetik tranzˈaməˌnayz) an enzyme found in cardiac muscle and the liver. Raised serum levels (SGOT) may indicate an acute MYOCARDIAL INFARCTION or the presence of liver disease.

glutamic pyruvic transaminase (glooˈtamik pieˈroovik tranzˈ-aməˌnayz) an enzyme found in the liver. Measurement of serum levels (SGPT) is used in the study and diagnosis of liver diseases.

glutaraldehyde (ˌglootəˈraldəˌhied) a disinfectant active against all viruses, fungi, vegetative bacteria and spores. Used in aqueous solution for sterilisation of non-heat-resistant equipment.

glutaric aciduria type 1 (ˌglooˈtarikˌ asəˈdyooreeə ˌtiep wun) a rare inherited condition characterised by an inability to process certain amino acids, such as lysine, hydroxylysine and tryptophan. Babies are tested for the condition as part of newborn screening. The condition can be treated with diet and medication.

gluteal (ˈglooteeəl, glooˈti·əl) relating to the buttocks. *G. muscles* three muscles that form the fleshy part of the buttocks.

gluten (ˈglootən) a sticky protein found in wheat and other cereals, e.g. rye and barley. Gluten consists of two proteins: gliadin and glutenin. Some people are sensitive to gluten, which causes in them intestinal malabsorption (gluten-induced enteropathy). *G.-induced enteropathy* COELIAC DISEASE.

glycaemia (glieˈsee·miə) the presence of glucose in the blood. Hyperglycaemia and hypoglycaemia imply higher and lower blood glucose levels than usual, respectively.

glycaemic index (GI) (glieˈseemik ˈindeks) the classification of carbohydrate foods based on their overall effects on blood glucose levels. Carbohydrate foods are ranked from 1 to 100. Foods with a low GI factor, e.g. wholegrain cereals, raise blood glucose levels a little and are absorbed more slowly and evenly, whereas those with a high GI factor, e.g. refined flours and sugars, raise blood glucose levels sharply and considerably. Low-level GI diets have been shown to improve blood glucose and lipid levels in people with type 1 and type 2 diabetes mellitus.

glycerin (ˈglisəˌrin) a colourless syrupy substance obtained from fats and fixed oils. It has a hygroscopic action. As an emollient, it is an ingredient of many skin preparations. *G. suppository* one composed of glycerin and gelatin, used as an evacuant. *G. of thymol* an antiseptic mouthwash and gargle.

glycine (ˈglieseen) a non-essential amino acid.

glycogen (ˈgliekəjən) the form in which carbohydrate is stored in the liver and muscles; animal starch. *G. storage disease* inherited disease in which there is a deficiency in the synthesis of glycogen. This accumulates in the liver, causing enlargement.

glycogenesis (ˌgliekohˈjenəsəs) the process of glycogen formation from the blood glucose.

glycogenolysis (ˌgliekəjəˈnoləsəs) the breakdown of glycogen to glucose in the body so that it may be utilised.

glycosuria (ˌgliekohˈsyoo·ri·ə) an excess of glucose in the urine, a symptom of DIABETES MELLITUS. *Renal g.* sugar in the urine, in an otherwise healthy person, due to a rare inherited inability to reabsorb glucose normally.

glycosylated haemoglobin (GHb or HbA_{1c}) (glieˈkohsəlaytəd ˌheeməˈglohbən) a haemoglobin A molecule with a glucose group on the terminal amino acid unit of the beta chain. The HbA_{1c} concentration represents the average blood glucose level over the previous 3 months. It is used to assess the level of blood glucose control of people with DIABETES MELLITUS.

gnathic (ˈnathik) pertaining to the jaw.

goal (gohl) a statement of what a nursing intervention or activity is expected to achieve in either the short or the longer term. May also be referred to as an outcome. *See* NURSING.

goblet cell (ˈgoblət ˌsel) a goblet-shaped cell, found in the intestinal epithelium, which produces mucus.

goitre (ˈgoytə) an enlarged thyroid gland usually evident as a pronounced swelling in the front of the neck. The thyroid gland may enlarge (without any disturbance of its function) at puberty, during pregnancy or as a result of taking oral contraceptives. In many parts of the world the main cause of a goitre is a lack of iodine in the diet. *Exophthalmic g.* hyperthyroidism with marked protrusion of the eyeballs (exophthalmos). GRAVES' DISEASE may lead to thyrotoxicosis and weight loss is often reported.

gold (gohld) *symbol* Au. A metallic element used in treating rheumatoid arthritis. *Radioactive g.* an isotope that gives off beta and gamma rays. Used in the form of small grains or seeds in some malignant conditions.

Golgi apparatus (ˈgoljee, ˈgolgee ˌapəˈrahtəs) *Camillo Golgi, Italian histologist, 1844–1926.* Specialised structures seen near the nucleus of a cell on microscopic examination.

Golgi's organ (golgees awgən) the sensory end-organs in muscle tendons that are sensitive to stretch.

gonad (ˈgohnad, ˈgonad) a reproductive gland; the testicle or ovary.

gonadotrophic (ˌgonədəˈtrohfik) having influence on the gonads. *G. hormone* GONADOTROPHIN.

gonadotrophin (ˌgonədəˈtrohfən) any hormone having a stimulating effect on the gonads. Two such hormones are secreted by the anterior pituitary: follicle-stimulating hormone (FSH) and luteinising hormone (LH), both of which are active, but with differing effects, in the two sexes. *Chorionic g.* a gonad-stimulating hormone produced by CYTOTROPHOBLASTIC cells of the placenta; used in the treatment of underdevelopment of the gonads and to induce ovulation in infertile women.

gonioscope (ˈgohneeohˌskohp) an apparatus for examining the angle of the anterior chamber of the eye.

goniotomy (ˌgohneeˈotəmee) an operation for glaucoma; it consists in opening Schlemm's canal under direct vision.

gonococcus (ˌgonəˈkokəs) *Neisseria gonorrhoeae*, a diplococcus which causes GONORRHOEA.

gonorrhoea (ˌgonəˈreeə) a common sexually transmitted disease caused by *Neisseria gonorrhoeae* infecting the genital tract and most often transmitted during sexual activity, including anal and oral sex. An infected woman may also transmit the disease to her baby during childbirth. Spread by the bloodstream, it may give rise to iritis or arthritis. Scar tissue formation may bring about urethral stricture or infertility owing to occlusion of the uterine tubes. Gonorrhoea has an incubation period of 2–10 days. In men, symptoms include a discharge from the urethra and dysuria. Many infected women have no symptoms.

gonorrhoeal (ˌgonəˈreeəl) relating to gonorrhoea. *G. arthritis* intractable infection of joints, causing great pain and disability.

goose-flesh (goos flesh) the reaction of the skin to cold and fear. The blood vessels and hair follicles in the skin contract causing the hair to stand up giving the impression of plucked poultry skin. Also known as goose pimples.

GORD *see* GASTRO-OESOPHAGEAL REFLUX.

gout (gowt) a hereditary form of arthritis with an excess of uric acid in the blood. It is characterised by painful inflammation and swelling of the smaller joints, especially those of the big toe and thumb. Inflammation is accompanied by the deposit of urates around the joints.

GP *see* GENERAL PRACTITIONER.

Graafian follicle (ˈgrahfi·ən ˈfolikəl) *Regnier de Graaf, Dutch physician*

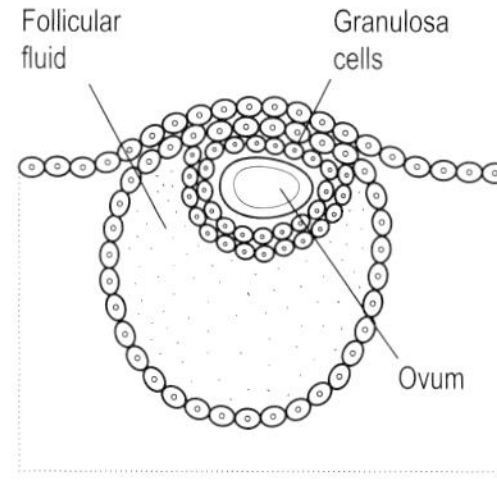

Graafian follicle.

and anatomist, 1641–1673. A follicle which is formed in the ovary and contains an ovum (*see* figure). A follicle matures during each menstrual cycle, ruptures and releases the ovum (ovulation), which is then picked up by the fimbriated end of the uterine tube.

graft (grahft) 1. any tissue or organ for implantation or transplantation. 2. to implant or transplant such tissue. *Allogenic g.* a graft from a compatible donor. Also known as allograft or homograft. *Autogenous g.* a graft taken from and given to the same individual. *Bone g.* a portion of bone transplanted to repair another bone. *Corneal g.* a portion of cornea, usually from a recently deceased person, used to repair a diseased cornea. *Homologous g.* tissue obtained from the body of another animal of the same species but with a genotype differing from that of the recipient; a homograft or allograft. *Pedicle g.* a skin graft, one end of which remains attached to its original site until the grafting has become established.

graft-versus-host disease (GvHD) (ˌgrahftvərsəzˈhohst diˈzeez) may follow a successful transplant. A condition that occurs when immunologically competent cells or their precursors are transplanted into an immunologically incompetent recipient (host) that is not histocompatible with the donor. Characteristic signs include skin lesions, ulceration, alopecia, painful joints and haemolytic anaemia. G_VHD disease is a frequent complication of bone marrow transplants, but can be prevented by the giving of immunosuppressant drugs and use of corticosteroid drugs. Human leucocyte antigen (HLA) matching of the donor and recipient reduces the possibility of G_VHD. G_VHD does not occur with stem cell transplants. Also called graft-versus-host reaction (G_VHR).

gram (gram) *symbol* g. The fundamental SI unit of weight, equal to one-thousandth of a kilogram

Gram stain (gram stayn) *Hans Gram, Danish physician, 1853–1938*. A method of staining bacteria which is used to classify them into Gram-negative and Gram-positive.

grand mal (ˌgronh ˈmal) [Fr.] former name for tonic clonic seizures. *See* EPILEPSY.

grand multipara (grand multeepahrah) a woman who has borne five or more children. Increasing parity can lead to an increased risk of problems in pregnancy, labour and the puerperium.

granular (ˈgranyələ) containing small particles. *G. casts* the degenerated cells from the lining of renal tubules excreted in the urine in certain kidney disorders.

granulation (ˌgranyəˈlayshən) 1. the division of a hard solid substance into small particles. 2. the growth of new tissue by which ulcers and wounds heal when the edges are not in apposition. It consists of new capillaries and fibroblasts which fill in the space and later form fibrous tissue. The resulting scar is often unsightly.

granulocyte (ˈgranyələˌsiet) any cell containing granules in its cytoplasm, especially POLYMORPHONUCLEAR leucocytes which contain neutrophilic, basophilic and eosinophilic granules in their cytoplasm.

granulocytopenia (ˌgranyəloh-ˌsietəˈpeeni·ə) a marked reduction in the number of granulocytes in the blood. The condition may precede AGRANULOCYTOSIS.

granuloma (ˌgranyəˈlohmə) a tumour composed of granulation tissue, usually due to chronic infection or invasion by a foreign body.

granulomatosis (ˌgranyəˌlohməˈ-tohsəs) an infection producing GRANULOMATA. *Lipoid g.* xanthomatosis; Hand–Schüller–Christian disease. *Malignant g.* lymphadenoma; Hodgkin's disease.

gravel (ˈgravəl) small 'sandy' calculi formed in the kidneys and bladder, and sometimes excreted with the urine. They can also form in the gallbladder, where they may accumulate or cause low-grade CHOLECYSTITIS.

Graves' disease (grayvz diˈzeez) *Robert Graves, Irish physician, 1796–1853.* An autoimmune disease that affects the thyroid gland leading to hyperthyroidism. Formally known as exophthalmic goitre.

gravid (ˈgravəd) pregnant.

gravida (ˈgravidə) a woman who is pregnant.

gravity (ˈgravətee) weight. *Specific g.* the weight of a substance compared with that of an equal volume of water.

gray (gray) *symbol* Gy. The SI unit used to denote the absorbed dose in radiation therapy.

grey-scale display (ˈgrayˌskayl dəˈsplay) a method to show the texture of tissue on ULTRASOUND display. The amplitude of each echo is represented by varying shades of grey. A bright white outline is seen from specular surfaces, a mottled grey outline from various tissue areas, and a black outline from collections of fluid, such as the bladder and AMNIOTIC sac.

grey syndrome (ˈgrayˌ sinˌdrohm) a potentially fatal condition seen in preterm babies caused by a reaction to the drug chloramphenicol. Characterised by ashen grey cyanosis, vomiting, abdominal distension, hypothermia and shock.

grid (grid) a chart with horizontal and vertical lines on which curves may be plotted.

grief (greef) *see* BEREAVEMENT.

groin (groyn) the junction of the upper thigh with the abdomen. The groins slope outwards and upwards from the pubic region.

grounded theory (ˈgrowndəd ˌthiəree) a qualitative research approach which emphasises the process of theory generation from systematically collected and stored data, the concept being that the theory remains 'grounded in' the data, demonstrating the fit between the theory and the supporting empirical evidence.

group practice (groop praktis) a team of healthcare professionals working together in a local setting including general practitioners, nurses, midwives, pharmacists and counsellors.

group therapy (groop ˈtherəpee) a form of psychotherapy in which a group of patients meets regularly with a therapist in order to discuss and share problems, anxieties and fears in a psychotherapeutic setting. The group also provides emotional support for self-revelation and a structured environment for trying out new ways of relating to people.

growing pains (ˈgroh·ing paynz) recurrent quasi-rheumatic limb pains peculiar to early youth, once believed to be caused by the growing process. It is now recognised that growth does not cause pain and that these pains can be a symptom of many different disorders.

growth (grohth) 1. the progressive development of a living thing, especially the process by which the body reaches its point of complete physical development. 2. an abnormal formation of tissue, such as a tumour. *G. hormone* a substance that stimulates growth, especially a secretion of the anterior lobe of the PITUITARY gland that directly influences protein, carbohydrate and lipid metabolism, and controls the rate of skeletal and visceral growth.

guanine (ˈgwahneen) a purine base, one of the constituents of all nucleic acids.

guardian *ad litem* (ˈgahdi·ən ad ˈleetəm) a person, usually from the local authority social service department, who is appointed by a court to look after the interests of a child before the child's full Adoption Order is granted. Meanwhile the prospective adoptive parents have continuous possession of the child, and are visited and interviewed by the guardian *ad litem* to ensure that the home will be satisfactory.

guided imagery (giedəd iməjəree) a complementary therapy that uses pleasant mental images of events, feelings or sensations as a distraction method in coping with pain.

Guillain-Barré syndrome (ˌgiyanhˈ-baray sinˌdrohm) *Georges Guillain, French neurologist, 1876–1961; Jean Barré, French neurologist, 1880–1967.* Acute infective POLYNEURITIS. After an infection, usually respiratory, there is a general weakness or paralysis which frequently affects the respiratory muscles as well as the peripheral muscles.

guilt (gilt) feelings of self-blame and reproach causing distress to the individual, who believes that they have contravened accepted cultural, moral and ethical standards of behaviour. A deep, lasting and sometimes seemingly inappropriate sense of guilt is often a feature of psychiatric disorder.

guinea-worm (ˈgineeˌwərm) a nematode worm, *Dracunculus medinensis*, which burrows into human tissues, particularly into the legs or feet.

Gulf War syndrome (gulf waw ˈsinˌdrohm) experienced by military personnel during the Gulf War and later wars as a variety of symptoms including chronic fatigue, muscle and joint pains, headaches, memory loss, depression and irritability. Possibly due to chemical exposure (e.g. to insecticides or nerve gas) or the interaction of multiple vaccinations and drugs given to protect personnel from the perceived threat of chemical or biological warfare combined with prolonged fatigue and stress. Also known as Gulf War illness.

gumboil (ˈgumˌboyl) the opening on the gum of an abscess at the root of a tooth.

gumma (ˈgummə) a soft, degenerating tumour characteristic of the tertiary stage of syphilis. It may occur in any organ or tissue.

gustatory (gu'staytə·ree) relating to taste.

gut (gut) the intestine.

Guthrie test ('guthree ˌtest) *Robert Guthrie, microbiologist, 1916–1995.* 1. a sensitive screening test for phenylketonuria. 2. test performed on a small amount of blood, usually taken from the heel stab and carried out on a neonate between the 6th and 14th days of life to diagnose PHENYLKETONURIA.

gutta ('gutə) a drop. *G. percha* the juice of a tropical tree which, when dried, forms an elastic semisolid substance. Used in dentistry as a root filler.

GvHD *see* GRAFT-VERSUS-HOST DISEASE.

Gy symbol for *gray*.

gynaecologist (ˌgienə'koləˌjəst) one who specialises in the healthcare of women, including diseases of the female reproductive organs and breasts.

gynaecology (ˌgienə'koləjee) the science of those diseases that are peculiar to the female reproductive organs including the breasts.

gynaecomastia (ˌgienəkoh'masti·ə) excessive growth of the male breast.

gypsum ('jipsəm) plaster of Paris (calcium sulphate).

gyrus ('jierəs) a convolution, as of the cerebral cortex.

Hh

H symbol for *hydrogen*.

H5N1 virus that causes a virulent strain of AVIAN INFLUENZA.

habit (habit) automatic response to a specific situation acquired as a result of repetition and learning. *Drug h.* drug addiction. *H. forming* drugs that may lead to physiological addiction. *H. retraining* technique used by nurses to retrain patients in the process for control of micturition. The patient is encouraged to void at set times according to an agreed baseline chart, but may use the toilet at other times. *H. training* a method used in psychiatric nursing whereby deteriorated patients can be rehabilitated and taught personal hygiene by constant repetition and encouragement.

habilitation (ˌhəˈbilətayshən) the process of assisting a person with a disability, with the means to keep, learn or improve skills to maximum independence in activities of daily living. Services may include occupational therapy, speech pathology, pain management, audiology and other services that are offered in a variety of hospitals and outpatient settings.

habituation (həˌbichyooˈayshən) the gradual adaptation to a stimulus or to the environment. The acquisition of a habit, e.g. a condition resulting from the repeated consumption of a drug, but with little or no tendency to increase the dose; there may be psychological but no physical dependence on the drug.

haemangioblastoma (heeˌman-jeeohblaˈstohmə) a brain tumour consisting of a proliferation of capillaries and of disorganised clusters of capillary cells or angioblasts, usually occurring in the cerebellum.

haemangioma (ˌheemanjeeˈohmə) a benign tumour formed by dilated blood vessels. *Strawberry h.* a birthmark, which may become very large, but frequently disappears in a few years.

haemarthrosis (ˌheemahˈthrosəs) an effusion of blood into a joint.

haematemesis (ˌheeməˈteməsəs) vomiting of blood. If it has been in the stomach for some time and become partially digested by gastric juice, it is of a dark colour and contains particles resembling coffee grounds.

haematin (ˈheemətən) the iron-containing part of haemoglobin.

haematocele (ˈheemətohˌseel) a swelling produced by effusion of blood, e.g. in the sheath surrounding a testicle or a broad ligament.

haematocrit (ˈheemətohˌkrit, hiˈ-mətə-) the volume of red cells in the blood. Usually expressed as a percentage of the total blood volume.

haematology (ˌheeməˈtoləjee) the science dealing with the nature, functions and diseases of blood.

haematoma (ˌheeməˈtohmə) a swelling containing clotted blood.

haematomyelia (ˌheemətohmie-ˈeeli·ə) an effusion of blood into the spinal cord.

haematuria (ˌheemə'tyoo·ri·ə) the presence of blood in the urine due to injury or disease of any of the urinary organs.

haemochromatosis (ˌheemohˌkroh-mə'tohsəs) a condition in which there is high absorption and deposition of iron leading to a high serum level, pigmentation of the skin and liver failure. Also known as bronze diabetes.

haemoconcentration (ˌheemoh-ˌkonsən'trayshən) a loss of circulating fluid from the blood resulting in an increase in the proportion of red blood cells to plasma. The viscosity of the blood is increased.

haemodialysis (ˌheemohdie'aləsəs) the removal of waste material from the blood of a patient with acute or chronic renal failure by means of a dialyser or artificial kidney. The apparatus is coupled to an artery and dialysis is achieved by the blood and rinsing fluid (dialysate) passing through a semipermeable membrane. Blood is returned through a vein.

haemoglobin (Hb) (ˌheemə'glohbən) the complex protein molecule contained within the red blood cells which gives them their colour and by which oxygen is transported.

haemoglobinopathy (ˌheeməˌgloh-bə'nopəthee) any one of a group of hereditary disorders, including sickle-cell ANAEMIA and THALASSAEMIA, in which there is an abnormality in the production of haemoglobin.

haemolysin (hee'moləsən) a substance that destroys red blood cells.

haemolysis (hee'moləsəs) the disintegration of red blood cells. Excessive haemolysis, which may produce anaemia, may be caused by injection with viruses or bacteria, drugs, chemicals and incompatible blood transfusions.

haemolytic (ˌheemə'litik) having the power to destroy red blood cells. *H. disease of the newborn* a condition associated with an Rh-negative pregnant woman with an Rh-positive fetus. *See* RH FACTOR.

haemophilia (ˌheemoh'fili·ə) a condition characterised by impaired coagulability of the blood and a strong tendency to bleed. Over 80% of all patients with haemophilia have haemophilia A (classic haemophilia), which is characterised by a deficiency of clotting factor VIII (8). Haemophilia B (Christmas disease), which affects about 15% of all haemophiliac patients, results from a deficiency of factor IX (9). Inherited as an X-linked recessive trait, it is transmitted by females only, to their male offspring. Bleeding episodes are common and may occur spontaneously, without an obvious cause, or as a result of trauma or injury. In these situations specialised medical treatment with the deficient clotting factor is required to stop the bleeding. Over a period of time bleeding into joints and muscles can cause permanent damage, such as arthritis, chronic pain and joint damage requiring surgery. Before surgery or dental treatment, the patient must be given an infusion of the appropriate clotting factor.

Haemophilus (hee'mofələs) a genus of Gram-negative rod-like bacteria. *H. ducreyi* the cause of soft chancre. *H. influenzae* bacterium that causes various infectious diseases in humans. *H. pertussis* the cause of whooping cough; Bordet-Gengou bacillus.

haemophthalmia (ˌheemofˈthalmi·ə) bleeding into the vitreous of the eye, usually the result of trauma; haemophthalmos.

haemopneumothorax (ˌheemohˌnyoomohˈthaw·raks) the presence of blood and air in the pleural cavity, usually the result of injury.

haemopoiesis (ˌheemohpoyˈeesəs) the formation of red blood cells, which normally takes place in the bone marrow and continues throughout life. *Extramedullary h.* the formation of blood cells other than in the bone marrow, e.g. in the liver or spleen.

haemopoietic (ˌheemohpoyˈetik) relating to red blood cell formation. *H. factors* those necessary for the development of red blood cells, e.g. vitamin B_{12} and folic acid.

haemoptysis (heeˈmoptəsəs) the coughing up of blood from the lungs or bronchi. Being aerated, it is bright red and frothy.

haemorrhage (ˈhemə·rij) an escape of blood from a ruptured blood vessel, externally or internally. Arterial haemorrhage. It involves bright red blood which escapes in rhythmic spurts, corresponding to the beats of the heart. Venous haemorrhage involves dark red blood which escapes in an even flow. Haemorrhage may also be: (a) *primary*, at the time of operation or injury; (b) *reactionary* or recurrent, occurring later when the blood pressure rises and a ligature slips or a vessel opens up; and (c) *secondary*, may be several days after injury, and usually due to sepsis. Special types are as follows. *Antepartum h.* that which occurs before labour starts (*see* PLACENTA PRAEVIA). *Cerebral h.* an episode of bleeding into the cerebrum; one of the three main forms of STROKE. *Concealed h.* collection of the blood in a cavity of the body. *Intracranial h.* bleeding within the cranium, which may be extradural, subdural, subarachnoid or cerebral. *Intradural h.* bleeding beneath the dura mater. It may be due to injury and causes signs of compression. The cerebrospinal fluid will be bloodstained. *Postpartum h.* that which occurs within 12–24 hours of delivery, from the genital tract, and which either measures 500 mL or more or which adversely affects the woman's condition. Secondary postpartum haemorrhage is excessive bleeding more than 24 hours after delivery. *Subgaleal h. (SGH)* a condition found in newborns as a result of rupture of the emissary veins causing blood to accumulate between the epicranial aponeurosis of the scalp and the periosteum. It is a very serious complication of instrumental delivery and is associated with significant morbidity and mortality.

haemorrhagic (ˌheməˈrajik) pertaining to or characterised by haemorrhage. *H. disease of the newborn* a self-limited haemorrhagic disorder of the first days of life, caused by deficiency of vitamin K dependent blood clotting factors II, VII, IX and X. It should be prevented by the prophylactic administration of vitamin K to all newborn babies. *Viral h. fevers* a group of notifiable virus diseases of diverse aetiology but with similar characteristics of fever, headache, myalgia, prostration and haemorrhagic symptoms. They include dengue haemorrhagic fever. *See* MARBURG DISEASE, EBOLA VIRUS DISEASE, LASSA FEVER and YELLOW FEVER.

haemorrhoid (ˈheməˌroyd) a 'pile' or locally dilated rectal vein. Piles may be either external or internal to the anal sphincter. Pain is caused on defecation, and bleeding may occur.

haemorrhoidectomy (ˌhemə·roy-ˈdektəmee) the surgical removal of haemorrhoids.

haemosiderosis (ˌheemohˌsidəˈ-rohsəs) iron deposits in the tissues resulting from excessive haemolysis of red blood cells.

haemostasis (ˌheemohˈstaysəs, heeˈmostəsis) the arrest of bleeding or the slowing up of blood flow in a vessel.

haemostatic (ˌheemohˈstatik) a drug or remedy for arresting haemorrhage; a styptic.

haemothorax (ˌheemohˈthor·raks) blood in the thoracic cavity, e.g. from injury to soft tissues as a result of fracture of a rib.

HAI *see* HEALTHCARE-ASSOCIATED INFECTION.

hair (hair) a delicate, keratinised epidermal filament growing out of the skin. The root of the hair is enclosed beneath the skin in a tubular follicle. Erect hair has a minimal role in thermoregulation of the body. If the body is too cold arrector pili muscles contract in the skin, pulling the hairs upright and trapping an insulating layer of air. *See* GOOSE-FLESH. *H. analysis* used as an adjunct to other tests in preconception care of women to assess nutritional status and detect the concentration of up to 18 metals. High levels of some metals, such as lead, may be associated with congenital abnormalities. Deficiencies of substances such as zinc can be treated with dietary advice and/or supplements. *H. ball see* BEZOAR. *H. loss see* ALOPECIA.

halal (ˈhalˌlal) meat from an animal that has been killed according to Islamic law and is therefore lawful to be eaten by Muslims.

half-life (hahf lief) 1. the time it takes for a substance to decay to one-half of its original value. 2. in pharmacology, the time it takes for the level of a drug to decrease to one-half in the blood. This is used to determine the dosing level required for therapeutic treatment.

half-way house (hahfway hows) a specialised treatment facility, usually for clients with a mental health illness who no longer require complete hospitalisation but who need some care and time to adjust to living independently.

halitosis (ˌhaləˈtohsəs) foul-smelling breath.

hallucination (həˌloosəˈnayshən) a sensory impression (sight, touch, sound, smell or taste) that has no basis in external stimulation. Hallucinations can have psychological causes, as in mental illness, or they can result from drugs, alcohol or organic illnesses, such as brain tumour or senility. People subjected to sensory deprivation or overwhelming physical stress sometimes suffer from temporary hallucinations.

hallucinations rating scale (HRS) (həˌloosəˈnayshəns ˈrayting skayl) a scale that uses 11 items to determine auditory hallucinations in patients. It also assesses the way in which the hallucinations are experienced and controlled by the patient.

hallucinogen (həˈloosənəˌjen) an agent that causes hallucinations, e.g. LSD and cannabis.

hallux (ˈhaləks) the big toe. *H. valgus* a deformity in which the big toe is bent towards the other toes. *H. varus* a deformity in which the big toe is bent outwards away from the other toes.

halo (ˈhayloh) a circular structure, such as a luminous circle seen surrounding an object or light. *Glaucomatous h., h. glaucomatosus* a narrow light zone surrounding the optic disc in glaucoma.

halo effect (ˈhayloh əˈfekt) a beneficial effect noted after a healthcare intervention, visit or research project. The halo effect cannot be attributed to the content of the interview, visit or project, but is the outcome of indefinable factors as a result of the intervention.

halogen (ˈhaləjən) any of the five non-metallic elements: chlorine, iodine, bromine, astatine and fluorine.

halo splint (hayloh splint) an orthopaedic device used to immobilise the head and neck, to assist in the healing of cervical injuries and postoperatively after cervical surgery.

hamartoma (ˌhaməˈtohmə) a benign nodule which is an overgrowth of mature tissue.

hammer (ˈhamə) the malleus. *H. toe* a deformity in which the first phalanx is bent upwards, with plantar flexion of the second and third phalanx.

hamstring (ˈhamˌstring) the flexors of the knee joint that are situated at the back of the thigh.

hand (hand) the terminal part of the arm below the wrist. *Claw h.* a paralytic condition in which the hand is flexed and the fingers contracted, caused by injury to nerves or muscles. *Cleft h.* a congenital deformity in which the cleft between the third and fourth fingers extends into the palm. *H., foot and mouth disease* a mild infectious disease in children, caused by Coxsackie virus, which results in vesicle formation on all three sites. Not the same as foot and mouth disease. *H. washing see* figure p. 212 and Appendix 10. *5 Moments of H. Hygiene* these steps have been identified as some of the most critical times when hand washing needs to be performed, e.g. Step 1 before touching a patient; Step 2 before a procedure; Step 3 after procedures or body fluid exposure risk; Step 4 after touching a patient; and Step 5 after touching a patient's surroundings.

hand–arm vibration syndrome (hand arm ˌvieˈbrayshən ˈsinˌdrohm) pain and numbness with blanching in the hand and arm due to the use of vibrating tools, usually in the workplace. The syndrome tends to develop slowly over time and gangrene may develop. Exposure to cold tends to aggravate the condition.

Hand–Schüller–Christian disease (ˌhandˌ shoolə ˈkrischən diˈzeez) *Alfred Hand, American paediatrician, 1868–1949*; *Arthur Schüller, Austrian neurologist, 1874–1958*; *Henry Christian, American physician, 1876–1951*. A disease of the reticuloendothelial system in which GRANULOMA containing cholesterol is formed, chiefly in the skull.

handicap (ˈhandeeˌkap) a disadvantage for a given individual, resulting from an impairment or a disability that limits or prevents the fulfilment of a role that is normal (depending on age, sex and social and cultural factors) for that individual.

handover (handovə) the transfer of information from the nurses on a shift to the nurses on the following

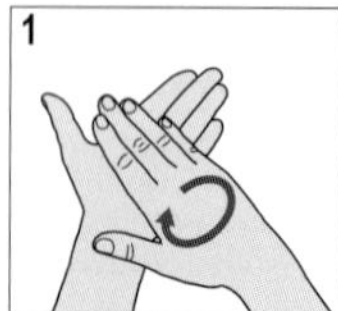

Rub hands palm to palm

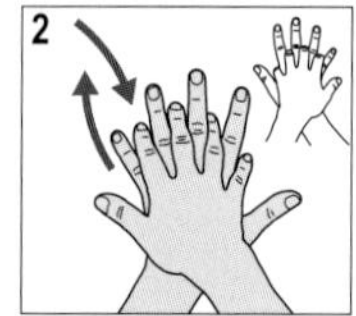

Rub back of each hand with the palm of other hand with fingers interlaced

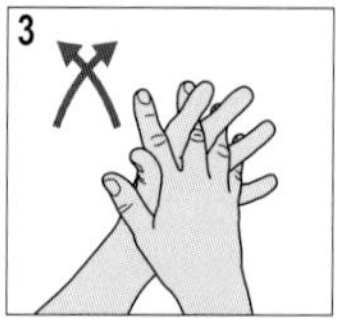

Rub palm to palm with fingers interlaced

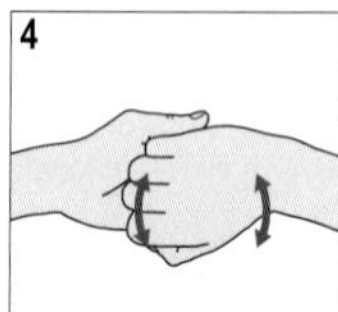

Rub with backs of fingers to opposing palms with fingers interlaced

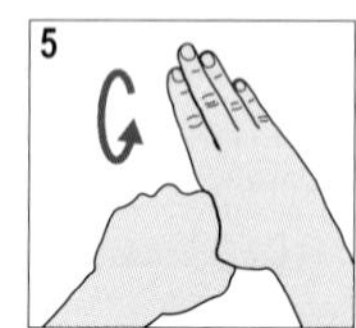

Rub each thumb clasped in opposite hand using rotational movement

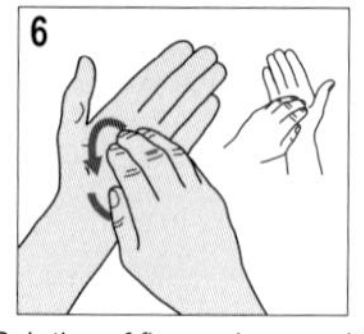

Rub tips of fingers in opposite palm in a circular motion

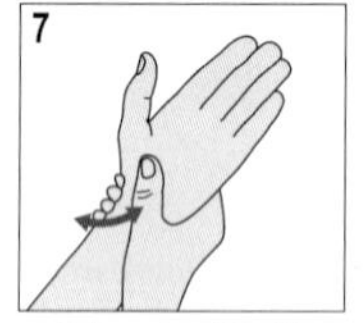

Rub each wrist with opposite hand

Handwashing technique.

shift or before transfer of a patient from one unit to another.

Hansen's disease (ˈhansənz diˈzeez) *Gerhard Hansen, Norwegian physician, 1841–1912.* Leprosy, caused by Hansen's bacillus, *Mycobacterium leprae. See* LEPROSY.

haploid (ˈhaployd) having one set of chromosomes after division instead of two.

harassment (ˌhəˈrasmənt) any repetitive physical or verbal conduct that causes another person alarm or distress, including physically threatening, humiliating, offensive or derogatory acts or utterances. Harassment is unlawful and examples include bullying, workplace violence, sexual harassment, racial, age or gender discrimination and cyberstalking. Harassment can occur in healthcare settings and this may take many forms, but an example is when a consultant, manager or senior professional repeatedly makes derisory or critical comments to another member of staff in front of patients or colleagues, leading to that person losing confidence and feeling powerless in the workplace.

hard drugs (hard drugz) an imprecise term used in relation to drugs that are highly addictive, e.g. heroin or cocaine, and therefore prone to misuse.

Harrison's groove or sulcus (ˈhari-sənz groohv aw ˈsulkəs) *Edward Harrison, British physician, 1789–1838.* A horizontal groove along the lower border of the thorax corresponding to the costal insertion of the diaphragm; seen in rickets.

Hartmann's solution (hartmənz ˌsəˈlooshən) a saline solution containing sodium lactate used intravenously in treating acidosis.

Hartnup disease (ˈhahtnup diˈzeez) a hereditary defect in amino acid metabolism which may produce learning difficulties (named after the first person found to suffer from it).

Hashimoto's disease (ˌhashiˈmoh-tohz diˈzeez) *Hakaru Hashimoto, Japanese surgeon, 1881–1934.* A lymphoadenoid goitre caused by the formation of antibodies to thyroglobulin. It is an autoimmune condition giving rise to HYPOTHYROIDISM.

hashish (ˈhasheesh, -ish) Indian hemp. *See* CANNABIS.

haustration (hawˈstrayshən) a HAUSTRUM or the process of forming one.

haustrum (ˈhawstrəm) any one of the pouches formed by the sacculations of the colon.

Haversian canal (həˈvərsi·ən, -shən kəˈnal) *Clopton Havers, British physician and anatomist, 1650–1702.* One of the minute canals that permeate compact bone, containing blood and lymph vessels to maintain its nutrition. *See* BONE.

Hawthorne effect (ˈhawthawn əˈfekt) the term given to the alteration of behaviour by the subjects of a study due to their awareness of being observed. It was named after an industrial management study in the United States, where the effect was first identified.

hay fever (ˈhayfeevə) an atopic ALLERGY characterised by sneezing, itching, watery eyes, running nose and a burning sensation of the palate and throat. It is a localised reaction to an extrinsic allergen, most commonly pollens and the spores of moulds. When the allergen comes in contact with mast cell bound IgE immunoglobulin in the tissues of the conjunctiva, nasal mucosa and bronchial tree, the cells release mediators such as histamine, which produce the characteristic symptoms of hay fever, including swelling of tissues, itching and sneezing. Also known as allergic rhinitis. *See* ATOPY.

HCA *see* HEALTHCARE ASSISTANT.

HCG human chorionic gonadotrophin. *See* GONADOTROPHIN.

HCl *see* HYDROCHLORIC ACID.

HDU *see* HIGH-DEPENDENCY UNIT.

He *symbol* for *helium*.

head (hed) the anterior or superior part of a structure or organism, in vertebrates containing the brain and the organs of special sense. *H. injury* traumatic injury to the head resulting from a fall or violent blow. Such an injury may be open or closed and may involve a brain CONCUSSION, skull fracture or contusions of the brain. All head injuries are potentially dangerous because there may be a slow leakage of blood from damaged blood vessels into the brain, or the formation of a blood clot which gradually increases pressure against brain tissue. Long-term effects of head injury may include chronic headache, disturbances in mental and motor function and a host of other symptoms that may or may not be psychogenic. Organic brain damage and post-traumatic epilepsy resulting from scar formation are possible sequels to head injury. *H. lice see* PEDICULUS. *H. tilt* or *chin lift* a method of opening the airway in an unconscious patient. One hand is placed upon the forehead to gently tilt the head back. The fingers of the other hand lift the chin. If head or spinal injury is suspected this manoeuvre should NOT be used. (*See* Appendix 6.)

headache (ˈhedˌayk) a pain or ache in the head. A symptom rather than a disorder. It accompanies many diseases and conditions, including emotional distress. *See also* MIGRAINE.

Heaf test (heef ˌtest) *Frederick Heaf, British physician, 1894–1973.* A form of tuberculin testing which has now been replaced by the more commonly used Tuberculin Skin Test (TST); also known as the MANTOUX TEST.

healing (ˈheeling) the process of return to normal function after a period of disease or injury. *H. by first intention* signifies union of the edges of a clean incised wound without visible granulations, and leaving only a faint linear scar. *H. by second intention* union of the edges of an open wound by the formation of granulations from the bottom and sides. *H. by third intention* union of a wound that is closed surgically several days after the injury.

health (helth) the World Health Organisation (WHO) states that 'Health is a state of complete physical, mental and social wellbeing and not merely the absence of disease or infirmity'. *H. assessment* an evaluation made by a healthcare professional of an individual's health status, which takes account of the health history and lifestyle together with the findings of a physical examination. *H. centre* a primary community healthcare organisation for providing ambulatory healthcare and coordinating the efforts of all health agencies, commonly focused around the general practitioner's services. *H. culture* a system that attempts to explain and treat health problems and illness and to maintain health. Part of the wider culture to which people belong, it may be a traditional or a biomedical system. *H. education officer* an officer appointed to make health education resources available to the community. *H. food* used to indicate food thought to promote health. *H. literacy* the degree to which individuals understand essential health information and how they can successfully make use of this information to promote and maintain good health, and make appropriate health decisions. Health literacy is central to an individual's life as low levels of health literacy contribute to poorer health outcomes, increased risk of an adverse event and higher healthcare cost. *H. promotion* a process of enabling people to increase control over, and to improve, their health. It moves beyond individual behaviour to focus on a wide range of social and environmental interventions. Supported by WHO as a process of orientating communities to move health services from a treatment approach to one of prevention. The three key elements defined by WHO are good governance for health, health literacy and healthy cities. *H. services* the term usually employed to signify the system or program by which healthcare is made available to the population and financed by government or private enterprise, or both. *H. statistics* summated data on any aspect of the health of populations, e.g. mortality, morbidity, use of health services, treatment outcome and costs of healthcare. *Holistic h.* a system of preventative medicine that takes into account the whole individual, and that person's own responsibility for wellbeing, with the total influences (social, psychological, environmental) that affect health, including nutrition, exercise and mental relaxation. *Public h.* the organised response by a society to prevent illness, injury and disability and to protect and promote the health of the community as a whole.

health and safety obligation (helth and sayftee obluh'gayshən) the duty of care an employer has under common law to provide employees with a safe work environment. Marked similarities with occupational health and safety (OHS) legislation, which exists in each state and territory of Australia.

healthcare assistant (HCA) (helth kair ˌəsistənt) a support worker in the clinical area who works with the supervision of a registered practitioner responsible for the quality of care delivered by the HCA.

healthcare-associated infection (HAI) (helthkair uh'sohseeaytəd in'fekshən) also known as a nosocomial infection. An infection acquired during an episode of healthcare in either acute (hospital) or non-acute settings, usually as a result of a clinical intervention, such as urinary catheterisation or the insertion of a vascular access device.

healthcare system (helth kair sistəm) an organised plan of health services. The term is usually employed to denote the system or program by which healthcare is made available to the population and financed by government or private enterprise or both. *H. facilities* employ health professionals to manage and treat health-related problems. May include community care, private and public hospitals, home care, day-stay centres and residential aged-care services.

Health Care Complaints Commission (helth kair complayntz kuh'mishən) a statutory body that investigates and conciliates complaints from clients concerning healthcare that they perceive to be harmful.

health education (helth ˌedyoo'kayshən) various methods of education aimed at the prevention of disease; includes the changing of behaviours that have been identified as risk factors for particular diseases. All nurses and midwives have particular responsibilities and opportunities to promote good health.

Health Practitioner Regulation National Law (helth prak'tishənə

ˌregyoo'layshun 'nashnəl law) came into effect in July 2010 and is state- and territory-based legislation. This law applies to those professions regulated under that law and aims to protect the public by establishing a national system for the regulation of health practitioners and students undertaking programs of study leading to registration as a health professional. Also known as the National Law.

hearing ('hiəˌring) the reception of sound waves and their transmission onwards to the brain in the form of nerve impulses. *H. aid* an apparatus, usually electronic, to amplify sounds before they reach the inner ear. *H. screening test* a program to screen infants to detect hearing loss. This program is offered in some states and territories in Australia as soon as possible after birth. The Australian Government also offers screening tests for eligible clients later in life to access hearing services and hearing devices to assist with hearing loss. *H. therapy* the support and rehabilitation of people with hearing difficulties, tinnitus or vertigo. It includes the teaching of lip reading, the use of hearing aids and providing tinnitus retraining therapy.

heart (haht) a hollow, muscular organ which pumps the blood throughout the body, situated behind the sternum slightly towards the left side of the thorax. *H. attack* MYOCARDIAL INFARCTION. *H. block* impairment of conduction in heart excitation; often applied specifically to atrioventricular heart block. *H. failure* a condition in which the heart cannot pump sufficient blood to meet the metabolic requirements of body tissues. *H.–lung machine* an apparatus used to perform the functions of both the heart and the lungs during heart surgery. *H. murmur* an abnormal sound heard in the heart, frequently caused by disease of the valves. Occurs when the blood flow through the heart exceeds a certain velocity. *H. rate* the number of heart beats per minute. The normal resting heart rate is 60–100 beats per minute, and should be monitored for rate, strength and rhythm. *H. sounds* the normal heart sounds correspond to the closure of the four valves of the heart. First heart sound = 'LUB' sound corresponding to the closure of the mitral and tricuspid valves. Second heart sound = 'DUP' sound with closure of the aortic and pulmonary valves. *Maximum h. rate* used in sports medicine to assess an individual's heart during exercise. It is equal to 220 minus the age of the person.

heartburn ('hahtˌbərn) indigestion marked by a burning sensation in the oesophagus, often with regurgitation of acid fluid.

heat (heet) warmth; a form of energy, which may cause an increase in temperature or a change of state, e.g. the conversion of water into steam. *H. exhaustion* a rapid pulse, anorexia, dizziness and cramps in arms, legs or abdomen, sometimes followed by sudden collapse, caused by loss of body fluids and salts under very hot conditions. *H. stroke* a severe, life-threatening condition resulting from prolonged exposure to heat. *See* SUNSTROKE. *Prickly h.* MILIARIA. *H. rash* acute itching caused by blocking of the ducts of the sweat glands following profuse sweating.

hebephrenia (ˌhebə'freeni·ə) a form of schizophrenia characterised by thought disorder and emotional incongruity. Delusions and hallucinations are common.

Heberden's nodes (ˈhebəˌdənz nohdz) *William Heberden, British physician, 1710–1801.* Bony or cartilaginous outgrowths causing deformity of the terminal finger joints in OSTEOARTHRITIS.

hebetude (ˈhebətyood) emotional dullness. A common symptom in dementia and schizophrenia.

hectic (ˈhektik) occurring regularly. *H. fever* a regularly occurring increase in temperature. It is frequently observed in pulmonary tuberculosis. *H. flush* a redness of the face accompanying a sudden rise in temperature.

hedonism (ˈheedəˌnizəm, ˈhed-) excessive devotion to pleasure.

Hegar's sign (ˈhaygərz sien) *Alfred Hegar, German gynaecologist, 1830–1914.* A softening of the isthmus of the uterine cervix that occurs early in gestation. It is a probable sign of pregnancy.

Heimlich manoeuvre (ˈhiemlik mənoovə) *Henry Heimlich, US surgeon, 1920–2016.* Now referred to as ABDOMINAL THRUST.

Helicobacter (helikohbaktə) a genus of spiral and flagellated Gram-negative bacteria. *H. pylori* a species found in the stomach. May cause damage to the prostaglandins protecting the mucosal cells in the stomach wall, leading to progressive gastritis and ulceration.

heliotherapy (ˌheeleeohˈtherəpee) treatment of disease by exposure of the body to sunlight.

helium (ˈheelee·əm) *symbol* He. An inert gas sometimes used in conjunction with oxygen to facilitate respiration in obstructional types of DYSPNOEA and for decompressing deep-sea divers.

helix (ˈheeliks) 1. a spiral twist. Used to describe the configuration of certain molecules, e.g. deoxyribonucleic acid (DNA). 2. the outer rim of the auricle of the ear.

Hellin's law (helinz law) one in about 89 pregnancies ends in the birth of twins; one in 89^2, or 7921, in the birth of triplets; one in 89^3, or 704, 969, in the birth of quadruplets. Assisted reproduction techniques have raised the rate of multiple pregnancies, therefore the formula is less indicative of true incidence.

helminthiasis (ˌhelminˈthieəsəs) an infestation with worms.

hemeralopia (ˌhemə·rəˈlohpi·ə) day blindness. The vision is poor in a bright light but is comparatively good when the light is dim. *See* NYCTALOPIA.

hemianopia (ˌhemi·əˈnohpi·ə) partial blindness, in which the patient can see only half of the normal field of vision. It arises from disorders of the optic tract and of the occipital lobe.

hemicolectomy (ˌhemeekohˈlek-təmee) the removal of the ascending and part of the transverse colon with an ileotransverse colostomy (*see* figure, p. 218).

hemiparesis (ˌhemeepəˈreesəs) paralysis on one side of the body; HEMIPLEGIA.

hemiplegia (ˌhemeeˈpleeji·ə, -jə) paralysis of one-half of the body, usually due to cerebral disease or injury. The lesion is on the side of the brain opposite to the side paralysed.

hemisphere (ˈheməsˌfiə) a half sphere; in anatomy, one of the two halves of the cerebrum or CEREBELLUM.

hemp *see* CANNABIS.

Henle's loop (ˈhenleez loop) *Friedrich Henle, German anatomist,*

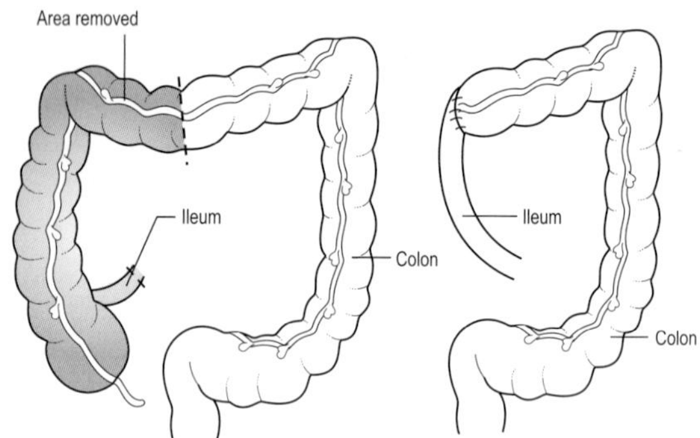

Hemicolectomy and transverse ileocolostomy.

1809–1885. The U-shaped loop of the uriniferous tubule of the kidney.

Henoch -Schönlein purpura (henokh ˈshərnlien ˈpərpyərə) *Eduard Henoch, German paediatrician, 1820–1910. Johann Schönlein, German naturalist/physician, 1793–1864*. Allergic purpura. *See* PURPURA.

heparin (ˈhepə·rən) an anticoagulant formed in the liver and circulated in the blood. Injected intravenously, it prevents the conversion of prothrombin into thrombin, and is used in the treatment of THROMBOSIS.

hepatectomy (ˌhepəˈtektəmee) excision of a part or the whole of the liver.

hepatic (heˈpatik) relating to the liver. *H. flexure* the angle of the colon that is situated under the liver.

hepaticojejunostomy (heˌpatikoh-ˌjejəˈnostəmee) the anastomosis of the hepatic duct to the JEJUNUM, usually created after extensive excision for carcinoma of the pancreas.

hepaticostomy (heˌpateeˈkostəmee) a surgical opening into the hepatic duct.

hepatisation (ˌhepətieˈzayshən) the alteration of lung tissue into a solid mass resembling the liver, which occurs in acute lobar pneumonia.

hepatitis (ˌhepəˈtietəs) inflammation of the liver, characterised by the presence of inflammatory cells in the tissue of the organ. The condition can be self-limiting or can progress to fibrosis and cirrhosis. Hepatitis is acute when it lasts less than 6 months and chronic when it lasts for longer. Worldwide most commonly caused by one of a group of hepatitis viruses, but it can also be due to toxins (alcohol, certain medications, some industrial organic solvents and plants), other infections and autoimmune diseases such as cytomegalovirus infection or Legionnaires' disease. Hepatitis may present with limited or no symptoms, but often leads to jaundice, fever, anorexia and general malaise. *Viral h.* an acute, notifiable, infectious hepatitis caused by one of several different viruses that infect human liver cells, e.g. hepatitis A virus (HAV), hepatitis B virus (HBV), hepatitis C virus (HCV), hepatitis D (Delta virus) and hepatitis E virus (HEV).

hepatogenous (ˌhepəˈtojənəs) arising in the liver. Applied to jaundice in which the disease arises in the parenchymal cells of the liver.

hepatolenticular (ˈhepətohlen-ˈtikyələ) pertaining to the liver and the lentiform nucleus. *H. degeneration* Wilson's disease; a progressive condition, usually occurring between the ages of 10 and 25 years. There are tremors of the head and limbs, pigmentation of the cornea and sometimes defective twilight vision.

hepatoma (ˌhepəˈtohmə) a primary malignant tumour arising in the liver cells.

hepatomegaly (ˌhepətohˈmegəlee) an enlargement of the liver.

hepatosplenomegaly (ˌhepətoh-ˌspleenohˈmegəlee) enlargement of the liver and spleen, such as may be found in KALA-AZAR.

hepatotoxic (ˌhepətohˈtoksik) applied to drugs and substances that cause destruction of liver cells, e.g. alcohol.

herbal medicine (herbəl medəsən) a form of complementary or alternative medicine in which plants are used for their therapeutic properties.

herd immunity (hərd iˈmyoonətee) the immunity of a population. When there is a high enough number of persons in a population immune to a particular infection, the infection fails to spread because of the absence of enough susceptibles. For example, in measles, this could probably be achieved by vaccination of 90–95% of the population.

hereditary (həˈredətree) derived from ancestry; inherited.

heredity (həˈredətee) the transmission of both physical and mental characteristics to the offspring from the parents. Recessive characteristics may miss one or two generations and reappear later.

hermaphrodite (hərˈmafrəˌdiet) an individual whose gonads contain both testicular and ovarian tissue. These may be combined as an ovotestis or there may be a testis on one side and an ovary on the other. The external genitalia may be indeterminate or of either sex. *Pseudo h.* one whose gonads are histologically of one sex, but in whom the genitalia have the appearance of the opposite sex. *True h.* one who possesses both male and female gonads.

hermeneutics (ˌhərməˈnyootiks) the study of meanings in social behaviour and experience. Denotes the art, skill or theory of interpreting human behaviour, speech and writings in terms of intentions and meanings.

hermetic (hərˈmetik) airtight. A wound dressing may be sealed to ensure that the wound is not exposed to air.

hernia (ˈhərni·ə) a protrusion of any part of the internal organs through the structures enclosing them. *Cerebral h.* a protrusion of brain through the skull. *Diaphragmatic h.* and *hiatus h.* a protrusion of a part of the stomach through the oesophageal opening in the diaphragm. *Femoral h.* a loop of intestine protruding into the femoral canal; more common in females.

Hiatus h. see DIAPHRAGMATIC HERNIA. *Incisional h.* a hernia occurring at the site of an old wound. *Inguinal h.* protrusion of the intestine through the inguinal canal. This may be congenital or acquired, and is commoner in males. A rupture. *Irreducible h.* a hernia that cannot be replaced by manipulation. *Reducible h.* a hernia that can be returned to its normal position by manipulative measures. *Strangulated h.* a hernia of the bowel in which the neck of the sac containing the bowel is so constricted that the venous circulation is impeded and gangrene will result if not treated promptly (*see* figure). *Umbilical h.* protrusion of bowel through the umbilical ring. This may be congenital or acquired. *Vaginal h.* RECTOCELE OR CYSTOCELE.

hernioplasty (ˈhərneeohˌplastee) a surgical repair of the abdominal wall performed after reduction of a hernia.

herniorrhaphy (ˌhərneeˈo·rəfee) removal of a hernial sac and repair of the abdominal wall.

herniotomy (ˌhərneeˈotəmee) an operation to remove a hernial sac.

heroin (ˈheroh·ən) a diacetate of morphine used as an analgesic and abused illicitly for its euphoriant effects. The drug readily induces physical dependence and may be sniffed, smoked or injected subcutaneously or intravenously ('shooting up' or 'mainlining'). Street names for heroin include 'smack', 'H' and 'horse'.

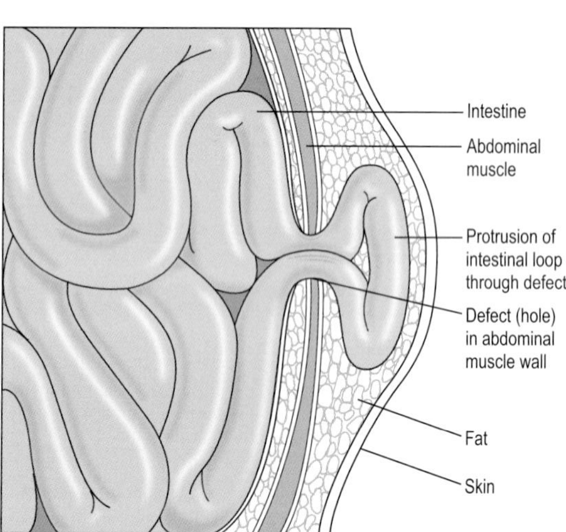

Strangulated hernia.

H. baby a baby that has received regular heroin (morphine) via the placenta before birth and who shows signs of withdrawal after birth. Withdrawal symptoms may persist for 1–4 weeks and include vomiting, abdominal cramps, diarrhoea, sweating, breathing difficulties and hyperactivity.

herpes (ˈhərpeez) an inflammatory skin eruption showing small vesicles caused by a herpes virus. *H. simplex* a viral infection which gives rise to localised vesicles in the skin and mucous membranes and is characterised by latency and subsequent recurrence. It is caused by herpes simplex viruses types 1 and 2. Type 1 infection is common in children and is often symptomless. Type 2 infection is common in older age groups and is associated with sexual activity. Recurrent attacks may occur. Lesions appear on the cervix, vulva and surrounding skin in women, and on the penis in men. In homosexual men, rectal lesions are common. Once the virus enters the body, it stays there for the rest of the person's life. Recurrent attacks are common. To prevent neonatal herpes, caesarean section is usually recommended for women presenting with clinical genital tract herpes within 2 weeks of delivery to avoid genital herpes being passed on to the baby. *Congenital h. simplex* a serious neonatal condition with a generalised vesicular rash, causing encephalitis and death. *H. zoster* a local manifestation of reactivation of infection of the varicella-zoster virus, the causative agent of chickenpox, characterised by a vesicular rash in the area of distribution of a sensory nerve. Also called shingles.

herpes virus (ˈhərpeez ˌvierəs) one of a group of DNA-containing viruses. They include the causative agents of herpes simplex, herpes zoster, chickenpox, cytomegalic inclusion disease and infective mononucleosis.

heterochromia (ˌhetə·rohˈkroh-mi·ə) a difference in colour in the irises of the two eyes or in different parts of one iris. It may be congenital or secondary resulting from inflammation.

heterogeneous (ˌhetə·rohˈjeeni·əs) composed of diverse constituents.

heterogenous (ˌhetəˈrojənəs) derived from different sources.

heterosexual (ˌhetə·rohˈseksyooəl) 1. pertaining to, characteristic of or directed towards the opposite sex. 2. a person with erotic interests directed towards the opposite sex.

heterotropia (ˌhetə·rohˈtrohpi·ə) a marked deviation of the eyes; STRABISMUS or squint.

heterozygous (ˌhetə·rohˈziegəs) possessing dissimilar alternative genes for an inherited characteristic, one gene coming from each parent. One gene is dominant and the other is recessive. *See* HOMOZYGOUS.

hexachlorophene (ˌheksəˈklor·rəˈ-feen) a detergent and germicidal compound commonly incorporated in soaps and dermatological agents. Topical preparations have been associated with severe neurotoxicity and should not be used on children under 2 years of age except on medical advice.

Hg symbol for MERCURY [L. *hydrargyrum*].

hiatus (hieˈaytəs) a space or opening. *H. hernia* a protrusion of a part of the stomach through the oesophageal opening in the diaphragm.

Hib (hib / aych ie bee) an injectable vaccine which protects against

Haemophilus influenzae type B, which causes severe respiratory and ear infections, and meningitis. Offered to infants at ages of 2, 3 and 4 months. (*See* Appendix 7.)

hiccup (ˈhikup) hiccough; a spasmodic contraction of the diaphragm causing an abrupt inspiratory sound. Also known as myoclonic jerk.

Hickman line® (ˈhikmən lien) trade name for a central venous line catheter.

hidrosis (hiˈdrohsəs) the excretion of sweat.

high-altitude sickness (hieˈaltət-yood ˈsiknəs) the condition resulting from difficulty in adjusting to diminished oxygen pressure at high altitudes. It may take the form of mountain sickness, high-altitude pulmonary oedema or cerebral oedema.

high-dependency unit (HDU) (hie dəpendənsee yoonit) for those patients who do not need intensive care in the clinical situation but require a greater degree of specialist monitoring and observation than in a general ward, nursing and medical care is provided in the high-dependency unit.

highly active antiretroviral therapy (HAART) (hieˈlee ˈaktiv ˌanteeˈretrohˌvierəl ˈtherəpee) a treatment regimen that incorporates a combination of different antiviral drugs for human immunodeficiency viral infection. Sometimes also called ART, antiretroviral therapy.

hilum (ˈhieləm) hilus; a recess in an organ by which blood vessels, nerves and ducts enter and leave.

hindbrain (ˈhiendˌbrayn) that part of the brain consisting of the MEDULLA OBLONGATA, the PONS and the CEREBELLUM.

hip (hip) 1. the region of the body at the articulation of the femur and the innominate bone at the base of the lower trunk. These bones meet at the hip joint. Also called *coxa*. 2. loosely, the hip joint. *Total h. replacement* replacement of the femoral head and acetabulum with prostheses that are cemented into the bone. Also called *total h. arthroplasty*. The procedure is done to replace a severely damaged arthritic hip joint.

hippus (ˈhipəs) alternate contraction and dilatation of the pupils. This occurs in various diseases of the nervous system, e.g. MULTIPLE SCLEROSIS.

Hirschsprung's disease (ˈhərsh-spruhngz diˈzeez) *Harald Hirschsprung, Danish physician, 1831–1916.* A congenital abnormality (birth defect) of the bowel in which there are missing nerve cells in the muscles starting at the anus and extending up the colon. This may result to obstruction and MEGACOLON

hirsute (ˈhərsyoot) hairy.

hirsutism (ˈhərsyooˌtizəm) excessive hairiness.

hirudin (hiˈroodin) the active principle in the secretion of the leech and certain snake venoms that prevents clotting of blood.

Hirudo (hiˈroodoh) a genus of leeches. *H. medicinalis* the medical leech.

histamine (ˈhistəmeen) an enzyme that causes local vasodilatation and increased permeability of the blood vessel walls. Readily released from body tissues, it is a factor in allergy response, greatly increases gastric secretion of hydrochloric acid and increases the heart rate.

histidine (ˈhistəˌdeen) one of the 10 essential amino acids formed by the digestion of dietary protein. Histamine is derived from it.

histiocyte (ˈhisteeohˌsiet) a stationary macrophage of connective tissue. Derived from the reticuloendothelial cells, it acts as a scavenger, removing bacteria from the blood and tissues.

histiocytosis (ˌhisteeohsieˈtohsəs) a group of diseases of bone in which granulomata containing HISTIOCYTES and eosinophil cells appear. *See* LETTERER–SIWE DISEASE and HAND–SCHÜLLER–CHRISTIAN DISEASE.

histocompatibility (ˌhistohkəmˌpatəˈbilətee) the ability of cells to be accepted and to function in a new situation. Tissue typing reveals this and ensures a higher success rate in organ and tissue transplantation.

histogram (ˈhistəˌgram) a bar chart. Statistical values are expressed as blocks on a graph.

histology (hiˈstoləjee) the science dealing with the minute structure, composition and function of tissues.

histolysis (hiˈstoləsəs) the disintegration of tissues.

histoplasmosis (ˌhistohplazˈmohsəs) infection caused by inhalation of the spores of a yeast-like fungus, *Histoplasma capsulatum*. Usually symptomless, the infection may progress and produce a condition resembling tuberculosis.

HIV *see* HUMAN IMMUNODEFICIENCY VIRUS.

HIV disease (HIV diˈzeez) the entire spectrum of cellular and clinical disease, from initial infection and asymptomatic disease to early and late symptomatic disease (AIDS) and death, caused by human immunodeficiency virus (HIV) infection. *See* HUMAN IMMUNODEFICIENCY VIRUS.

hives (hievz) URTICARIA.

Hodgkin's disease (ˈhojkənz diˈzeez) *Thomas Hodgkin, British physician, 1798–1866.* LYMPHADENOMA, a malignant condition of the reticuloendothelial cells. There is progressive enlargement of lymph nodes and lymph tissue all over the body. Treated by radiotherapy and cytotoxic drugs. This disease has a good prognosis.

holism (ˈhohlizəm) a philosophy in which the person is considered as a functioning whole rather than as a composite of several systems. May be spelt wholism.

holistic (həˈlistik) pertaining to holism. *H. healthcare* a comprehensive approach to healthcare that implies body–mind–spirit consideration in all actions and interventions for the patient, while recognising the concept of the uniqueness of the individual and the influence of external and internal environmental factors on health.

Holter monitor (ˈholtə ˈmonətə) *Norman Holter, American biophysicist, 1914–1983.* A non-invasive wearable device used in ambulatory electrocardiography or ECG to record the heart's electrical activity continuously for 12–24 hours. The monitor records by means of electrodes to the chest. The electrodes are placed over bones to minimise artefacts from muscular activity. The extended recording period is useful for noting cardiac arrhythmias that are often difficult to identify in a shorter period of time.

Homans' sign (ˈhohmənz sien) *John Homans, American surgeon, 1877–1954.* Pain elicited in the calf when the foot is dorsiflexed. A Homans' sign is no longer considered reliable for diagnosing deep venous thrombosis.

home (hohm) the place where a person lives. *H. assessment* made by an occupational therapist to assess the home environment for a patient, in order to determine the need for any adaptations appropriate to the patient's needs, to maintain independent living at home. *H. and Community Care (HACC)* Australian programs that provide funding for services such as home nursing, home help, assistance with meals. Other services provided may include respite care and transport which are designed to support frail older people, younger people with disabilities and their carers. These services also provide support to people living at home who may be at risk of premature admission to long-term residential care. *H. birth* the delivery of a baby in the mother's home. Women may choose to deliver their babies and receive care from a community or independent midwife and general practitioner. *H. Care Package Program* assists older Australians to live independently in their homes. The Australian Government, under the *Aged Care Act (1997)*, provides a subsidy towards a package of care, including services and case management that meets a client's needs. *H. carers* members of community care teams organised by local authority social services who provide care in the home for older and/or disabled people as part of an agreed care package. Formerly called home help. *H. page* the first page of an internet website.

homeopathy (ˌhohmeeˈopəthee) a system of medicine promulgated by *Samuel Hahnemann (German physician, 1755–1843)* based on the principle that 'like cures like'. Remedies are given which can produce in the patient the symptoms of the disease to be cured, but they are administered in minute doses.

homeostasis (ˌhohmeeohˈstaysəs, ˌhom-) a tendency of biological systems to maintain stability while continually adjusting to conditions that are optimal for survival.

homogeneity (ˌhohməjəˈneeətee) similarity of conditions; also called INTERNAL CONSISTENCY.

homogeneous (ˌhohməˈjeeni·es) uniform in character. Similar in nature and characteristics.

homogenise (həˈmojəˌniez) to make homogeneous. To reduce to the same consistency.

homogenous (həˈmojənəs) derived from the same source.

homograft (ˈhoməˌgrahft, ˈhomoh-) a tissue or organ transplanted from one individual to another of the same species. An ALLOGRAFT.

homolateral (ˌhoməˈlatəˌrəl, ˌhoh-moh-) on the same side; ipsilateral.

homologous (həˈmoləgəs) 1. in anatomy, having the same embryological origin, although performing a different function. 2. in chemistry, possessing a similar structure. *H. chromosomes* those that pair during meiosis and contain an identical arrangement of genes in the DNA pattern.

homologue (ˈhoməˌlog) a part or organ which has the same relative position or structure as another one.

homoplasty (ˈhomohˌplastee, ˈhohm-) surgical replacement of defective tissues with a homograft.

homosexual (ˌhomohˈsekshooəl, ˌhohm-) 1. of the same sex. 2. a person who is sexually attracted to a person of the same sex.

homosexuality (ˌhomohˌsekshoo-ˈalətee, ˌhohm-) sexual and emotional orientation towards persons of the same sex.

homozygous (ˌhomohˈziegəs) possessing an identical pair of genes for an inherited characteristic. *See* HETEROZYGOUS.

hookworm (ˈhookwerm) *see* ANCYLOSTOMA.

hordeolum (hordeeˈohləm) a stye; inflammation of the sebaceous glands of the eyelashes.

hormone (ˈhawmohn) a chemical substance that is generated in one organ and carried by the blood to another, in which it excites activity. *H. replacement therapy* (abbreviated as HRT) the giving of prepared hormones, orally or by implant, skin patch, gel or nasal spray, as a substitute for those hormones that the body no longer produces or that have been lost as a result of surgery. A combination of oestrogenic hormones is commonly given to women for the relief of menopausal symptoms and the prevention of osteoporosis.

Horner's syndrome (ˈhawnəz ˈsinˌdrohm) *Johann Horner, Swiss ophthalmologist, 1831–1886.* A rare condition in which there is a lesion on the path of sympathetic nerve fibres in the cervical region. The symptoms include ENOPHTHALMOS, PTOSIS, a contracted pupil and a decrease in sweating.

Horton's syndrome (ˈhawtənz ˈsinˌdrohm) *Bayard Horton, American physician, 1895–1980.* Severe headache caused by the release of histamine in the body.

hospice (ˈhospəs) the concept of a hospice is that of a caring community of professional and non-professional people, together with the family. Emphasis is on dealing with emotional and spiritual problems, as well as the medical problems of the terminally ill. Of primary concern is control of pain and other symptoms, keeping the patient at home for as long as possible or desirable, and making the person's remaining days as comfortable and meaningful as possible. After the patient dies, family members are given support throughout their period of bereavement.

hospital (ˈhospət'l) an institution for the care, diagnosis and treatment of the sick and injured. *H.-acquired infection see* HEALTHCARE-ASSOCIATED INFECTIONS. *H. information system (HIS)* a comprehensive information system designed to manage financial and clinical aspects of a hospital to improve patient outcomes and provide the most up-to-date patient management records. Also called clinical information system (CIS).

host (hohst) the animal, plant or tissue on which a parasite lives and multiplies. *Definitive* or *final h.* one that harbours the parasite during its adult sexual stage. *Intermediate h.* one that shelters the parasite during a non-reproductive period.

hourglass contraction (ˈowəˌglahs kənˌtrakshən) a contraction near the middle of a hollow organ, such as the stomach or uterus, producing an outline resembling an hourglass shape.

housemaid's knee (ˈhowsmaydz nee) prepatellar bursitis; inflammation of the prepatellar bursa, which becomes distended with serous fluid.

HRT *see* HORMONE REPLACEMENT THERAPY.

HSN1 virus that causes a virulent strain of avian influenza.

human chorionic gonadotrophin *see* GONADOTROPHIN.

human immunodeficiency virus (HIV) (hyoomən imunohdəfishənsee vierəs) a lentivirus that belongs to a group of viruses known as retroviruses and causes AIDS in humans. There are two main types of HIV: HIV-1, the predominant AIDS-causing virus in the world, and HIV-2, also an AIDS-causing virus that is found more commonly in countries on the west coast of Africa. HIV is transmitted sexually, parenterally, from mother to child (during pregnancy, at time of birth or in the postnatal period from breastfeeding) and, more rarely, iatrogenically. Most people become infected sexually through unprotected penetrative vaginal or anal sexual intercourse. Unprotected means that the male insertive partner has not worn a good-quality, intact rubber latex condom. Parenteral transmission is usually associated with injecting drug users sharing contaminated injection equipment. Blood tests to identify HIV infection detect antibodies to the virus and may not be positive for 8 to 12 weeks following primary infection. Because it is not possible to detect all HIV-infected patients, all healthcare workers in direct patient contact should practise standard and transmission-based control precautions.

humidity (hyoo'midətee) the degree of moisture in the air. *H. therapy* the therapeutic use of water to prevent or correct a moisture deficit in the respiratory tract. The principal reasons for employing humidity therapy are: (a) to prevent drying and irritation of the respiratory mucosa; (b) to facilitate ventilation and diffusion of oxygen and other therapeutic gases being administered; and (c) to aid in the removal of thick and viscous secretions that obstruct the air passages. Another important use of water aerosol therapy is to aid in obtaining an induced sputum specimen.

humour ('hyoomə) any fluid of the body, such as lymph or blood. *Aqueous h.* the fluid filling the anterior chamber of the eye. *Vitreous h.* the jelly-like substance that fills the chamber of the eye between the lens and the retina.

humour and laughter therapy ('hyoomə and 'lahftuh 'therəpee) an amusing intervention used by a health professional or patient and designed to benefit the patient.

Huntington's chorea (disease) ('huntingtənz ko'reeə (di'zeez)) *George Huntington, American physician, 1850–1916.* A rare, degenerative inherited disorder of the brain in which there is progressive CHOREA and mental deterioration (dementia).

Hurler's syndrome ('hərləz 'sin,drohm) *Gertrud Hurler, Austrian paediatrician, 1889–1965.* A rare inherited disorder caused by a lack of specific lysosomal enzymes involved in the degradation of glycosaminoglycans (GAGs). Clinical features include learning difficulties, short stature and other physical abnormalities. Also known as mucopolysaccharidosis type IH (MPS IH).

Hutchinson's teeth ('hutchənsənz teeth) *Sir Jonathan Hutchinson, British surgeon, 1828–1913.* Typical notching of the borders of the permanent incisor teeth occurring in congenital syphilis.

hyaline ('hieə,lien) resembling glass. *H. degeneration* a form of deterioration that occurs in tumours and is due to deficiency of blood supply. It precedes cystic degeneration. *H. membrane* *disease see* RESPIRATORY DISTRESS SYNDROME OF NEWBORN.

hyaluronidase (ˌhieəlyəˈroniˌdayz) an enzyme that facilitates the absorption of fluids in subcutaneous tissues.

hydatid (ˈhiedətəd) a cystic swelling containing the embryo of *Echinococcus granulosus*. It may be found in any organ of the body, e.g. in the liver. 'Daughter cysts' are produced from the original. Infection is from contaminated foods, e.g. salads. *H. disease* the result of the presence of hydatids in the lungs, liver or brain.

hydatidiform (ˌhiedəˈtidəˌfawm) resembling a hydatid cyst. *H. mole see* MOLE.

hydraemia (hieˈdreemi·ə) a modification of the blood in which there is an excess of plasma in relation to the cells. A degree of hydraemia is physiological in pregnancy.

hydramnios (hieˈdramnee·os) an excessive amount of amniotic fluid in the uterus during pregnancy. It is associated with maternal diabetes mellitus, congenital abnormalities especially of the central nervous system and with uniovular twins. Sometimes used synonymously with polyhydramnios.

hydrarthrosis (ˌhiedrahˈthrohsəs) a collection of fluid in a joint.

hydrate (ˈhiedrayt) a compound of an element with water, to combine with water.

hydroa vacciniforme (ˈhiedrohˌah ˈvaksəˌnifawm) a rare and chronic childhood hypersensitivity of the skin to sunlight, resulting in the formation of a vesicular eruption on the exposed parts, with intense irritation.

hydrocarbon (ˈhiedrohˌkahbən) a compound of hydrogen and carbon. Fats are of this type.

hydrocele (ˈhiedrəˌseel) a swelling caused by accumulation of fluid, especially in the TUNICA VAGINALIS surrounding the testicle.

hydrocephalus (ˈhiedrohˌkefələs, -ˈsef-) 'water on the brain'. Enlargement of the skull due to an abnormal collection of cerebrospinal fluid around the brain or in the ventricles. It may be either congenital or acquired from infection, trauma or tumour. The most effective treatment is surgical correction employing a shunting technique.

hydrochloric acid (ˈhiedrəˌklo·rik, -ˈklaw·rik ˈasəd) (HCl) a colourless compound of hydrogen and chlorine. It is present (in 0.2% solution) in gastric juice, and aids digestion.

hydrocolloid dressings (hiedroh-koloyd drəsəngz) absorbent dressings with a soft, spongy consistency that are applied to wounds that are subject to pressure, e.g. those in the sacral area or on heels. They relieve pain from the site, rehydrate and encourage debridement and healing.

hydrogel dressings (hiedrohjel dresəngz) wound dressings that rehydrate dry necrotic tissue, reduce pain and promote healing.

hydrogen (ˈhiedrəjən) *symbol* H. A combustible gas, present in nearly all organic compounds, which, in combination with oxygen, forms water. *H. ion concentration* the amount of hydrogen in a liquid, which is responsible for its acidity. The degree of acidity is expressed in pH values: the higher the hydrogen ion concentration, the greater the acidity and the lower the pH value. The concentration in the blood is of importance in acidosis. *H. peroxide* H_2O_2, a strong disinfectant, cleansing and bleaching liquid used, diluted in water, for cleansing wounds.

hydrolysis (hie'droləsəs) the process of splitting up into smaller molecules by uniting with water.

hydrometer (hie'dromətə) an instrument for estimating the specific gravity of fluids, e.g. a urinometer.

hydromyelia (ˌhiedrohmie'eeli·ə) a dilatation of the central canal of the spinal cord caused by an accumulation of cerebrospinal fluid.

hydronephrosis (ˌhiedrohnə'frohsəs) an accumulation of urine in the pelvis of the kidney, resulting in atrophy of the kidney structure due to an obstruction to the flow of urine from the kidney. The condition may be: (a) congenital, due to malformation of the kidney or ureter; or (b) acquired, due to an obstruction of the ureter by tumour or stone, or to back pressure from stricture of the urethra or an enlarged prostate gland.

hydropathy (hie'dropəthee) the treatment of disease by the use of water internally and externally. HYDROTHERAPY.

hydropericarditis (ˌhiedrohˌpereekah'dietəs) inflammation of the pericardium resulting in serous fluid in the pericardial sac.

hydroperitoneum (ˌhiedrohˌperitə'neeəm) *see* ASCITES.

hydrophobia (ˌhiedrə'fohbi·ə) 1. rabies. 2. irrational fear of water.

hydropneumothorax (ˌhiedrohˌnyoomoh'thor·raks) the presence of fluid and air in the pleural space.

hydrops ('hiedrops) [L.] abnormal accumulation of serous fluid in the tissues or in a body cavity; previously called dropsy. *Fetal h., h. fetalis* gross oedema of the entire body of the newborn infant, occurring in haemolytic disease of the newborn.

hydrosalpinx (ˌhiedroh'salpingks) distension of the fallopian tubes by fluid.

hydrotherapy (ˌhiedroh'therəpee) the treatment of disease by means of water. For example douching or bathing.

hydrothorax (ˌhiedroh'thor·raks) fluid in the pleural cavity due to serous effusion, as in cardiac, renal and other diseases.

hydroureter ('hiedroh·yə'reetə) an accumulation of urine in a ureter.

hygiene ('hiejeen) 1. the science of health and its preservation. 2. a condition of practice, such as cleanliness, that is conducive to preservation of health. *Communal h.* the maintenance of the health of the community by the provision of a pure water supply, efficient sanitation, good housekeeping, etc. *Industrial h.* (occupational health) care of the health of workers in an industry. *Mental h.* the science dealing with development of healthy mental and emotional reactions and habits. *Oral h.* the proper care of the mouth and teeth. *Personal h.* individual measures taken to preserve one's own cleanliness and wellbeing.

hygroma (hie'grohmə) a swelling caused by fluid. *Cystic h.* a cystic LYMPHANGIOMA of the neck. *Subdural h.* a collection of clear fluid in the subdural space.

hygrometer (hie'gromətə) an instrument for measuring the water vapour in the air.

hygroscopic (ˌhiegrə'skopik) readily absorbing moisture. An example is glycerin, which is used in suppositories as a means of aiding evacuation by moistening the faeces.

hymen (ˈhiemən) a fold of mucous membrane partially closing the entrance to the vagina. *Imperforate h.* a membrane which completely occludes the vaginal orifice.

hyoid (ˈhieoyd) shaped like a U. *H. bone* a U-shaped bone above the thyroid cartilage, to which the tongue is attached.

hyperacidity (ˌhiepə·eˈsidətee) excessive acidity. *Gastric h.* HYPERCHLORHYDRIA.

hyperactive (ˌhiepəˈraktiv) exhibiting HYPERACTIVITY; hyperkinetic.

hyperactivity (ˌhiepə·rakˈtivətee) abnormally increased activity. Developmental hyperactivity of children (hyperkinesia) is characterised by very restless, impulsive behaviour. These children are usually aged between 2 and 4 years, inattentive and have a poor concentration span. Other features that may be associated with hyperactivity include aggression, anxiety, poor eating and sleeping patterns, and social and learning difficulties. Persistent hyperactivity is known as attention deficit hyperactivity disorder (ADHD), which may require assessment and treatment. *See* ATTENTION DEFICIT SYNDROME.

hyperaemia (ˌhiepə·reemi·ə) excess blood in an organ or tissues in the body.

hyperaesthesia (ˌhiepə·rəsˈtheezi·ə) excessive sensitiveness to touch or to other sensations, e.g. taste or smell.

hyperalimentation (ˌhiepə·rălə-menˈtayshən) a program of parenteral administration of all nutrients for patients with gastrointestinal dysfunction; also called total parenteral alimentation (TPA) and total parenteral nutrition (TPN). Although the term hyperalimentation is commonly used to designate total or supplementary nutrition by intravenous feedings, it is not technically correct inasmuch as the procedure does not involve an abnormally increased or excessive amount of feeding. *See* NUTRITION (PARENTERAL).

hyperasthenia (ˌhiepə·rəsˈtheeni·ə) extreme weakness.

hyperbaric (ˌhiepəˈbarik) at a greater pressure than normal; applied to gases under greater than atmospheric pressure. *H. oxygenation* exposure to oxygen under conditions of greatly increased pressure. The patient is placed in a sealed enclosure, called a hyperbaric chamber. Compressed air is introduced; at the same time, the patient is given pure oxygen through a face mask. Patients suffering from tetanus and gas gangrene and infections caused by bacteria that are resistant to antibiotics but vulnerable to oxygen are helped by hyperbaric oxygenation. The technique is also useful in radiotherapy for cancer. When full of oxygen, cancer cells seem more vulnerable to radiation. Carbon monoxide poisoning can be treated by hyperbaric oxygenation. Carbon monoxide molecules, displacing the oxygen in the erythrocytes, usually cause asphyxiation, but hyperbaric oxygenation can often keep the patient alive until the carbon monoxide has been eliminated from the body's system.

hyperbilirubinaemia (ˌhiepəˈbilee-ˌroobəˈneemi·ə) an excess of bilirubin in the blood.

hypercalcaemia (ˌhiepəkalˈseemi·ə) an excess of calcium in the blood. May rarely be caused by over administration of vitamin D, HYPERPARATHYROIDISM, THYROTOXICOSIS, prolonged immobility, breakdown of bone by malignant disease or impaired renal function.

hypercalciuria (ˌhiepəˌkalseeˈyoo·-ri·ə) a high level of calcium in the urine, leading to renal stone formation.

hypercapnia (ˌhiepəˈkapni·ə) an increased amount of carbon dioxide in the blood, causing over-stimulation of the respiratory centre. Also known as hypercarbia.

hypercatabolism (ˌhiepəkəˈtabəˌli-zəm) an excessive rate of catabolism leading to wasting or destruction of a part of tissue.

hyperchloraemia (ˌhiepəˌklaw-ˈreemi·ə) an excess of chloride in the blood.

hyperchlorhydria (ˌhiepəklaw-ˈhiedri·ə) an excess of hydrochloric acid in the gastric juice.

hypercholesteraemia, hyper-cholesterolaemia (ˌhiepəkəˈlestəˌ-reemi·ə; ˌhiepəkəˈlestəˌrərleemi·ə) excess of cholesterol in the blood. Predisposes to ATHEROMA and gallstones.

hyperacusis (ˌhiepəˈkyoosəs) excessive sensitivity to sound.

hyperdynamia (ˌhiepədieˈnami·ə) excessive muscle activity. *H. uteri* excessive uterine contractions in labour.

hyperemesis (ˌhiepəˈreməsəs) excessive vomiting. *H. gravidarum* an uncommon, serious complication of pregnancy, characterised by severe and persistent vomiting, necessitating medical intervention. It is associated with fluid and electrolyte imbalance and a 10% weight loss of the pre-pregnant weight. The aetiology is not fully understood.

hyperextension (ˌhiepə·rekˈstenshən) the forcible extension of a limb beyond the normal. It is used to correct orthopaedic deformities.

hyperflexion (ˌhiepəˈflekshən) the forcible bending of a joint beyond the normal.

hypergalactia, hypergalactosis (ˌhiepəgəˈlakti·ə; ˌhiepəˌgaləkˈtohsəs) excessive secretion of milk.

hyperglycaemia (ˌhiepəglieˈsee-mi·ə) excess of glucose in the blood (normal 3.5–5.5 mmol/L when fasting); a sign of DIABETES MELLITUS. *See* HYPOGLYCAEMIA and table on p. 138.

hyperhidrosis (ˌhiepəhiˈdrohsəs) excessive perspiration; hyperidrosis.

hyperinsulinism (ˌhiepəˈinsyələ·-nizəm) 1. excessive secretion of insulin. 2. shock produced by an overdose of insulin.

hyperkalaemia (ˌhiepəkəˈleemi·ə) an excess of potassium in the blood. If untreated, this will lead to cardiac arrest.

hyperkeratosis (ˌhiepəˈkerəˌtohsəs) hypertrophy of the horny layers of the skin.

hyperkinesis (ˌhiepəkəˈneesəs) a condition in which there is excessive motor activity. *See* HYPERACTIVITY.

hyperlipaemia (ˌhiepəliˈpeemi·ə) an excess of fat or lipids in the blood.

hypermastia (ˌhiepəˈmasti·ə) 1. the presence of one or more supernumerary breasts. 2. overdevelopment of one or both breasts.

hypermetropia (ˌhiepəmeˈtrohpi·ə) hyperopia; long-sightedness. The light rays entering the eye converge beyond the retina. Clear vision can be obtained by the wearing of spectacles or contact lenses.

hypermobility (ˌhiepəmohˈbilətee) some or all joints have an unusually large range of movement. *Joint h. syndrome* is a common benign childhood condition involving hyperflexible joints that can move beyond the normal range of motion. Also referred to as loose joints or double-jointed.

hypermotility (ˌhiepəmohˈtilətee) excessive movement. *Gastric h.* increased muscle action of the stomach wall, associated with increased secretion of hydrochloric acid.

hypernatraemia (ˌhiepənəˈtreemi·ə) an excess of sodium in the blood, usually diagnosed when the plasma sodium is above 145 mmol/L. It is the result of loss of water and electrolytes from the body caused by diarrhoea, POLYURIA, excessive sweating or inadequate fluid intake.

hypernephroma (ˌhiepəneˈfrohmə) a malignant tumour of the kidney; renal cell carcinoma.

hyperostosis (ˌhiepə·roˈstohsəs) a thickening of bone; a bony outgrowth; exostosis.

hyperparathyroidism (ˌhiepəˌparəˈthieroyˌdizəm) excessive activity of the parathyroid glands, causing drainage of calcium from the bones, with consequent fragility and liability to spontaneous fracture.

hyperphagia (ˌhiepəˈfayji·ə) overeating.

hyperphasia (ˌhiepəˈfayzi·ə) excessive talkativeness.

hyperpituitarism (ˌhiepəˈpətyooətəˌrizəm) overactivity of the pituitary gland.

hyperplasia (ˌhiepəˈplayzi·ə) excessive formation of normal cells in a tissue or organ, which increases in size.

hyperpnoea (ˌhiepəˈneeə, -pəpˈneeə) over-breathing; hyperventilation; an abnormal increase in the rate and depth of breathing.

hyperprolactinaemia (ˌhiepəprohˌlaktəˈneemi·ə) increased levels of prolactin in the blood; in women, it is associated with infertility and may lead to GALACTORRHOEA. In men, it may cause impotence and loss of libido.

hyperpyrexia (ˌhiepəpieˈreksi·ə) an excessively high body temperature, i.e. over 41°C.

hypersensitivity (ˌhiepəˌsensəˈtivətee) abnormal sensitivity, especially to a particular antigen. The reactions include allergies (such as asthma) and ANAPHYLAXIS. *Contact h.* produced by contact of the skin with a chemical substance having the properties of an antigen or hapten; it includes CONTACT DERMATITIS. *Delayed h.* a slowly developing increase in cell-mediated immune response (involving T-lymphocytes) to a specific antigen, as occurs in graft rejection, autoimmune disease, etc. *Immediate h.* antibody-mediated hypersensitivity characterised by lesions resulting from release of histamine and other mediators of hypersensitivity from reagin-sensitised mast cells, causing increased vascular permeability, oedema and smooth muscle contraction; it includes ANAPHYLAXIS and ATOPY.

hypersplenism (ˌhiepəˈsplenizəm) overactivity of an enlarged spleen resulting in the depression of blood cells and platelets.

hypertelorism (ˌhiepəˈteləˌrizəm) abnormally increased distance between two organs or parts. *Ocular h.*, *orbital h.* increase in the interocular distance, often associated with craniofacial DYSOSTOSIS and sometimes with intellectual disabilities.

hypertension (ˌhiepəˈtenshən) persistently high BLOOD PRESSURE. In adults, it is generally agreed that blood pressure is abnormally high when the resting, supine arterial systolic pressure is equal to or greater than 140 mmHg and the diastolic pressure is equal to or greater than 90 mmHg. A diagnosis of hypertension should be based on a series of readings rather than a single measurement and will vary with age. Hypertension is very common and usually symptomless but may cause headaches and visual disturbances when severe. Its incidence is highest in men, the middle-aged and older people. Associated factors are smoking, high-salt diet, obesity, a family history, lack of exercise and a high degree of stress. Lifestyle changes are recommended, e.g. losing weight, giving up smoking, exercising, adopting a low-salt diet. Antihypertensive drugs may be needed to maintain blood pressure readings within reasonable levels. Hypertension is considered to be a risk factor for the development of cardiovascular disease. *Essential h.* high blood pressure without demonstrable change in kidneys, blood vessels or heart. *Malignant h.* severe, fulminant, life-threatening high blood pressure. *Portal h.* raised pressure in the portal system. *Pulmonary h.* increased pressure in the arteries of the lung, usually as a result of EMPHYSEMA or FIBROSIS.

hyperthermia (ˌhiepəˈthərmi·ə) an exceedingly high body temperature. *Malignant h.* a serious condition, sometimes arising during general anaesthesia.

hyperthyroidism (ˌhiepəˈthieroy-ˌdizəm) excessive activity of the thyroid gland. *See* THYROTOXICOSIS.

hypertonic (ˌhiepəˈtonik) 1. showing excessive tone or tension, as in a blood vessel or muscle. 2. describing a solution that has greater osmotic pressure than normal physiological tissue fluid.

hypertrichosis (ˌhiepətriˈkohsəs) excessive growth of hair on any part of the body.

hypertrophy (hieˈpərtrəfee) an increase in the size of a tissue or a structure caused by an increase in the size of the cells that compose it (as opposed to an increase in the number of cells). *See* HYPERPLASIA.

hyperuricaemia (ˌhiepəˌyoo·rəˈseemi·ə) an excess of uric acid in the blood. *See* GOUT.

hyperventilation (ˌhiepəˌventə-ˈlayshən) 1. increase of air in the lungs above the normal amount. 2. abnormally prolonged and deep breathing, usually associated with acute anxiety or emotional tension. HYPERPNOEA. Also occurs in uncontrolled diabetes mellitus, kidney failure and in some lung disorders. Symptoms occur as a result of an abnormal loss of carbon dioxide from the blood and include faintness, tetany and a tense feeling of not being able to take a full breath.

hypervitaminosis (ˌhiepəˌvitəmə-ˈnohsəs) a condition caused by the intake of an excessive quantity of vitamins.

hypervolaemia (ˌhiepəvoˈleemi·ə) abnormal increase in the volume of circulating fluid (plasma) in the body.

hyphaema (hieˈfeem·ə) haemorrhage into the anterior chamber of the eye.

hypnosis (hipˈnohsəs) an artificially induced passive state in which there is increased amenability and responsiveness to suggestions and commands. In hypnosis, a drowsy phase is followed by a sleep. It may also be used to produce painless childbirth and tooth extraction.

hypnotherapy (ˌhipnohˈtherəpee) treatment by hypnosis or by the induction of prolonged sleep.

hypnotic (hipˈnotik) an agent that causes sleep; a soporific.

hypnotism (ˈhipnəˌtizəm) the practice of hypnosis.

hypocalcaemia (ˌhiepohkalˈseemi·ə) a deficiency of calcium in the blood.

hypocapnia (ˌhiepohˈkapni·ə) a deficiency of carbon dioxide in the blood.

hypochloraemia (ˌhiepohkloˈreemi·ə) a deficiency of chloride in the blood.

hypochlorhydria (ˌhiepohklawˈhiedri·ə) a lower than normal amount of hydrochloric acid in the gastric juice.

hypochlorite (ˌhiepohˈklaw·riet) any salt of hypochlorous acid used in solution to yield chlorine, a disinfecting and germicidal agent. Milton, a proprietary preparation, is used in solution for the disinfection of equipment and infant feeding utensils.

hypochondria (ˌhiepohˈkondri·ə) a morbid preoccupation or anxiety about one's health. The sufferer feels that first one part of the body and then another part is the seat of some serious disease.

hypochondriac (ˌhiepohˈkondriˌak) one affected by hypochondria. *H. region* the hypochondrium.

hypochondrium (ˌhiepohˈkondri·əm) the upper region of the abdomen on each side of the EPIGASTRIUM.

hypodermic (ˌhiepohˈdərmik) beneath the skin; applied to subcutaneous injections and to the syringes used for such injections.

hypofibrinogenaemia (ˌhiepohfieˌbrinəjəˈneemi·ə) a lack of fibrinogen in the blood. This may occur in severe trauma or haemorrhage or as an inherited condition.

hypogammaglobulinaemia (ˌhiepohˌgaməˌglobyəliˈneemi·ə) a deficiency of gamma globulin in the blood, rendering the person susceptible to infection.

hypogastrium (ˌhiepohˈgastri·əm) the lower middle area of the abdomen, immediately below the umbilical region.

hypoglossal (ˌhiepohˈglosəl) under the tongue. *H. nerve* the 12th cranial nerve.

hypoglycaemia (ˌhiepohglieˈseemi·ə) a condition in which the blood sugar level is less than normal. Usually arising in people with diabetes mellitus as a result of insulin over-dosage, delay in eating or a rapid combustion of carbohydrate. *See* HYPERGLYCAEMIA; table on p. 1.

hypokalaemia (ˌhiepohkəˈleemi·ə) a low potassium level in the blood. This is likely to be present in dehydration and with the repeated use of diuretics.

hypomania (ˌhiepohˈmayni·ə) a degree of elation, excitement and activity higher than normal but less severe than that present in mania.

hypometropia (ˌhiepohməˈtrohpi·ə) myopia; short-sightedness.

hypomotility (ˌhiepohmohˈtilətee) deficient power of movement in any part.

hyponatraemia (ˌhiepohnəˈtreemi·ə) a deficiency of sodium in the blood.

hypoparathyroidism (ˌhiepohparəˈthieroy·dizəm) a lack of parathyroid secretion, leading to a low blood calcium and tetany.

hypophysis (hieˈpofəsəs) an outgrowth. *H. cerebri* the PITUITARY gland.

hypopituitarism (ˌhiepohpiˈtyooətəˌrizəm) deficiency of secretion from the anterior lobe of the pituitary gland, causing excessive deposition of fat in children. *See* FRÖLICH'S SYNDROME. Dwarfism may result. In adults, asthenia, drowsiness and adiposity may occur, together with an impairment of sexual activity and premature senility.

hypoplasia (ˌhiepohˈplayzi·ə) imperfect development of a part or organ.

hypopnoea (ˌhiepohˈneeə, -ˈpopnee·ə) shallow breathing.

hypoproteinaemia (ˌhiepohˌprohtə-ˈneemi·ə) a deficiency of serum proteins in the blood.

hypoprothrombinaemia (ˌhiepoh-prohˌthrombəˈneemi·ə) a deficiency of prothrombin in the blood, leading to a tendency to bleed. *See* HAEMOPHILIA.

hyposecretion (ˌhiepohsəˈkreeshən) a deficiency in secretion from any glandular structure or secreting cells.

hyposensitivity (ˌhiepohˌ-sensəˈtivətee) a lack of sensitivity, especially to a particular allergen to which the patient may have been exposed over a period of time.

hypospadias (ˌhiepohˈspaydi·əs) a developmental anomaly in the male in which the urethra opens on the underside of the penis or on the perineum.

hypostasis (ˌhieˈpostəsəs) 1. a sediment or deposit. 2. congestion of blood in a part, due to slowing of the circulation.

hypostatic (ˌhiepohˈstatik) relating to hypostasis. *H. pneumonia see* PNEUMONIA.

hypotension (ˌhiepohˈtenshən) abnormally low arterial blood pressure; hypopiesis. *Controlled* or *induced h.* an artificially produced lowering of the blood pressure so that an operation field is rendered practically bloodless. *Orthostatic* or *postural h.* temporary hypotension when the patient stands up, producing giddiness and sometimes a faint.

hypotensive (ˌhiepohˈtensiv) producing a reduction in blood pressure, especially pertaining to a drug that lowers the blood pressure.

hypothalamus (ˌhiepohˈthaləməs) in the brain a portion of grey matter lying beneath the THALAMUS at the base of the CEREBRUM and forming the floor and part of the lateral wall of the third ventricle. It influences peripheral autonomic mechanisms, endocrine activity and many somatic functions, e.g. a general regulation of water balance, body temperature, sleep, thirst and hunger, and the development of secondary sexual characteristics. It plays an important role in the regulation of protein, fat and carbohydrate metabolism, body fluid volume and electrolyte content and internal secretion of endocrine hormones.

hypothermia (ˌhiepohˈthərmi·ə) 1. a severe reduction in the core body temperature to below 35°C. The condition usually arises gradually and may prove fatal if untreated. It is most common among babies and frail older people. 2. artificial cooling of the body to reduce the oxygen requirements of the tissues. Generalised lowering of the body temperature is used in three main situations: (a) to control fever, as in malignant HYPERTHERMIA; (b) to enable certain cardiac and neurological operations to be carried out; and (c) to protect the brain from raised intracranial pressure in patients with head injuries or following drowning.

hypothesis (hieˈpothəsəs) a supposition that appears to explain a group of phenomena and is assumed as a basis of reasoning and experimentation; a starting point for further investigations from known facts.

hypothrombinaemia (ˌhiepoh-ˌthrombəˈneemi·ə) a diminished amount of thrombin in the blood, with a consequent tendency to bleed.

hypothyroidism (ˌhiepohˈthie-roydizəm) an insufficiency of thyroid secretion. Hypothyroidism is diagnosed by measuring the level of thyroid hormones in the blood. Babies are screened for the condition shortly after birth as part of the newborn screening program. In adults, it leads to MYXOEDEMA.

hypotonia (ˌhiepohˈtohni·ə) 1. deficient muscle tone. 2. deficient tension in the eyeball.

hypotonic (ˌhiepohˈtonik) describing a solution that has a lower osmotic pressure than another one. *See* HYPERTONIC.

hypoventilation (ˌhiepohˌventəˈlay-shən) hypopnoea; shallow breathing, usually at a very slow rate. It may cause a build-up of carbon dioxide in the blood.

hypovolaemia (ˌhiepohˈvoleemi·ə) a reduction in the circulating blood volume due to external loss of body fluids or to loss from the blood into the tissues, as in shock.

hypoxaemia (ˌhiepokˈseemi·ə) an insufficient oxygen content in the blood.

hypoxia (hieˈpoksi·ə) a diminished amount of oxygen in the tissues. *Anaemic h.* low oxygen content due to deficiency of haemoglobin in the blood.

hysterectomy (ˌhistəˈrektəmee) removal of the uterus. *Abdominal h.* removal via an abdominal incision. *Subtotal h.* removal of the body of the uterus only. *Total h.* removal of the body of the uterus and the cervix. *Vaginal h.* removal through the vagina. *Wertheim's h.* additional excision of the PARAMETRIUM, upper vagina and lymph glands. Radical abdominal hysterectomy.

hysteria (hisˈtiə·ri·ə) a psychoneurosis in which the individual converts anxiety created by emotional conflict into physical symptoms, e.g. tics, mutism or paralysis of an arm or leg, that have no organic basis; formally called conversion reaction or conversion hysteria. The term hysteria is also used to describe a state of tension or excitement in which there is a temporary loss of control over the emotions.

hysterical (hiˈsterikəl) relating to hysteria.

hystero-oophorectomy (ˌhistə·rohˌoofəˈrektəmee) excision of the uterus and the ovaries.

hysterosalpingography (ˌhistə·roh ˌsalpingˈgogrəfee) radiographic examination of the uterus and uterine tubes after the injection of a radio-opaque dye. Uterosalpingography.

hysterosalpingostomy (ˌhistə·rohˌsalpingˈgostəmee) the operation of forming an anastomosis, or opening, between the distal portion of the uterine tube and the uterus in an effort to overcome infertility when the medial portion is occluded or excised.

hysterotomy (ˌhistəˈrotəmee) incision of the uterus, usually in order to remove a fetus in mid-pregnancy when it is too late to perform a therapeutic abortion. *See* CAESAREAN SECTION.

Ii

I symbol for *iodine*.

iatrogenesis (ie͵atroh'jenəsis) additional patient problems, complications or disease brought about by the activities of physicians, surgeons or other healthcare professionals, including new infections, unwanted effects of drug therapy and psychological distress.

IBD *see* INFLAMMATORY BOWEL DISEASE.

ICD *see* INTERNATIONAL CLASSIFICATION OF DISEASES.

ice (ies) 1. water in a solid state, at or below freezing point. *Dry i.* a solid form of carbon dioxide. *I. pack therapy* a portable rubber or plastic bag half-filled with crushed ice or a specially formulated gel placed on or near the affected area. It works by reducing blood flow to the area, inflammation and swelling, but does not treat the underlying cause. Also known as cold pack or cryotherapy. 2. Street name for METHAMPHETAMINE HYDROCHLORIDE.

ichthyosis (͵ikthee'ohsəs) a congenital abnormality of the skin in which there is dryness and roughness, the horny layer is thickened and large scales appear.

ICM INTERNATIONAL CONFEDERATION OF MIDWIVES.

ICN *see* INTERNATIONAL COUNCIL OF NURSES.

ICP *see* INTRACRANIAL PRESSURE.

ICSH *see* INTERSTITIAL CELL STIMULATING HORMONE.

icterus (iktə·rəs) jaundice. *I. gravis* a rare but fatal form of jaundice occurring in pregnancy. Acute yellow atrophy. *I. gravis neonatorum* haemolytic disease of the newborn. *See* RH FACTOR.

ICU *see* INTENSIVE CARE UNIT.

id (id) that part of the personality, containing the instinctive drives, which leads to gratification of primitive needs and which exists in the unconscious.

idea (ie'diə) a mental impression or conception. *Autochthonous i.* a strange idea that comes into the mind in some unaccountable way, but is not a hallucination. *Compulsive i.* an idea that persists despite reason and will and that drives one to action, usually inappropriate. *Dominant i.* a morbid or other impression that controls or colours every action and thought. *Fixed i.* a persistent morbid impression or belief that cannot be changed by reason. *I. of reference* the incorrect idea that the words and actions of others refer to one's self, or the projection of the causes of one's own imaginary difficulties upon someone else.

identical (ie'dentikəl) exactly alike. *I. twins* twins of the same sex developing from a single fertilised ovum. Monozygotic.

identification (ie͵dentəfə'kayshən) a mental mechanism by which an individual adopts the attitudes and ideas of another, often admired, person.

identity (ie'dentətee) part of the 'self-concept' of being distinguishable and separate from others and who they are in relation to their group or society. *I. crisis* a period of uncertainty and confusion concerning a person's sense of self and role in society. Occurs most often in the transition from one stage of life to the next. Often expressed by isolation, negativism and rebelliousness.

ideology (ˌiedee'oləjee) 1. the science of the development of ideas. 2. the body of ideas characteristic of an individual or of a social unit.

ideomotion (ˌiedeeoh'mohshən) the association of ideas and muscle action, as in involuntary acts.

idiopathic (ˌideeoh'pathik) self-originated; applied to a condition for which the cause is not known.

idiosyncrasy (ˌideeoh'singkrəsee) 1. a habit or quality of body or mind peculiar to any individual. 2. an abnormal susceptibility to an agent (e.g. a drug) that is peculiar to the individual.

Ig immunoglobulin of any of the five classes: IgA, IgD, IgE, IgG and IgM.

ileal ('ili·əl) referring to the ileum. *I. conduit* a surgical procedure in which the ureters are transplanted into the ileum, an isolated loop of which is then brought to the surface of the abdomen in order to allow the urine to drain into a bag.

ileitis (ˌilee'ietəs) inflammation of the ILEUM. *Regional i.* Crohn's disease. A chronic condition of the terminal portion of the ileum in which granulation and oedema may give rise to obstruction.

ileocolitis (ˌileeohkə'lietəs) inflammation of the ileum and colon.

ileocolostomy (ˌileeohkə'lostəmee) the making of a permanent opening between the ileum and some part of the colon.

ileocystoplasty (ˌileeoh'sistohˌplastee) repair of the wall of the urinary bladder with an isolated segment of the ileum.

ileoproctostomy (ˌileeohprok'tostəmee) surgical anastomosis between the ileum and the rectum; ILEORECTAL ANASTOMOSIS.

ileorectal (ˌileeoh'rekt'l) referring to the ileum and rectum. *I. anastomosis* ILEOPROCTOSTOMY.

ileosigmoidostomy (ileeohsigmoy'dostəmee) an operation carried out when most of the colon has to be removed and an anastomosis is made between the ileum and the sigmoid colon.

ileostomy (ˌilee'ostəmee) an artificial opening (stoma) created from the ileum and brought to the surface of the abdomen for the purpose of evacuation. Ileostomy is an inevitable part of proctocolectomy. An ileostomy may be temporary or permanent. *I. bags* disposable stoma bags to collect the liquid faecal matter discharged from an ileostomy. The bags can be adhesive or worn on a belt.

ileum ('ili·əm) the last part of the small intestine, terminating at the caecum.

ileus ('ili·əs) functional obstruction of the bowel caused by impaired peristalsis. Most commonly occurs after abdominal or pelvic surgery and is one of the causes for readmission to hospital following surgery. The principal symptoms of ileus are abdominal pain and distension, vomiting (the vomitus may contain faecal material) and constipation. If the intestinal obstruction does not resolve or is not relieved, the patient becomes extremely ill with SHOCK and DEHYDRATION.

iliac ('ileeˌak) pertaining to the ilium. *I. artery* the right and left arteries form the terminal branches of the abdominal aorta and supply blood to the pelvic region and the lower limbs. *I. crest* the crest of the hip bone. *I. fossa* the depression on the concave surface of the iliac bone. *I. vein* the right and left veins join to form the inferior VENA CAVA and drain the blood from the lower limbs and pelvis.

ilium (ˈili·əm) the haunch bone; the upper part of the hip bone.

illness (ˈilnəs) a condition marked by pronounced deviation from the normal healthy state; sickness. *I. behaviour* the way in which ill individuals regard the structure and function of their own body, interpret symptoms and seek treatment for their condition. *I. experience* the process of being ill.

illusion (iˈloozhən) a mistaken perception due to a misinterpretation of a sensory stimulus; believing something to be what it is not.

image (ˈimij) 1. the mental recall of a former precept. 2. the optical picture transferred to the brain cells by the optic nerve.

imaging (iməjing) diagnostic techniques that are used to produce images of organs or tissues within the body. These may be plain X-rays used to view dense structures such as bone, or contrast X-rays to view internal organs, e.g. barium X-rays to examine the oesophagus, stomach and small intestine. Techniques include ultrasonography. Computerised tomography (CT) uses X-rays and a scanner, and is particularly useful in examination of the head, chest and abdomen; other techniques include radionuclide scans and magnetic resonance and positron emission tomography. *See* MAGNETIC RESONANCE IMAGING and RADIONUCLIDE. Some of these techniques use computers to process the data and produce the image.

imago (iˈmaygoh, iˈmahgoh) [L.] 1. in psychoanalysis, a childhood memory or fantasy of a loved person that persists in adult life. 2. the adult or definitive form of an insect.

imbalance (imˈbaləns) lack of balance, e.g. of endocrine secretions, between water and electrolytes, or of muscles.

immature (ˌiməˈtyooə, -chyooə) unripe; not fully developed, as in a cataract when only a part of the lens is opaque.

immiscible (iˈmisəbəl) incapable of being mixed, e.g. oil and water.

immobilise (iˈmohbəˌliez) to render incapable of being moved, as by a plaster of Paris cast.

immune (iˈmyoon) protected against a particular infection or allergy. *I. response* the (in general) helpful events that follow activation of the immune system, including T-lymphocyte activity (cell-mediated responses) and B-lymphocyte activity (humoral responses). Immune responses are involved in protecting persons from disease following infection and are also involved in the rejection of transplanted organs and tissues that the body recognises as foreign, or non-self.

immunisation (ˌimyənieˈzayshən) the act of creating immunity by artificial means. *National I. Program Schedule* a standard schedule for immunisation against infectious diseases. (*See* Appendix 7.)

immunity (iˈmyoonətee) the resistance possessed by the body to infectious diseases, foreign tissues, foreign non-toxic substances and other ANTIGENS. The opposite of susceptibility. *Acquired i.* is produced specifically in response to an antigen. It involves a change in the behaviour of cells and in the production of antibody. Antibody is produced as a primary response and, after a short time, the body becomes sensitised. The secondary response is produced more quickly and is more marked. *Active i.* may be (a) natural, i.e. from infectious diseases; or (b) artificial, i.e. from injection of living or dead organisms or their products in the form of toxins and toxoids. *Passive i.* may be: (a) natural, e.g. maternal IMMUNOGLOBULIN G (IgG) via the placenta protects the infant from various infectious diseases for a few months, but undesirable antibodies such as anti-D immunoglobulin may also be transmitted to the fetus; or (b) acquired, e.g. the temporary immunity that follows the injection of antibodies of human origin (gamma globulin) or, more rarely, animal origin. *Natural or innate i.* is mainly non-specific. It is provided by intact cellular barriers of epithelium and by humoral substances such as COMPLEMENT and LYSOZYME. It is affected by genetic factors, age, race and hormone levels.

immunoassay (ˌimyənohˈasay) a quantitative estimate of the proteins contained in the blood serum.

immunodeficiency (ˌimyənohdəˈfishənsee) a deficiency of the immune response, either mediated by a humoral antibody or by a cell-mediated response involving a deficiency of T-lymphocytes. *I. disorders* acquired or congenital conditions in which the body's immune system fails to protect against infection, foreign material and some forms of cancer.

immunoglobulin (ˌimyənohˈglobyələn) antibody. A variety of chemical compounds found mainly in gamma globulin (*see* GAMMA). Immunoglobulins are major components of the humoral immune response system. They are synthesised by lymphocytes and plasma cells and found in the serum and in other body fluids and tissues. The five classes of immunoglobulin (Ig) are: IgA, IgD, IgE, IgG and IgM. There are two types of IgA and both are known to have antiviral properties. Secretory IgA is present in non-vascular fluids such as colostrum and breast milk. IgD is found in trace quantities in serum. It serves as a B-lymphocyte surface receptor. IgE is called the reaginic antibody and may be increased in persons with allergy. IgG is the most abundant of the five classes of immunoglobulin and is the major antibody in the secondary humoral response of immunity. It is the only immunoglobulin to cross the placenta. IgM is principally concerned with the primary antibody response.

immunology (ˌimyəˈnoləjee) the study of immunity and the body's defence mechanisms.

immunosuppression (ˌimyənohsəˈpreshən) inhibition of the formation of antibodies to antigens that may be present; used in transplantation procedures to prevent rejection of the transplanted organ or tissue.

immunosuppressive (ˌimyənohsəˈpresiv) 1. pertaining to or inducing immunosuppression. 2. an agent that induces immunosuppression.

immunotherapy (ˌimyənohˈtherəpee) 1. treatment by immunisation. Sometimes used in the treatment of leukaemia. 2. the establishing of passive immunity.

immunotransfusion (iˌmyoonohtranzˈfyoozhən, -trahns-) transfusion of blood from a donor previously rendered immune to the disease affecting the person.

impaction (im'pakshən) a state of being wedged. *Dental i.* the condition in which a tooth, usually a molar, is unable to erupt through the gum because it is lodged in position by bone or the other teeth. *Faecal i.* a collection of putty-like or hardened faeces in the rectum or colon.

impairment (im'pairmənt) any loss or abnormality of psychological, physiological or anatomical structure or function.

impalpable (im'palpəbəl) incapable of being felt by manual examination. May apply to an organ or a tumour.

imperforate (im'pərfə·rət) without an opening. *I. anus* a congenital defect in which this opening is closed. *I. hymen* complete closure of the vaginal opening by the hymen.

impermeable (im'pərmi·əbəl) not permitting the passage of fluid or molecules.

impetigo (ˌimpə'tiegoh) an acute contagious inflammation of the skin marked by pustules and scabs; of streptococcal or staphylococcal origin. It occurs most commonly on the face and scalp, particularly those of children.

implant (im'plahnt, 'implahnt, -ant) any substance grafted into the tissues; may be living cells or inert materials. *Hormone i.* a hormonal pellet which may be implanted subcutaneously. *Intraocular lens i.* a plastic lens which may be implanted in the eye after lens extraction. *Plastic i.* a silicone implant which may be used in plastic surgery, e.g. to reshape the breast.

implantable cardioverter-defibrillator (ICD) (ˌim'plahntəbuhl kahdeeoh-vərtə ˌdə'fibrəlaytə) an implanted device that automatically terminates life-threatening arrhythmias by delivering low-energy shocks to the heart, restoring normal rhythm. Some devices now have inbuilt pacing capabilities.

implantation (ˌimplahn'tayshən, -plan-) the act of planting or setting in. 1. the embedding of the fertilised ovum in the wall of the uterus. 2. the placing of a drug within the tissues. 3. the surgical introduction of healthy tissue to replace tissue that has been damaged.

implementation (ˌimpləmen'tayshən) one of the phases of the nursing process, signifying the giving of care in relation to defined nursing interventions and goals. During implementation, the nursing care plan is tested for effectiveness and accuracy. Data gathering continues and plans may change on the basis of new information obtained. The implementation phase concludes with the recording of the activities performed and the response of the person. *See* ASSESSMENT AND EVALUATION.

implementation science (ˌimpləmen'tayshən sie'əns) the study of methods and strategies to promote the systematic uptake of research findings and other evidence-based recommendations into routine practice with the aim of improving the quality of health care and services. Implementation science also examines the influences that act on the patient, healthcare professionals and organisational behaviours to ensure any intervention is accessible and equitable.

implosion (im'plohzhən) in behaviour therapy, a form of desensitisation used in the treatment of phobias and related disorders. *See* FLOODING.

impotence (ˈimpətəns) an outdated term commonly used of erectile dysfunction and/or premature ejaculation. The inability in a man to carry out sexual intercourse from either psychological or physical causes.

impregnation (ˌimpregˈnayshən) insemination; rendering pregnant.

impression (imˈpreshən) an imitation of a person or thing. In dentistry, a mould made of a toothless jaw or of the teeth and surrounding tissues, used in the construction of dentures and dental braces.

impulse (ˈimpuls) 1. a sudden pushing force. 2. a sudden uncontrollable act. 3. nerve impulse. *Cardiac i.* movement of the chest wall caused by the heartbeat. *Nerve i.* the electrochemical process propagated along nerve fibres.

IMV *see* INTERMITTENT MANDATORY VENTILATION.

inaccessibility (ˌinəkˌsesəˈbilətee) state of unresponsiveness characteristic of certain psychiatric people, e.g. schizophrenics.

inarticulate (ˌinahˈtikyələt) 1. without joints. 2. unable to speak intelligibly.

inborn error of metabolism (inbawn erə ov məˈtabəˌlizəm) one of many abnormal metabolic conditions caused by an inherited defect of a single enzyme or other protein. Although people with such diseases are defective in only one protein, they generally display a large number of physical signs that are characteristic of the genetic trait. Examples include phenylketonuria, TAY-SACHS DISEASE and galactosaemia.

incarcerated (inˈkahsə·raytəd) held fast. Applied to: (a) a hernia that is immovable, and therefore only curable by operation; and (b) a pregnant uterus held under the sacral brim.

incentive spirometry (inˈsentiv spieˈromətree) a method of encouraging voluntary deep breathing by promoting visual feedback about inspiratory volume. Incentive spirometry may reduce pulmonary complications such as atelectasis and pulmonary consolidation.

incest (ˈinsest) sexual intercourse between close blood relatives, e.g. brothers and sisters; marriage between them is legally or culturally prohibited. Some form of incest taboo is found in all known societies, although the relationships that are prohibited vary.

incidence (ˈinsədəns) the number of particular new events which occur in a population in a given period of time, e.g. the number of new cases of a disease, such as measles, expressed per 1000 of population per year.

incident report (insədənt repawt) a report, the completion of which is required of all healthcare facilities following any accident or untoward incident involving a patient, visitor or member of staff. These incidents may be clinical, e.g. cardiac arrest or the incorrect administration of a medication, but can also include such issues as the loss of a patient's belongings. Also known as a critical incident report.

incipient (inˈsipi·ənt) beginning to exist.

incision (inˈsizhən) 1. in surgery, a cut into soft tissue. 2. the act of cutting.

incisor (inˈsiezə) one of the four front teeth in the centre of each jaw.

inclusion (ingˈkloozhən) something that is enclosed or the act of enclosing. *I. bodies* particles that are temporarily enclosed in the cytoplasm of a cell. For example, in trachoma, virus particles can be seen in the conjunctival epithelial cells.

incoherent (ingkoh'hiə·rənt) 1. unconnected; inconsistent. 2. uttering speech that is disconnected and rambling.

incompatibility (ˌingkəmpatə'bilətee) the state of two or more substances being antagonistic, or destroying the efficiency of each other. Applied to mixtures of drugs, and to blood. *See* BLOOD GROUPS.

incompetence (ing'kompətəns) inefficiency. *Aortic i.* failure of the aortic valves to regulate the flow of blood. *Mitral i.* failure of the mitral valve to close properly.

incompetent cervix (incompətənt sərviks) a condition characterised by painless dilation of the cervical os of the uterus before term without labour or contractions of the uterus. Miscarriage or premature delivery result.

incontinence (ing'kontənəns) inability to control natural functions or discharges. *Faecal i.* inability to control the movements of the bowels. *Overflow i.* that from an overfull bladder, most common in older men with urinary obstruction. *Paralytic i.* loss of control of anal and urethral sphincters due to injury to nerve centres. *Stress i.* that which is due to a defect in the urethral sphincters and is liable to occur when intra-abdominal pressure is increased, as in coughing or lifting heavy weights; most common in women with weak pelvic muscles. *Urinary i.* inability to control the outflow of urine.

incoordination (ˌingkohˌawdə-nay'shən) inability to adjust various muscle movements harmoniously.

increment (incrəmənt) 1. an increase or addition. 2. the amount of an increase or gain in intrauterine pressure as uterine contractions begin in labour.

incremental (incrə'mentəl) to build up as in the contractions of labour or to add in stages.

incrustation (ˌinkrə'stayshən) the formation of a crust or scab on a wound.

incubation (ˌingkyə'bayshən) the development and growth of microorganisms and animal embryos. *I. period* the period between the date of infection and the appearance of symptoms of an infectious disease.

incubator ('ingkyə'baytə) 1. an apparatus providing a suitable environment for preterm and ill babies. 2. an apparatus used in a laboratory to develop bacteria at a uniform temperature suitable to their growth.

incurable (ˌin'kyoorəbuhl) unresponsive to medical or surgical treatment.

incus ('ingkəs) the small anvil-shaped bone of the middle ear. The second auditory ossicle.

indicator ('ində'kaytə) 1. the index finger, or the extensor muscle of the index finger. 2. any substance that indicates the appearance or disappearance of a chemical by a colour change or attainment of a certain pH.

indigenous (in'dijənəs) occurring naturally in a certain locality.

indigestion (ˌindi'jeschən) *see* DYSPEPSIA.

indolent ('indələnt) slow growing. Reluctant to heal. Largely painless. *I. ulcer* a chronic ulcer of the skin or mucous membrane.

indomethacin (ˌindoh'methəsən) an anti-inflammatory analgesic used in the treatment of arthritis and of acute attacks of gout.

induction (in'dukshən) the act of initiating something. *Electromagnetic i.* the production of an electric current in a body because of its nearness to an electrified (or magnetised) body. *I. of abortion* the intentional bringing about of an abortion. *I. of anaesthesia* the start of the administration of a general anaesthetic. *I. of labour* the artificial starting of the process of childbirth.

induration (ˌindyə'rayshən) the abnormal hardening of a tissue or organ.

industrial (in'dustree'l) referring to industry. *I. or occupational diseases* those that are caused by the nature of the work. *Prescribed i. diseases* those for which sickness benefit is payable, including those that are notifiable under Acts such as the *Workers Compensation (Dust Diseases) Amendment Act 1967* (NSW) which covers dust diseases such as asbestos-related diseases (asbestosis, mesothelioma and lung cancer).

indwelling catheter (IDC) (indweling kathətə) any catheter designed to be left inside the body, either temporarily or permanently.

inebriation (iˌneebree'ayshən) the condition of being intoxicated by alcohol; drunkenness.

inert (i'nərt) having no action. *I. gas* a gas which does not react with other elements, e.g. neon.

inertia (i'nərshə) sluggishness; inability to move except when stimulated by an external force. *Uterine i.* lack of muscle contraction during the first and second stages of labour.

infant ('infənt) a child under 1 year of age. Educationally, a child under 7 years of age. *Floppy i., floppy i. syndrome* a congenital myopathy of infants, marked clinically by MYOTONIA and muscle weakness. *I. feeding* the supplying of nutrition to an infant. Breast milk is the ideal food for the baby, and if breastfeeding is established satisfactorily for the first few months, can aid physical and emotional development. Where it is not possible, an infant food formula can be given. *I. mortality rate* the number of deaths of children under 1 year of age per 1000 live births in any one year. *Premature i.* one born before the state of maturity. *See* PRETERM INFANT.

infanticide (in'fantəˌsied) the killing of a child during the first year of its life by the natural mother while she may be psychologically disturbed. Occurs in association with some mental health illnesses, e.g. depressive disorders.

infantile ('infənˌtiel) concerning an infant; childish. *I. paralysis* POLIOMYELITIS.

infantilism (in'fantəˌlizəm) persistence of the characteristics of childhood into adult life, marked by underdevelopment of the reproductive organs, and often short stature.

infarct ('infahkt) the wedge-shaped area of necrosis in an organ usually the lung or myocardium, produced by the blocking of a blood vessel, usually due to an embolism, atheroma or thrombosis. *Red i.* a haemorrhage infarct. Red blood cells infiltrate the area. *White i.* an anaemic infarct. The area is suddenly deprived of blood and is pale.

infarction (in'fahkshən) the formation of an infarct. *Myocardial i.* an infarct of the heart muscle following a coronary THROMBOSIS. *Pulmonary i.* an infarct resulting from obstruction of a branch of the pulmonary artery by EMBOLISM or thrombosis.

infection (in'fekshən) 1. invasion and multiplication of microorganisms in body tissues, especially that causing local cellular injury due to competitive metabolism, toxins, intracellular replication or antigen–antibody response. 2. an infectious disease. *Aerobic i.* infection caused by an aerobe. *Airborne i.* infection by inhalation of organisms suspended in air on water droplets, droplet nuclei or dust particles. *Anaerobic i.* infection caused by an ANAEROBE. *Cross i.* infection transmitted between patients infected with different pathogenic microorganisms. *Droplet i.* infection due to inhalation of respiratory pathogens suspended on liquid particles exhaled by someone already infected. *Dustborne i.* infection by inhalation of pathogens that have become affixed to particles of dust. *Healthcare-associated i. (HAI)* those acquired during episodes of healthcare, usually but not exclusively in hospitals. Also known as hospital-acquired infection. The most common causative agents are *Escherichia coli*, *Proteus*, *Pseudomonas* and *Klebsiella*, among the Gram-negative organisms, and *Staphylococcus aureus*, *Clostridium difficile* and *Enterococcus* among the Gram-positive organisms. *National I. Control Guidelines.* Guidelines that outline principles and practices of infection prevention and control with the aim of creating a safe healthcare environment. The responsibility for implementing the guidelines applies to everybody working and visiting a healthcare facility, including administrators, staff, patients and carers. *Opportunistic i.* an infection with a microorganism that does not usually cause disease but may do so when the patient's resistance to infection is lowered, e.g. after surgery. *Secondary i.* infection by a pathogen superimposed upon an infection by a pathogen of another kind. *Sexually transmitted i.* an infection transmitted by sexual intercourse or by intimate contact with the genitals, mouth and rectum. *See* SEXUALLY TRANSMITTED INFECTION. *Subclinical i.* infection associated with no detectable symptoms but caused by microorganisms capable of producing easily recognisable diseases, such as poliomyelitis or mumps; it is detected by the production of antibody, or by delayed hypersensitivity exhibited in a skin test reaction to such antigens as tuberculoprotein.

infectious (in'fekshəs) caused by or capable of being communicated by infection (*see* table, p. 245). *I. disease* disease caused by specific pathogenic microorganisms capable of transmission to another individual by direct and indirect contact. *See also* COMMUNICABLE DISEASE. *I. mononucleosis* (glandular fever). An acute virus infection, characterised by sore throat and glandular enlargement, caused by the Epstein-Barr (EB) virus. A common infection worldwide. Particularly prevalent in older children and young adults in Western countries. The source of infection is human and spread is by oropharyngeal secretions, e.g. during kissing. The incubation period is 4–6 weeks and infectivity after the disease may be prolonged.

infective (in'fektiv) infectious, capable of producing infection; pertaining to or characterised by the presence of pathogens.

inferior (in'fie͵ri·ə͵) lower. *I. vena cava* the lower large vein.

Common Infectious Diseases		
Disease	Incubation period (days)	Period of infectivity
Chicken pox (varicella)	10–20	2–3 days before until 10 days after onset of rash
Diphtheria	2–7	Until culture of three consecutive nose swabs proves negative
Enteric fevers Typhoid Paratyphoid	6–21	Until at least 1 month after onset of disease and after six consecutive negative stools
Measles (morbilli)	6–12	4 days before until 4 days after onset of rash
Mumps (parotitis)	12–28	2 days before onset until resolution of symptoms
Pertussis (whooping cough)	7–14	7 days before until 3 weeks after onset of cough
Rubella (German measles)	14–21	During incubation period until 2 days after resolution of symptoms

inferiority (in͵fiə·ri'orətee) lesser rank, stature, position or ability. *I. complex see* COMPLEX.

infertility (͵infər'tilətee) inability of a woman to conceive or of a man to bring about conception.

infestation (͵infe'stayshən) the presence of animal parasites, e.g. mites, ticks or worms, in or on the body, in clothing or in a house.

infibulation ('infibyoo͵layshən) an extensive form of female circumcision performed in some cultures in which the clitoris and labia are removed and the vaginal entrance narrowed. *See* CIRCUMCISION.

infiltration (͵infəl'trayshən) the entrance and diffusion of some substance not usually found there, either fluid or solid, into tissues or cells. *I. analgesia* the injection into tissues of a local analgesic solution.

inflammation (͵inflə'mayshən) a localised protective response elicited by injury or destruction of tissues, which serves to destroy, dilute or wall off both the injurious agent and the injured tissue. The cardinal signs are heat, swelling, pain and redness. *Acute i.* sudden onset of inflammation, with marked and progressive symptoms. *Catarrhal i.* inflammation in which mucous surfaces are attacked, with stimulation of exudation. *Chronic i.* inflammation that develops slowly. Granulation tissue forms and tends to localise the infection. *Diffuse i.* extensive inflammation, as in NEPHRITIS and CELLULITIS. *Suppurative i.* one marked by pus formation. *Traumatic i.* that which follows an injury.

inflammatory bowel disease (IBD) (inflamətree bowl di'zeez) collective term for a group of chronic disorders affecting the small and/or large intestines that result in pain, bleeding and diarrhoea. *See* CROHN'S DISEASE.

influenza (ˌinfloo'enzə) an acute viral infection of the respiratory tract, occurring in isolated cases, epidemics and pandemics. Also called flu. Transmission is by droplet inhalation and the period of infectivity lasts from 1 day before the onset of symptoms until up to 7 days later. Most cases occur in winter. There is fever, headache, pain in the back and limbs, anorexia, and sometimes nausea and vomiting. The fever subsides in 2–3 days, leaving a feeling of lassitude. There is no specific drug cure for influenza, but an influenza vaccine is available, the formulation of which is changed annually to include recently circulating strains of viruses on recommendation of the World Health Organisation (WHO). *I. vaccination* the most important measure available to prevent influenza and reduce the number of flu infections, complications and deaths. Under the National Immunisation Program (NIP) people who are eligible for a free influenza vaccine injection include those 65 years and over, pregnant women, those who suffer chronic conditions, as well as, for the first time, all Aboriginal and Torres Strait Islander people from 6 months of age. People not eligible under the NIP are able to purchase the vaccine on the private market. Annual flu injection is necessary as the virus changes each year. Influenza seasons and severity are unpredictable; however, influenza usually occurs from June, with the peak around August. Vaccinating from mid-April will allow people to develop immunity before influenza transmission is at its peak. (*See* Appendix 7.)

informatics (infawmatiks) discipline that integrates science, computer science and information science in systematising, identifying, collecting, processing and managing data. *Nursing i.* the way in which nurses, managers, researchers and practitioners use information systems in their work, enabling technology to develop a body of readily available knowledge to support the practice of nursing and the delivery of healthcare.

informed choice (in'fawmd choys) in order to make decisions about their own healthcare and treatment, mentally competent people need to be given information regarding their own condition that is accurate, non-judgemental and valid, in language that is jargon-free and understandable. This enables the person to make an informed choice from the treatment options. In some situations an interpreter may be required.

informed consent (in'fawmd kən'-sent) an ethical principle that requires a researcher to obtain voluntary participation of subjects in research, or a healthcare practitioner to obtain voluntary consent from a patient before undergoing a clinical or surgical procedure. In both cases, the person providing consent must be given full advice regarding the nature of the research or procedure, the risks involved, the chances of success and the alternative methods of research or treatment that are available. *See also* CONSENT.

infrared (ˌinfrə'red) rays of a lower wavelength than those in the visible spectrum. They can produce radiant heat which is used in the treatment of rheumatic conditions. *See* ULTRAVIOLET RAYS.

infundibulum (ˌinfuhnˈdibyələm) *pl.* infundibula. A general anatomical term for a funnel-shaped structure or passage, such as the cavity formed by the fimbriae tubae at the distal end of the fallopian tube; the stalk that extends from the hypothalamus to the posterior lobe of the pituitary gland; passage connecting the middle meatus of the nose with the frontal sinus.

infusion (inˈfyoozhən) 1. the process of extracting the soluble principles of substances (especially drugs) by soaking in water. 2. the solution thus produced. 3. the slow therapeutic introduction by gravity of fluid other than blood into a vein.

infusion pump (inˈfyoozhən pump) a device designed to administer intermittent or continuous measured amounts of fluids, medications or nutrients. Infusion pumps can be gravitational, electric or mechanically driven.

ingestion (inˈjeschən) the taking in of food and drugs by mouth.

inguinal (ˈing·gwin'l) relating to the groin. *I. canal* the channel through the abdominal wall, above POUPART'S LIGAMENT, through which the spermatic cord and vessels pass to the testis in the male, and which contains the round ligament of the uterus in the female. *I. ligament* Poupart's ligament; that connecting the anterior superior spine of the ilium to the tubercle of the pubis.

inhalation (ˌinhəˈlayshən) 1. the drawing of air or other substances into the lungs. 2. any drug or solution of drugs, administered (by means of nebulisers or aerosols) by the nasal or oral respiratory route.

inhaler (inˈhaylə) a device used for administering an inhalation of a drug in powder or as a vapour. Used mainly in the treatment of respiratory disorders, e.g. asthma and chronic respiratory disorders.

inherent (inˈhiə·rənt, -ˈher-) a characteristic that is innate or natural and essentially a part of the person.

inheritance (inˈherətəns) the acquisition of qualities and characteristics from parents and ancestors.

inhibition (ˌinhəˈbishən) arrest or restraint of a process. In psychiatry, the unconscious restraining of an instinctual drive.

injection (inˈjekshən) 1. the forcing of a liquid into a part, as into the subcutaneous tissues, the vascular tree or an organ (*see* figure, p. 248). 2. a substance so forced or administered. In pharmacy, a solution of a medicament suitable for injection. 3. prominence of small blood vessels on the surface of an organ or tissue, frequently indicating the vascular phase of an inflammatory response. *Hypodermic i.* that made just below the skin; a subcutaneous injection. *Intradermal i.* that made into the dermis just below the epidermis. *Intramuscular i.* that made into a muscle. *Intrathecal i.* that made into the subarachnoid space of the spinal cord. *Intravenous i.* that made into a vein. *Subcutaneous i.* that made into the subcutaneous tissues; a hypodermic injection. *Z-track i.* an intramuscular injection technique which allows a medication, e.g. an iron preparation, to be given but which prevents the leakage and the staining of tissues surrounding the site.

inlay (ˈinˌlay) material inserted to replace a defect in a tissue, e.g. a bone graft or a filling cast in metal to fit a hole in a tooth.

innate (iˈnayt) inborn; present in the individual at birth.

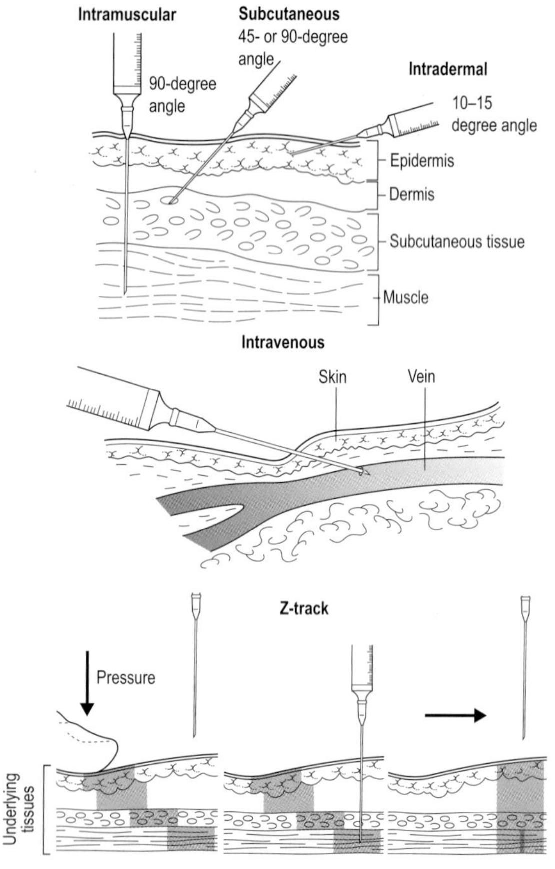

Intramuscular, subcutaneous, intradermal, intravenous and Z-track injections.

innervation (ˌinəˈvayshən) nerve supply to a part.

innocent (ˈinəsənt) as applied to a tumour, benign or non-malignant.

innocuous (iˈnokyooəs) harmless.

innominate (iˈnomənət) unnamed. *I. artery* a branch of the aorta, now termed the brachiocephalic trunk. *I. bone* the hip bone, formed by the union of the ilium, ischium and pubis.

inoculation (iˌnokyəˈlayshən) 1. introduction of pathogenic microorganisms, injected material, serum or other substances into tissues of living organisms or into culture media. 2. introduction of a disease agent (usually a live infectious agent) into a healthy individual to produce a mild form of the disease, followed by IMMUNITY.

inorganic (ˌinawˈganik) of neither animal nor vegetable origin.

inositol (iˈnohsəˌtol) a form of muscle or plant carbohydrate that has the same formula as simple sugar but not its other properties. *I. nicotinate* a vasodilator used in peripheral vascular disease.

inotropic (ˌinəˈtrohpik, -tropik) affecting the force or energy of muscular contractions, particularly the heart muscle. Beta-blocking drugs are said to be inotropic.

inquest (ˌingkwest) a legal inquiry held by a coroner, with or without a jury, into the cause of sudden or unexpected death.

insanity (inˈsanətee) a legal term for mental illness, roughly equivalent to PSYCHOSIS and implying inability to be responsible for one's actions.

insecticide (inˈsektəˌsied) one of a large group of chemical compounds that kill insect pests.

insemination (inˌseməˈnayshən) 1. fertilisation of an ovum by a SPERMATOZOON. 2. introduction of semen into the vagina. *Artificial i.* insemination by means other than sexual intercourse. The semen can be either the partner's (AIH) or some other donor's (AID). Also known as intrauterine insemination (IUI).

insensible (inˈsensəbəl) 1. unable to perceive with the senses. 2. unconscious. 3. imperceptible to the senses.

insertion (inˈsərshən) 1. the act of implanting. 2. something that is implanted. 3. the attachment of a muscle to the bone that it moves.

insidious (inˈsidi·əs) approaching by stealth. A term applied to any disease that develops imperceptibly. For example, symptoms develop gradually and are undetected by the person until the disease is well established.

insight (ˈinˌsiet) mental awareness. The capacity of individuals to estimate a situation or their own behaviour, or the connection between their present attitudes and past experiences. In psychiatry, a recognition by people that they are ill. Insight in this context may be complete, partial or absent, and may alter during the course of the illness.

in situ (inˈsityoo) [L.] in the original position.

insoluble (inˈsolyəbəl) not capable of being dissolved in a liquid.

insomnia (inˈsomni·ə) inability to sleep.

inspiration (inspəˈrayshən) the act of drawing in the breath.

inspissated (inˈspisaytəd) thickened, through evaporation, the absorption of fluid (and withdrawal of water) applied to culture medium in the laboratory and sputum.

instillation (ˌinstəˈlayshən) the act of inserting a liquid into a cavity drop by drop, e.g. into the eye.

instinct (ˈinstingkt) a complex of unlearned responses characteristic of a species. *Death i.* in psychoanalysis, the latent instinctive impulse towards death; the drive to reduce tensions by reaching the ultimate tensionless state of death. *Herd i.* the instinct or urge to be one of a group and to conform to its standards of conduct and opinion.

institutionalisation (instəˌtyoo-shənalieˈzayshən) a condition of apathy and withdrawal occurring in residents of long-stay institutions, prisons, etc., as a result of rigid routines and lack of independence. The person may resist leaving because the routine has become predictable and familiar, making minimal demands.

insufficiency (ˌinsəˈfishənsee) inadequacy. Used to describe the failure of function of an organ, such as the heart, stomach, liver or muscles.

insufflation (ˌinsəˈflayshən) the act of blowing air, gas or powder into a cavity of the body.

insulin (ˈinsyələn) a protein hormone formed in the beta cells of the PANCREATIC ISLETS OF LANGERHANS. The major fuel-regulating hormone, it is secreted into the blood in response to a rise in concentration of blood glucose or amino acids. A deficiency results in DIABETES MELLITUS. Various types of commercially prepared insulin are available. There are three main groups: rapid acting, intermediate acting and long acting. People with diabetes mellitus react differently in the rate at which they absorb and utilise insulin; therefore the duration of action varies from person to person. Insulin is measured in units. The concentration used is 100 units/mL. This strength allows for accurate measurement of dosage and reduces the possibility of error in calculating an individual dose. *I. pump* a device consisting of a syringe filled with a predetermined amount of short-acting insulin, a plastic cannula and a needle, and a pump that periodically delivers the desired amount of insulin. *See* DIABETES.

insulinase (ˈinsyələˌnayz) an enzyme that destroys the action of insulin.

insulinoma (ˌinsyələˈnohmə) a benign adenoma of the islet cells of the pancreas, causing HYPOGLYCAEMIA.

insulin sensitivity test (insyoolən ˌsensəˈtivətee test) a test used to determine the body's response to HYPOGLYCAEMIA induced by a small intravenous dose of insulin. It is used to test anterior pituitary function, particularly the ability to secrete growth hormone.

insult (ˈinsult) any trauma, irritation, poisoning or injury to the body.

integrated care (ˈintəgraytəd kair) a way of working that enables care to be provided that reflects the whole of a person's health needs; from prevention through to end of life, across both physical and mental health, and in partnership with the individual, their carers and family. The aim is to have care centred around the person, rather than organisations, to help people with complex needs get the care they need.

integrated models of care (ˈintəgraytəd modəlz ov kair) an approach to health care that aims to improve patient experience and achieve greater efficiency by nurses, physicians and other healthcare professionals working collaboratively in multidisciplinary teams. This approach also involves collaboration across disciplines, across organisations and across the primary–secondary care continuum.

integrated therapy (ˈintəgraytəd therəpee) a combination of complementary therapies with orthodox medicine to facilitate healing and promote the wellbeing of the patient. A biopsychosocial approach to care.

integument (ˈinˈtegyəmənt) 1. the skin. 2. a layer of tissue covering a part or organ of the body.

intellect (ˈintəˌlekt) the mind, thinking faculty, reasoning or understanding.

intelligence (inˈteləjəns) 1. the capacity to understand. 2. general mental ability. *I. quotient (IQ)* the ratio of the mental age to the chronological age expressed as a percentage. *I. test* a test designed to measure the level of intelligence, usually expressed as an IQ.

intensive care unit (ICU) (inˈtensiv kair ˈyoonət) a hospital unit in which are concentrated special equipment and specially trained personnel for the care of seriously ill patients requiring immediate and continuous monitoring and treatment. Also called critical care unit (CCU) or intensive therapy unit (ITU). *Neonatal ICU (NICU)* an intensive care unit that is designated solely for small, preterm neonates and those neonates requiring surgery or other specialised care. *Paediatric ICU (PICU)* a unit providing intensive care solely for seriously ill children.

intention (inˈtenshən) a process of healing.

intercellular (ˌintəˈselyələ) between the cells of a structure. May be applied to the connective tissue or to fluid bathing the cells.

intercostal (ˌintəˈkost'l) between the ribs. *I. muscles* muscles situated between the ribs and controlling their movements during inspiration and expiration.

intercourse (ˈintəˌkaws) 1. social exchange. 2. sexual intercourse or COITUS.

intercurrent (ˌintəˈkurənt) occurring at the same time. Describes a disease occurring during the course of another disease in the same person.

interdisciplinary (ˌintəˈdisəplənəree) joint working between professional disciplines: nursing, social work, clergy, medical staff, physiotherapy and other allied health professions.

interferon (ˌintəˈfie·ron) a protein, produced by cells infected by a virus, which has an inhibitory effect on the multiplication of the invading viruses thus preventing uninfected cells from becoming infected and hastening recovery from viral disease. Human interferon preparations, products of genetic engineering, are used in the treatment of some cancers, multiple sclerosis and hepatitis B and C.

interlobular (ˌintəˈlobyələ) between lobules. *I. veins* branches of the portal vein in the liver.

intermediate care (intəmeedyət kair) the purpose of services designed to assist the transition for a patient or client from medical and social dependence to day-to-day independence. A range of services having the potential to fulfil this function as people move from hospital to home, where the objectives of care are not primarily medical, the patient's discharge destination is anticipated, and a clinical outcome of recovery (or restoration of health) is desired. Intermediate care is also used to prevent hospital admission through provision of care in the home.

intermenstrual (ˌintəˈmenstrooəl) occurring between two menstrual periods.

intermission (ˌintəˈmishən) a temporary interruption, particularly of a feverish condition.

intermittent (ˌintəˈmitənt) occurring at intervals. *I. claudication* See CLAUDICATION. *I. fever* one in which the temperature drops to normal or lower, at times. *I. mandatory ventilation (IMV)* a type of mechanical ventilation in which the VENTILATOR is set to deliver a prescribed tidal volume at specified intervals and a high-flow gas system permits the patient to breathe spontaneously between cycles. *I. pneumatic compression hose* a stocking worn to prevent deep vein thrombosis of the upper and lower leg. *I. positive pressure breathing (IPPB)* a form of assisted or controlled mechanical ventilation that delivers a preset pressure of a gas into the airway until the desired pressure is reached. Passive exhalation is allowed through a valve, and the cycle begins again as the flow of gas is triggered by ventilation. Also known as intermittent positive pressure ventilation (IPPV). *I. self-catheterisation* a procedure carried out by the patient or their carer to drain urine from the bladder. This procedure is recommended for patients who cannot empty their bladder completely but can retain urine for 2–4 hours at a time and who have mental cognition, some manual dexterity and the ability to insert a catheter into the urethra. It can be used successfully by women, men and children. This is a clean rather than a sterile procedure.

internal (inˈtərn'l) situated on the inside. *I. consistency* the extent to which items within a scale reflect or measure the same concept. *I. haemorrhage* one occurring in a cavity or into the tissues. *I. secretion* one in which the hormones pass directly into the bloodstream from the secreting gland.

International Classification of Diseases (ICD) (intənashnəl ˌklas-ifəˈkayshən ov diˈzeezəs) a publication of the World Health Organisation produced about every 10 years listing all known disease categories.

International Council of Nurses (ICN) (intənashnəl kownsəl ov nərsəs) founded in 1899 to represent worldwide international nurses' associations as a corporate organisation.

internet (intənet) sometimes abbreviated to 'the net'. A global computer network with millions of connected computers. By connecting to this network, it is possible to access a wide range of information including health-related information, and to provide for the transmission of electronic mail. *I. addiction disorder* compulsive internet use which may lead to financial hardship, sleep deprivation, isolation and job or relationship breakdown, related to excessive hours spent on the internet. Management may include cognitive behavioural therapy and internet addiction support groups. Also known as problematic internet use.

interphase (ˈintəˌfayz) the period between two cell divisions during which the chromosomes are not easily visible.

intersex (ˈintəˌseks) 1. a congenital abnormality in which anatomical features of both sexes are evident. 2. a person displaying INTERSEXUALITY.

intersexuality (ˌintəˌseksyoo'alətee, -seksh-) an intermingling of the characters of each sex (including physical form, reproductive tissue and sexual behaviour) in one individual, as a result of some flaw in embryonic development.

interstitial (ˌintə'stishəl) situated within the tissue spaces or between the tissues. *I. cell-stimulating hormone (ICSH)* luteinising hormone. *I. fluid* the fluid in which body cells are bathed. It acts as an intermediary between the cells and the blood. Extracellular fluid. *I. keratitis see* KERATITIS. *I. nephritis* chronic NEPHRITIS associated with fibrosis and hypertension.

intertrigo (ˌintə'triegoh) an irritating, eczematous skin eruption caused by chafing of two moist skin surfaces.

intervention (ˌintə'venshən) in healthcare, any act carried out to prevent harm to patients, or to improve, promote or enhance their physical, mental or spiritual wellbeing.

intervertebral (ˌintə'vərtəbrəl) between the vertebrae. *I. disc* the pad of fibrocartilage between the bodies of the vertebrae. Protrusion of the contents of the disc may give rise to SCIATICA by exerting pressure on the nerve roots.

interviewing (intə'vyooing) process involving a structured, semi-structured or conversational style interview that allows the interviewer to probe for further information. This technique is also used at the initial stage of patient assessment in developing a nursing care plan. Interviews are also used as a method of data collection involving face-to-face or telephone questioning by the researcher; most often used in qualitative research.

intestinal (in'testən'l) referring to the INTESTINE.

intestine (in'testən) that part of the alimentary canal that extends from the stomach to the anus. *Small i.* the first 6 m from the pylorus to the caecum, consisting of the duodenum, the jejunum and the ileum. *Large i.* the final 2 m, consisting of the caecum, ascending colon, transverse and descending colon and the rectum.

intima ('intəmə) the innermost coat of an artery or vein.

intolerance (in'tolə·rəns) lack of power to endure. Applied to the effect of some drugs on individuals, e.g. iodine and quinine. *See* IDIOSYNCRASY.

intoxication (inˌtoksə'kayshən) 1. poisoning by drugs or harmful substances. 2. the condition produced by excessive use of alcohol.

intra-abdominal (ˌintrə·əb'domən'l) within the abdomen.

intra-articular (ˌintrə·ah'tikyələ) within a joint capsule. *I-a. injection* injection into a joint capsule, applicable to hydrocortisone, e.g. into a joint.

intracapsular (ˌintrə'kapsyələ) within a capsule, usually of a joint. *I. extraction* the removal of the whole lens with its capsule in the treatment of cataract.

intracellular (ˌintrə'selyələ) within a cell. *I. fluid* the water and its dissolved salts found within the cells.

intracerebral (ˌintrə'serəbrəl) within the brain substance. *I. haemorrhage* an escape of blood in the CEREBRUM, most often arising from the middle cerebral artery or from an ANEURYSM.

intracranial (ˌintrə'krayni·əl) within the skull. *I. abscess* one arising within the brain or meninges. *I. aneurysm* dilatation of one of the cerebral vessels. It may be congenital or acquired. *I. pressure (ICP)* the pressure exerted by the cerebrospinal fluid within the subarachnoid space and ventricles of the brain.

intractable (inˈtraktəbəl) not able to be relieved, controlled or cured.

intradermal (ˌintrəˈdərməl) between the layers of the skin.

intradural (ˌintrəˈdyoo·rəl) within the DURA MATER. *I. haemorrhage see* HAEMORRHAGE.

intragastric (ˌintrəˈgastrik) within the stomach.

intrahepatic (ˌintrəhəˈpatik) within the liver. Referring to a condition of the liver cells or connective tissue.

intralobular (ˌintrəˈlobyələ) within a lobule. *I. veins* veins that collect blood from within the lobules of the liver or kidneys.

intramedullary (ˌintraməˈduləree) 1. within the MEDULLA oblongata. 2. within the bone marrow. *I. nail* a metal pin used for the internal fixation of fractures.

intramuscular (ˌintrəˈmuskyələ) within muscle tissue.

intranasal (ˌintrəˈnayzəl) within the nose.

intranet (intrənet) a computer network designed to meet the internal needs of a single organisation. It is not necessarily open to the INTERNET and is not accessible by individuals from outside the organisation. *Healthcare i.* a well-designed healthcare intranet can improve the patient care experience by improving communications between staff, centralising resources such as diagnostic results and staff education.

intraocular (ˌintrəˈokyələ) within the eyeball.

intraorbital (ˌintrəˈawbət'l) within the orbit of the eye.

intraosseous (ˌintrəˈosi·əs) within a bone.

intraperitoneal (ˌintrəˌperətəˈneeəl) within the peritoneal cavity.

intrathecal (ˌintrəˈtheekəl) within the meninges of the spinal cord, usually in the subarachnoid space.

intratracheal (ˌintrəˈtraki·əl, -trəˈkeeəl) endotracheal; within the trachea. *I. anaesthesia* inhalation anaesthesia. *See* ANAESTHESIA.

intrauterine (ˌintrəˈyootə·rien) within the uterus. *I. contraceptive device* a contraceptive device introduced into the uterine cavity. *I. douche* irrigation of the uterine cavity. A special grooved nozzle is used, so that the fluid may return and is not forced into the uterine tubes. *I. growth restriction* associated with a poor blood supply to the placenta or with maternal disease. Other factors include infection during pregnancy, maternal smoking or drug addiction. The infant at birth is 'small for dates' and falls below the 10th percentile appropriate gestational age for infants. *I. insemination (IUI)* following the induction of ovulation fresh sperm are introduced into the uterus with ultrasound supervision; allows fertilisation to take place naturally in the uterine tubes. *See* IN VITRO FERTILISATION. *I. life* fetal development in the uterus.

intravenous (ˌintrəˈveenəs) within a vein. *I. flow rate* the rate at which fluids, medications and blood products flow into the bloodstream during intravenous infusion. The flow rate is usually ordered by the doctor as total volume (mL) per total hours or, in the case of drugs, total dose per total hours. *I. infusion* the therapeutic introduction of a fluid, such as saline, into a vein. The infusion works by gravity, in that the container of fluid is higher than the blood vessel into which the fluid is being introduced. *I. urography (IVU)* radiographic examination of the urinary tract after the injection of a radio-opaque contrast medium into a vein.

intravenous catheter (intrəveenəs kathətə) a catheter that is inserted into the vein for supply of fluids, medications or nutrients directly into the bloodstream.

intraventricular (ˌintrəvenˈtrikyələ) within a ventricle; may apply to a cerebral or a cardiac ventricle.

intrinsic (inˈtrinsik, -zik) particular to or contained within an organ. *I. factor* a glycoprotein, contained in the gastric juices, which is necessary for the absorption of the EXTRINSIC factor (vitamin B_{12}).

introitus (inˈtroh·itəs, ˌinˈtroytəs) [L.] an opening or entrance into a hollow organ or cavity. *I. vaginae* the vulva.

introjection (ˌintrəˈjekshən) a mental process by which individuals take into themselves the personal characteristics of another person, usually those of someone much loved or admired.

introspection (ˌintrəˈspekshən) a subjective study of the mind and its processes, in which individuals study their own reactions.

introversion (ˌintrəˈvərshən) 1. a turning inwards within itself of a hollow organ. 2. preoccupation with oneself, with reduction of interest in the outside world.

introvert (ˈintrəˌvərt) a person whose interests are turned inwards upon the self. *See* EXTROVERT.

intubation (ˌintyəˈbayshən) the introduction of a tube into a part of the body, particularly into the air passages to allow air to enter the lungs.

intumescence (ˌintyooˈmesəns) a swelling or increase in bulk, as of nasal mucous membrane in catarrh.

intussusception (ˌintəsəˈsepshən) prolapse of one part of the intestine into the lumen of an immediately adjacent part, causing OBSTRUCTION (intestinal) (*see* figure).

inunction (inˈungkshən) 1. rubbing an oily or fatty preparation containing a medicinal ingredient into the skin, with absorption of the drug. 2. any preparation so applied.

invagination (inˌvajəˈnayshən) 1. the folding inwards of a part, thus forming a pouch. 2. INTUSSUSCEPTION.

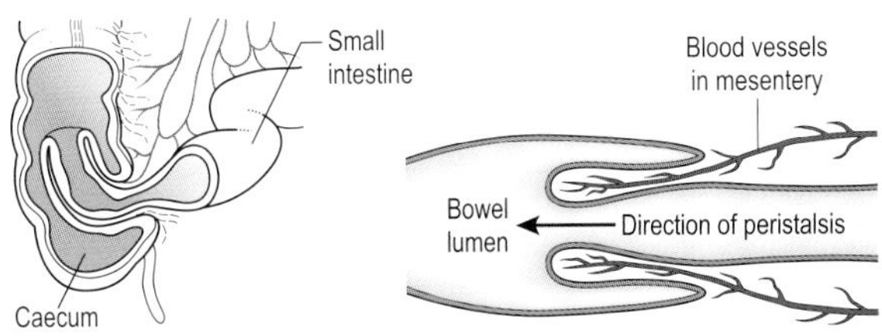

Example of intussusception.

invasion (in'vayzhən) 1. the entry of bacteria into the body. 2. the entrance of parasites into the body of a host.

invasive (in'vaysiv, -ziv) 1. having the quality of invasiveness. 2. involving puncture or incision of the skin or insertion of an instrument or foreign material into the body; said of diagnostic or therapeutic techniques.

invasiveness (in'vaysivnəs) 1. the ability of microorganisms to enter the body and spread in the tissues. 2. the ability to infiltrate and actively destroy surrounding tissue, a property of malignant tumours.

inversion (in'vərshən) a turning upside down or inside out. *Sexual i.* homosexuality. *Uterine i.* the condition of the uterus after parturition when a part of its upper segment protrudes through the cervix.

investigations (investəgayshənz) procedures performed to establish a diagnosis, to monitor a person's health, disease or the effectiveness of treatment. They are classified as non-invasive where there is no direct entry into the body, e.g. recording body weight, or as invasive, e.g. endoscopy or blood sampling.

in vitro (in vee'troh) the occurrence of a phenomenon in laboratory experiments (literally 'within a glass', e.g. test tube) and not necessarily reflecting what happens within the human body. For example, a drug may exhibit certain characteristics in vitro that may or may not occur inside the body. *I. v. fertilisation* a technique used to treat infertility for women who have blocked uterine tubes. The woman is given hormone therapy that promotes the maturity of more than one egg at a time. These eggs are harvested by laparoscopy and fertilised with sperm in the laboratory until a blastocyte is formed. Usually two of the fertilised eggs are implanted into the woman's uterus; if these become safely embedded pregnancy continues normally.

in vivo (in'veevoh) [L.] within the living body. *Compare* IN VITRO.

involucrum (ˌinvo'lookrəm) new bone which forms a sheath around necrosed bone, as in chronic OSTEOMYELITIS.

involuntary (in'voləntree) independent of the will. *I. muscle* one that acts without conscious control, e.g. the heart and stomach muscles.

involution (ˌinvə'looshən) 1. turning inwards; describes the contraction of the uterus after labour. The process whereby the uterus returns to its normal size. 2. the progressive degeneration occurring naturally with advancing age, resulting in shrivelling of organs or tissues.

iodine ('ieəˌdeen, -ien) *symbol* I. A non-metallic element with a distinctive odour obtained from seaweed. Iodine is essential in nutrition, being especially prevalent in the colloid of the THYROID (gland). Iodine is bactericidal and is used as povidone iodine for skin disinfection prior to invasive procedures. Iodine is opaque to X-rays and can be combined with other compounds for use as contrast media in diagnostic radiology.

iodopsin (ˌieə'dopsən) a violet pigment found in the retinal cones of the eyes.

iodoxyl (ˌieə'doksəl) a radio-opaque contrast medium. *See* INTRAVENOUS UROGRAPHY.

ion ('ieən) an atom or group of atoms having a positive (cation) or negative (anion) electric charge by virtue of having gained or lost one or more electrons. Substances forming ions are ELECTROLYTES. *See* HYDROGEN.

ionisation (ˌieənieˈzayshən) the breaking up of molecules into electrically charged particles or ions when an electric current is passed through an electrolytic solution.

iontophoresis (ieˌontohfəˈreesəs) the introduction through the skin of therapeutic ions by ionisation.

IPPB *see* INTERMITTENT POSITIVE PRESSURE BREATHING.

IPPV intermittent positive pressure ventilation.

ipsilateral (ˌipseeˈlatəˌrəl) occurring on the same side. Term applied particularly to paralysis or other symptoms occurring on the same side as the cerebral lesion causing them.

IQ intelligence quotient. *see* INTELLIGENCE.

IRDS infant respiratory distress syndrome.

iridectomy (ˌirəˈdektəmee) excision of a part of the iris, usually for the treatment of GLAUCOMA.

iridencleisis (ˌirədenˈkliesəs) an operation to make a drain out of a part of the iris, used in the treatment of GLAUCOMA.

iridium (iˈridi·əm) *symbol* Ir. *I.-192* A radioisotope used in brachytherapy to treat superficial malignancies such as those of the prostate, biliary tract, cervix and some head and neck.

iridocele (iˌridohˈseel) herniation of a part of the iris through a corneal wound.

iridocyclitis (ˌiridohsieˈklietəs) inflammation of the iris and ciliary body.

iridodonesis (ˌiridohdəˈneesis) trembling of the iris due to lack of support from the lens in dislocation of the lens or after a cataract extraction.

iridoptosis (ˌirədopˈtohsəs) prolapse of the iris.

iridotomy (ˌirəˈdotəmee) the making of a hole in the iris to form an artificial pupil.

iris (ˈierəs) the coloured part of the eye, made of two layers of muscle, the contraction of which alters the size of the pupil and so controls the amount of light entering the eye. *I. bomb* a bulging forwards of the iris due to pressure of the AQUEOUS HUMOUR when its passage into the anterior chamber is obstructed.

iritis (ieˈrietəs) inflammation of the iris, causing pain, photophobia, contraction of the pupil and discolouration of the iris. *See* UVEITIS.

iron (ˈieən) *symbol* Fe. A metallic element, present in the body in small quantities and essential to life. A deficiency may produce ANAEMIA.

irradiation (iˌraydeeˈayshən) the treatment of disease by electromagnetic radiation.

irreducible (ˌirəˈdyoosəbəl) incapable of being replaced in a normal position. Applied to a fracture or a hernia.

irrigation (ˌirəˈgayshən) the washing out of a cavity or wound with a stream of lotion or water.

irritable (ˈirətəbəl) reacting excessively to a stimulus. *I. bowel syndrome* mucous COLITIS; spastic colon. The person complains of disordered bowel function with abdominal pain, but no organic disease can be found.

irritant (ˈirətənt) an agent causing stimulation or excitation.

irritation (ˌirəˈtayshən) 1. a condition of undue nervous excitement resulting from abnormal sensitiveness. *Cerebral i.* a stage of excitement present in many brain conditions and typical of the recovery stage of concussion. 2. itching of the skin.

ischaemia (is'keemi·ə) a deficiency in the blood supply to a part of the body. *Myocardial i.* ischaemia of the heart muscles, which causes ANGINA PECTORIS.

ischiorectal (ˌiskeeoh'rekt'l) concerning the ischium and the rectum. *I. abscess* a collection of pus in the ischiorectal connective tissue. An anal fistula may result.

ischium ('iski·əm) the lower posterior bone of the pelvic girdle.

Ishihara colour charts (ˌishee'hahrə 'kulə chahtz) *Shinobu Ishihara, Japanese ophthalmologist, 1879–1963.* Patterns of dots of the primary colours on similar backgrounds which make numbers or patterns. The numbers or patterns can be seen by a normal sighted person, but one who is colour blind will be able to identify only some of them, depending on the type of colour blindness.

islet of Langerhans (ˌielet ov 'langəˌhanz) *Paul Langerhans, German pathologist, 1847–1888.* One of a group of cells in the pancreas that produce insulin and glucagon; islet of the pancreas.

isograft ('iesohˌgrahft) a tissue graft from one identical twin to another.

isoimmunisation (ˌiesohˌimyə-nie'zayshən) the development of antibodies against an antigen derived from an individual of the same species, e.g. a Rh-negative woman may immunise herself against her fetus, if it is Rh-positive, by forming specific ANTIBODY.

isolation (ˌiesə'layshən) the separation of a person with an infectious disease from those non-infected. *I. period* quarantine; the length of time during which a patient with an infectious fever is considered capable of infecting others by contact.

isoleucine (ˌiesoh'looseen) one of the 10 essential amino acids that are vital for health in the adult.

isometric (ˌiesə'metrik) having equal dimensions. *I. exercises* the contraction and relaxation of muscles without producing movement; used to maintain muscle tone after a fracture.

isotonic (ˌiesə'tonik) having uniform tension. *I. solution* a solution of the same osmotic pressure as the fluid with which it is compared. Normal saline (0.9% solution of salt in water) is isotonic with blood plasma.

isotope ('iesəˌtohp) one of the several forms of an element with the same atomic number but different atomic weights. *Radioactive i.* an unstable isotope which decays and emits alpha, beta or gamma rays. May be used in diagnostic and therapeutic procedures.

isovaleric acidaemia ('iesəˌvol'erik ˌasə'deemi·ə) a rare hereditary condition where the body cannot process the amino acid leucine. Screening for the condition takes place as part of newborn bloodspot screening.

isthmus ('isməs, 'isthməs) a narrow connection between two larger bodies or parts, e.g. the band of tissue between the two lobes of the thyroid gland.

itch (ich) a skin eruption. A skin sensation that makes the person want to scratch the part. Often associated with eczema and other skin conditions. Also known as pruritus. Generalised itching. May occur as a result of excessive bathing or using irritant detergent soaps, bath gels or foams. Itching is common in the older person who often has dry skin, and also commonly occurs in pregnancy. Generalised itching may also occur as a result of an allergic reaction to medications such as antibiotics. *Baker's i.* eczema of the hands due to the proteins of flour. *Barber's i.* sycosis; TINEA BARBAE. *Dhobie i.* TINEA CRURIS. The name is derived from the belief in India that the spread of infection was due to washermen (dhobies) wearing their clients' clothes. *I. mite* the cause of scabies, *Sarcoptes scabiei*. *Washerwomen's i.* dermatitis of the hands due to the constant use of detergents. Some people experience general itching as a result of taking certain drugs.

ITP idiopathic thrombocytopenic purpura.

IUCD *see* INTRAUTERINE CONTRACEPTIVE DEVICE.

IUI *see* INTRAUTERINE INSEMINATION.

IVF in vitro fertilisation. *See* FERTILISATION.

IVP *see* UROGRAPHY.

IVU *see* INTRAVENOUS UROGRAPHY.

Jj

J symbol for *joule*.

Jacksonian epilepsy (jak'sohni·ən 'epə,lepsee) *John Jackson, British neurologist, 1835–1911.* Focal motor EPILEPSY.

Jacquemier's sign ('zhahkmi·ayz sien) *Jean-Marie Jacquemier, French obstetrician, 1806–1879.* Blueness of the lining of the vagina seen from the early weeks of pregnancy.

jactitation (,jaktə'tayshən) the extreme restlessness of a severely ill person.

jargon ('jahgən) the terminology used and generally understood only by those who have knowledge of that specialty, e.g. medical jargon, legal jargon.

jaundice ('jawndəs) icterus; a yellow discolouration of the skin and conjunctivae, due to the presence of bile pigment in the blood often associated with pruritus. It may be one of the following types: (a) *haemolytic j.* due to excessive destruction of red blood cells, causing increase of bilirubin in the blood. The liver is not involved. *Acholuric j.* is of this type. It is characterised by increased fragility of the red blood cells; (b) *hepatocellular j.* in which the liver cells are damaged by either infection or drugs; (c) *obstructive j.* or *cholestatic j.* in which the bile is prevented from reaching the duodenum owing to obstruction by a gallstone, a growth or a stricture of the common bile duct; (d) *physiological j.* (icterus neonatorum), which occurs within the first few days of life, and is caused by the breakdown of the excessive number of red blood cells present in the newborn.

jaw (jor) a bone of the face in which the teeth are embedded. *Lower j.* the mandible. *Upper j.* the two maxillae.

JBI *see* JOANNA BRIGGS INSTITUTE.

jealousy (jeləsee) intense concern for the loss of affection or attention of another person; may also be exhibited as being envious of someone else's achievements or advantages. *Morbid j.* preoccupation with the potential sexual infidelity of one's partner. Morbid jealousy is usually caused by a personality disorder, but may also occur in those suffering from organic brain disease or alcohol dependency.

jejunal biopsy (jejoonəl bieopsee) removal of a small piece of the jejunum for histological and enzyme examination. Used to confirm Crohn's disease, coeliac disease and other malabsorption syndromes. The biopsy is taken using a flexible endoscope passed down through the mouth into the jejunum.

jejunectomy (,jejoo'nektəmee) excision of a part or the whole of the JEJUNUM.

jejunoileostomy (jə,joonoh,ilee'ostəmee) the making of an anastomosis between the JEJUNUM and the ILEUM.

jejunostomy (,jejoo'nostəmee) the making of an opening into the JEJUNUM through the abdominal wall.

jejunotomy (ˌjejooˈnotəmee) an incision into the JEJUNUM.

jejunum (jəˈjoonəm) the portion of the small intestine from the DUODENUM to the ILEUM; about 2.4 m in length.

jelly (ˈjelee) a soft, coherent, resilient substance; generally, a colloidal semisolid mass. *Contraceptive j.* a non-greasy jelly containing spermicide used in the vagina for prevention of conception (*see also* CONTRACEPTION). *Petroleum j.* a purified mixture of semisolid hydrocarbons obtained from petroleum (also called petrolatum). *Wharton's j.* the soft, jelly-like intracellular substance of the umbilical cord which insulates the vein and arteries, preventing occlusion and fetal hypoxia.

jellyfish sting (jeleefish sting) a dermal injury resulting from direct contact with a jellyfish. In Australia, the box jellyfish has caused deaths in humans.

jerk (jərk) a sudden muscular contraction. *Knee j.* also known as the patellar reflex is a kicking movement produced by tapping the tendon below the patella. Used with other jerks such as the ankle jerk to test the nervous reflexes.

jet lag (jet lag) the lack of balance that occurs between the local time and the person's biological rhythms that results from air travel over a long distance, especially in an easterly direction and to a lesser extent westwards. Sleep, memory and concentration are disturbed and there is a persistent feeling of tiredness usually lasting 2–3 days as the body adjusts to the time change.

jigger (ˈjigə) a sand flea, found in the tropics, which burrows into the soles of the feet and causes severe irritation.

Joanna Briggs Institute (JBI) (ˌjoˈanə brigz instətyoot) a group of collaborating centres that aim to promote evidence-based healthcare. Established in 1996 and based in Adelaide, South Australia.

jogger's heel (jogəz heel) a painful condition of the heel caused by repeatedly striking the heel against the ground or road surface when running or jogging.

jogger's nipple (jogəz nipəl) soreness of the nipple(s) caused by friction of clothing against them; occurs in runners and athletes. Prevention is achieved by applying petroleum jelly before running.

jogging (joging) running at a slow, even pace. A popular form of street exercise.

joint (joynt) an articulation; the point of junction of two or more bones, particularly one which permits movement of the individual bones relative to each other.

joint appointment (joynt ˌaˈpoyntmənt) a faculty appointment of a person to two institutions, e.g. to a university and a healthcare organisation.

joint practice (joynt praktis) the practice of one or more doctors, nurses and other health professionals who work as a team, sharing responsibility for a group of patients.

Jordan's frame (jawˈdəns fraym) a type of stretcher used to lift and transport patients with suspected or actual spinal injuries.

joule (jool) *symbol* J. The SI unit of energy.

JRA *see* JUVENILE RHEUMATOID ARTHRITIS.

judgement (ˈjujmənt) the ability of an individual to estimate a situation, to arrive at reasonable conclusions and to decide on a course of action.

jugular (ˈjugyələ) relating to the neck. *J. veins* several veins in the neck which drain the blood from the head.

Jungian theory (ˈyuhngee·ˌən thiəree) *Carl Jung, Swiss psychologist and psychiatrist, 1875–1961*. The concept that certain ideas from past experiences are present in the unconscious and controlled by the way in which the person views the world. Jung called these shared ideas the 'collective unconscious' as an entity common to all human beings. Jung considered that each person also had a 'personal unconscious' containing personal life experiences. Jung separated individuals into personality types: the externally sensitive type who directs energy outwards, and the introvert whose energies are inwardly directed. The goal of Jungian psychotherapy is to permit the individual to become what they essentially are, i.e. to encourage individual development.

junk food (junk food) convenience food or fast food, usually high in monosodium glutamate, fat and/or salt.

jurisprudence (ˈjoorisˌproodəns) the science of law. *Medical j.* is another name for forensic medicine.

juvenile (ˈjoovəˌniel) relating to young people.

juvenile rheumatoid arthritis (JRA) (joovəniel roomətoyd ˌahˈthrietəs) a rare form of inflammatory arthritis affecting children, most often girls, between the ages of 2 and 4 years or at puberty; usually affects four or more joints. Management is based around the relief of pain, suppression of the inflammatory process and the prevention of deformity. Also referred to as juvenile chronic arthritis or juvenile arthritis. In the systemic form of the disorder, known as Still's disease, features include a characteristic pink evanescent rash, high fever and cardiac involvement.

juxta-articular (ˌjukstə·ahˈtikyələ) near a joint.

juxtaglomerular (ˌjukstəglo-ˈmeryələ) near to a GLOMERULUS of the kidney. *J. cells* specialised cells found in the kidney which appear to play an important part in the control of aldosterone release.

juxtaposition (ˌjukstəpəˈzishən) an adjacent or side-by-side position.

Kk

K symbol for *potassium*.

Kahn test (kahn test) *Reuben Kahn, American bacteriologist, 1887–1979*. An agglutination test for syphilis.

kala-azar (ˌkahlə·əˈzah) visceral LEISHMANIASIS. A tropical disease caused by the protozoan parasite *Leishmania donovani*, which is carried by the sandfly. Symptoms include enlargement of the liver and spleen, anaemia and wasting. The disease is often fatal.

kangaroo care (kangəroo kair) the use of skin-to-skin contact between the premature but stable infant and parent or caregiver. The infant in nappy and cap rests on the mother's or father's exposed chest. The skin contact has a soothing effect, calming and warming the infant while promoting bonding between the parent and baby.

Kaposi's sarcoma (ˈkapohˌseez sahˈkohmə) *Moritz Kaposi, Austrian dermatologist, 1837–1902*. A multifocal, metastasising, malignant reticulosis with angiosarcoma-like features, chiefly involving the skin and mainly seen in people with poorly controlled or severe HIV infection or others with weakened immune systems. It is characterised by the development of blueish-red cutaneous nodules usually on the lower extremities, most often on the toes or feet, increasing in size and number and spreading to more proximal sites, especially on the face and nose.

Kaposi's spots (kapohseez spotz) a serious complication of atopic eczema occurring on exposure to HERPES SIMPLEX virus infection. More commonly known as Kaposi's varicelliform eruption.

karaya (kəˈrie·ə) a gum made from certain species of *Sterculia*, a genus of tropical trees and shrubs. Used as an aid to applying ostomy bags to the skin.

karyotype (ˈkareeohˌtiep) 1. the chromosomal constitution and arrangement of a cell of an individual. 2. the pattern that is seen when human chromosomes are photographed during metaphase. The pictures are then enlarged and paired according to the length of their short arm.

Kawasaki disease (kawasahkee diˈzeez) *Tomisaku Kawasaki, Japanese paediatrician, 1925–*. A rare, acute inflammatory disorder of young children. Cause and mode of transmission are not known but may be a sequela of a viral infection. Symptoms include fever, rash, sore throat, erythema of the lips and oral mucosa, and cervical lymphadenopathy and, in some children, cardiac complications. Occurs mainly in Japan and the United States. Also called mucocutaneous lymph node syndrome.

kcal kilocalorie.

Kegel exercises (ˈkaygəl ˈeksəˌsiezs) *Arnold Kegel, US gynaecologist, 1894–1981*. Specific exercises to strengthen the pelvic–vaginal muscles as a means of controlling stress incontinence in women.

Keller's operation ('keləz ˌopə'rayshən) *William Keller, American surgeon, 1874–1959*. An operation for correcting HALLUX VALGUS.

keloid ('keeloyd) hard, raised scar tissue in the skin, common in people with dark skins. A type occurs in a healed wound due to overgrowth of fibrous tissue, causing the scar to be raised above the skin level.

Kennedy's syndrome ('kenədeez 'sinˌdrohm) *Foster Kennedy, American neurologist, 1884–1952*. Ipsilateral optic atrophy caused by a frontal lobe tumour which involves one of the optic nerves.

keratectasia (ˌkerətek'tayzi·ə) protrusion of the cornea following inflammation.

keratectomy (ˌkerə'tektəmee) excision of a portion of the cornea.

keratic (kə'ratik) 1. horny. 2. relating to the cornea. *K. precipitates* inflammatory exudates adhering to the back of the cornea; a sign of IRITIS and IRIDOCYCLITIS.

keratin ('kerətən) one of a family of fibrous proteins which forms the main constituent of hair and nails.

keratinise (kə'ratəˌniez) to make or become horny.

keratitis (ˌkerə'tietəs) inflammation of the cornea. The causes may be physical (trauma, or exposure to dust, vapours or ultraviolet light) or due to infectious conditions such as corneal and dendritic ulcers. *Interstitial k.* deep chronic keratitis, usually arising in congenital syphilis. *Striate k.* inflammation that appears in lines due to the folding over of the cornea after injury or operation, particularly one for cataract.

keratocele ('keratohˌseel) protrusion of Descemet's membrane through the base of a corneal ulcer.

keratoconjunctivitis (ˌkeratohkənˌjungktə'vietəs) inflammation of both the cornea and the conjunctiva of the eye.

keratoconus (ˌkeratoh·konus) progressive thinning of the cornea.

keratoiritis (ˌkerətoh·ie'rietis) inflammation of both the cornea and the iris.

keratoma (ˌkerə'tohmə) KERATOSIS; a hard, thick epidermal growth caused by hypertrophy of the horny layer of the skin. Also called callus.

keratomalacia (ˌkerətohmə'layshi·ə) ulceration and softening of the cornea due to a deficiency of vitamin A.

keratometer (kerə'tomətə) ophthalmometer. An instrument by which the amount of corneal astigmatism can be measured accurately.

keratophakia (ˌkerətoh'fayki·ə) KERATOPLASTY, in which a slice of a donor's cornea is shaped to a desired curvature and inserted between layers of the recipient's cornea to change its curvature and to correct hypermetropia.

keratoplasty ('keratohˌplastee) a plastic operation on the cornea, including corneal grafting.

keratoscope ('keratohˌskohp) an instrument for examining the eye to detect keratoconus. Also known as Placido's disc.

keratosis (ˌkerə'tohsəs) a skin disease marked by excessive growth of the epidermis or horny tissue.

keratotomy (ˌkerə'totəmee) incision of the cornea.

kerion ('keeri·ən) a complication of ringworm of the scalp, with formation of pustules.

kernicterus (kər'niktə·rəs) a condition in the newborn marked by severe neural symptoms, associated with high levels of BILIRUBIN in the blood; it is commonly a sequela of ICTERUS GRAVIS NEONATORUM and may result in learning disabilities.

Kernig's sign (ˈkərnigz sien) *Vladimir Kernig, Russian physician, 1840–1917.* A sign of meningitis. When the thigh is supported at right angles to the trunk, the person is unable to straighten the leg at the knee joint (either actively or passively).

ketoacidosis (ˌkeetohˌasəˈdohsəs) acidosis accompanied by an accumulation of ketone bodies, resulting from extensive breakdown of fats because of faulty carbohydrate metabolism. In this condition, urinary loss of water, potassium, ammonium and sodium results in hypovolaemia, electrolyte imbalance, extremely high blood glucose levels and breakdown of free fatty acids, causing acidosis. It occurs primarily as a complication of DIABETES MELLITUS, and is characterised by a fruity odour of acetone on the breath, mental confusion, dyspnoea, nausea, vomiting, dehydration, weight loss and, if untreated, coma. Emergency treatment includes the administration of insulin and intravenous fluids and the evaluation and correction of electrolyte imbalance.

ketogenic (ˌkeetəˈjenik) forming or capable of being converted into ketone bodies. *K. diet* one that contains large amounts of fat, with minimal amounts of protein and carbohydrate. The object of such a diet is to produce KETOSIS. It is occasionally used in the treatment of certain types of epilepsy in young children.

ketone (ˈkeetohn) an organic compound containing the carbonyl group (CO) attached to two hydrocarbon groups. Ketones are produced by the CATABOLISM of fats.

ketonuria (ˌkeetəˈnyoo·ri·ə) the presence of ketones in urine; ACETONURIA.

ketosis (keeˈtohsəs) the condition in which ketones are formed in excess in the body and accumulate in the blood. Severe ACIDOSIS may occur.

ketosteroid (ˌkeetohˈstiə·royd) a steroid hormone which contains a ketone group attached to a carbon atom. *17-k.s* are excreted in the urine and formed from the adrenal corticosteroids, testosterone and, to a lesser extent, oestrogens.

kick chart (kik chaht) a method of fetal assessment carried out by the mother. The number of kicks or movements felt during the day is counted and noted. If fewer than 10 kicks are felt in a 12-hour daytime period on two consecutive occasions, the mother is advised to contact her midwife or doctor immediately. This is a subjective assessment, and is usually combined with other tests of fetal wellbeing. Also known as a fetal movement chart.

kidney (ˈkidnee) one of two organs situated in the lumbar region which purify the blood and secrete urine. The kidney secretes renin and renal erythropoietic factor. *Artificial k.* the apparatus used to remove retained waste products from the blood when kidney function is impaired. *Granular k.* the small fibrosed kidney of chronic NEPHRITIS. *Horseshoe k.* a congenital defect producing a fusion of the two kidneys into a horseshoe shape. *K. dish* a kidney-shaped dish commonly used to hold instruments, dressings and injection equipment. *K. failure* the condition in which renal function is severely impaired and the organs are unable to maintain the fluid and electrolyte balance of the body. *K. transplant* the surgical implantation of a kidney taken from a live donor or from one who has recently died. Used in the treatment of renal failure. *Polycystic k.* a congenital bilateral condition of multiple cysts replacing kidney tissue.

kilocalorie (ˈkiləˌkalə·ree) *symbol* kcal. One thousand calories; a unit of food energy.

kilojoule (ˈkiləˌjool) *symbol* kJ. One thousand joules; a unit of food energy (1 kcal = 4.184 kJ).

Kimmelstiel-Wilson syndrome (ˌkiməlsteelˈwilsən ˈsinˌdrohm) *Paul Kimmelstiel, German pathologist, 1900–1970; Clifford Wilson, British physician, 1906–1997.* A degenerative complication of DIABETES MELLITUS, with albuminuria, oedema, hypertension, renal insufficiency and retinopathy; may lead to kidney failure. Also called intercapillary glomerulosclerosis.

kinaesthesia (ˌkinəsˈtheezi·ə) the combined sensations by which position, weight and muscular position are perceived.

kinanaesthesia (ˌkinanəsˈtheezi·ə) an inability to perceive the sensation of movements of parts of the body.

kinase (ˈkienayz) an enzyme activator; *see* enterokinase and thrombokinase.

kineplasty (ˈkinəˌplastee) a form of amputation; amputation in which the stump is so formed as to be used for producing motion of the prosthesis. Also called cineplastic or kineplastic amputation.

kinetic (kəˈnetik) producing or pertaining to motion.

kinin (ˈkienən) a polypeptide which occurs naturally and is a powerful vasodilator.

kinship (ˈkinˌship) relationship. *K. studies* in anthropology, the study of kin (relatives) and their patterns of marriage, descent, inheritance, habitation, social values, health beliefs and economics.

Kirschner wire (ˈkiəshnəˈwier) *Martin Kirschner, German surgeon, 1879–1942.* A thin wire that may be passed through a bone to apply skeletal traction.

kiss of life (ˌkis ov ˈlief) the expired air method of artificial respiration, by either mouth-to-nose or mouth-to-mouth breathing.

kJ *symbol* for *kilojoule*.

Klebs-Löffler bacillus (ˌklebzˈlərflə bəˈsiləs) *Edwin Klebs, German bacteriologist, 1834–1913; Friedrich Löffler, German bacteriologist, 1852–1915.* Former name for *Corynebacterium diphtheriae*, the causative agent of diphtheria.

Klebsiella (ˌklebseeˈelə) a genus of Gram-negative bacteria (family *Enterobacteriaceae*).

Kleihauer test (ˈkliehowə test) a microscopic test to detect fetal cells in the maternal circulation, usually done immediately after delivery so that, if the mother is Rh-negative and the fetus Rh-positive, anti-D immunoglobulin may be given to prevent ISOIMMUNISATION.

kleptomania (ˈkleptəˌmayni·ə) an irresistible urge to steal when there is often no need and no particular desire for the objects. Often associated with depression.

Klinefelter's syndrome (ˈklienfeltəz ˈsinˌdrohm) *Harry Klinefelter, American physician, 1912–1990.* A congenital chromosome abnormality in which each cell has three sex chromosomes, XXY, rather than the usual XX or XY, making a total of 47 (normal is 46). Affected men have female breast development, small testes and are infertile.

Klippel-Feil syndrome (ˌklipəl'fiel 'sinˌdrohm) a congenital abnormality in which the neck is very short as a result of the absence or fusion of several vertebrae in the cervical region.

knee (nee) the joint between the femur and the tibia. *Housemaid's k.* prepatellar BURSITIS. *K. cap* the patella. *K. jerk* an upward jerk of the leg obtained by striking the patellar tendon when the knee is passively flexed. *Knock-k.* a condition in which the knees turn inwards towards each other; GENU VALGUM.

knee replacement (nee ˌrə'plays-mənt) the surgical incision of a prosthesis performed to relieve pain and restore motion to a knee severely affected by osteoarthritis, rheumatoid arthritis or trauma.

kneecap (neekap) the patella.

Koch's bacillus (koks bə'siləs) *Robert Koch, German bacteriologist, 1843–1910.* Former name for *Mycobacterium tuberculosis*, the causative organism of tuberculosis.

Köhler's disease ('kərləz di'zeez) *Alban Köhler, German physician and radiologist, 1874–1947.* OSTEOCHONDRITIS of the navicular bone of the foot, occurring in children.

koilonychia (ˌkoylə'niki·ə) the development of brittle, spoon-shaped nails, which may occur in iron-deficiency anaemia.

Koplik's spots ('kopliks spotz) *Henry Koplik, American paediatrician, 1858–1927.* Small white spots that sometimes appear on the mucous membranes inside the mouth in measles on the second day of onset, before the general rash.

Korotkoff's method (ko'rotkofs 'methuhd) *Nikolai Korotkoff, Russian physician, 1874–1920.* A method of finding the systolic and diastolic blood pressure by listening to the sounds produced in an artery while the pressure in a previously inflated cuff is gradually reduced.

Korsakoff's syndrome or psychosis ('kawsəkofs 'sinˌdrohm aw sie'kohsəs) *Sergei Korsakoff, Russian neurologist, 1854–1900.* A chronic condition in which there is impaired memory, particularly for recent events, and the person is disorientated for time and place. It may be present in psychosis of infective, toxic or metabolic origin, or in chronic alcoholism.

kosher (kohshə) food that is prepared and cooked in accordance with Jewish dietary laws; it is eaten by practising Jews.

kraurosis (kraw'rohsəs) dryness and shrinking of a part of the body. *K. vulvae* a degenerative condition of the vulva. May be treated by giving oestrogen preparations.

Kreb's cycle (krebz 'siekəl) *Sir Hans Krebs, German–British biochemist, 1900–1981.* A series of reactions during which the aerobic oxidation of pyruvic acid takes place. This is part of carbohydrate metabolism. Also known as the citric acid cycle or tricarboxylic acid cycle. *K. urea c.* the way in which urea is formed in the liver.

Küntscher nail ('koontshə nayl) *Gerhard Küntscher, German orthopaedic surgeon, 1902–1972.* Intramedullary nail used in treating fractures of long bones, especially the shaft of the femur.

Kupffer's cells ('kuhpfəz ˌsels) *Karl von Kupffer, German anatomist, 1829–1902.* Phagocytic reticuloendothelial cells of the liver which form bile from haemoglobin released by disintegrated ERYTHROCYTES.

kuru (ˈkooroo) (New Guinea shivering) a slow, progressive, fatal infection of the central nervous system found only in natives of New Guinea. The disease was transmitted by eating brain tissue during funeral rites. No new cases have been reported since cessation of cannibalism.

Kussmaul breathing (ˈkuhsmowl ˈbreething) deep, rapid and sighing respirations, associated with diabetic ketoacidosis.

Kveim test (ˈkvaym test) *Morten Kveim, Norwegian physician, 1892–1966.* A test for SARCOIDOSIS in which antigen from the lymph nodes or spleen of a person with sarcoidosis is injected intradermally.

kwashiorkor (ˌkwasheeˈawkaw) a condition of protein malnutrition occurring in children in underprivileged populations. Fatty infiltration of the liver arises and may cause cirrhosis.

kymograph (ˈkiemәˌgrahf, -ˌgraf) an instrument for recording variations or undulations in pressure, arterial or other.

kyphoscoliosis (ˌkiefohˌskohleeˈohsәs) an abnormal curvature of the spine in which there is forward and sideways displacement.

kyphosis (kieˈfohsәs) posterior curvature of the spine; humpback.

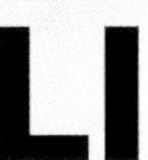

L symbol for *litre*.

label (laybəl) 1. a classifying name given to a person or object. When a label is given to someone there is a tendency for that person to be perceived by others and often by themselves as having the characteristics implied by the label, and being nothing more than that and therefore being undervalued. 2. a means of providing data when attached to an item, e.g. drugs, food or surgical dressings.

labia (ˈlaybi·ə) 1. the lips: the fleshy, lip-like edges of an organ or tissue. 2. the folds of skin at the opening of the vagina. *L. majora* two long lips of skin, one on each side of the vaginal orifice outside the labia minora. They extend from the anterior labial commissure to the posterior labial commissure and form the lateral boundaries of the pudendal cleft. Each labium contains areolar tissue, fat, and a thin layer of non-striated muscle. In some women the outer surface of each lip may be covered with coarse pubic hair. The embryonic derivations of the labia majora and the scrotum are homologous. *L. minora* two thin folds of skin between the labia majora, extending from the clitoris backwards on both sides of the vaginal orifice, ending between it and the labia majora. Anteriorly each labium divides into an upper and lower division. The upper divisions pass above the clitoris and meet to form the preputium clitoridis; the lower divisions pass beneath the clitoris and unite to form the frenulum of the clitoris. Opposed surfaces of the labia minora contain sebaceous follicles.

labial (ˈlaybi·əl) pertaining to the lips or LABIA.

labile (ˈlaybiel) unstable. Applied to those chemicals that are subject to change or readily altered by heat.

lability (ləˈbilətee) instability. *L. of mood* the tendency to sudden changes of mood of short duration.

labium (ˈlaybi·əm) a lip. *L. majus pudendi* the large fold of flesh surrounding the vulva. *L. minus pudendi* the lesser fold within the labium majus.

labor (ˈlaybə) *see* LABOUR.

labour (ˈlaybə) parturition or childbirth, which takes place in three stages: (a) dilatation of the cervix uteri; (b) passage of the child through the birth canal; and (c) expulsion of the placenta. *Induced l.* labour brought on by artificial means before term, as in cases of contracted pelvis, or if overdue. *Obstructed l.* labour in which there is a mechanical hindrance also known as labour dystocia. *Precipitate l.* labour in which the baby is delivered extremely rapidly. *Premature l.* labour which occurs after the 24th week of pregnancy and before full term. *Spontaneous l.* that which occurs without being artificially induced or accelerated. *Spurious l.* ineffective labour pains which sometimes precede true labour pains.

labyrinth (ˈlabə·rinth) the structures forming the internal ear, i.e. the cochlea, vestibule and semicircular canals. *Bony l.* the bony canals of the internal ear. *Membranous l.* the soft structure inside the bony canals.

labyrinthectomy (ˌlabə·rinˈthek-təmee) excision of the labyrinth.

labyrinthitis (ˌlabə·rinˈthietəs) inflammation of the labyrinth, causing vertigo.

laceration (ˌlasəˈrayshən) 1. the act of tearing or slashing. 2. a wound with torn and ragged edges. *Perineal l. see* PERINEAL.

lacrimal (ˈlakrəməl) relating to tears. *L. apparatus* the structures secreting the tears and draining the fluid from the conjunctival sac (*see* figure). *L. gland* a gland that secretes tears, which drain through two small openings in the eyelids (*l. puncta*) into a pair of ducts (*l. canaliculi*) into the sac and finally into the nasal cavity through the nasolacrimal duct. Situated in the outer and upper corner of the orbit.

lacrimation (ˌlakrəˈmayshən) an excessive secretion of tears.

lacrimator (ˈlakrəˌmaytə) a substance that causes excessive secretion of tears, e.g. tear gas.

lactagogue (ˈlaktəˌgog) any agent that promotes the secretion or flow of milk; galactagogue.

lactalbumin (lakˈtalbyəmən) an albumin of milk.

lactase (ˈlaktayz) an enzyme produced in the small intestine, which converts lactose into glucose and galactose.

lactate (ˈlaktayt) 1. any substance given to promote lactation. 2. any salt of lactic acid. 3. to secrete milk. *L. dehydrogenase* or lactic acid dehydrogenase, abbreviated LD or LDH. An enzyme that catalyses the interconversion of lactate and pyruvate. Widespread in tissues and particularly abundant in kidney, skeletal muscle, liver and myocardium. It has five isoenzymes, denoted LD_1 to LD_5. The 'flipped' pattern, in which the serum LD_1

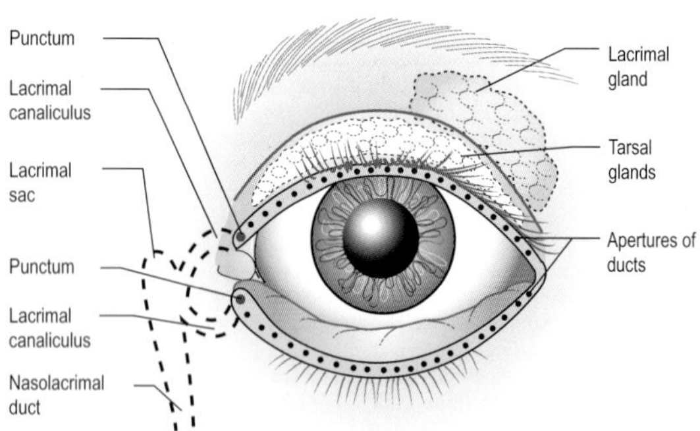

Lacrimal apparatus.

level is greater than the LD_2 level, is indicative of an acute myocardial infarction. This pattern occurs within 12–24 hours after the attack.

lactation (lakˈtayshən) 1. the period during which the infant is nourished from the breast. 2. the process of milk secretion by the mammary glands.

lacteal (ˈlakti·əl) 1. consisting of milk. 2. a lymphatic duct in the small intestine which absorbs CHYLE.

lactic (ˈlaktik) pertaining to milk. *L. acid* an acid formed by the fermentation of lactose or milk sugar. It is produced naturally in the body as a result of glucose metabolism. An excess of the acid accumulating in the muscles may cause cramp.

lactiferous (lakˈtifə·rəs) conveying or secreting milk. *L. duct* one of many channels that carry milk from the lobes of each breast or nipple. *L. glands* ones that secrete or convey milk, such as mammary glands.

lactifuge (ˈlaktəfyooj) a drug or agent that retards the secretion of milk.

Lactobacillus (ˌlaktohbəˈsiləs) a genus of Gram-positive, rod-shaped bacteria, many of which produce fermentation.

lactoferrin (ˌlaktohˈferən) an iron-binding protein found in neutrophils and bodily secretions (milk, tears, saliva, bile, etc.), having bactericidal activity and acting as an inhibitor of colony formation by GRANULOCYTES and MACROPHAGES.

lactogenic (ˌlaktəˈjenik) stimulating the production of milk. *See* LUTEOTROPHIN.

lactometer (lakˈtomətə) an instrument for measuring the specific gravity of milk.

lactose (ˈlaktohz, -tohs) milk sugar consisting of glucose and galactose. *L. intolerance* the ingestion of milk containing lactose results in the person experiencing severe abdominal colic and diarrhoea due to a deficiency of the lactose-splitting enzyme (beta-galactosidase) in the lining of the small intestine.

lactosuria (ˌlaktəˈsyoo·ri·ə) lactose in the urine.

lactovegetarian (ˌlaktohˌvejəˈtair·ri·ən) 1. a person who subsists on a diet of milk or milk products and vegetables. 2. pertaining to such a diet.

lactulose (ˈlaktyəlohz) a synthetic disaccharide which is used as a laxative.

lacuna (ləˈkyoonə) a small cavity or depression in any part of the body.

Laënnec's cirrhosis (ˌlie·əˈneks səˈrohsəs) *René Laënnec, French physician, 1781–1826.* The most common type of cirrhosis of the liver, frequently attributable to high alcohol consumption.

laevulose (ˈlevyəˌlohz) fruit sugar; fructose.

laking (ˈlayking) haemolysis of the red blood cells. The cells swell and burst and the haemoglobin is released.

lallation (laˈlayshən) a babbling, infantile form of speech.

Lamaze method (laˈmayz ˈmethuhd) *Fernand Lamaze, French obstetrician, 1890–1957.* A method of preparing for NATURAL CHILDBIRTH developed by Fernand Lamaze, and based on the technique of training the mind and body for the purpose of modifying perception of pain during labour and delivery.

lambdoid (ˈlamdoyd) shaped like the Greek letter lambda, L or l. *L. suture* the junction of the occipital bone with the parietals.

lambliasis (lamˈblieəsəs) GIARDIASIS.

lamella (ləˈmelə) 1. a thin layer, membrane or plate, as of bone.

2. a thin medicated disc of gelatin used in applying drugs to the eye. The gelatin dissolves and the drugs are absorbed.

lamina (ˈlamənə) a bony plate or layer. *L. air flow* a system of circulating filtered air in parallel flowing planes in hospitals or other healthcare facilities. The system may reduce the risk of airborne contamination and exposure to chemical pollutants in surgical theatres, food preparation areas, hospital pharmacies and laboratories.

laminectomy (ˌlaməˈnektəmee) excision of the posterior arch of a vertebra, sometimes performed to relieve pressure on the spinal cord or nerves.

Lancefield's groups (ˈlansfeeldz groops) *Rebecca Lancefield, American bacteriologist, 1895–1981.* Divisions of beta-haemolytic streptococci, which are classified on the basis of serological action into groups A–R. Most human infections are due to group A.

lancet (lahnsət) a pricking needle used to obtain a drop of blood for testing. It has a guard above the needle that prevents deep penetration, and is usually disposable.

landmark (landmark) a readily recognisable anatomical structure used as a point of reference in establishing the location of another structure or in determining certain measurements.

Landry's paralysis (lanˈdreez pəˈraləsəs) *Jean Landry, French physician, 1826–1865.* Guillain-Barré syndrome; acute ascending POLYNEURITIS.

Landsteiner's classification (ˈland-stienəz ˌklasifəˈkayshən) *Karl Landsteiner, Austrian biologist, 1868–1943.* A system of blood groups; the ABO system, consisting of groups A, B, AB and O. *See* BLOOD GROUPS.

Langerhans cells (ˈlangəˌhanz selz) *Paul Langerhans, German pathologist, 1847–1888.* Dendritically shaped cells located in the stratified squamous epithelium of mammals. Dendritic cells play an important role in local defence mechanisms in the epithelium.

Langerhans, islet of (ˈlangəˌhanz ˌielet ov) *Paul Langerhans, German pathologist, 1847–1888.* One of the group of cells in the pancreas that produce insulin. They constitute 1–2% of the pancreas volume.

Langhans' cell (ˈlanghanz sel) *Theodor Langhans, Swiss pathologist, 1834–1915.* Multinucleated giant cells seen in tuberculosis and other granulomas.

language (ˈlanˌgwij) the means of human communication consisting of the use of the spoken or written word in a structured way. Gestures of hands, head and even the body may be involved, although this is reflected differently from one setting to another, e.g. from a formal presentation to the greeting of a friend. Cultural background too plays a part in the use or absence of gestures. *L. disorders* problems affecting the ability to communicate and/or comprehend the spoken and/or written word. *See* SPEECH.

lanolin (ˈlanələn) a fat obtained from sheep's wool and used as a basis for ointments, salves, creams and cosmetics.

lanugo (ləˈnyoogoh, -noo-) the fine hair that covers the body of the fetus and newly born infants, especially those who are premature. Also called down.

laparoscopy (ˌlapəˈroskəpee) viewing of the abdominal cavity by passing an endoscope through the abdominal wall.

laparotomy (ˌlapəˈrotəmee) incision of the abdominal wall for exploratory purposes.

laryngeal (ləˈrinji·əl, ˌlarənˈjeeəl) pertaining to the larynx.

laryngectomy (ˌlarənˈjektəmee) excision of the larynx.

laryngismus (ˌlarənˈjizməs) a spasmodic contraction of the larynx. *L. stridulus* a crowing sound on inspiration, following a period of apnoea, due to spasmodic closure of the glottis. It occurs in children, particularly those suffering from rickets. CROUP.

laryngitis (ˌlarənˈjietəs) inflammation of the larynx causing hoarseness or loss of voice due to acute infection or irritation by gases.

laryngopharynx (laringohfarinks) the lower portion of the pharynx connecting with the larynx.

laryngoscope (ləˈring·gəˌskohp) an endoscopic instrument for examining the larynx or for aiding the insertion of endotracheal tubes or the bronchoscope.

laryngospasm (ləˈring·gohˌspazəm) a reflex, prolonged contraction of the laryngeal muscles that is liable to occur on insertion or withdrawal of an endotracheal tube.

laryngostenosis (ləˌring·goh-stəˈnohsəs) contraction or stricture of the larynx.

laryngostomy (ˌlaringˈgostəmee) the making of an opening into the larynx to provide an artificial air passage.

laryngotomy (ˌlaringˈgotəmee) an incision into the larynx to make a temporary opening in an emergency when the larynx is obstructed. TRACHEOSTOMY.

laryngotracheal (ləˌring·gohˈtraki əl) referring to both the larynx and the trachea.

laryngotracheitis (ləˌring·ohˌtrakee-ˈietəs) inflammation of both the larynx and the trachea.

laryngotracheobronchitis (ləˌring·-gohˌtrakeeohbrongˈkietəs) an acute viral infection of the respiratory tract which occurs particularly in young children. Also known as CROUP.

larynx (ˈlaringks) [Gr.] the muscular and cartilaginous structure, lined with mucous membrane, situated at the top of the trachea and below the root of the tongue and the hyoid bone. The larynx contains the vocal cords and is the source of the sound heard in speech. Also called the voice box.

laser (ˈlayzə) acronym for Light Amplification by Stimulated Emission of Radiation. An apparatus producing an extremely concentrated beam of light that can be used to cut metals. When used in the treatment of neoplasms, detached retina, diabetic RETINOPATHY and macular degeneration, and some skin conditions, eye protection must be worn by the operator. *L. assisted hair removal* the use of various light sources for hair removal. Treatment results in temporary hair loss for several months. Hair loss may be permanent.

Lassa fever (ˈlasə ˈfeevə) a highly contagious disease of West Africa caused by an arenavirus. It can also be transmitted by contact with or inhalation of excreta of infected rodents. Person-to-person transmission occurs through contact with infected blood, secretions or excreta or transmission may be via the airborne route. Prevention is dependent on the early detection of cases and their isolation, and strict precautions to protect healthcare staff caring for a febrile person.

lassitude (ˈlasəˌtyood) a feeling of extreme weakness and apathy.

latent (ˈlaytənt) temporarily concealed; not manifest. *L. heat* the heat absorbed by a substance during a change in state, e.g. from water into steam. When condensation occurs, this heat is released. *L. period* 1. the incubation period of an infectious disease. 2. the time between the application of a nerve stimulus and the reaction.

lateral (ˈlatə·rəl) situated at the side; therefore, away from the centre. *L. epicondylitis* tennis elbow. A condition which occurs after strenuous overuse of the muscles and tendons near the elbow joint.

lateroversion (ˌlatə·rohˈvərshən, -zhən) a turning to one side, such as may occur of the uterus.

latex (ˈlayteks) a milky fluid derived from tapping the rubber tree, *Hevea brasiliensis*, found mainly in Thailand, Indonesia and Malaysia. It comprises an aqueous suspension of globules of rubber hydrocarbon coated with proteins. *L. allergy* a reaction to latex proteins, varying in severity. It is a significant occupational health problem for healthcare workers and patients (especially children) with chronic conditions. Latex is a component of many medical products, e.g. various tubes, materials and gloves. Latex gloves have been frequently implicated due to either the latex or the proteins used in the powders that lubricate the gloves for ease of use.

lavage (ˈlavij, laˈvahzh) the washing out of a cavity. *Colonic l.* the washing out of the colon. *Gastric l.* the washing out of the stomach.

laxatives (ˈlaksətivs) a group of drugs used to treat constipation or to evacuate the bowel before surgery on the large bowel. May be used orally, in suppositories or in enemas. There are different categories of laxative based upon their method of working: (a) bulk forming, e.g. methyl cellulose, that increase volume, encouraging the passage of a softer and bulkier stool; (b) stimulant laxatives that cause the intestinal wall to contract and speed up the elimination of faeces, e.g. senna or bisacodyl; (c) softeners, e.g. liquid paraffin, that lubricate and facilitate the passage of faeces; (d) osmotic laxatives primarily used in enemas that increase the fluid in the bowel by osmosis, e.g. magnesium sulphate or lactulose. Laxatives may also be given in a combined form of softener and stimulant.

LE *see* LUPUS ERYTHEMATOSUS.

lead (led) *symbol* Pb. A metallic element, many of the compounds of which are highly poisonous. *L. lotion* lead subacetate solution used externally on bruises. *L. poisoning* a condition that usually occurs as the result of excessive lead in the atmosphere, or from chewing objects made from lead alloys or covered with paint containing lead. Lead can also be ingested as a result of drinking water contaminated by lead piping or cooking utensils. The symptoms and signs include malaise, diarrhoea and vomiting, and sometimes ENCEPHALITIS. There is often pallor and a blue line around the gums. The use of lead in paints is now controlled by legislation and safety regulations. The increasing use of lead-free petrol as motor car fuel has reduced previously high levels of lead in the environment.

Lean Six Sigma (leen siks sigˈmə) a methodology adopted in health services that relies on a collaborative team effort to improve performance by systematically minimising waste and reducing variation in practice.

learning (lərning) knowledge or skills gained, or behaviour modified through being taught or from study. *L. curve* a person's rate of progress in gaining experience or new skills which can be represented as a graph. *L. difficulties* problems with learning arising from a result of a range of mental and physical problems. *L. disability* the preferred term to the one formerly used of 'mental handicap'. Essentially, disorders are characterised by substantial deficits in scholastic or academic skills.

Leber's disease (ˈlaybərz diˈzeez) *Theodor Leber, German ophthalmologist, 1840–1917.* Hereditary optic atrophy.

Leboyer method (leˈboyə ˈmethuhd) a method of delivering an infant designed to minimise trauma and encourage maternal–infant bonding.

lecithin (ˈlesəthən) one of a group of phospholipids that are found in the cell tissues and are concerned in the metabolism of fat.

leech (leech) *Hirudo medicinalis*, an aquatic worm which sucks blood and secretes hirudin (an anticoagulant) in its saliva. Historically used to withdraw blood from a person. May now be used following some forms of surgery, e.g. plastic or microsurgery, to restore the patency of collapsed or blocked blood vessels. Leeches are also occasionally used to drain a haematoma from a wound.

left occipitoanterior (LOA) (left okˌsipətoh·anˈtiə·ri·ə) refers to a position that might be taken up by the fetus in the uterus.

leg (leg) the lower limb, from knee to ankle. May include the thigh, the hip or gluteal region; however, the precise definition refers to the lower limb. *Bow-l.* genu varum. *Scissor l.* condition in which the person is cross-legged, such as occurs in cerebral DIPLEGIA. *White l.* PHLEGMASIA ALBA DOLENS.

Legionella pneumophila (ˌleejəˈnelə nyooˈmofələ) a species of Gram-negative, non-acid-fast, rod-shaped bacteria which require both cysteine and iron for growth; it is the causative agent of LEGIONNAIRES' DISEASE and PONTIAC FEVER.

legionellosis (ˌleejəneˈlohsəs) disease caused by infection with *Legionella* species, such as *L. pneumophila*.

Legionnaires' disease (ˌleejənˈairz diˈzeez) a pulmonary form of legionellosis resulting from infection with *Legionella pneumophila*. It is a notifiable disease. It is contagious and may be fatal. Symptoms include fever, confusion, pain in the muscles and across the chest, a dry cough and a partial loss of kidney function. It is associated with an infected water supply in public buildings such as hotels, hospitals and large office blocks, a cause of both community and hospital acquired infection. The infective organism is spread by droplets; there is no person-to-person spread.

leiomyoma (ˌlieohmieˈohmə) a benign smooth muscle tumour (fibroid) most commonly found in the uterus.

leiomyosarcoma (ˌlieohˌmieohsahˈkohmə) a malignant muscle tumour.

Leishmania (leeshˈmayni·ə) a genus of parasitic flagellated protozoa which infect the blood of humans and are the cause of LEISHMANIASIS.

leishmaniasis (ˌleeshməˈnieəsəs) a group of diseases caused by one of the protozoan *Leishmania* parasites. *See* KALA-AZAR.

lens (lenz) 1. a piece of glass or other material shaped to transmit light rays in a particular direction. 2. the transparent crystalline body situated behind the pupil of the eye. It serves as a refractive medium for rays of light. *Contact l.* a thin sheet of glass or plastic moulded to fit directly over the cornea. Worn instead of spectacles.

lentigo (len'tiegoh) a brownish or yellowish spot on the skin. A freckle. *L. maligna* Hutchinson's melanotic freckle. *See* FRECKLE.

lentivirus ('lentee,vierəs) from the Latin *lentus* (slow) 1 virus. A group of retroviruses that cause disease in animals and humans, including HIV-1 and HIV-2 (*see* HUMAN IMMUNODEFICIENCY VIRUS). These viruses are associated with slowly progressive diseases.

leontiasis (,leeən'tieəsəs) an osseous deformity of the face which produces a lion-like appearance. It occurs sometimes in leprosy and rarely in OSTEITIS DEFORMANS.

Leopold's manoeuvre ('leeə,pohldz mənoovə) *Christian G. Leopold, German physician, 1846–1911.* A series of four steps used in palpating the abdomen of a pregnant woman to determine position and presentation of the fetus.

lepidosis (,lepə'dohsəs) any scaly eruption of the skin.

leprosy ('leprəsee) HANSEN'S DISEASE. A chronic granulomatous disease of peripheral verves, mucosa of the upper respiratory tract and skin. Left untreated, leprosy can be progressive with permanent damage to skin, nerves and eyes. Caused by *Mycobacterium leprae.* It is predominantly a disease of warm climates which is transmitted by prolonged contact with an incubation period of 1 to 30 years, the average being between 3 and 5 years. Leprosy is now treated with a combination of drugs including dapsone, rifampicin and clofazimine. None of these is used alone because of the risk of developing resistance.

leptomeningitis (,leptoh,menən'jietəs) inflammation of the PIA MATER and arachnoid membranes of the brain and spinal cord.

Leptospira (,leptoh'spierə) a genus of spirochaetes. *L. icterohaemorrhagiae* the cause of spirochaetal jaundice (WEIL'S DISEASE).

leptospirosis (,leptohspie'rohsəs) any of a group of rare notifiable infectious diseases due to serotypes of *Leptospira.* The best known is WEIL'S DISEASE, or leptospiral jaundice; others are mud fever, autumn fever and swineherd's disease. The aetiological agent is a spiral organism that is common in water. Initially, the symptoms include fever, rigors, vomiting, headache, and often jaundice. Diagnosis may be difficult because the symptoms resemble those of several other diseases. Jaundice is a key symptom. Sanitation measures can reduce the spread of the disease in both humans and animals.

Leriche's syndrome (lə'reeshiz 'sin,drohm) *René Leriche, French surgeon, 1879–1955.* A condition in which ATHEROSCLEROSIS of peripheral arteries is accompanied by obstruction of the lower end of the aorta.

lesbianism ('lezbi·ənizəm) sexual and emotional orientation of one woman to another; female homosexuality.

Lesch-Nyhan syndrome (,lesh'niehan 'sin,drohm) *Michael Lesch, American physician, 1939–2008; William Nyhan Jr, American physician, b. 1926.* A hereditary disorder of purine metabolism transmitted as an X-linked recessive trait with physical and learning disabilities, compulsive self-mutilation of fingers and lips by biting, spasticity, spastic cerebral palsy and impaired renal function.

lesion (ˈleezhən) any pathological or traumatic discontinuity of tissue or loss of function of a part. Lesion is a broad term, including wounds, sores, ulcers, tumours, cataracts and any other tissue damage. Lesions range from the skin sores associated with eczema to the changes in lung tissue that occur in tuberculosis.

let-down (letdown) a sensation in the breasts of lactating women that often occurs as the milk flows into the ducts. It may occur when the infant begins to suck or when the mother hears the baby cry, or even thinks of nursing the child.

lethargy (ˈlethəjee) a condition of drowsiness or stupor that cannot be overcome by the will.

Letterer-Siwe disease (ˌletə·rəˈ-seevə diˈzeez) *Erich Letterer, German physician, 1895–1982*; *Sture Siwe, German physician, 1897–1966*. Reticuloendotheliosis of early childhood, marked by a haemorrhagic tendency, eczematoid skin eruption, HEPATOSPLENOMEGALY with lymph node involvement and progressive anaemia.

leucine (ˈlooseen) a naturally occurring essential amino acid, vital for growth in infants and for nitrogen equilibrium in adults.

leuco-, leuko- (ˌlookoh) combining form meaning 'white', or 'white blood cell'.

leucocyte (ˈlookəˌsiet) a white blood corpuscle. There are three types: (a) granular (polymorphonuclear cells) formed in bone marrow, consisting of neutrophils, eosinophils and basophils; (b) lymphocytes (formed in the lymph glands); and (c) monocytes (*see* figure, p.278 and table above).

Normal Leucocyte Count	
Type of leucocytes	No. cells per litre
Neutrophils	$2.0–8.0 \times 10^9$
Eosinophils	$0.0–0.5 \times 10^9$
Basophils	$0.0–0.1 \times 10^9$
Lymphocytes	$1.0–4.0 \times 10^9$
Monocytes	$0.2–1.0 \times 10^9$

leucocytolysis (ˌlookohsieˈtoləsəs) destruction of white blood cells.

leucocytopoiesis (ˌlookohˌsietoh-poyˈeesəs) LEUCOPOIESIS.

leucocytosis (ˌlookohsieˈtohsəs) an increase in the number of leucocytes in the blood. Often a response to infection.

leucoderma (ˌlookohˈdərmə) an absence of pigment in patches or bands, producing abnormal whiteness of the skin. VITILIGO.

leucodystrophy (ˌlookohˈdistrəfee) a degenerative disorder of the brain which starts during the first few months of life and leads to mental, visual and motor deterioration.

leuconychia (ˌlookohˈniki·ə) white patches on the nails due to air underneath.

leucopenia (ˌlookohˈpeeni·ə) a decreased number of white cells, usually GRANULOCYTES, in the blood.

leucophoresis (ˌlookohfəˈreesəs) withdrawal of blood for the selective removal of leucocytes. The remaining blood is re-transfused.

leucoplakia (ˌlookohˈplayki·ə) a chronic inflammation, characterised

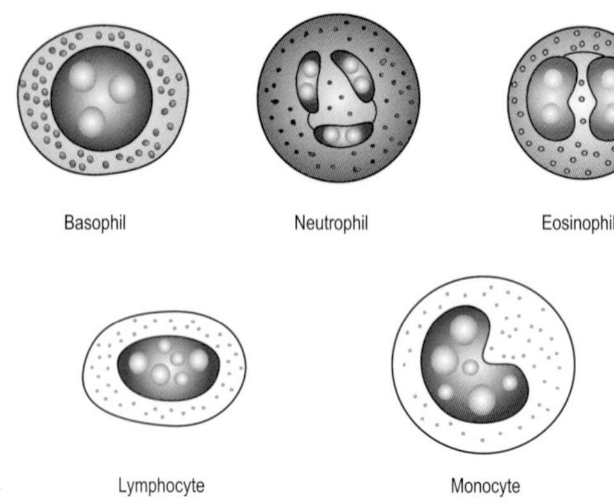

Types of leucocytes.

by white thickened patches on the mucous membranes, particularly on the tongue, gums and inside of the cheeks. *L. vulvae* thickening of the mucous membrane of the labia with the appearance of scattered white patches.

leucopoiesis (ˌlookohpoyˈeesəs) the formation of white blood cells. LEUCOCYTOPOIESIS.

leucorrhoea (ˌlookəˈreeə) a viscid, whitish discharge from the vagina.

leukaemia (looˈkeemi·ə) a progressive, malignant disease of the blood-forming organs, marked by abnormal proliferation and development of leucocytes and their precursors in the blood and bone marrow. It is accompanied by a reduced number of ERYTHROCYTES and blood platelets, resulting in anaemia and increased susceptibility to infection and haemorrhage. Other typical symptoms include fever, excessive bruising, breathlessness, pain in the joints and bones and swelling of the lymph nodes, spleen and liver. Leukaemia is classified clinically on the basis of: (a) the duration and character of the disease (acute or chronic); and (b) the cell line involved, i.e. myeloid (myelocytic, myeloblastic, granulocytic) or lymphoid (lymphatic, lymphoblastic, lymphocytic). The incidence of the disease is growing and the increase is only partially explained by increased efficiency of detection. Treatment options may include a combination of: chemotherapy, radiotherapy, steroid therapy, bone marrow or stem cell transplant. Antibiotics are commonly required to prevent infections.

leuko- (ˌlookoh) for words beginning thus, *see* LEUCO.

levator (ləˈvaytə) a muscle that raises a structure or organ of the body.

levels of care (ˈlevəlz ov kair) a classification of healthcare service levels by the kind of care provided, the number of people served and the people providing the care. Kinds of healthcare service levels are primary healthcare, secondary or acute healthcare and tertiary healthcare.

Levin tube (ˈlevən tyoob) a plastic catheter used in gastric intubation.

Lewy body dementia. *See* DEMENTIA.

LFT *see* LIVER *FUNCTION TEST*.

LH *see* LUTEINISING HORMONE.

Li symbol for *lithium*.

liaison (leeayzən) communication and contact between groups, units and/or agencies and organisations. *L. community nurse* appointed to facilitate communications between the hospital and the community services for the benefit of the person's care at home after discharge from the inpatient unit. *L. nursing* an arrangement with clinical specialists in psychiatry nursing whereby nurses and health professionals in other disciplines obtain consultation services in medical–surgical, parent–child and geriatric settings.

libido (ləˈbeedoh) 1. the vital force or impulse which brings about purposeful action. 2. sexual drive in Freudian psychoanalysis, the motive force of all human beings.

lice (lies) *see* PEDICULOSIS.

lichen (ˈliekən, ˈlichən) a group of inflammatory infections of the skin in which the lesions consist of papular eruptions. *L. planus* raised flat patches of dull, reddish purple colour with a smooth or scaly surface. *L. sclerosus* a long-term skin disorder with white patches and itching, mainly affecting the skins of the genitals.

lichenification (lieˌkenəfəˈkayshən) the stage of an eruption when it resembles lichen.

lid (lid) eyelid. *Granular l.* trachoma. *L. lag* jerky movement of the upper lid when it is being lowered. A sign of exophthalmic GOITRE (thyrotoxicosis).

lie (lie) a position or direction. *L. of fetus* the position of the fetus in the uterus. The normal lie is longitudinal.

Lieberkühn's glands (ˈleebəˌkoonz glandz) *Johann Lieberkühn, German anatomist, 1711–1756.* Tubular glands of the small intestine.

lien (ˈlie·ən) the spleen.

lienculus (lieˈengkyələs) an accessory spleen.

lienorenal (ˌlieənohˈreen'l) relating to the spleen and kidneys; splenorenal; splenonephric.

lientery (ˈlieəntə·ree) diarrhoea consisting mainly of undigested food.

life crisis (lief ˈkriesəs) an unpleasant experience which may often be unforeseen and sudden such as being robbed or mugged, redundancy, early retirement, divorce, bereavement and sudden and severe ill health.

life event (lief əˈvent) a sociological term used to describe major events in a person's life, e.g. leaving home for the first time, getting married, moving house, changing a job.

life expectancy (lief əkˈspektənsee) the average length of life based upon prevailing mortality trends. It is influenced by health status and illness record, but also by social factors such as education, occupation and ethnicity, and environmental factors such as sanitation and quality of housing.

lifelong learning (lieflong lərning) a process of personal, social and professional development throughout the life span of the individual.

lifestyle (lief stiel) the pattern of daily living that an individual develops. On the initial assessment of a person entering the healthcare services this is considered in relation to the delivery of healthcare by health professionals in order that the aims and objectives for care may be individualised.

life support system (lief sə'pawt sis,təm) the equipment and technology used to maintain the life of a person who is not otherwise able to survive.

lift assessment (lift ə'sesmənt) the choice of the most appropriate method to use when moving a person, as from bed to a chair. Factors that need to be taken into account include: (a) whether the person is conscious or unconscious; (b) whether there is a visual, hearing or cognitive impairment present; (c) other equipment such as urinary drainage, IV lines or monitors; and (d) the body weight of the person. No particular method is suggested as correct or appropriate in all situations, rather that safe moving and handling practices should be used at all times. Lifting devices are the first option when implementing manual handling activities. *See* MANUAL HANDLING.

ligament ('ligəmənt) 1. a band of fibrous tissue connecting bones, forming a joint. 2. a layer or layers of peritoneum connecting one abdominal organ to another or to the abdominal wall. *Annular l.* the ring-like band that fixes the head of the radius to the ulna. *Cruciate l.* crossed ligaments within the knee joint. *Inguinal l.* that between the pubic bone and anterior iliac crest. *Round l.* one of the two anterior ligaments of the uterus, passing through the inguinal canal and ending in the LABIA MAJORA. There are also round ligaments of the femur and of the liver.

ligation (lie'gayshən) the application of a ligature.

ligature ('ligəchə) a thread of silk, catgut or other material used for tying round a blood vessel to stop it bleeding.

light (liet) electromagnetic waves which stimulate the retina of the eye. *L. adaptation* the changes that take place in the eye when the intensity of the light increases or decreases. *L. coagulation* a method of treating retinal detachment by directing a beam of strong light (including laser) through the pupil to the affected area.

lightening ('lietəning) the relief experienced in pregnancy, 2–3 weeks before labour, when the uterus sinks into the pelvis and ceases to press on the diaphragm.

Likert-type scales ('likərt, 'lie- ,tiep ,skaylz) *Rensis Likert, American social psychologist (1903–1981).* Psychometric 5-point rating scale that allows people to respond to questions or statements of interest by specifying their level of agreement or disagreement.

limbus ('limbəs) an edge or border. *Corneal l.* the border where the cornea joins the SCLERA.

lime (liem) a citrus fruit with a high ascorbic acid content.

liminal ('limən'l) pertaining to the threshold of perception.

linctus ('lingktəs) a thick syrup, usually given to soothe and allay coughing.

linea ('lini·ə) [L.] a line. *L. alba* the tendinous area in the centre of the abdominal wall into which the transversalis and part of the oblique muscles are inserted. *L. albicantes* white streaks that appear on the abdomen when it is distended by pregnancy or a tumour. *L. aspera* the rough ridge on the back of the femur into which muscles are inserted. *L. nigra* the pigmented line that often appears in pregnancy on the abdomen between the umbilicus and the pubis.

linear (ˈlini·ə) pertaining to line. *L. accelerator* a megavoltage machine for accelerating electrons so that powerful X-rays are given off for use in the treatment of deep-seated tumours.

lingual (ˈling·gwəl) pertaining to the tongue.

lingula (ˈling·gyələ) a tongue-like structure, such as the projection of lung tissue from the left upper lobe.

liniment (ˈlinəmənt) a liquid applied externally by rubbing on to the skin.

lip (lip) 1. the upper or lower fleshy margin of the mouth. 2. any lip-like part; labium. *Cleft l.* congenital fissure of the upper lip.

lip reading (lip ˈreeding) understanding of speech through observation of the speaker's lip movements; called also speech reading.

lipaemia (liˈpeemi·ə) the presence of excess fat in the blood. Sometimes a feature of diabetes. *L. retinalis* condition in which the retinal blood vessels appear to be filled with milk owing to the presence of an excess of fat in the blood.

lipase (ˈlipayz, -pays) fat-splitting enzyme; any enzyme that catalyses the splitting of fats into glycerol and fatty acids. Measurement of the serum lipase level is an important diagnostic test for acute and chronic PANCREATITIS.

lipid (ˈlipəd) one of a group of fatty substances that are insoluble in water but soluble in alcohol or chloroform. They form an important part of the diet and are normally present in the body tissues, providing a source of energy and insulation. Lipids are also an important constituent of some cell structures. *L. disorders* metabolic disorders that result in abnormal amounts of lipids in the body, leading to hyperlipidaemia; this can cause atherosclerosis and pancreatitis. There are also some rare hereditary disorders. *See* TAY-SACHS DISEASE. *L.-lowering drugs* a group of drugs used in treating hyperlipidaemia to prevent or slow the progression of coronary heart disease and severe atherosclerosis.

lipochondrodystrophy (ˌlipohˌkon-drohˈdistrəfee) a congenital condition affecting the metabolism of fat and producing bone deformities, short stature, facial abnormalities and learning difficulties. HURLER'S SYNDROME.

lipodystrophy (ˌlipohˈdistrəfee) a disorder of fat metabolism. *Progressive l.* a rare condition occurring mainly in females in which there is progressive loss of fat over the upper half of the body.

lipoidosis (ˌlipoyˈdohsəs) a group of diseases in which there is an error in lipoid metabolism producing reticuloendothelial hyperplasia. XANTHOMA is common.

lipolysis (liˈpoləsəs) the breakdown of fats by the action of bile salts and enzymes to a fine emulsion and fatty acids.

lipoma (liˈpohmə) a benign tumour composed of fatty tissue arising in any part of the body and developing in connective tissue. *Diffuse l.* a tumour of fat in an irregular mass, without a capsule, occurring above the pelvis.

lipoprotein (ˌlipoh'prohteen) one of a group of fatty proteins present in blood plasma.

liposarcoma (ˌlipohsah'kohmə) a malignant tumour of the fat cells.

liposuction ('lipohˌsukshən) the removal by suction of excess fat in the body through a small skin incision; most commonly used cosmetically as a means of contour reduction or reshaping. Also called lipectomy.

lipuria (li'pyoo·ri·ə) the presence of fat in urine.

liquefaction (ˌlikwi'fakshən) reduction to liquid form.

liquid ('likwəd) 1. a substance that flows readily in its natural state. 2. flowing readily, neither solid nor gaseous. *L. diet* a diet limited to the intake of liquids or foods that can be changed to a liquid state. A liquid diet may be restricted to any liquids taken being clear liquids, or it may be a full liquid diet in which only liquids are taken.

liquor ('likə) a watery fluid; a solution. *L. amnii* the fluid in which the fetus floats; amniotic fluid.

Listeria (lis'tiə·ri·ə) *Baron Joseph Lister, British surgeon, 1827–1912.* A genus of Gram-negative bacteria which produce upper respiratory disease, septicaemia and encephalitic disease in humans. They can be transmitted by the consumption of infected, unpasteurised dairy produce or infected leafy vegetables, or by direct contact with infected animals or contaminated soil. Newborn infants, pregnant women, the older person and the immunosuppressed are more susceptible to infection.

listeriosis (lisˌtiə·ree'ohsəs) infection with organisms of the genus *Listeria*.

lithiasis (li'thieəsəs) the formation of calculi. *Conjunctival l.* the formation of small white chalky areas on the inner surface of the eyelids.

litholapaxy (li'tholəˌpaksee) the removal of fragments of a calculus from the bladder after LITHOTRIPSY.

lithonephrotomy (ˌlithohnə'frotəmee) incision into the kidney to remove a stone; NEPHROLITHOTOMY.

lithosis (li'thohsəs) PNEUMOCONIOSIS resulting from inhalation of particles of silica etc. into the lungs.

lithotomy (li'thotəmee) 1. incision into the bladder for the removal of calculi. 2. a position in the operating theatre for surgical procedures, medical examination and treatment of the pelvis and lower abdomen. Common position for childbirth in Western countries.

lithotripsy ('lithohˌtripsee) the crushing of calculi in the bladder typically using ultrasound shock waves; lithotrity.

lithotrite ('lithohˌtriet) an instrument used for LITHOTRIPSY.

lithuresis (ˌlithyə'reesəs) passage of small calculi or gravel in the urine.

litmus paper ('litməs 'paypə) a blotting paper impregnated with blue pigment obtained from lichen and used for testing the reaction of fluids. *Blue l.* is turned red by an acid. *Red l.* is turned blue by an alkali.

litre ('leetə) *symbol* L. The SI unit of capacity. One cubic decimetre.

Little's disease ('lit'lz di'zeez) *William Little, British surgeon, 1810–1894.* Spastic DIPLEGIA. A congenital muscle rigidity of the lower limbs causing 'scissor leg' deformity.

liver ('livə) the large gland situated in the right upper area of the abdominal cavity. It is essential to life. Its chief functions are: (a) formation of bile; (b) production of plasma proteins except gamma globulins; (c) storage of carbohydrates as glycogen, iron and vitamins A, D, E and K; (d) regulation of metabolism of fat, protein and carbohydrate; (e) detoxification of drugs and other substances; (f) the formation and destruction of erythrocytes; (g) production of prothrombin and fibrinogen; (h) heat production; and (i) phagocytic action on bacteria. *Cirrhotic l.* fibrotic changes which occur in the liver as the result of degeneration of the liver cells, often as a result of alcoholism. *L. biopsy* the taking of a small core of liver tissue through a liver biopsy needle under a local anaesthetic. Allows for microscopic examination to aid diagnosis of a wide range of disorders of the liver. *L. function tests* blood tests used to assess liver function including: alanine aminotransferase, alkaline phosphatase, aspartate aminotransferase, coagulation tests, gamma-glutamyl transferase, serum bilirubin and serum proteins. *L. transplant* the transplantation of a liver or a segment of a liver from a suitable donor in the treatment of liver failure.

livid (ˈlivəd) descriptive of the blueish-grey discolouration of the skin produced by congestion of blood.

living will (living wil) a statement signed by a person requesting and indicating what should be done in the event of becoming totally incapacitated or terminally ill. It enables the writer, while still alive, to refuse resuscitation or other measures to maintain life. Alternative name for ADVANCE CARE DIRECTIVE or advance care plan.

LMP last menstrual period.

LOA *see* LEFT OCCIPITOANTERIOR.

loading dose (lohding dohs) in pharmaco-therapeutics, the administration of a drug in larger doses than the body can eliminate in order to bring the concentration of the drug within the body to an effective level. After this, the dose is gradually reduced.

lobar (ˈlohbə) relating to a lobe.

lobe (lohb) a section of an organ separated from neighbouring parts by fissures. The liver, lungs and brain are divided into lobes.

lobectomy (lohˈbektəmee) removal of a lobe, e.g. of the lung.

lobular (ˈlobyələ) relating to a lobule.

lobule (ˈlobyool) a small lobe, particularly one making up a larger lobe.

local anaesthetic (ˈlohkəl ˌanəsˈthetik) numbing of a part of the body, with no loss of consciousness using medication administered by injection or topically which blocks pain signals from nerves to the brain.

localise (ˈlohkəˌliez) 1. to limit the spread, e.g. of disease or infection, to a certain area. 2. to determine the site of a lesion.

lochia (ˈlohki·ə) the discharge of blood and tissue debris from the uterus after childbirth and lasting for 2–3 weeks. Initially, lochia is bright red and gradually becomes paler.

lochiometra (ˈlokeeˌomətre) the retention of lochia in the uterus, causing its distension.

lockjaw (ˈlokˌjor) TETANUS.

locomotor (ˌlohkəˈmohtə) pertaining to movement from one place to another.

loculated (ˈlokyəˌlaytəd) divided into small locules or cavities.

loculus (ˈlokyələs) a small cystic cavity, one of a number.

locum tenens (ˈlohkəm ˈtenənz) [L.] holding the place. A person, usually a doctor, who substitutes for another over a period of time; usually referred to as a locum.

locus of control (lohkəs ov ˌkənˈtrohl) the ideas and beliefs that people have about the way in which they can control external events in their lives. Those with an internal locus of control tend to expect that any change or reinforcement is the result of their own efforts or behaviour and will want to be actively involved in any healthcare measures or decisions. Those with an external locus of control see themselves as being dependent upon luck, fate or the actions of 'powerful others' and are therefore fatalistic about any healthcare provisions or treatment.

logorrhoea (ˌlogəˈreeə) excessive and often unintelligible volubility.

log roll (ˈlog ˌrohl) a nursing technique used to turn a reclining person from one side to the other. The person lies on the back with arms folded across the chest, and legs extended. The nurses manipulate the underlying drawsheet so that the person is rolled on to one side or the other.

loiasis (lohˈieəsəs) infestation of the conjunctiva and eyelids with a parasite worm, *Loa loa*. A tropical condition.

loin (loyn) the area of the back on each side between the thorax and the pelvis.

longitudinal study (ˈlongətyoodən'l ˈstudee) an investigation that involves making observations of the sample group at sequential time intervals. Longitudinal studies are valuable as a means of studying human development or change and may also be used to observe change over time within an institution or organisation.

long QT syndrome (ˌlong kyoo ˈtee ˈsinˌdrohm) irregularity of the electrical activity of the heart as a result of a faulty gene which can cause blackouts, seizures, arrhythmia and cardiac arrest. It is a leading cause of sudden death in young and otherwise healthy people and is thought to be an underlying cause in cases of SUDDEN INFANT DEATH SYNDROME.

long sight (ˌlongˈsiet) HYPERMETROPIA.

loosening (ˈloosəning) in psychiatry, a disorder of thinking in which associations of ideas become so shortened, fragmented and disturbed as to lack logical relationship.

LOP left occipito-posterior a possible position of the fetus in the uterus.

lordosis (lawˈdohsəs) a form of spinal curvature in which there is an abnormal forward curve of the lumbar spine.

lotion (ˈlohshən) a medicinal solution for external application to the body. Lotions usually have a soothing or antiseptic effect. *Calamine l.* a soothing mixture containing calamine and zinc oxide. *Evaporating l.* a dilute alcoholic solution applied to bruises.

loupe (loop) a magnifying lens which may be used in eye examination.

louse (lows) *pl.* lice a general term covering a number of small insects that are parasitic to humans and to other mammals and birds. Three varieties are parasitic to humans: (a) *Pediculus humanus capitis*, the head louse; (b) *Pediculus humanus corporis*, the body louse; and (c) *Phthirus humanus pubis*, which infects the coarse hair on the body and also the eyebrows. Diseases known to be transmitted by lice are typhus fever, relapsing fever and trench fever.

lozenge (ˈlozinj) a medicated tablet with a sugar basis, used to treat mouth and throat conditions.

LSD lysergic acid diethylamide *see* LYSERGIDE.

lub-dup (lubˈdup) representation of the sounds heard through the stethoscope when listening to the normal heart: *lub* when the atrioventricular valves shut, and *dup* when the semilunar valves meet each other.

lucid (ˈloosəd) clear, particularly of the mind. *L. interval* period of clear thinking that may occur in cerebral injury between two periods of unconsciousness, or as a sane interval in a mental disorder.

Lugol's solution (ˈloogolz ˌsəˈlooshən) *Jean Lugol, French physician, 1786–1851.* A preparation of iodine and potassium iodide. It is best given in milk and is used in the treatment of toxic GOITRE.

lumbago (lumˈbaygoh) pain in the lower part of the back. It may be caused by muscular strain or by a prolapsed intervertebral disc ('slipped disc').

lumbar (ˈlumbə) pertaining to the loins. *L. puncture* insertion of a trocar and cannula into the spinal canal in the lower back and withdrawal of cerebrospinal fluid for diagnostic and sometimes treatment purposes.

lumbosacral (ˌlumbohˈsaykrəl) relating to both the lumbar vertebrae and the sacrum. *L. support* a corset aimed at both supporting and restricting movement in that region. *L. vertebra* one of the five vertebrae in the lower back, lying between the thoracic vertebrae and the sacrum.

lumen (ˈloomən) the space inside a tube.

lumpectomy (ˌlumpˈektəmee) the surgical excision of only the local lesion (benign or malignant) of the breast.

lunacy (ˈloonəsee) an obsolete term formerly applied to insanity.

Lund and Browder chart (luhnd ənd ˈbrowdə ˈchaht) a chart used for the calculation of the surface area of a burn. At birth the size and area of the head is large compared with the adult, and the legs and thighs constitute a much smaller proportion of the total body surface. On admission to a burns unit or ward, the area of the body burned is mapped on to the Lund and Browder chart and the area of the burn affecting each portion of the body surface is calculated (*see* figures, p. 286 and p. 287).

lung (lung) one of a pair of conical organs of the respiratory system, consisting of an arrangement of air tubes terminating in air vesicles (alveoli) and filling almost the whole of the thorax. The alveoli are the sites of gaseous exchange in the lungs. Atmospheric oxygen is absorbed and carbon dioxide from the pulmonary capillaries is released and excreted in expiration from the lungs. The right lung has three lobes and the left lung two. They are connected with the air by means of the bronchi and trachea. *L. capacity* a lung volume that is the sum of two or more of the four primary, non-overlapping lung volumes. Lung capacities are functional residual capacity, inspiratory capacity, total lung capacity and vital capacity (*see* figure, p. 287). *L. compliance* a measure of the ease of expansion of the lung and thorax. It is determined by pulmonary volume and capacity. A high degree of compliance indicates a loss of elastic recoil of the lungs, as in older age or emphysema.

lunula (ˈloonyələ) the white semicircle near the root of each nail.

lupus (ˈloopəs) a chronic skin disease having many manifestations. *L. vulgaris* a tuberculous disease of the skin producing brownish nodules, frequently on the nose or cheek, and severe scarring.

lupus erythematosus (LE) (loopəs erithəməˈtohsəs (el ee)) a collection of autoimmune diseases in which the immune system becomes hyperactive and attacks normal healthy tissues. Symptoms can affect many different body systems including joints, skin, kidneys, blood cells, heart and lungs. *LE cell* a mature neutrophilic POLYMORPHONUCLEAR leucocyte that has phagocytised a large, spherical inclusion derived from another

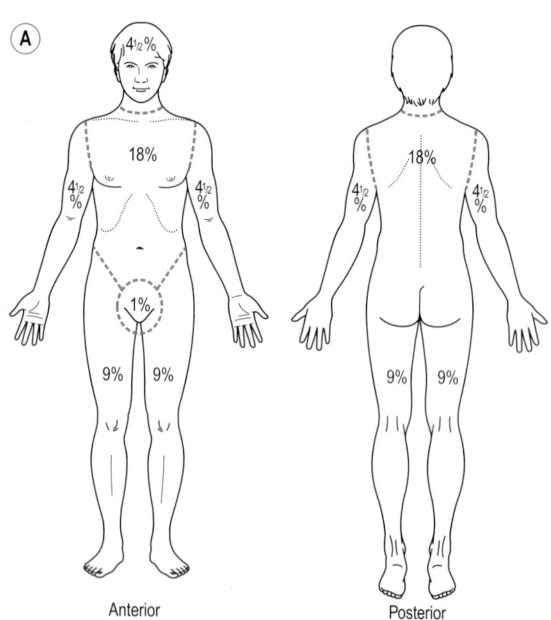

Lund and Browder burns chart for adults.

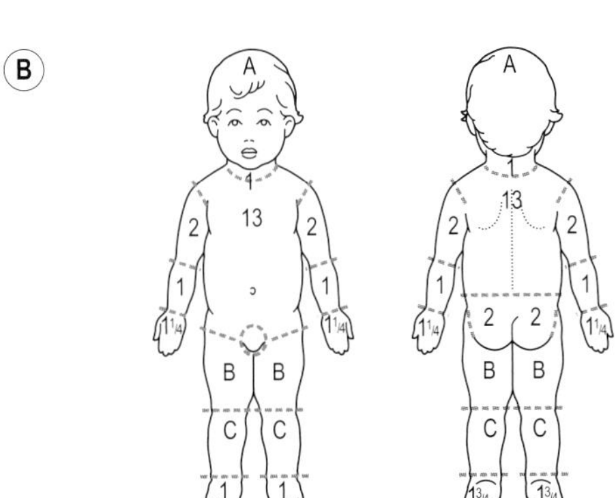

Relative percentages of areas affected by growth

AREA	BIRTH	AGE 1YR	AGE 5YR
A = $^1/_2$ of head	$9^1/_2$	$8^1/_2$	$6^1/_2$
B = $^1/_2$ of one thigh	$2^3/_4$	$3^1/_4$	4
C = $^1/_2$ of one leg	$2^1/_2$	$2^1/_2$	$2^3/_4$

Lund and Browder burns chart for children up to five years.

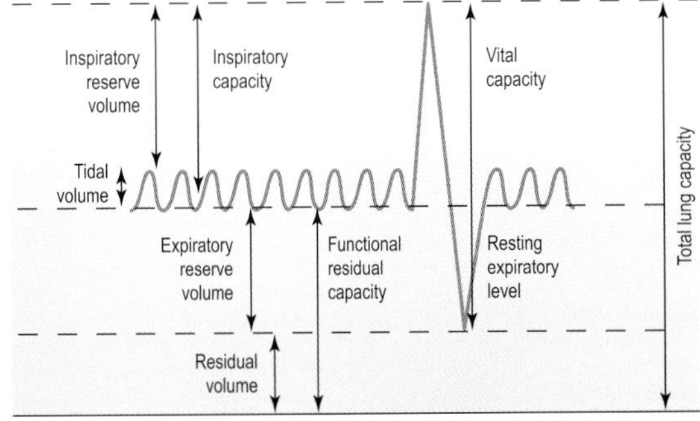

Lung volumes and capacities.

neutrophil; a characteristic of lupus erythematosus, but also found in analogous connective tissue disorders.

luteinising hormone (LH) (ˈlooteeəˌniezing ˈhawmohn) one of three hormones produced by the anterior pituitary gland which control the activity of the gonads.

luteotrophin (ˌlooteeohˈtrohfən) an anterior pituitary hormone which stimulates the formation of the corpus luteum and the production of milk. PROLACTIN.

luxation (lukˈsayshən) the dislocation of a joint. *L. of the lens* displacement of the lens of the eye into the anterior chamber or posteriorly into the vitreous humour.

Lyme disease (liem diˈzeez) a ZOONOSIS transmitted by ticks and characterised by a rash (erythema chronicum migrans), arthritis and aseptic meningitis, caused by the spirochaete *Borrelia burgdorferi*.

lymph (limf) the fluid from the blood which has transuded through capillary walls to supply nutriment to tissue cells. It is collected by lymph vessels which ultimately return it to the blood. *L. nodes* or *glands* structures placed along the course of lymph vessels, through which the lymph passes and is filtered of foreign substances, e.g. bacteria. These nodes also make lymphocytes. *Vaccine l.* a lymph preparation obtained from calves or other animals and used for vaccination.

lymphadenectomy (ˌlimfadəˈnektəmee) excision of a lymph gland or nodes.

lymphadenitis (ˌlimfadəˈnietəs) inflammation of a lymph gland. ADENITIS.

lymphadenoma (ˌlimfadəˈnohmə) lymphoma. *Multiple l.* HODGKIN'S DISEASE.

lymphadenopathy (ˌlimfadəˈnopəthee) any disease condition of the lymph nodes.

lymphangiectasis (ˌlimfanjeeˈektəsəs) dilatation of the lymph vessels due to some obstruction of the lymph flow.

lymphangiography (ˌlimfanjeeˈografee) radiographic examination of lymph vessels after the insertion of a radio-opaque contrast medium.

lymphangioma (ˌlimfanjeeˈohmə) a swelling composed of dilated lymph vessels.

lymphangioplasty (limˈfanjeeohˌplastee) a surgical operation with the aim of creating artificial lymph drainage.

lymphangitis (ˌlimfanˈjietəs) inflammation of lymph vessels manifested by red lines on the skin over them. It occurs in cases of severe infection through the skin.

lymphatic (limˈfatik) referring to lymph. *L. system* the system of vessels and glands through which the lymph is returned to the circulation. The vessels end in the thoracic duct and the right lymphatic duct.

lymphoblast (ˈlimfəˌblast) an early developmental cell that will mature into a LYMPHOCYTE.

lymphocyte (ˈlimfəˌsiet) a white blood cell formed in the lymphoid tissue. Lymphocytes produce immune bodies to overcome and protect against infection.

lymphocythaemia (ˌlimfohsieˈtheemi·ə) an excessive number of lymphocytes in the blood. LYMPHOCYTOSIS.

lymphocytopenia (ˌlimfohˌsietohˈpeeni·ə) absence or scarcity of lymphocytes in the blood. LYMPHOPENIA.

lymphocytosis (ˌlimfohsieˈtohsəs) LYMPHOCYTHAEMIA.

lymphoedema (ˌlimfohˈdeemə) a condition in which the intercellular spaces contain an abnormal amount of lymph due to obstruction of the lymph drainage.

lymphogranuloma (ˌlimfohˌgranyəˈlohmə) HODGKIN'S DISEASE. *L. venereum* a sexually transmitted disease, caused by a virus; primarily a tropical condition.

lymphoid (ˈlimfoyd) relating to the lymph.

lymphoma (limˈfohmə) lymphadenoma. Used to denote any malignant condition of the lymphoid tissue. Generally these diseases are classified as either Hodgkin's or non-Hodgkin's lymphomata. *Burkitt's l.* a type of lymphoma found predominantly in East Africa and affecting the jaws of children.

lymphopenia (ˌlimfohˈpeeni·ə) LYMPHOCYTOPENIA.

lymphopoiesis (ˌlimfohpoyˈeesəs) the production of lymphocytes. Occurs chiefly in the bone marrow, lymph nodes, thymus, spleen and gut wall.

lymphorrhagia (ˌlimfəˈrayji·ə) the escape of lymph from a ruptured lymphatic vessel. Lymphorrhoea.

lymphosarcoma (ˌlimfohsahˈkohmə) a term formerly used to denote a malignant lymphoma (with the exception of Hodgkin's disease).

Lynch syndrome (ˌlinch ˈsinˌdrohm) *Henry Lynch, American physician, 1928–2019* also known as hereditary nonpolyposis colorectal cancer (HNPCC), is an inherited disorder that increases the risk of developing many types of cancers, particularly cancers of the colon. Women with this disorder have a higher risk of ovarian and endometrial cancer.

lyophilisation (lieˌofəlieˈzayshən) a method of preserving biological substances in a stable state by freeze drying. It may be used for plasma, sera, bacteria, viruses and tissues.

lysergide (lieˈsərjied) lysergic acid diethylamide (LSD). A hallucinogenic drug that may cause visual hallucinations and increased auditory acuity, but may prove to be very disruptive to personality and can affect mental ability.

lysin (ˈliesən) a specific antibody present in the blood that may destroy cells. *See* BACTERIOLYSIN.

lysine (ˈlieseen) an essential amino acid formed by the digestion of dietary protein. It is vital for normal health.

lysis (ˈliesəs) 1. the gradual decline of a disease, especially of a fever. The temperature falls gradually, as in typhoid. *See* CRISIS. 2. the destruction of cells.

lysosome (ˈliesəˌsohm) a particle found in the cytoplasm of cells which causes the breakdown of metabolic substances and foreign particles (e.g. bacteria) within the cell.

lysozyme (ˈliesəˌziem) an enzyme present in tears, nasal mucus and saliva that may kill most bacteria coming into contact with it.

Mm

m symbol for *metre* and *misce* (mix).

M symbol for *molar*.

maceration (ˌmasəˈrayshən) softening of a solid by soaking it in liquid. *Neonatal m.* the natural softening of a dead fetus in the uterus.

Mackenrodt's ligaments (ˈmakenˌrohts ˈligəmənts) *Alwin Mackenrodt, German gynaecologist, 1859–1925.* The transverse or cardinal ligaments that support the uterus in the pelvic cavity.

macrocephaly (ˌmakrohˈsefəlee) a congenital anomaly characterised by abnormal largeness of the head and brain in relation to the rest of the body, resulting in some degree of intellectual disability and delayed growth. The head is more than two standard deviations above the average circumference size for age, sex, race and period of gestation, with excessively wide fontanels: the facial features are usually normal.

macrocheilia (ˌmakrohˈkieli·ə) a congenital condition in which there is excessive development of the lips.

macrocyte (ˈmakrohˌsiet) an abnormally large red corpuscle found in the blood in some forms of anaemia.

macrocythaemia (ˈmakrohsieˌtheemi·ə) the presence of abnormally large red cells in the blood. Macrocytosis.

macrocytic anaemia (makrohsitək ˌaˈneemyə) a disorder of the blood characterised by impaired erythropoiesis and the presence of large red blood cells in the circulation. Macrocytic anaemia is most often the result of a deficiency of folic acid or vitamin B_{12}.

macrodrip (ˌmakrohˈdrip) intravenous giving set which delivers an infusion at the rate of 20 drops per 1 mL.

macromastia (ˌmakrohˈmasti·ə) abnormal increase in the size of the breast.

macronutrient (ˌmakrohˈnyootri·ənt) an essential nutrient that has a large minimal daily requirement (greater than 100 mg). Calcium, phosphorus, magnesium, potassium, sodium and chloride are macronutrients.

macrophage (ˈmakrohˌfayj) a large reticuloendothelial cell which has the power to ingest cell debris and bacteria. It is present in connective tissue, especially when there is inflammation.

macrophthalmia (ˌmakrofˈthalmi·ə) a congenital condition of abnormally large eyes.

macroscopic (ˌmakrohˈskopik) discernible with the naked eye. The opposite of microscopic.

macrosomia *see* GIGANTISM. *Fetal m.* a complication of several conditions including DIABETES MELLITUS and prolonged pregnancy. A macrosomic fetus is defined as weighing more than 4000 g.

macrostomia (ˌmakrohˈstohmi·ə) an abnormal development of the mouth in which the mandibular and maxillary processes do not fuse and the mouth is excessively wide.

macula (ˈmakyələ) a spot or discoloured area of the skin, not raised above the surface; a macule. *M. corneae* a small area of opacity in the cornea, seen through an ophthalmoscope as a deeper red. *M. hole* a small gap in the centre of the macula resulting in blurred and distorted vision. *M. lutea* the yellow central area of the retina where vision is clearest.

macular (ˈmakyələ) pertaining to the macula. *M. degeneration* the loss of retinal pigment cells and damage to the macula. Occurs with ageing and results in the loss of colour vision and progressive visual impairment.

maculopapular (ˌmakyəlohˈpapyələ) displaying both maculae and papules. *M. eruption* a rash comprised of both maculae and papules as in measles.

Madurafoot (məˈdyoo·rə fuht) MYCETOMA of the foot.

Madurella (ˌmadyəˈrelə) a genus of fungi causing MYCETOMA.

maduromycosis (məˌdyoo·rohmie-ˈkohsəs) a chronic disease caused by *Madurella mycetoma*. The most common form is Madura foot.

Magendie's foramen (ˌmazhonˈdeez fəˈraymən) *François Magendie, French physiologist, 1783–1855*. Aperture in the roof of the fourth ventricle of the brain through which cerebrospinal fluid passes into the subarachnoid space.

magnesium (magˈneezi·əm) *symbol* Mg. A blueish-white metallic element. It occurs widely in mineral sources and is present in some of the body tissues. *M. carbonate* and *m. hydroxide* neutralising antacids used in hyperacidity. *M. sulphate* a saline purgative. Epsom salts. *M. trisilicate* an antacid powder taken after food for dyspepsia and peptic ulceration.

magnet (ˈmagˌnət) in ophthalmology, an instrument used for removing metallic foreign bodies that have penetrated the eye.

magnetic resonance imaging (MRI) (magˈnetik ˈrezənəns iməjəng) a non-invasive imaging technique based on the NUCLEAR MAGNETIC RESONANCE properties of the hydrogen nucleus. Cross-sectional images in any plane of the body for examination may be obtained.

Makaton (ˈmakəton) one of the sign languages.

mal (mal) [Fr.] disease. *Grand m., petit m.* former name for forms of epilepsy. *M. de mer* seasickness.

malabsorption (ˌmaləbˈsawpshən, -ˈzaw-) inability of the small intestine to absorb certain substances. It may be the cause of a deficiency disease due to the lack of an essential factor.

malacia (məˈlayshi ə) softening of tissues. *Keratomalacia* softening of the cornea. *Osteomalacia* softening of bone tissue.

maladaptation (ˌmaladəpˈtayshən) the inability to make normal adjustments in personal relationships and in society which may result in stress, ill health and abnormal behaviour.

maladjustment (ˌmaləˈjustmənt) in psychiatry, a failure to adjust to the environment.

malaise (maˈlayz) a feeling of general discomfort and illness.

malalignment (ˌmaləˈlienmənt) displacement, especially of the teeth from their normal relation to the line of the dental arch.

malaria (məˈlair·ri·ə) a serious, notifiable infectious illness which is a mosquito-borne disease of humans (and other animals). The symptoms of the disease vary according to the protozoa of the genus *Plasmodium* and begin with a bite from an infected female mosquito. This introduces the microorganism into the circulatory system and ultimately the liver where they mature and reproduce. The disease is characterised by chills and fever, anaemia, an enlarged spleen, myalgia, arthralgia, weakness and vomiting. Splenomegaly, anaemia, thrombocytopenia, hypoglycaemia, pulmonary or renal dysfunction and neurosis may occur. Malaria is widespread in tropical and subtropical regions around the equator, including sub-Saharan Africa, Asia and Central and South America, and travellers to these regions are at risk of infection. A vaccine RTS,S/AS01 has been developed and trialled and is being further piloted in sub-Saharan Africa. Various anti-malarial drugs are used for treatment and chemoprophylaxis. Prevention of malaria includes the use of medication, vector control with insecticide-treated mosquito nets and indoor residual spray. Health education measures are important to promote an awareness of malaria and control measures are important for the populations and travellers to affected areas. *Airport m.* a term sometimes used to describe malaria occurring at or near an airport, in a country normally free of the disease, and spread by infected mosquitoes brought in on an aeroplane from an endemic area. Control measures include disinfection of aircraft where appropriate.

malformation (ˌmalfawˈmayshən) deformity; a structural defect.

malignant (məˈlignənt) tending to become progressively worse and to result in death if untreated; having the properties of ANAPLASIA, INVASIVENESS and METASTASIS; said of tumours.

malingering (məˈling·gə·ring) wilful, deliberate and fraudulent feigning or exaggeration of the symptoms of illness or injury to attain a consciously desired end.

malleolus (ˈmaleeohˌləs) one of the two protuberances on either side of the ankle joint. *Lateral m.* that on the outer surface at the lower end of the fibula. *Medial m.* that on the inner surface at the lower end of the tibia.

malleus (ˈmali·əs) the hammer-shaped bone in the middle ear.

Mallory-Weiss syndrome (ˌmaləriˈ-vais ˈsinˌdrohm) massive bleeding caused by a tear in the oesophagus, usually associated with protracted vomiting.

malnutrition (ˌmalnyooˈtrishən) any disorder of nutrition. It may result from an unbalanced, insufficient or excessive diet or from impaired absorption.

malocclusion (ˌmaləˈkloozhən) an abnormality of dental development which causes overlapping of the bite.

Malpighian body (malˈpigi·ən bodee) *Marcello Malpighi, Italian anatomist, physician and physiologist, 1628–1694.* The GLOMERULUS and Bowman's capsule of the kidney.

malposition (ˌmalpəˈzishən) an abnormal position of any part of the body.

malpractice (malˈpraktəs) failure to maintain accepted standards and cause harm. Professional misconduct.

malpresentation (ˌmalprezən-ˈtayshən) any abnormal position of the fetus at birth that renders delivery difficult or impossible.

Malta fever (ˈmawltə ˈfeevə) BRUCELLOSIS; undulant fever.

maltase (ˈmawltayz) a sugar-splitting enzyme which converts maltose to glucose. Present in pancreatic and intestinal juice.

maltose (ˈmawltohz, -tohs) the sugar formed by the action of digestive enzymes on starch.

malunion (malˈyooni·ən) faulty repair of a fracture.

mamilla (məˈmilə) a nipple.

mamma (ˈmamə) a breast; a milk-secreting gland.

mammary (ˈmamə·ree) relating to the breasts.

mammography (məˈmogrəfee) radiographic or infrared examination of the breast to detect abnormalities.

mammoplasty (ˈmamohˌplastee) a plastic operation to reduce the size of abnormally large, pendulous breasts or augment the size of very small breasts.

mammothermography (ˌmamoh-thərˈmogrəfee) an examination of the breast that depends on the more active cells producing heat that can be shown on a thermograph; it may indicate abnormalities of the breast tissue.

mandatory notification (ˈman·dat·oree ˈnohtəˌfiˈkayˌshun) a requirement under the HEALTH PRACTITIONER REGULATION NATIONAL LAW Act 2009 for registered health practitioners, employers and education providers to report certain conduct if they have formed a reasonable belief that a registered health practitioner has behaved in a way that constitutes NOTIFIABLE CONDUCT.

mandatory reporting (ˈman·dat·oree ˌreˈporˌting) a state and territory legislative requirement in Australia imposed to protect at-risk groups, such as children and young people.

mandible (ˈmandəbəl) the lower jawbone.

manganese (ˈmang·gəneez) a common metallic element found in trace amounts in the body, where it aids in the function of various enzymes.

mania (ˈmayni·ə) a disordered mental state of extreme excitement; especially, the manic type of bipolar disorder psychosis. Also used as a word termination to denote obsessive preoccupation with something, as in kleptomania.

maniac (ˈmayniˌak) colloquial term for one suffering from a violent or extreme form of insanity.

manic (ˈmanik) pertaining to mania. *M. depressive psychosis* a mental illness characterised by mania and endogenous depression. The attacks may alternate between mania and depression or the person may have recurrent attacks of mania or depression. A bipolar disorder.

manipulation (məˌnipyəˈlayshən) use of the hands to produce a desired movement, such as in reducing a fracture or a hernia or changing the position of a fetus. Its use is important in orthopaedics, physiotherapy, osteopathy and in chiropractic.

mannitol (ˈmanəˌtol) a sugar alcohol occurring widely in nature; an osmotic diuretic used for forced diuresis in drug overdose and in cerebral oedema.

manometer (məˈnomətə) an instrument for measuring the pressure of liquids or gases.

Mantoux test (manˈtoo test) *Charles Mantoux, French physician, 1877–1947*. A tuberculin skin test in which a solution of purified protein derivative (PPD) tuberculin is injected intradermally into either the anterior or the posterior surface of the forearm. The test is read 48–72 hours after injection. It is considered positive when the induration at the site of injection is more than 10 mm in diameter.

manual (ˈmanyoo·əl) involving the use of the hands. *M. evacuation of the bowel* a nursing technique used to evacuate the bowel following use of faecal softening agents (*see* LAXATIVE) in a severely constipated person. This procedure is less commonly used now due to the possibility of causing rectal trauma and distress to the person. *M. expression of urine* pressure placed upon the abdomen by using the hands at regular intervals to encourage the person to void when the bladder is paralysed. *M. handling see* MOVING AND HANDLING.

manubrium (məˈnyoobri·əm) the upper part of the sternum to which the clavicle is attached.

MAOI *see* MONOAMINE OXIDASE INHIBITOR.

MAP mean arterial pressure.

maple syrup urine disease (ˈmaypəl ˈsirəp ˈyoo·rən diˈzeez) an inborn error of metabolism in which there is an excess in the urine of certain amino acids; the urine smells like maple syrup. There are learning difficulties, lethargy and convulsions.

marasmus (məˈrazməs) severe and chronic malnutrition producing a gradual wasting of the tissues, owing to insufficient or unassimilated food, occurring especially in infants. It is not always possible to discover the cause.

marble bone disease (ˌmahbəl ˈbohn diˈzeez) a condition in which there is increased density of bone, which is visible on radiographic examination. Albers-Schönberg's disease. OSTEOPETROSIS.

Marburg virus disease (ˈmahbərg vierəs diˈzeez) a severe and acute, often fatal, haemorrhagic viral disease. Similar to Ebola virus disease, principally seen in central African countries caused by the Marburg virus, of the family *Filoviridae*. The incubation period ranges from 5 to 10 days and people present with abrupt onset of high fever, weakness, muscle pain, headache and sore throat. This is quickly followed by more severe symptoms including vomiting, diarrhoea, rash, decreased kidney and liver functioning and, in some cases, both internal and external bleeding and death in up to 90% of cases. It occurs in sporadic outbreaks, frequently centred in healthcare settings in developing countries, where social and economic conditions often favour the spread of the virus. Marburg virus can be transmitted in several ways, the most significant being person-to-person through direct contact with body fluids (e.g. blood, semen, vaginal fluid) of an infected person. *See* EBOLA VIRUS DISEASE.

Marfan's syndrome (mahˈfanhz ˈsinˌdrohm) *Antoine Marfan, French paediatrician, 1858–1942.* A hereditary disorder in which there is excessive height with very long digits, a high arched palate, hypertonus and dislocation of the lens of the eyes; heart disease commonly occurs.

marijuana (ˌmarəyəˈwahnə, ˌmarəˈ-wahnə) *Cannabis sativa*; Indian hemp or hashish. *See* CANNABIS.

marrow (ˈmaroh) the substance contained in the middle of long bones and in the cancellous tissue of all bones. *M. puncture* investigatory procedure in which marrow cells are aspirated from the sternum or iliac crest. *Red m.* that found in all cancellous tissue at birth. Blood cells are made in it. *Yellow m.* the fatty substance contained in the centre of long bones in later life.

Marshall-Marchetti operation (ˈmahˌshəl marˈketee ˌopəˈrayshən) a surgical procedure performed to control stress incontinence.

masculinisation (ˌmaskyələnieˈ-zayshən) the development in a woman of male secondary sexual characteristics.

mask (mahsk) 1. to cover up or conceal. 2. a covering for the mouth and nose (sometimes for the whole face), designed to protect the wearer or person in preventing the inhalation of pathogenic organisms or toxic substances. Masks are also used in the administration of oxygen and other aerosol medications. 3. a facial expression characteristic of a certain disorder or condition. *Aerosol m.* used with a nebuliser that humidifies the inspired air or oxygen. *M. of pregnancy* a brownish patchy discolouration on the face and neck occurring during pregnancy in some women and disappears after delivery. *Parkinson's m.* an unblinking, fixed facial expression characteristic of people with Parkinson's disease. *Venturi m.* *see* VENTURI MASK.

Maslow's hierarchy of needs (ˈmazlohz ˌhie·rahkee ov needz) *Abraham Maslow, American psychologist, 1908–1970.* A hierarchical ranking, in ascending order of importance, concerning human needs and motivation, and the aim of realising one's full potential. Physiological needs (for oxygen, nutrition, shelter, sleep, etc.) are the most basic and need to be met first, before one is able to deal, in successive order, with the need for safety, security, love and belonging, self-esteem and, ultimately, the need for self-actualisation. (*See* figure above.)

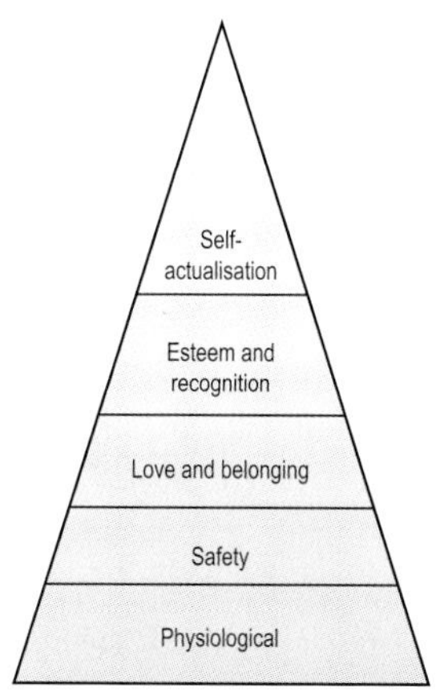

Maslow's hierarchy of needs.

masochism (ˈmasəˌkizəm) a sexual perversion in which pleasure is derived from suffering mental or physical pain.

mass (mas) 1. the quantity of material in an object or body. Can be measured in terms of the force that is needed to accelerate it. 2. a lump of undefined shape. *M. number* the total mass of protons and neutrons in an atom.

massage (ˈmasahzh, -sahj) the application of diverse manual techniques of touch, stroking, rubbing, kneading and manipulating the body to stimulate circulation and to promote a sense of wellbeing. Used in physiotherapy and as a complementary therapy. *External cardiac m.* the application of rhythmic pressure to the lower sternum to cause expulsion of blood from the ventricles and restart circulation in cases of cardiac arrest.

masseter (maˈseetə) the muscle of the cheek chiefly concerned in mastication.

MAST medical anti-shock trousers.

mastalgia (maˈstalji·ə) pain in the breast.

mastatrophia (ˌmastəˈtrohfeeə) atrophy of the breast.

mast cell (mahst sel) a large connective tissue cell found in many body tissues including the heart, liver and lungs. Most cells contain granules which release heparin, serotonin and histamine in response to inflammation or allergy.

mastectomy (maˈstektəmee) amputation of the breast. *Radical m.* removal of the breast, axillary lymph glands and the pectoral muscle.

mastication (ˌmastəˈkayshən) the act of chewing food.

mastitis (maˈstietəs) inflammation of the breast, usually due to bacterial infection.

mastocytosis (ˌmastohˈsieˌtohsis) a rare condition caused by excessive numbers of mast cells in body tissues.

mastodynia (ˌmastohˈdini·ə) pain in the breast, which frequently occurs during the premenstrual phase.

mastoid (ˈmastoyd) breast- or nipple-shaped. *M. antrum* the cavity in the mastoid process which communicates with the middle ear and contains air. *M. cells* hollow spaces in the mastoid bone. *M. operation* drainage of mastoid cells when infection spreads from the middle ear. *M. process* the breast-shaped prominence on the temporal bone which projects downwards behind the ear and into which the sternocleidomastoid muscle is inserted.

mastoidectomy (ˌmastoyˈdektəmee) removal of diseased bone and drainage of the mastoid antrum in severe purulent MASTOIDITIS.

mastoiditis (ˌmastoyˈdietəs) inflammation of the mastoid antrum and cells.

masturbation (ˌmastəˈbayshən) the production of sexual excitement by friction of the genitals.

materia medica (məˈtiə·ri·ə ˈmedikə) the science of the source and preparation of drugs used in medicine.

maternal (məˈtərn'l) pertaining to the mother. *M. mortality rate* the number of deaths in childbirth per 1000 births.

matrix (ˈmaytriks) 1. that tissue in which cells are embedded. 2. in research, a matrix is an arrangement of data which may consist of numbers or text in rows and columns. Matrices are used as part of overall data management, for accessing important data, retaining data for analysis throughout (and after) a research study.

matter (ˈmatə) substance. *Grey m.* a collection of nerve cells or non-medullated nerve fibres. *White m.* medullated nerve fibres massed together, as in the brain.

maturation (ˌmatyəˈrayshən, ˌmachuh-) ripening or developing.

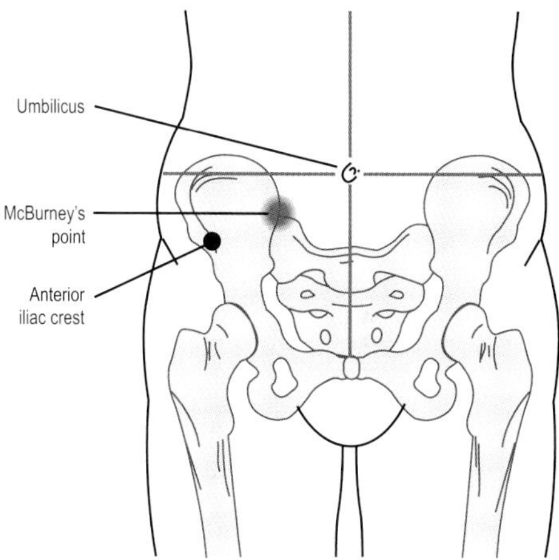

McBurney's point.

maxilla (mak'silə) one of the pair of bones forming the upper jaw and carrying the upper teeth.

maxillary (mak'silə·ree) pertaining to the upper jawbones.

maxillofacial (ˌmaksiloh'fayshəl) pertaining to the maxilla and the face.

McBurney's point (mək'bərneez poynt) *Charles McBurney, American surgeon, 1845–1913.* The spot midway between the anterior iliac spine and the umbilicus where pain is felt on pressure if the appendix is inflamed (*see* figure, above).

McDonald cerclage (mək'donawld sər'klahzh) *Ian McDonald, Australian gynaecologist, 1922–1990.* A purse-string suture placed in the uterine cervix to treat cervical incompetence.

MCHC mean corpuscular haemoglobin concentration.

MCV mean corpuscular volume.

ME myalgic encephalomyelitis. *See* CHRONIC FATIGUE SYNDROME.

mean (meen) a measure of central tendency; the arithmetic average of all scores.

measles ('meezəlz) morbilli; rubeola. An acute, infectious, statutorily notifiable disease of childhood caused by a virus spread by droplets. Endemic and worldwide in distribution. Onset is catarrhal before the rash appears on the fourth day. KOPLIK'S SPOTS are diagnostic earlier. Secondary infection may give rise to the serious complication of OTITIS MEDIA or BRONCHOPNEUMONIA. Vaccination provides a high degree of immunity and may be offered with protection against mumps and rubella (MMR). *German m. see* RUBELLA.

measles, mumps and rubella vaccine (MMR) (ˈmeezəlz, mumps ənd rooˈbelə vakˈseen) an injectable vaccine offered to children aged 12–18 months.

measures of central tendency (ˈmezhəz ov ˈsentrəl ˈtendənsee) descriptive statistical procedure that describes the average member of a sample (mean, median and mode).

meatus (meeˈaytəs) an opening or passage. *Auditory m.* the opening leading into the auditory canal. *Urethral m.* the opening of the urethra to the exterior.

mechanism of labour (ˈmekəˌnizəm ov ˈlaybə) the sequence of movements whereby the fetus adapts itself to pass through the maternal passages during the process of birth.

Meckel's diverticulum (ˈmekəlz dievəˈtikyələm) *Johann Meckel, German anatomist and surgeon, 1781–1833.* The remains of a passage which, in the embryo, connected the yolk sac and intestine; evident as an enclosed sac or tube in the region of the ileum.

meconium (məˈkohni·əm) the first intestinal discharges of a newly born child. It is dark green and consists of epithelial cells, mucus and bile. *M. aspiration* the inhalation by a fetus or newborn of amniotic fluid contaminated by meconium. It may block the air passages, interfere with gas exchange and cause severe respiratory distress. *M. ileus* intestinal obstruction due to blockage of the bowel by a plug of meconium in a neonate with CYSTIC FIBROSIS. *M.-stained amniotic fluid* a sign of fetal distress.

median (ˈmeedi·ən) 1. placed in the centre. 2. in a series of values, the value middle in position. *M. tibial stress* syndrome pain in the front of the legs caused by exercise. Also known as shin splints.

mediastinum (ˌmeedi·əˈstienəm) the space in the middle of the thorax, between the two pleurae; contains all the thoracic viscera other than the lungs.

mediation (meediˈayshən) is a way of resolving disputes between two or more parties. It is a confidential process where an independent and neutral third party facilitates the parties to negotiate their own settlement. In mediation a variety of techniques are used to open and improve communications between parties as a way of assisting them to reach an agreement.

medical (ˈmedikəl) pertaining to medicine. *M. audit*, also known as clinical audit, is an evaluative process applied to the quality of clinical practice, often by peer review of routine or specially collected records of individual cases. Judgements are frequently made on the appropriateness of the processes carried out during the management of the case, in the light of outcomes. *See* AUDIT. *M. model* the traditional approach to the diagnosis and treatment of disease in the Western world. The medical practitioner, using a problem-solving approach, focuses on the disease process and the deficits identified in the organs and tissues. *M. social worker* a professionally qualified worker who looks after the patient's socioeconomic and welfare needs. *M. statistics* that branch of statistics concerned with data relating to health and health services. Traditionally these include the use of routine data relating to death, illness and use of hospitals, clinics, etc. The term is also often used to encompass statistics derived from aspects of medical research, such as the conduct of trials of new drugs or procedures.

medicalisation (ˌmedikəlieˈzayshən) 1. the extension of medical authority into areas previously regarded as being non-medical, where the lay or a popular approach prevailed, e.g. pregnancy and childbirth. 2. the tendency to view undesirable conduct as illness and therefore requiring medical intervention. Medically unexplained symptoms, also known as functional symptoms. Various symptoms, such as pain or dizziness, for which no cause can be found.

medicament (məˈdikəmənt) any medicinal substance used in treatment.

Medicare (ˈmedikair) the name given to Australia's publicly funded national health scheme. The broad objective of the scheme is to make healthcare accessible according to need to all Australian citizens and those holding citizenship or visa status from countries with which Australia has signed a reciprocal healthcare agreement. The scheme covers all public hospital expenses. It also covers general practitioner visits to a prescribed rebate. Medicare is funded by an income surcharge which is calculated at the rate of 2% of each individual's taxable income. Individuals are permitted to supplement their public insurance by taking out additional healthcare coverage through the private sector.

medicated (ˈmedəˌkaytəd) impregnated with a medicinal substance.

medication (ˌmedəˈkayshən) 1. a substance administered to a person for therapeutic purposes. 2. the treatment of a person by means of drugs. *M. error* any incorrect or wrongful administration of a medication. *The six rights of m. administration* emphasise areas of safe practice when checking and giving a medication. They are: right dose, right patient, right route, right drug, right time and right documentation. The six rights also highlight areas where potential errors can occur during medication administration.

medicinal (məˈdisən'l) 1. having therapeutic qualities. 2. pertaining to a medicine. *M. error* any incorrect or wrongful administration of a medication, such as a mistake in dosage or route of administration, failure to prescribe or administer the correct medication or formulation for a particular disease or condition, use of outdated medications, failure to observe the correct time for administration, lack of knowledge or skills related to medication administration. *M. order* a written order by a doctor, dentist, nurse practitioner or other designated health professional for a medication to be dispensed by a pharmacy for administration to a patient.

medicine (ˈmedəsən, ˈmedsən) 1. any drug or remedy. 2. the art and science of the diagnosis and treatment of disease and the maintenance of health. 3. the non-surgical treatment of disease. *Community m.* that specialty which deals with all aspects of medical care in the community, including notification and control of infectious diseases, preschool and school healthcare, and factors affecting the health of the population as a whole. *Emergency m.* that specialty which deals with the acutely ill or injured who require immediate medical treatment. *Family m.* family practice; the medical specialty concerned with the provision of comprehensive primary healthcare. *Forensic m.* the application of medical knowledge to questions of law; medical jurisprudence; also called legal medicine. *Group m.* the practice of medicine by a group of doctors, usually representing various specialties, who are associated together for the cooperative diagnosis, treatment and prevention of disease. *Legal m.* forensic medicine. *Nuclear m.* that branch of medicine concerned with the use of radionuclides in the diagnosis and treatment of disease. *Physical m.* that branch of medicine using physical agents in the diagnosis and treatment of disease. It includes the use of heat, cold, light, water, electricity, manipulation, massage, exercise and mechanical devices. *Preventive m.* science aimed at preventing disease. *Proprietary m.* any chemical, drug or similar preparation used in the treatment of diseases, if such article is protected against free competition as to name, product, composition or process of manufacture by secrecy, patent, trademark, copyright or by other means. *Psychosomatic m.* the study of the interrelations between bodily processes and emotional life. *Space m.* that branch of aviation medicine concerned with conditions to be encountered in space. *Sports and Exercise m.* the field of medicine concerned with injuries sustained in exercise and athletic endeavours, including their prevention, diagnosis and treatment.

medicosocial (ˌmedəkohˈsohshəl) applying to both medicine and the social factors involved.

meditation (ˌmedəˈtayshən) an altered state achieved by concentrating on an object, word or idea. *Transcendental m.* an exercise in contemplative relaxation that promotes a feeling of wellbeing and calmness. It also induces changes in physiological functions, e.g. lowering of the metabolic rate, decreased cardiac output and reduced oxygen consumption, and is used in various complementary therapies.

medium (ˈmeedi·əm) in bacteriology, a preparation for the culture of microorganisms. *Contrast m.* a substance used in radiography to make visible structures that could not otherwise be seen.

MEDLINE (ˈmedˌlien) the print or computerised database of standard medical literature analysis and retrieval system online; it is also available on DVD-ROM.

medulla (məˈdulə) 1. bone marrow. 2. the innermost part of an organ, particularly the kidneys, lymph glands and suprarenal glands. *M. oblongata* that portion of the spinal cord that is contained inside the cranium. In it are the nerve centres that govern respiration, the action of the heart, etc.

medullary (məˈdulə·ree) pertaining to the marrow or a medulla. *M. cavity* the hollow in the centre of long bones.

medullated (ˈmedəˌlaytəd) having a myelin covering. *M. nerve fibre* one enclosed in a myelin sheath.

medulloblastoma (mə͵dulohbla'stohmə) a rapidly growing tumour of neuroepithelial origin occurring in childhood and appearing near the fourth ventricle of the brain. The tumour is highly radiosensitive.

mega (megə) a combining form meaning large, enlarged or of abnormally large size.

megacolon (͵megə'kohlon) extreme dilatation and hypertrophy of the large intestine. When the condition is congenital, it is known as HIRSCHSPRUNG'S DISEASE.

megakaryocyte (͵megə'kareeə͵siet) a large cell of the bone marrow, responsible for blood platelet formation.

megaloblast (͵megəloh'blast) an abnormally large nucleated cell from which mature red blood cells are derived.

megalocephaly (͵megəloh'kefəlee, -'sef-) 1. abnormal largeness of the head. 2. LEONTIASIS ossea.

megalomania (͵megəloh'mayni·ə) delusions of grandeur or self-importance characteristic of general paralysis of the insane.

megaureter (͵megəyə'reeta) dilatation of the ureter.

Meibomian cyst (mie'bohmi·ən sist) *Heinrich Meibom, German anatomist, 1638–1700*. A small swelling of the Meibomian gland caused by obstruction of its duct. If untreated, it may become infected.

Meibomian glands (mie'bohmi·ən glandz) small sebaceous glands situated beneath the conjunctiva of the eyelid; tarsal glands.

meibomianitis (mie͵bohmi·ə'nietəs) a bilateral chronic inflammation of the MEIBOMIAN GLANDS.

meiosis (mie'ohsəs) 1. a stage of reduction cell division when the chromosomes of a GAMETE are halved in number ready for union at fertilisation. 2. contraction of the pupil of the eye; miosis.

melaena (mə'leenə) abnormal, black, tarry faeces that have a distinctive odour and contain digested blood. The condition usually results from bleeding in the upper GI tract.

melancholia (͵melən'kohleeə) a state of extreme depression. *See* DEPRESSION.

melanin ('melənən) a dark pigment found in the hair, the choroid of the eye, the skin and melanotic tumours.

melanism ('melə͵nizəm) a condition marked by an abnormal deposit of dark pigment in the skin or other tissue. Melanosis.

melanocyte ('melənoh͵siet) a cell of the skin pigment melanin. *M.-stimulating hormone (MSH)* hormone produced in the pituitary gland which stimulates the formation of melanin.

melanoderma (͵melənoh'dərmə) a patchy pigmentation of the skin.

melanoma (͵melə'nohmə) a malignant tumour arising in any pigment-containing tissues, especially the skin and more rarely the eye. The incidence of melanoma is rising worldwide amongst light skinned people due to increased exposure to sunlight. Preventative measures should be taken such as limiting exposure to sunlight especially between 10:00 and 14:00 hours, avoiding sunburn and tanning. Protective clothing should also be worn with the use of an effective sunscreen of SPF (Sun Protection Factor) of 30 or higher for children and adults. Australia has the highest incidence of melanoma in the world with an estimated 15 000 new cases of melanoma and approximately 17 000 deaths per year. *Amelanotic m.* an unpigmented malignant melanoma. *Juvenile m.* a benign lesion which usually occurs on the face before puberty; may be mistaken for a malignant melanoma.

melanosis (ˌmelə'nohsəs) *see* MELANISM.

melanotic (ˌmelə'notik) pertaining to melanosis. *M. sarcoma see* SARCOMA.

melanuria (ˌmelə'nyoo·ri·ə) the presence of black pigment in the urine. Occurs in melanotic SARCOMA and PORPHYRIA.

melasma (me'lazma) dark discolouration of the skin; CHLOASMA.

membrane ('membrayn) a thin elastic tissue covering the surface of certain organs and lining the cavities of the body. *Basement m.* the interface between epithelial cells and the underlying connective tissue. *Mucous m.* a membrane that secretes mucus and lines all cavities connected directly or indirectly with the skin. *Serous m.* membrane lining the abdominal cavity and thorax and covering most of the organs within.

memory ('memə·ree) the mental faculty that enables one to register, retain and recall previously experienced sensations, impressions, information and ideas. The ability of the brain to retain and to use knowledge gained from past experience is essential to the process of learning. Short-term memory involves the registration of received information but this is lost quickly unless the information is repeated constantly. Important information that needs to be retained is stored in long-term memory and can be recalled. Memory provides a person with life history which is central to the concept of the 'individual self'. The exact way in which the brain remembers is not completely understood; it is believed that a portion of the temporal lobe of the brain acts as a memory centre, drawing on memories stored in other parts of the brain. *M. disturbance* any disorder of the memory functions whether of registration, retention, recall or recognition. The disorders are varied in character and in causation. The most common problem is difficulty in recall, i.e. short-term memory, that develops with age. More severe loss of memory may be an early symptom of dementia. *Procedural m.* that part of memory that stores information needed to do routine tasks that involve a sequence of steps, e.g. switching on a computer.

menarche ('menahk, 'menahkee) the first appearance of menstruation.

Mendel's theory ('mend'lz thiəree) *Gregor Mendel, Abbot of Brünn, 1822–1884.* The theory that the characters of sexually reproducing organisms are handed on to the offspring in fixed ratios and without blending.

Mendelson's syndrome ('mend'lˌsənz 'sinˌdrohm) *Curtis Mendelson, American obstetrician and cardiologist, 1913–2002.* A condition in which there is severe oedema and spasm of the bronchioles due to the inhalation of acid gastric contents.

Ménière's disease or syndrome ('meneeˌairz di'zeez aw 'sinˌdrohm) *Prosper Ménière, French physician, 1799–1862.* A disease of the inner ear causing attacks of vertigo and TINNITUS with progressive deafness.

meninges (mə'ninjeez, 'menin-) the membranes covering the brain and spinal cord. There are three:

the dura mater (outer), arachnoid mater (middle) and pia mater (inner).

meningioma (məˌninjeeˈohmə) a slow-growing, usually benign tumour developing from the arachnoid and pia mater.

meningism (ˈmeninˌjizəm) a condition in which there are signs of cerebral irritation similar to meningitis, including photophobia and neck stiffness due to either haemorrhage or infection.

meningitis (ˌmenənˈjietəs) inflammation of the meninges, due to organisms such as bacteria, viruses and fungi. Meningitis causes fever, intense headache, intolerance to light and sound, with rigidity of muscles, especially those in the neck (*see* KERNIG'S SIGN). Convulsions with severe vomiting and delirium may also occur in the more severely ill person. A petechial rash that does not disappear when pressure is applied may also occur in some people with meningococcal septicaemia. Therapy involves the use of appropriate antimicrobial drugs, together with intensive care interventions if required, combined with skilled nursing care and support. Meningitis is a notifiable disease and its causal organism, if known, should also be stated. *Meningococcal m. see* MENINGOCOCCAL DISEASE. *Tuberculous m.* inflammation of tuberculous origin.

meningocele (məˈning·gohˌseel) a protrusion of the meninges through the skull or spinal column, appearing as a cyst filled with cerebrospinal fluid. *See* SPINA BIFIDA.

meningococcal disease (məˌninjəˈkokəl diˈzeez) a rare but potentially fatal bacterial infection. The disease manifests as either meningococcal meningitis (inflammation of the membranes surrounding the brain) or meningococcal septicaemia (bacteria in the blood). Caused by the bacterium *Neisseria meningitidis*. The most common groups are A, B, C (W135) and Y. In Australia, groups B and C are common. Transmitted either through the air by droplets of respiratory secretions or by direct contact with an infected person. Early signs and symptoms include fever, severe headache, stiff neck, rash (tiny red or purple spots), nausea and vomiting. Disease progression is rapid and urgent medical care is required if two or more of the signs and symptoms are experienced concurrently. Immunisation (except for group B) is available to reduce the risk of meningococcal meningitis.

meningococcus (məˌning·gəˈkokəs) *Neisseria meningitides*. A diplococcus, the microorganism of cerebrospinal meningitis.

meningoencephalitis (məˌning·goh·enˌkefəˈlietəs, -ˌsef-) inflammation of the brain and meninges.

meningomyelocele (məˌning·gohˈmie·əlohˌseel) a protrusion of the spinal cord and meninges through a defect in the vertebral column; myelomeningocele. *See* SPINA BIFIDA.

meniscectomy (ˌmenəˈsektəmee) surgical removal of a semilunar cartilage from the knee joint.

meniscus (məˈniskəs) 1. the convex or concave surface of a liquid as observed in its container. 2. a lens having one convex and one concave surface. 3. a semilunar cartilage of the knee joint.

menopause (ˈmenəˌpawz) the span of time during which the menstrual cycle wanes and gradually stops;

also called change of life and climacteric. It is the period when the ovaries stop functioning and, therefore, when menstruation and childbearing cease. Usually occurs between the 45th and 55th years of life. There may be an associated hormonal imbalance which causes symptoms such as night sweats, hot flushes, diminished libido and extreme lethargy. *Artificial m.* an induced cessation of menstruation by surgery or by irradiation.

menorrhagia (ˌmenəˈrayji·ə) an excessive flow of the menses; menorrhoea.

menses (ˈmenseez) the discharge from the uterus during menstruation.

men's health clinic (menz helth klinək) a health promotion clinic available for men to screen for health problems and to promote health, e.g. self-examination of the testicles. *See* TESTICULAR SELF-EXAMINATION.

menstrual (ˈmenstrooəl) relating to the menses. *M. cycle* the monthly cycle commencing with the first day of menstruation, when the ENDOMETRIUM is shed, proceeding through a process of repair and hypertrophy until the next period. It is governed by the anterior pituitary gland and the ovarian hormones, oestrogen and progesterone.

menstruation (ˌmenstrooˈayshən) the monthly discharge of blood and ENDOMETRIUM from the uterus, starting at the age of puberty and lasting until the menopause. *Anovular m., anovulatory m.* periodic uterine bleeding without preceding ovulation. *Vicarious m.* discharge of blood at the time of menstruation from some organ other than the uterus, e.g. epistaxis, which is not uncommon.

mental (ˈment'l) 1. pertaining to the mind. 2. pertaining to the chin. *M. age* a measurement based on testing a person's intellectual development usually compared to standardised data for a chronological age. For example, a 13-year-old child with learning difficulties may have a mental age of 5. *M. disorder* a temporary or permanent change in an individual's mental state which makes the person unable to function in daily life as well as they would normally do. *M. handicap* a former term for learning difficulties. *See* LEARNING DIFFICULTIES. *M. health* a state of wellbeing characterised by the absence of mental or behaviour disorder whereby the person has made a satisfactory adjustment as an individual, and to the community, in relation to emotional, personal, social and spiritual aspects of their life.

menthol (ˈmenthol) a crystalline substance derived from oil of peppermint and used in neuralgia and rhinitis, and as a local anodyne and antiseptic.

mentor (ˈmentaw) 1. a wise or trusted adviser or guide. 2. in nursing, a professional colleague who assists with the career development of a colleague and who facilitates and encourages that person's professional growth and awareness; mentorship.

mercury (ˈmərkyə·ree) *symbol* Hg. Quicksilver; a heavy liquid metallic element, the salts of which are used occasionally as antiseptics and disinfectants. Also used in the manufacture of various types of thermometers and manometers. Poisoning from mercury (mercurialism) may occur in people in close contact with the metal over time. This may present with a variety of symptoms including gastrointestinal and dental problems, ataxia, visual and auditory disturbances.

meridian (mə'ridiən) a conceptual channel along which qi energy flows in the body.

mesarteritis (ˌmesahtə'rietəs) inflammation of the middle coat of an artery.

mesencephalon (ˌmesən'kefəˌlon, -'sef-) the middle brain.

mesenchyme ('mesəngˌkiem) in the embryo, the connective tissue developed from the MESODERM.

mesentery ('mesəntə·ree, 'mez-) a fold of the peritoneum which connects the intestine to the posterior abdominal wall.

mesh graft (mesh grahft) a partial or split-thickness skin graft that has multiple slits cut into it. The slits allow the graft to be stretched to several times its original size for coverage of a larger area on the recipient where skin has been lost due to burns, trauma or surgical removal of diseased tissue. Acceptance of the graft is facilitated by the graft permitting fluids to flow from beneath the graft.

mesmerism ('mezməˌrizəm) *Franz Mesmer, Austrian physician, 1734–1815.* HYPNOTISM.

mesoderm ('mesohˌdərm) the middle of the three primary layers of cells in the embryo from which the connective tissues develop.

mesometrium (ˌmesoh'meetri·əm) the broad ligament connecting the uterus with the abdominal wall.

mesomorph ('mesohˌmawf) a stocky individual of medium height with well developed muscles.

mesothelioma (ˌmesohˌtheelee'-ohmə) a rapidly growing tumour of the pleura, peritoneum or pericardium which may be seen in people with ASBESTOSIS. However, this tumour may also occur in people who have no history of exposure to asbestos. There is no effective treatment for large tumours, although radiotherapy, chemotherapy, surgery or a combination of these therapies may alleviate symptoms.

messenger RNA (MRNA) (ˌmesənjə ˌah'enˌay) the ribonucleic acid which acts as a template for the linking of amino acids during the formation of protein in the cells.

mestranol ('mestrəˌnol) a synthetic oestrogen commonly used in combination with a progesterone in contraceptive pills.

meta-analysis (ˌmetə·ə'naləsəs) a research method that takes the results of multiple studies in a specific area and synthesises the findings to make conclusions regarding the area of focus.

metabolic (ˌmetə'bolik) referring to metabolism. *M. syndrome* term for a combination of diabetes, high blood pressure and obesity.

metabolism (mə'tabəˌlizəm) the sum of the physical and chemical processes by which living organised substance is built up and maintained (ANABOLISM), and by which large molecules are broken down into smaller molecules to make energy available to the organism (CATABOLISM). Essentially, these processes are concerned with the disposition of the nutrients absorbed into the blood after digestion. *Basal m.* the minimal energy expended for the maintenance of respiration, circulation, peristalsis, muscle tonus, body temperature, glandular activity and the other vegetative functions of the body. *Inborn error of m.* a genetically determined biochemical disorder in which a specific enzyme defect produces a metabolic block that may have pathological consequences at birth, as in PHENYLKETONURIA, or in later life.

metabolite (mə'tabə,liet) any product or substance taking part in metabolism. *Essential m.* a substance that is necessary for normal metabolism, e.g. a vitamin.

metacarpal (,metə'kahpəl) one of the five bones of the hand which join the fingers to the wrist.

metacarpophalangeal (,metə,kahpohfə'lanji·əl) relating to the metacarpal bones and the phalanges.

metacarpus (,metə'kahpəs) the five bones of the hand uniting the carpus with the phalanges of the fingers.

metal (metəl) any element that is generally a good conductor of heat and electricity, it is malleable and ductile and forms positively charged ions (cations).

metamorphosis (,metə'mawfəsəs) a structural change or transformation.

metaphase ('metə,fayz) the second stage of mitosis or cell division.

metaphysis (mə'tafəsəs) the junction of the EPIPHYSIS with the DIAPHYSIS in a long bone.

metaplasia (,metə'playzi·ə) abnormal change in the structure of a tissue. May be indicative of malignant change.

metastasis (mə'tastəsəs) the transfer of a disease from one part of the body to another, through the blood vessels, via the lymph channels or across the body cavities. Secondary deposits may occur from a primary malignant growth. Septic infection may arise in other organs from some original focus.

metatarsal (,metə'tahsəl) one of the five bones of the foot which join the tarsus to the toes.

metatarsalgia (,metətah'salji·ə) pain in the metatarsal bones.

metatarsus (,metə'tahsəs) the five bones of the foot uniting the tarsus with the phalanges of the toes.

Metazoa (,metə'zoh·ə) the division of the animal kingdom that includes the multicellular animals, i.e. all animals except the PROTOZOA.

methadone ('methə,dohn) a powerful analgesic with no sedative action. Similar in action to morphine, it is used to relieve pain in terminal illness and also in withdrawal programs for heroin addicts. Methadone is addictive, but less socially disabling than heroin.

methaemalbumin (,met·heem'albyoomən) a compound of haem with plasma albumin found in the blood in some types of anaemia.

methaemoglobin ('met·heemə'glohbən) an altered form of haemoglobin found in the blood and usually produced by the action of a drug on the red blood corpuscles, causing a reduction in their oxygen-carrying ability. May be associated with the use of phenacetin and other aniline derivatives.

methaemoglobinaemia (,met·heemə,glohbə'neemi·ə) CYANOSIS and inability of the red blood cells to transport oxygen owing to the presence of methaemoglobin.

methamphetamine (,meth'amfetəmeen) a very addictive central nervous system psycho-stimulant drug. It is chemically related to amphetamine, but the effects of methamphetamine are much more potent, long-lasting and harmful to the brain. Methamphetamine has a high potential for abuse and is often referred to as speed, meth and chalk. *M. hydrochloride* refers to the crystalline smokeable form of the drug. Street methamphetamine hydrochloride is referred to by many names, such as ice, crystal, glass and tina.

methane (ˈmeethayn) marsh gas; an inflammable explosive gas produced by decomposition of organic matter.

methicillin-resistant *Staphylococcus aureus* (MRSA) (methəsilən resistənt ˌstafəlohˈkokəs ˌawreeəs) a strain of *S. aureus* that is resistant to beta-lactam antibiotics which include methicillin and flucloxacillin. Treatment depends upon the sensitivity of the particular strain of MRSA to anti-bacterial drugs and the site of infection. MRSA can affect people in different ways. People can carry the organism in the nose or on the skin without showing any symptoms of illness. This is called MRSA colonisation. MRSA can also cause infections, especially in hospitalised patients and particularly in the older person, those with impaired immune systems, e.g. those living with HIV/AIDS or transplant recipients, those who are seriously ill or who have an open wound or an indwelling urinary or intravenous catheter. Various types of infections occur, including skin, wound and surgical site infections, bone infections, pneumonia and severe life-threatening bloodstream infections. MRSA is almost always transmitted by direct physical contact and not through the air. Transmission may also occur through indirect contact by touching objects (fomites) contaminated by the infected skin of a person with MRSA, e.g. towels, sheets, wound dressings or medical equipment. The most common means by which MRSA is transmitted between patients in hospital is by the contaminated hands of nurses, doctors and other healthcare workers. Standard precautions and transmission-based precautions, including meticulous attention to hand decontamination, can effectively reduce the risk of MRSA transmission during healthcare activities.

methionine (meˈthieəˌneen) 1. a sulfur-containing essential amino acid occurring in proteins that is a vital component of the diet. 2. a drug used orally in the treatment of paracetamol poisoning.

methylated spirit (ˌmethəˌlaytəd ˈspirət) a mixture of 95% ethyl alcohol and 5% methyl alcohol. An industrial spirit which, taken as a drink, is poisonous.

methylene blue (ˈmethəˌleen bloo) a synthetic organic compound, in dark green crystals or lustrous crystalline powder, used in treatment of METHAEMOGLOBINAEMIA, as an antidote in cyanide poisoning, as a stain in pathology and bacteriology and as an antiseptic.

metra (ˈmeetrə) the uterus.

metre (ˈmeetə) *symbol* m. The fundamental SI unit of length.

metritis (məˈtrietəs) inflammation of the uterus.

metrocolpocele (ˌmetrohˈkolpəˌ-seel) the protrusion of the uterus into the vagina, the wall of the latter also being pushed forwards.

metropathia (ˌmetrohˈpathi·ə) any disorder affecting the uterus; metropathy. *M. haemorrhagica* excessive loss of blood from the uterus due to disease; uterine haemorrhage.

metroptosis (ˌmetropˈtohsəs) prolapse of the uterus.

metrorrhagia (ˌmetrəˈrayji·ə) irregular uterine bleeding not associated with menstruation.

metrostaxis (ˌmetrohˈstaksəs) persistent slight haemorrhage from the uterus.

mg milligram(s).

Mg symbol for *magnesium*.

Michel's suture clips (miˈshelz ˈsoochə klips) *Gaston Michel, French surgeon, 1875–1937*. Small metal clips used for suturing wounds.

microalbuminuria (ˌmiekrohˌalbyə-mənˈyoo·ri·ə) the urinary excretion of small amounts of albumin, below the detection level of routine dipstick analysis. The condition is an early indicator of altered glomerular permeability in diabetes mellitus.

microbe (ˈmiekrohb) a minute living organism, especially one causing disease. A microorganism.

microbiology (ˌmiekrohbieˈoləjee) the study of microorganisms and their effect on living cells.

microcephaly (ˌmiekrohˈkəfalee, -sə-) a congenital anomaly characterised by abnormal smallness of the head and brain in relation to the rest of the body, resulting in some degree of intellectual disability. The head is more than two standard deviations below the average circumference size for age, sex, race and period of gestation. It has a narrow, receding forehead, a flattened occiput and a pointed vertex: the facial features are generally normal. The condition may be caused by a variety of genetic and environmental conditions.

Micrococcus (ˌmiekrohˈkokəs) a genus of bacteria, each of which has a spherical shape. The bacteria occur in pairs or in groups and are Gram-positive. Found in soil and water.

microcornea (ˌmiekrohˈkawni·ə) a condition in which the cornea is smaller than normal, producing HYPERMETROPIA and sometimes causing GLAUCOMA.

microcythaemia (ˌmiekrohsie-ˈtheemi·ə) the presence of abnormally small red cells in the blood; microcytosis.

microdrip (ˌmiekrohˈdrip) an intravenous giving set that delivers an infusion rate of 60 drops per 1 mL.

micrognathia (ˌmiekrohˈnathi·ə) failure of development of the lower jaw, causing a receding chin.

microgram (ˈmiekrohˌgram) One-millionth of a gram. The Australian Commission on Safety and Quality in Health Care recommend microgram is written in full as the previously used abbreviation (mcg) can be mistaken for milligram (mg).

micrometre (ˈmiekrohˌmeetə) *symbol* μm. One-millionth of a metre. Formerly called micron.

micron (ˈmiekron) *see* MICROMETRE.

micronutrient (ˌmiekrohˈnyootri·ənt) a dietary element essential only in small quantities.

microorganism (ˌmiekrohˈawgəˌ-nizəm) a minute animal or vegetable, particularly a virus, a bacterium, a fungus, a rickettsia or a protozoon.

microphage (ˌmiekrohˈfayj) a minute PHAGOCYTE.

microphthalmos (ˌmiekrofˈthalməs) a condition in which one or both eyes are smaller than normal. Their function may or may not be impaired.

microscope (ˈmiekrəˌskohp) an instrument which produces a greatly enlarged image of objects that are normally invisible to the human eye. *Electron m.* a microscope in which a beam of electrons is used instead of a light beam, allowing magnification of as much as 500,000 diameters.

microscopic (ˌmiekrəˈskopik) visible only by means of the microscope. The opposite of macroscopic.

Microsporum (ˌmiekrohˈspaw·rəm) a genus of fungi. The cause of some skin diseases, especially ringworm.

microsurgery (ˌmiekrohˈsərjə·ree) the carrying out of surgical procedures using a binocular microscope with magnification and focusing ability. Microsurgery has been developed to enable operating, e.g. on the eye or in the ear, or other delicate and previously inaccessible tissues, nerves and blood vessels, in orthopaedics, gynaecology and neurosurgery.

micturition (ˌmiktyəˈrishən) the act of passing urine.

midbrain (ˈmidbrayn) that portion of the brain that connects the CEREBRUM with the pons and the CEREBELLUM.

midlife crisis (ˌmidˌlief ˈkriesəs) experienced by many people, usually during the fifth decade of life, resulting in doubt, anxiety and, sometimes, depression. During this time, men and women may reflect on their lives, review the past and be aware of physiological deterioration associated with ageing. Some children are growing up, moving away from home and establishing their own adult relationships; the empty nest syndrome.

midwife (ˈmidˌwief) qualified in the art and science of midwifery and meets certain prescribed standards of education and clinical competence and, if practising in Australia, is registered with the Nursing and Midwifery Board of Australia (NMBA).

midwifery (midˈwifə·ree, ˈmidˌwifə-ree) the art and science of caring for women undergoing pregnancy, labour and the period following childbirth (usually 6–8 weeks). *M. process* the application of the nursing process to midwifery. It is the systematic, cyclical method of organising midwifery care, and is carried out by the assessment of actual and potential problems, and the planning, implementation and evaluation of care. *M. Group Practice (MGP)* sometimes known as 'Caseload Midwifery', MGP enables women to be cared for by the same midwife (primary midwife) and supported by a small group of midwives throughout their pregnancy, during childbirth and in the early weeks at home with a new baby. Midwifery care focuses on women's individual needs (woman-centred care).

migraine (ˈmeegrayn, ˈmie-) paroxysmal attacks of severe headache, often with nausea, vomiting and visual disturbance.

milestone (ˈmielˌstohn) one of the norms against which the motor, social and psychological development of a child is measured.

milia (milyə) small white spots usually occurring in clusters around the nose and cheeks resulting from obstruction of a sebaceous gland. May occur in young adults. *M. neonatorum* milia occurring in the newborn which are harmless and quickly disappear if left alone.

miliaria (ˌmileeˈair·ri·ə) prickly heat, an acute itching skin eruption common among white people in tropical and subtropical areas.

miliary ('milyə·ree) resembling millet seed. *M. tuberculosis see* TUBERCULOSIS.

milieu (mil'yər) the environment or setting. *M. interieur* the internal physical and chemical environment experienced by individual cells. *M. therapy* a psychiatric intervention in which the physical surroundings and social setting are used as important elements in the therapeutic process.

milium ('mili·əm) [L.] a whitish nodule in the skin, especially of the face, usually 1–4 mm in diameter. Milia are spheroidal, epithelial cysts of lamellated keratin lying just under the epidermis, often associated with vellus hair follicles. Popularly called 'whitehead'.

milk (milk) 1. secretion of the mammary gland. 2. a liquid (emulsion or suspension) resembling the secretion of the mammary gland. *Human breast m.* contains lipids, 98% as triglycerides, which provide more than 50% of the calorific requirements; carbohydrates, mainly lactose, giving 40% of the calorific needs; whey-dominant protein; vitamins; minerals; trace elements; and anti-infective factors, such as leucocytes, immunoglobulins, lysozyme, lactoferrin, bifidus factor, hormones and growth factor. *Pasteurised m.* a process whereby milk is held at 72°C for 30 minutes and then rapidly cooled and bottled, this method kills non-spore-bearing pathogenic organisms without affecting flavour or food properties of the milk. *Sterilised m.* milk heated to 100°C for 15 minutes to render it free from bacteria. *M. sugar* lactose, a disaccharide present in the milk of all mammals. *M. teeth* the first set of a child's teeth. *Witch's m.* milk secreted from the breast of a newborn child.

Miller-Abbott tube (ˌmilə'abət tyoob) *T. Grier Miller, American physician, 1886–1981; William Abbott, American physician, 1902–1943.* A double-channel intestinal tube for treating obstruction, especially that due to paralytic ileus of the small intestine. It has an inflatable balloon at its distal end.

milliequivalent (ˌmileeə'kwivələnt) the amount of a substance that balances or is equivalent in combining power to 1 mg of hydrogen. A method of assessing the body's acid–base balance or needs during electrolyte upset.

milligram ('milee͵gram) *symbol* mg. One thousandth of a gram.

millilitre ('milee͵leetə) *symbol* mL. One thousandth of a litre (one cubic centimetre).

millimetre ('milee͵meetə) *symbol* mm. One thousandth of a metre.

millimole ('milee͵mohl) *symbol* mmol. The amount of a substance that balances or is equivalent in combining power to 1 mg of hydrogen. A method of assessing the body's acid–base balance or needs during electrolyte upset.

Millipore® filter ('milee͵paw 'filtə) trade name for a device used to filter nutrient solutions as they are administered intravenously.

Milwaukee brace (mil'wawkee brays) a brace consisting of a leather girdle and neck ring connected by metal struts; used to brace the spine in the treatment of SCOLIOSIS.

mind (mien'd) 1. the part of the brain that is the seat of mental activity and that enables one to know, reason, understand, remember, think, feel, react to and adapt to external and internal stimuli. 2. the totality of all conscious and unconscious processes of the individual that influences and directs mental and physical behaviour. 3. the faculty of the intellect or understanding, in contrast to emotion and will. *M. map* a way to brainstorm thoughts and ideas without concern about order and structure. It allows a visual diagram to be created that expresses ideas to assist with analysis and recall.

mindfulness (miend͵fuhlˈness) the process of bringing one's attention to the present moment in a non-judgemental and accepting way, with the aim of training the mind to become aware of awareness; noticing in a detached way. *M. of breathing* the act of focusing attention on your breath without trying to influence it; a way to achieve this is to concentrate on the rise and fall of the chest or the movement of air through the nostrils. *M. meditation* a form of meditation in which participants develop enhanced awareness of their moment-to-moment experience, but do not respond to their thoughts or mental images. It is used for stress management, spiritual growth, healing, deepening concentration and promoting creativity.

mineralocorticoid (͵minə·rəloh-ˈkawtə͵koyd) a hormone produced by the adrenal cortex. Its function is to maintain the salt and water balance in the body.

miosis (mieˈohsəs) contraction of the pupil of the eye, as in reaction to a bright light; MEIOSIS.

miotic (mieˈotik) a drug which causes contraction of the pupil.

miscarriage (ˈmis͵karij) abortion; the expulsion of the fetus before the 20th week of pregnancy, i.e. before it is legally viable.

mite (miet) a minute animal, frequently parasitic on humans and animals, which causes various forms of dermatitis.

mitochondrion (͵mietohˈkondri·ən) a body which is found in the cytoplasm of cells and is concerned with energy production and the oxidation of food.

mitosis (mieˈtohsəs) a method of multiplication of cells by a specific process of division.

mitral (ˈmietrəl) shaped like a mitre. *M. incompetence* the result of a defective mitral valve, when there is a back flow, or regurgitation, after closure of the valve. *M. stenosis* the formation of fibrous tissue causing a narrowing of the valve; usually due to rheumatic heart disease and ENDOCARDITIS. *M. valve* the bicuspid valve between the left atrium and left ventricle of the heart. *M. valvotomy* an operation for overcoming stenosis by dividing the fibrous tissue to free the cusps.

mittelschmerz (ˈmit'l͵shmərts) pain occurring between the menses, accompanying ovulation.

MMR abbreviation for measles, mumps and rubella vaccine, an injectable vaccine offered to children. (*See* Appendix 7.)

Mn symbol for *manganese*.

mobilisation (͵mobəlieˈzayshən) the bringing back into mobility of a limb, joint or person following illness or injury.

modality (mohˈdalətee) the number of peaks in a frequency distribution.

mode (mohd) a measure of central tendency; most frequent score or result.

model (modəl) a conceptual paradigm, framework or theory which can be used as an example to illustrate a problem, process or situation.

modelling (modəling) providing an example that may be imitated, and used as a means of teaching others to learn new behaviour.

modem (mohdəm) a device for converting digital and analogue signals to enable access to the internet. The device converts data into a format suitable for a transmission medium so that it can be transmitted from computer to computer.

MODS *see* MULTIPLE ORGAN DYSFUNCTION SYNDROME.

molar (ˈmohlə) a back tooth used for grinding. There are three on either side of each jaw, making 12 in all (only eight in children).

mole (mohl) 1. the molecular weight of a substance expressed in grams. 2. a pigmented naevus or dark-coloured growth on the skin. Moles are of various sizes and are sometimes covered with hair. 3. a uterine tumour. *Carneous m.* an organised blood clot surrounding a shrivelled fetus in the uterus. *Hydatidiform m.* (*vesicular m.*) a condition in pregnancy in which the chorionic villi of the placenta degenerate into clusters of cysts like hydatids. Malignant growth may follow if any remnants are left in the uterus. *See* CHORIOCARCINOMA.

molecular (məˈlekyələ) pertaining to or composed of molecules. *M. weight* the weight of a molecule of a substance compared with that of an atom of carbon.

molecule (ˈmoləˌkyool) the chemical combination of two or more atoms which form a specific chemical substance, e.g. H_2O (water). The smallest amount of a substance that can exist independently.

molluscum (moˈluskəm) a skin disease characterised by the development of soft, round tumours. *M. contagiosum* a benign tumour arising in the epidermis caused by a virus, transmitted by direct contact or FOMITES.

monarticular (ˌmonahˈtikyələ) referring to one joint only.

Mongolian spot (mongˈgohli·ən spot) blue-grey birth marks present from birth, usually appearing on the lower back and buttocks. They will usually disappear by the time the child is five years old. They resemble bruises.

mongolism (ˈmong·gəˌlizəm) outdated term for Down syndrome.

Monilia (moˈnili·ə) former name for the genus of fungi now known as *Candida*.

monitor (ˈmonətə) 1. to check constantly on a given condition, state or phenomenon, e.g. blood pressure, heart, respiration rate or standards of care. 2. an apparatus by which such conditions or phenomena can be constantly observed and recorded. *Patient m.* the use of electrodes or transducers attached to the patient so that information such as temperature, pulse, respiration and blood pressure can be seen on a screen or automatically recorded.

monoamine oxidase (ˌmonohˌameen ˈoksədayz) an enzyme that breaks down noradrenaline and serotonin in the body. *M. o. inhibitor (MAOI)* a drug that prevents the breakdown of serotonin and leads to an increase in mental and physical activity.

monochromatism (ˌmonohˈkromə-ˌtizəm) colour blindness. The person sees all colours as black, grey or white.

monoclonal (ˌmonohˈklohn'l) derived from a single cell. *M.*

antibodies antibodies derived from a single clone of cells. All the antibody molecules are identical and will react with the same antigenic site.

monocular (mo'nokyələ) pertaining to or affecting one eye only.

monocyte ('monoh,siet) a white blood cell having one nucleus, derived from the reticular cells, and having a phagocytic action.

mononucleosis (,monoh,nyooklee-'ohsəs) an excessive number of monocytes in the blood; monocytosis. *Infectious m.* an infectious disease due to the EPSTEIN-BARR VIRUS; glandular fever.

monoplegia (,monoh'pleeji·ə) paralysis of one limb or of a single muscle or a group of muscles.

monosaccharide (,monoh'sakə,ried) a simple sugar. The end result of carbohydrate digestion. Examples are glucose, fructose and galactose.

monosodium glutamate (MSG) (,monoh,sohdi·əm 'glootə,mayt) a chemical food flavour enhancer commonly added to Chinese dishes. May result in nausea, faintness, facial flushing and headache. It is sometimes called the Chinese restaurant syndrome.

monosomy (,monoh'sohmee) a congenital defect in the number of human chromosomes. There is one less than the normal 46.

monozygotic twins (,monoh'-ziegotək twinz) two offspring born of the same pregnancy and developed from a single fertilised ovum that splits into two equal halves during an early cleavage phase in embryonic development, giving rise to separate fetuses. Such twins are always of the same sex, have the same genetic constitution, possess identical blood groups and closely resemble each other in physical, psychological and mental characteristics.

mons (monz) a prominence or mound. *M. pubis* or *m. veneris* the eminence, consisting of a pad of fat, that lies over the pubic symphysis in the female.

Montgomery's glands or tubercles (mənt'gumə·reez glandz aw 'tyoobəkəlz) *William Montgomery, Irish obstetrician, 1797–1859.* Sebaceous glands around the nipple, which grow larger during pregnancy. Also known as areolar glands.

mood (mood) emotional reaction. Variations in mood are natural, but in certain psychiatric conditions there is severe depression in some cases and wild excitement in others, or alternations between both.

moon face ('moon,fays) a condition characterised by a rounded, puffy face. It occurs in people treated with large doses of corticosteroids. The features return to normal when the medication is stopped. Moon face is symptomatic of Cushing's disease and Cushing's syndrome.

morbid ('mawbəd) diseased, or relating to an abnormal or disordered condition.

morbidity (maw'bidətee) the state of being diseased. *M. rate* a figure that shows the susceptibility of a population to a certain disease. Usually shown statistically as the number of cases which occur annually per 1000 or other unit of population.

morbilli (maw'bilie) measles.

morbilliform (maw'bilə,fawm) resembling measles.

moribund ('mo·rə,bund) in a dying condition.

morning sickness ('mawning 'siknəs) nausea and vomiting

which sometimes occurs in early pregnancy.

Moro reflex (ˈmo·roh ˈreefleks) *Ernst Moro, Austrian paediatrician, 1874–1951*. The reaction to loud noise or sudden movement which should be present in the newborn. Startle reflex.

morphine (ˈmawfeen) the principal alkaloid obtained from opium and given mainly to relieve severe pain. It is a drug of addiction. Morphia.

mortality (mawˈtalətee) the state of being liable to die. *M. rate* the number of deaths, per 1000 or other unit of population, occurring annually from a certain disease or condition.

mortification (ˌmawtəfəˈkayshən) gangrene or death of tissue; NECROSIS.

morula (ˈmo·roolə) an early stage of development of the ovum when it is a solid mass of cells.

mosaic (mohˈzayək) an individual who has cells of varying genetic composition.

motile (ˈmohtiel) capable of movement.

motion (ˈmohshən) 1. the process of moving. 2. evacuation of the bowels; defecation. *M. sickness* sickness occurring as the result of travel by land, sea or air. Appears to be caused by excessive stimulation of the vestibular apparatus within the inner ear.

motivation (ˌmohtəˈvayshən) the reason or reasons, conscious or unconscious, behind a particular attitude or behaviour.

motive (ˈmohtiv) the incentive that determines a course of action or its direction.

motor (ˈmohtə) something that causes movement. *M. endplate* the nuclei and cytoplasm of muscle fibres at the termination of motor nerves. *M. nerve* one of the nerves which convey an impulse from a nerve centre to a muscle or gland to promote activity. *M. neurone disease* a disease in which there is progressive degeneration of the anterior cells in the spinal cord, the motor nuclei of cranial nerves and the corticospinal tracts. The cause is unknown.

mould (mohld) 1. a species of fungus. 2. the plastic shell used to immobilise a part of the body, usually the head, during radiotherapy.

moulding (ˈmohlding) the alteration in shape of the infant's head as it is forced through the maternal passages during labour.

mountain sickness (ˈmowntən ˈsiknəs) DYSPNOEA, headache, rapid pulse and vomiting, which occur on sudden change to the rarefied air of high altitudes.

mourning (ˈmawning) *see* BEREAVEMENT.

mouth (mowth) an opening, particularly the external opening (in the face) of the alimentary canal. *M. ulcers* painful, greyish white sores occurring inside the mouth. Most are of unknown cause and usually disappear after a few days. Those that persist should be reported. Aphthous ulcers. *M. wash* a solution for rinsing the mouth.

movement (ˈmoovmənt) 1. an act of moving; motion. 2. an act of defecation. *Active m.* movement produced by the person's own muscles. *Associated m.* movement of parts that act together, as the eyes. *Passive m.* a movement of the body or of the extremities of a person performed by another person without voluntary motion on the part of the person. *Vermicular m.s* the wormlike movements of the intestines in peristalsis.

moving and handling (ˈmooˈving and hanˈdling) technically the moving, lifting or supporting of a load. In the work environment this is now subject to regulations and guidelines to reduce the risk of back injuries for nurses and healthcare workers; these regulations are enforced by the healthcare facility. *M. and handling equipment* any piece of equipment that facilitates the transfer of persons or objects, e.g. monkey bars, mechanical lifters/hoists, slide sheets, Patslides®. *M. and handling risk* following an initial assessment, any hazard or risk that has the potential to cause harm or illness to the person during the manoeuvre.

MRI *see* MAGNETIC RESONANCE IMAGING.

MRNA *see* MESSENGER RNA.

MRSA *see* METHICILLIN-RESISTANT STAPHYLOCOCCUS AUREUS.

MSH *see* MELANOCYTE-STIMULATING HORMONE.

mucinase (ˈmyoosəˌnayz) an enzyme which acts upon mucin. Contained in some aerosols and useful in the treatment of CYSTIC FIBROSIS.

mucocele (ˈmyookohˌseel) a mucous tumour. *M. of the gallbladder* occurs if a stone obstructs the cystic duct. *Lacrimal m.* a distension of the lacrimal sac caused by a blockage of the nasolacrimal duct.

mucocutaneous (ˌmyookohkyoo-ˈtayni·əs) pertaining to mucous membrane and skin.

mucoid (ˈmyookoyd) resembling mucus.

mucolytic (ˌmyookohˈlitik) a drug that has a mucus softening effect and so reduces the viscosity of the bronchial secretion in chest disorders.

mucopurulent (ˌmyookohˈpyoo·rələnt) containing mucus and pus.

mucosa (ˌmyooˈkohsə) mucous membrane.

mucositis (ˌmyookohˈsietəs) pain and inflammation of the mucous membrane. A common side effect of chemotherapy and radiotherapy.

mucous (ˈmyookəs) pertaining to or secreting mucus. *M. membrane* a membrane that secretes mucus and lines many of the body cavities, particularly those of the respiratory and alimentary tracts.

mucoviscidosis (ˌmyookohˌvisəˈ-dohsəs) fibrocystic disease of the pancreas. *See* CYSTIC FIBROSIS.

mucus (ˈmyookəs) the viscous secretion of the mucous membrane.

multicellular (ˌmulteeˈselyələ) consisting of many cells.

multidisciplinary (ˌmulteeˈ-disəplənree) involving two or more professional disciplines.

multigravida (ˌmulteeˈgravəda) a pregnant woman who has had two or more pregnancies.

multilocular (ˌmulteeˈlokyələ) having many locules. *M. cyst* a cyst, usually in the ovary, containing many compartments.

multinuclear (ˌmulteeˈnyookli·ə) possessing many nuclei.

multipara (ˈmulteeˈpahrə) a woman who has had two or more children.

multiple (ˈmultəpəl) manifold, occurring in many parts of the body at once. *M. myeloma* malignant disease of the plasma cells which invade the bone marrow and suppress its functioning. *M. regression* measure of the relationship between one interval level dependent variable and several independent variables. *M. sclerosis see* SCLEROSIS.

multiple organ dysfunction syndrome (MODS) (multəpəl awgən ˌdis'funkshən 'sinˌdrohm) a situation usually precipitated by shock or trauma in which the functioning of interdependent body systems is severely affected, e.g. respiration, gastrointestinal tract, kidneys, blood circulation and coagulation. This multiple organ failure causes physiological disturbance requiring vital system support to maintain life. Other systems too may be compromised.

multivariate analysis (ˌmultee-ˌvaireeət ə'naləsəs) the analysis of data collected on several different variables but all having a relevance to the study; e.g. in a survey of the provision of community nursing services for a specific population, data may be collected on age, family size and previous use of the services. In analysing the data, the effect of each of these variables and their interaction can be examined and considered.

multivitamin (ˌmultee'vietəmən, -vit-) a tablet containing a combination of different vitamins.

mumps (mumps) a communicable paramyxovirus disease mainly of children, which is statutorily notifiable. Incubation period 2–3 weeks. Attacks one or both of the parotid glands, which are the largest of the three pairs of salivary glands; also called epidemic PAROTITIS or epidemic parotiditis. Most common among children; characterised by inflammation and swelling of the parotid glands. The symptoms are fever and a painful swelling in front of the ears making mastication difficult.

Münchhausen's syndrome ('muhn-ˌchowzənz 'sinˌdrohm) *Baron von Münchhausen, 16th century German traveller noted for his lying tales.* Habitual seeking of medical treatment for apparent acute illness, the person giving a plausible and dramatic history, all of which is false. *M. s. by proxy* an uncommon situation in which a parent (usually the mother) or both parents fabricate symptoms or signs in a child, who is then presented for hospital treatment; overlaps with other forms of child abuse, and fatal outcomes have been reported.

murmur ('mərmə) a sound, heard on auscultation, usually originating in the cardiovascular system. *Aortic m.* one indicating disease of the aortic valve. *Diastolic m.* one heard after the second heart sound. *Friction m.* one present when two inflamed surfaces of serous membrane rub on each other. *Mitral m.* a sign of incompetence of the mitral valve. *Systolic m.* one heard during systole.

Murphy's sign ('mərfeez sien) *John Murphy, American surgeon, 1857–1916.* A sign denoting inflammation of the gallbladder. Continuous pressure over the organ causes the person to 'catch' his or her breath at the zenith of inspiration.

muscae volitantes ('muskie ˌvolə-tanteez) [L] flying flies. Black spots floating before the eyes. They do not obscure the sight. Floaters.

muscarine ('muskə·reen) a poisoning alkaloid that is found in certain fungi and causes muscle paralysis.

muscle ('musəl) strong tissue composed of fibres which have the power of contraction, and thus produce movements of the body. *Cardiac m.* muscle composed of partially striped interlocking cells. Not under the control of the will. *M. relaxant* one of a group of drugs used to reduce muscular spasm and also to relax the muscles during surgery. *Smooth* or *nonstriated m.* involuntary muscle of spindle-shaped cells, e.g. that of the intestinal wall. Contracts independently of the will. *Striped* or *striated m.* voluntary muscle. Transverse bands across the fibres give the characteristic appearance. It is under the control of the will.

muscular (ˈmuskyələ) 1. pertaining to muscle. 2. well provided with strong muscles. *M. dystrophy* one of a number of inherited diseases in which there is progressive muscle wasting. *See* DUCHENNE DYSTROPHY.

musculocutaneous (ˌmuskyəloh-kyooˈtayni·əs) referring to the muscles and the skin. *M. nerve* one of the nerves which supply the muscles and the skin of the arms and legs.

musculoskeletal (ˌmuskyəloh-ˈskelət'l) referring to both the osseous and muscular systems.

mutant (ˈmyootənt) 1. any organism with genetic material that has undergone mutation. 2. produced by MUTATION.

mutation (myooˈtayshən) a chemical change in the genes of a cell causing it to show a new characteristic. Some produce evolutional changes, others produce disease.

mute (myoot) without the power of speech. *Deaf m.* one who cannot hear and therefore cannot speak.

mutilation (ˌmyootəˈlayshən) deliberate infliction of bodily injury.

mutism (ˈmyootizəm) inability or refusal to speak. In almost all cases, individuals are unable to speak because deafness has prevented them from hearing the spoken word. Speech is learned by imitating the speech of others. May also result from disease, the most common being a stroke. *Selective m.* failure to speak in specific situations; strongly associated with social anxiety disorder.

myalgia (mieˈalji·ə) pain in the muscles.

myalgic encephalomyelitis (ME) (mieˈaljik enˌkefəlohˌmieəˈlietəs, -ˌsef-) *see* CHRONIC FATIGUE SYNDROME.

myasthenia (ˌmieəsˈtheeni·ə) muscle weakness. *M. gravis* an extreme form of muscle weakness which is progressive. There is a rapid onset of fatigue, thought to be due to the rapid destruction of acetylcholine at the neuromuscular junction. Commonly affected muscles are those of vision, speaking, chewing and swallowing.

mycetoma (ˌmiesəˈtohmə) a chronic fungus infection of the tissues, both external and internal, but most commonly affecting the hands and feet. There is swelling and the formation of sinuses. Madura foot.

Mycobacterium (ˌmiekohbakˈtiə·ri·əm) a genus of slender, rod-shaped, acid-fast, Gram-positive bacteria that cause a variety of diseases. *M. leprae* the causative organism of leprosy. *M. tuberculosis* the cause of tuberculosis.

mycology (mieˈkoləjee) the study of fungi.

mycosis (mieˈkohsəs) any disease that is caused by a fungus. *M. fungoides* a rare malignant lymphoreticular neoplasm of the skin which later progresses to the lymph nodes and viscera.

mydriasis (məˈdrieəsəs, mie-) abnormal dilatation of the pupil of the eye. Usually caused by injury to the pupil sphincter or by the use of MYDRIATIC drugs.

mydriatic (ˌmidreeˈatik) any drug that causes mydriasis. Used in examination of the eye and in the treatment of inflammatory conditions.

myelin (ˈmieələn) the fatty covering of medullated nerve fibres.

myelitis (ˌmieəˈlietəs) 1. inflammation of the spinal cord, causing pain in the back and sometimes numbness and paralysis of the legs and the lower part of the trunk. 2. inflammation of the bone marrow; OSTEOMYELITIS.

myeloblast (ˈmieəlohˌblast) a primitive cell in the bone marrow, from which develop the granular leucocytes.

myelocyte (ˈmieəlohˌsiet) a cell of the bone marrow, derived from a myeloblast.

myelography (ˌmieəˈlogrəfee) radiographic examination of the spinal cord after the introduction of a radio-opaque substance into the subarachnoid space by means of lumbar puncture.

myeloid (ˈmieəˌloyd) 1. pertaining to, derived from or resembling bone marrow. 2. pertaining to the spinal cord. 3. having the appearance of MYELOCYTES, but not necessarily derived from bone marrow. *M. leukaemia* a malignant disease in which there is excessive production of LEUCOCYTES in the bone marrow. *M. tissue* red bone marrow.

myeloma (ˌmieəˈlohmə) a tumour composed of plasma cells. *Multiple m.* a primary malignant tumour of plasma cells usually arising in bone marrow and usually associated with anaemia.

myelomatosis (ˌmieəlohməˈtohsəs) a malignant disease of the bone marrow in which multiple myelomas are present.

myelomeningocele (ˌmieəlohməˈ-ning·gəˌseel) MENINGOMYELOCELE.

myiasis (mieəsəs) infestation of wounds or body openings by fly larvae (maggots); more commonly seen in the tropics.

myocardial (ˌmieohˈkahdi·əl) pertaining to the MYOCARDIUM. *M. infarction* necrosis of a part of the myocardium caused by a blockage in the blood supply. Associated with chest tightness and severe pain that may radiate down, most usually, the left arm. Men are more likely to have a heart attack than women. Risk factors include family history of the condition, obesity, history of smoking, hypertension, diabetes mellitus and raised cholesterol level together with sedentary lifestyle. Diagnosis is confirmed by ECG and the measurement of cardiac enzymes. A myocardial infarction is a medical emergency and initial treatment includes: aspirin, early thrombolytic therapy, oxygen therapy and analgesia. Increasingly, people with this condition are treated with an angioplasty, with the insertion of one or more stents to create a passage through the occluded artery for the flow of blood to be re-established. After treatment, preventative lifestyle changes are recommended: increase exercise, reduce weight, stop smoking and commence a more healthy diet.

myocarditis (ˌmieohkahˈdietəs) inflammation of the MYOCARDIUM.

myocardium (ˌmieohˈkahdi·əm) the muscle tissue of the heart.

myocele (ˈmieoh͵seel) protrusion of muscle through a rupture of its sheath.

myoclonus (͵mieohˈklohnəs) spasmodic contraction of the muscles; includes HICCUPS.

myoelectric (͵mieoh·əˈlektrik) pertaining to the electric properties of muscle.

myofibrosis (͵mieohfieˈbrohsəs) a degenerative condition in which there is some replacement of muscle tissue by fibrous tissue.

myogenic (͵mieohˈjenik) originating in myocytes or muscle tissue.

myoglobin (͵mieohˈglohbən) MYOHAEMOGLOBIN.

myohaemoglobin (͵mieoh͵heeməˈglohbən) a substance, resembling haemoglobin, which is present in muscle cells. It is a pigment and is responsible for the colour of muscle. It acts as an oxygen store. Myoglobin.

myohaemoglobinuria (͵mieoh͵heemə͵glohbəˈnyoo·ri·ə) the presence of myohaemoglobin in the urine.

myokymia (͵mieohˈkimi·ə) a benign condition in which there is persistent quivering of the muscles.

myoma (mieˈohmə) a benign tumour of muscle tissue. *See* FIBROMYOMA.

myomectomy (͵mieəˈmektəmee) removal of a myoma; usually referring to a uterine FIBROMA.

myometrium (͵mieohˈmeetri·əm) the muscular tissue of the uterus.

myoneural (͵mieohˈnyoo·rəl) relating to both muscle and nerve. *M. junction* the point at which nerve endings terminate in a muscle; neuromuscular junction.

myopathy (mieˈopəthee) any disease of the muscles. MUSCULAR DYSTROPHY is one of a group of inherited myopathies in which there is wasting and weakness of the muscles.

myopia (mieˈohpi·ə) shortsightedness. The light rays focus in front of the retina and a biconcave lens is needed to focus them correctly.

myoplasty (ˈmieoh͵plastee) any operation in which muscle is detached and used, as may be done to correct deformities.

myosarcoma (͵mieohsahˈkohmə) a sarcomatous tumour of muscle.

myosin (ˈmieəsən) muscle protein.

myositis (͵mieohˈsietəs) inflammation of a muscle. *M. ossificans* a condition in which bone cells deposited in muscle continue to grow and cause hard lumps. It may occur after fractures.

myotomy (mieˈotəmee) the division or dissection of a muscle.

myotonia (͵mieɔˈtohni·ɔ) lack of muscle tone. *M. congenita* a hereditary disease in which the muscle action has a prolonged contraction phase and slow relaxation.

myringa (miˈring·gə) the eardrum or tympanic membrane.

myringitis (͵mirinˈjietəs) inflammation of the tympanic membrane.

myringoplasty (məˈring·goh͵plastee) a plastic operation to repair the tympanic membrane; TYMPANOPLASTY.

myringotome (məˈring·gə͵tohm) an instrument for puncturing the tympanic membrane in MYRINGOTOMY.

myringotomy (͵miringˈgotəmee) incision of the tympanic membrane to drain fluid from an infected middle ear.

myxoedema (ˌmiksəˈdeemə) a condition caused by HYPOTHYROIDISM which is marked by mucoid infiltration of the skin. There is oedematous swelling of the face, limbs and hands, dry and rough skin, loss of hair, slow pulse, subnormal temperature, slowed metabolism and mental dullness. *Congenital m.* CRETINISM.

myxoma (mikˈsohmə) a benign mucous tumour of connective tissue.

myxosarcoma (ˌmiksohsahˈkohmə) a SARCOMA containing mucoid tissue.

myxovirus (ˌmiksohˈvierəs) the group name of a number of related viruses, including the causal viruses of influenza, parainfluenza, mumps and Newcastle disease (of fowl).

Nn

N symbol for *nitrogen* and *newton*.

N_2O symbol for *nitrous oxide*.

Na symbol for *sodium*.

naboth's follicle or cyst ('nayboths 'folikəl aw sist) *Martin Naboth, German anatomist, 1675–1721.* Cystic swelling of a cervical gland, the duct of which has become blocked by regenerating SQUAMOUS epithelium.

nadir ('naydiə) the lowest out of a series of measurements, e.g. the lowest level to which the viral load falls after starting antiretroviral treatment. The opposite is ZENITH.

naevus ('neevəs) a birthmark; a circumscribed area of pigmentation of the skin due to dilated blood vessels. A HAEMANGIOMA. *N. flammeus* a flat, blueish-red area, usually on the neck or face; popularly known as 'port wine stain'. *N. pilosus* a hairy naevus. *Spider n.* a small red area surrounded by dilated capillaries. *Strawberry n.* a raised tumour-like structure of connective tissue containing spaces filled with blood.

Nägele's rule ('naygələz rool) rule for calculating the estimated date of labour: add 1 year, subtract 3 months and add 7 days to first day of the last menstrual period.

NAI *see* NON-ACCIDENTAL INJURY.

nail (nayl) the keratinised portion of epidermis covering the dorsal extremity of the fingers and toes. *Hang n.* a strip of epidermis hanging at one side or at the root of a nail. *Ingrowing n.* a condition in which the flesh overhangs the edge of the nail, a sharp corner of which may pierce the skin causing a wound which may become septic. *N. bed* the skin underlying a nail. *N. biting* a sign of nervousness or tension which occurs in childhood and may persist into adult life. It is a common problem and the most frequent habitual manipulation of the body but is rarely of psychopathological significance. *Spoon n.* a nail with a depression in the centre and raised edges. KOILONYCHIA.

NANDA *see* NORTH AMERICAN NURSING DIAGNOSIS ASSOCIATION.

nanometre (ˌna'nomətə) *symbol* nm. A unit of measurement equal to one billionth (10^{-9}) of a metre, or more commonly used to describe a measure equal to one thousandth (10^{-3}) of a micrometre. Nanometres are used to describe the smallest particles in nature, e.g. atoms, small molecules, viruses, electromagnetic radiation. A nanometre is approximately the length of three to six atoms placed side by side, or the width of a single strand of DNA; the thickness of a human hair is between 50,000 and 100,000 nm and represents the smallest feature an unaided human eye can see.

nape (nayp) the back of the neck.

nappy rash (napee rash) an erythematous rash which may occur in infants in the nappy area. The many causes include the passage of frequent loose stools, thrush and ammoniacal dermatitis.

narcissism (ˈnahsiˌsizəm) the stage of infant development when children are mainly interested in themselves and their own bodily needs. In adults, it may be a symptom of mental disorder. The term is derived from the Greek myth of Narcissus.

narcoanalysis (ˌnahkoh·əˈnaləsəs) a controversial form of psychotherapy in which an injection of a narcotic drug produces a drowsy, relaxed state during which a person will talk more freely and in this way, much repressed material may be brought to consciousness. Also known as narcosynthesis.

narcolepsy (ˈnahkəˌlepsee) a rare condition in which there is an uncontrollable desire for sleep.

narcosis (nahˈkohsəs) a state of unconsciousness produced by a narcotic drug. *Basal n.* a reversible state of unconsciousness produced prior to surgical anaesthesia.

narcotic (nahˈkotik) a drug that produces narcosis or unnatural sleep.

nares (ˈnair·reez) the nostrils. *Posterior n.* the opening of the nares into the nasopharynx.

nasal (nayzəl) pertaining to the nose. *N. cannula* a device for delivering oxygen by way of a plastic tube with two prongs that are inserted into the nares. *N. polyp* swelling of the nasal lining inside the nasal passages and sinuses.

nascent (ˈnasənt, ˈnay-) 1. at the time of birth. 2. incipient.

nasoduodenal (ˌnaysohdyoo·ohˈdeenəl) related to the nose and duodenum. *N. tube* a fine-bore tube passed through the nose into the duodenum and used for enteral nutrition.

nasogastric (ˌnayzohˈgastrik) referring to the nose and stomach. *N. tube* one passed into the stomach via the nose. *N. intubation* the placement of a nasogastric tube through the nose into the stomach to relieve gastric distension by removing gas, gastric secretions or food; to instil medication, food or fluids or to obtain a specimen for laboratory analysis.

nasojejunal feeding (ˌnayzoh-jəˈjoonəl feeding) a method in which a silicone-coated catheter is passed through the nose into the JEJUNUM to provide sufficient nutrition to a sick baby on a ventilator or receiving continuous inflating pressure (CIP) by mask or nasal tube. It is used to prevent the dangers of aspiration with a nasogastric tube feed.

nasolacrimal (ˌnayzohˈlakrəməl) concerning both the nose and the lacrimal apparatus. *N. duct* the duct draining the tears from the inner aspect of the eye to the inferior meatus of the nose.

nasopharynx (ˌnayzohˈfaringks) the upper part of the pharynx; that above the soft palate.

nasosinusitis (ˌnayzohˌsienyəˈsietəs) inflammation of the nose and adjacent sinuses.

nasotracheal tube (ˌnayzohˈ trəˌkeel tyoob) a catheter inserted into the trachea via the nose and pharynx.

National law *see* HEALTH PRACTITIONER REGULATION NATIONAL LAW.

natriuresis (ˌnatreeyəˈreesəs) the excretion of abnormally high amounts of sodium in the urine.

natural childbirth (ˈnachərəl ˈchieldˌbərth) a term used to describe an approach to LABOUR and delivery in which there is little or no medical intervention. It is generally considered the optimal way of giving birth and being born, safest for the baby and most satisfying for the mother. Prerequisites include normal gestation, an adequate birth canal, strong maternal motivation, physical and emotional motivation and constant and intensive support of the mother during labour and birth.

natural killer cells (NK cells) (natchərəl kilə sels) a type of lymphocyte involved in natural killing (apoptosis) and forming part of the non-specific body defences. NK cells target viral infected cells and tumour cells.

nature–nurture debate (naychə–nərchə dəbayt) the debate surrounding the issue of to what extent human behaviour is the result of hereditary or innate influences (nature) or is determined by the environment and learning (nurture).

naturopathy (ˌnachəˈropəthee) combines conventional health sciences with a range of natural therapies and traditional medicines. Treatment considers the person in a holistic manner which includes mental, emotional, spiritual and physical states within the context of their living environment. Naturopathy encompasses a range of modalities to assist in the healing process, e.g. herbal medicine, diet and lifestyle recommendations, vitamin and mineral supplementation and positive thinking.

nausea (ˈnawzi·ə) a sensation of sickness with an inclination to vomit.

navel (ˈnayvəl) the UMBILICUS.

navicular (nəˈvikyələ) boat shaped. *N. bone* one of the tarsal bones of the foot.

NBM *see* NIL BY MOUTH.

near death experience (niə deth ˌekˈspiəreeənts) the subjective observations of people who either have been close to clinical death or may have recovered after being declared dead.

near drowning (niə ˈdrowning) survival, at least temporarily, from immersion in a liquid medium.

nebula (ˈnebyələ) a slight opacity or cloudiness of the cornea, caused by injury or by corneal ulceration.

nebuliser (ˈnebyəˌliezə) an apparatus for reducing a liquid to a fine spray; an atomiser.

NEC *see* NECROTISING ENTEROCOLITIS.

neck (nek) 1. the narrow part of an organ or bone. 2. the part of the body which connects the head and the trunk. *Wry n.* TORTICOLLIS.

necrobiosis (ˌnekrohbieˈohsəs) localised death of a part as a result of degeneration.

necropsy (ˈnekropsee) autopsy; a postmortem examination of a body.

necrosis (nəˈkrohsəs) death of a portion of tissue.

necrotising enterocolitis (NEC) (ˈnekrəˌtiezing ˌentə·rohkəˈlietəs) inflammatory bowel disease of the preterm and low birth-weight infants, associated with septicaemia, especially where there is a history of asphyxia, respiratory distress, hypoglycaemia, hypothermia or cardiovascular disease. Possibly due to bacterial proliferation and penetration of the bowel wall in areas of ischaemic damage. May lead to perforation and peritonitis. Treatment is with parenteral nutrition, antibiotics and surgery for perforation.

necrotising fasciitis (nekrohtiezing fashee·ietəs) a bacterial infection of *Streptococcus* type A underneath the skin in the fascia layer; produces necrosis and toxins, resulting in shock and organ failure. Urgent treatment is required with antibiotics and surgical excision of the infected tissues.

needlestick injury (ˈneedˈlstik injəree) an accidental injury with a needle that is contaminated with blood or body fluids. The term is also used sometimes to include other sharps injuries. Such injuries can be dangerous, particularly if the needle has been used in treatment of a person with blood-borne infections such as hepatitis viruses (hepatitis B or C) or human immunodeficiency virus (HIV). A risk assessment procedure, training policies and clinical guidelines should be in place in all healthcare situations for staff to follow, should such an injury occur.

needling (ˈneedling) discission; the operation for cataract of lacerating and splitting up the lens so that it may be absorbed.

needs analysis (needz əˈnaləsəs) exercise often undertaken by healthcare personnel, service organisations and agencies of a target population to assess a service or situation with a view to change, e.g. alteration to clinic times. Multiple research methods and techniques for data collection and analysis may be used in the process.

negative (ˈnegətiv) the opposite of positive; the absence of some quality or substance.

negativism (ˈnegətiˌvizəm) a symptom of mental illness in which the person does the opposite of what is required and so presents an uncooperative attitude. Common in SCHIZOPHRENIA.

negligence (ˈneglijəns) in law, the failure to do something that a reasonable person of ordinary prudence would do in a certain situation and may provide the basis for a lawsuit when there is a legal duty as in nursing and midwifery to provide reasonable care to patients/clients and when negligence results in damage to the patient or client.

Neisseria (nieˈsiə·ri·ə) *Albert Neisser, German bacteriologist, 1855–1916.* A genus of paired, spherical, Gram-negative bacteria. *N. gonorrhoeae* the causative organism of GONORRHOEA. *N. meningitidis* the cause of MENINGOCOCCAL MENINGITIS.

Nelson's syndrome (ˈnelsənz ˈsinˌdrohm) *Donald Nelson, American physician, 1925–2010.* The development of an ACTH-producing tumour after bilateral adrenalectomy in CUSHING'S SYNDROME; it is characterised by aggressive growth of the tumour and hyperpigmentation of the skin.

Nematoda (ˌneməˈtohdə) a phylum of worms, including the genus *Ascaris* or roundworm and the genus *Enterobius* or threadworm.

neoadjuvant therapy (ˌneeohˈajəvənt ˈtherəpee) a preliminary cancer treatment such as chemotherapy or radiation to reduce the size of a tumour. Usually precedes another phase of treatment.

neocerebellum (ˌneeohˌserəˈbeləm) the middle lobe of the CEREBELLUM.

neocortex (ˌneeohˈkawteks) the cerebral cortex, excluding the hippocampal formation and piriform aperture.

neoglycogenesis (ˌneeohˌgliekə-ˈjenəsəs) the formation of liver glycogen from non-carbohydrate sources. Glyconeogenesis.

neologism (neeˈoləˌjizəm) the formation of new words, either completely new ones or ones formed by contraction of two separate words. This is done particularly by schizophrenic people.

neonatal (ˌneeəˈnayt'l) referring to the first 28 days of life. *N. intensive* *care unit (NICU) see* INTENSIVE CARE UNIT. *N. mortality rate* the number of deaths of infants up to 4 weeks old per 1000 live births in any one year. *N. period* the interval from the birth to 28 days of age and the period of greatest risk to the infant. *N. respiratory distress syndrome* occurs when newborn babies' lungs are not fully developed and there is a lack of surfactant in the lungs.

neonate (ˈneeəˌnayt) newborn; specifically pertaining to an infant from birth to 28 days of age.

neonatologist (ˌneeohnayˈtoləjəst) a medically qualified person specialising in the management, assessment, diseases and intensive care of newborn babies, especially those of low birth weight and those with congenital abnormalities.

neonatology (ˌneeohnayˈtoləjee) the branch of medicine dealing with disorders of the newborn infant.

neoplasia (ˈneeohˌplazi·ə) the new and abnormal growth of cells that may be benign or malignant.

neoplasm (ˈneeohˌplazəm) a morbid new growth; a tumour. It may be benign or malignant.

nephrectomy (nəˈfrektəmee) excision of a kidney.

nephritis (nəˈfrietəs) inflammation of the kidney; a focal or diffuse proliferative or destructive disease that may involve the GLOMERULUS, tubule or interstitial renal tissue. The most usual form is GLOMERULONEPHRITIS.

nephroblastoma (ˌnefrohblaˈstohmə) a rapidly developing malignant mixed tumour of the kidneys, made up of embryonic cells and occurring chiefly in children before the fifth year; WILMS' TUMOUR.

nephrocalcinosis (ˌnefrohˌkalsəˈnohsəs) a condition in which there is deposition of calcium in the renal tubules resulting in calculi formation and renal insufficiency.

nephrocele (ˈnefrohˌseel) hernia of the kidney.

nephrogram (ˈnefrohˌgram) a radiograph of the kidney with contrast medium in the renal tubules. It is usually the immediate film in an excretion urogram.

nephrolith (ˈnefrohˌlith) stone in the kidney; renal calculus.

nephrolithiasis (ˌnefrohləˈthieəsəs) the presence of a calculus or of gravel in the kidney.

nephrolithotomy (ˌnefrohləˈthotəmee) removal of a renal calculus by incising the kidney or by extracorporeal shock wave LITHOTRIPSY.

nephroma (neˈfrohmə) tumour of the kidney.

nephron (ˈnefron) the functional unit of the kidney, comprising Bowman's capsule, the proximal and distal tubules, the loop of Henle and the collecting duct which conveys urine to the renal pelvis.

nephropexy (ˈnefrohˌpeksee) the fixation of a floating (mobile) kidney, usually by sutures to neighbouring muscle.

nephroptosis (ˌnefropˈtohsəs) downward displacement or undue mobility of a kidney.

nephropyeloplasty (ˌnefrohˈpieəlohˌplastee) any plastic operation on the pelvis of the kidney performed in cases of HYDRONEPHROSIS.

nephropyosis (ˌnefrohpieˈohsəs) suppuration in the kidney.

nephrosclerosis (ˌnefrohskləˈrohsəs) constriction of the arterioles of the kidney. Seen in benign and malignant hypertension and in ARTERIOSCLEROSIS in old age.

nephrosis (ne'frohsəs) any disease of the kidney, especially that characterised by oedema, proteinuria and a low plasma albumin. Caused by non-inflammatory degenerative lesions of the tubules.

nephrostomy (nə'frostəmee) creation of a permanent opening into the renal pelvis.

nephrotic (nə'frotik) referring to or caused by nephrosis. *N. syndrome* a clinical syndrome in which there is proteinuria, low plasma protein and gross oedema. The result of increased capillary permeability in the GLOMERULI. It may occur as a result of acute GLOMERULONEPHRITIS, in subacute NEPHRITIS, DIABETES MELLITUS, amyloid disease, systemic LUPUS ERYTHEMATOSUS and renal vein thrombosis.

nephrotomogram (ˌnefroh'tohmə-ˌgram) a tomogram of the kidney obtained by NEPHROTOMOGRAPHY.

nephrotomography (ˌnefrohtə'mo-grəfee) radiological visualisation of the kidney by tomography after introduction of a contrast medium.

nephrotomy (nə'frotəmee) incision of the kidney.

nephrotoxic (ˌnehfroh'toksik) poisonous or destructive to the cells of the kidney.

nephroureterectomy (ˌnefroh·yəˌreetə'rektəmee) surgical removal of the kidney and the ureter.

nerve (nərv) a bundle of conducting fibres enclosed in a sheath called the EPINEURIUM. Its function is to transmit impulses between any part of the body and a nerve centre. *Motor* (efferent) *n.* one that conveys impulses, causing activity from a nerve centre to a muscle or gland. *N. block* a method of producing regional anaesthesia by injecting a local anaesthetic into the nerves supplying the area to be operated on. *N. fibre* the prolongation of the nerve cell, which conveys impulses. Each fibre has a sheath. Medullated nerve fibres have an insulating myelin sheath. *N. gas* a gas that interferes with the functioning of the nerves and muscles. Such gases may cause death from respiratory paralysis; some of them act through the skin and cannot be avoided by the use of gas masks. *Sensory* (afferent) *n.* one that conveys sensation from an area to a nerve centre.

nervous ('nərvəs) 1. pertaining to or composed of nerves. 2. apprehensive. *N. breakdown* a popular and misleading term for any type of mental illness that interferes with a person's normal activities. A so-called 'nervous breakdown' can include any of the mental disorders, including NEUROSIS, PSYCHOSIS or DEPRESSION, but is usually used to describe neurosis.

nervousness ('nərvəsnəs) excitability of the nervous system, characterised by a state of mental and physical unrest.

nesting (nesting) the provision of an enclosed space bounded by a small blanket roll encircling the sick or preterm infant in a cot or incubator. This helps to provide a supportive, calming environment for the infant.

nettle rash ('net'l ˌrash) an allergic skin condition; URTICARIA.

network ('netˌwərk) 1. an interconnected group or system of voluntary organisations or of colleagues with similar interests. 2. a system of interconnected computer terminals in which the user has access to others using the system for sharing data, etc. *Clinical n.* a group of health professionals and organisations from primary, secondary and tertiary care working together in a managed and coordinated way that is not constrained by existing organisational or professional boundaries. The aim is to deliver a person-focused service that highlights quality care and clinical effectiveness. These networks may be grouped by client group (maternity, children, young people), or by disease (cancer, coronary heart disease) or specialty (vascular surgery, cardiology). Other networks may be developed according to local need.

networking (ˈnetˌwərking) 1. forming and maintaining professional connections and contacts through informal social meetings. 2. the interconnection of two or more computer networks in different places.

neural (ˈnyoo·rəl) pertaining to the nerves. *N. arch* the bony arch on each vertebra which encloses the spinal cord. *N. tube defect* any of a group of congenital malformations involving the neural tube, including ANENCEPHALY and SPINA BIFIDA.

neuralgia (nyəˈraljə, -ji·ə) a sharp stabbing pain, usually along the course of a nerve owing to neuritis or functional disturbance.

neurapraxia (ˌnyoo·rəˈpraksi·ə) an injury to a nerve resulting in temporary loss of function and paralysis. It is usually caused by compression of the nerve and there is no lasting damage.

neurectomy (nyəˈrektəmee) excision of part of a nerve.

neurilemma (ˌnyoo·rəˈlemə) the membranous sheath surrounding a nerve fibre.

neurinoma (ˌnyoo·rəˈnohma) a benign tumour arising in the NEURILEMMA of a nerve fibre.

neuritis (nyəˈrietəs) inflammation of a nerve, with pain, tenderness and loss of function. *Multiple n.* that involving several nerves; POLYNEURITIS. *Nutritional* (alcoholic) *n.* that which may be caused by alcoholism or lack of vitamin B complex. *Optic n.* that affecting the optic disc or nerve. *Peripheral n.* that involving the terminations of nerves. *Sciatic n.* SCIATICA. *Tabetic n.* a type occurring in TABES DORSALIS. *Traumatic n.* that which results from an injury to a nerve.

neuroblast (ˈnyoo·rohˌblast) an embryonic nerve cell.

neuroblastoma (ˌnyoo·rohbla-ˈstohmə) a malignant tumour of immature nerve cells, most often arising in the very young.

neurodermatitis (ˌnyoo·rohˌdər-məˈtietəs) a localised PRURIGO of somatic and psychogenic origin. It irritates, and rubbing causes thickening and pigmentation of the skin.

neurodevelopmental therapy (nyoorohˈdəvelopmentəl therəpee) a non-invasive approach to the rehabilitation of people with neurological problems based on current research findings into motor development and neurophysiology.

neuroepithelioma (ˌnyoo·rohˌepee-ˌtheeleeˈohmə) a malignant tumour of the retina of the eye which may spread into the brain.

neurofibroma (ˌnyoo·rohfieˈbrohmə) a usually benign tumour of nerve and fibrous tissue.

neurofibromatosis (ˌnyoo·rohˌfie-brohməˈtosəs) von Recklinghausen's disease. A generalised hereditary disease in which there are numerous fibromas of the skin and nervous system.

neurogenic (ˌnyoo·rəˈjenik) derived from or caused by nerve stimulation. *N. bladder* a disorder of the urinary bladder caused by a lesion of the nervous system. *N. shock* shock originating in the nervous system.

neuroglia (nyəˈrogli·ə) the special form of connective tissue supporting nerve tissues also known as glial cells.

neurohypophysis (ˌnyoo·roh·hieˈpofəsəs) the posterior lobe of the pituitary gland.

neuroleptic (ˌnyoo·rohˈleptik) a drug which acts on the nervous system.

neurological assessment (ˌnyoo·rəˈlojikəl əˈsesmənt) evaluation of the health status of a person with a nervous system disorder or dysfunction. Purposes of the assessment include establishing nursing goals to guide the nurse in planning and implementing nursing measures to help the person cope effectively with daily living activities. Nursing assessment of a person's neurological status is concerned with identifying functional disabilities that interfere with the person's ability to provide self-care and lead an active life. A functionally oriented nursing assessment includes: (a) consciousness; (b) mental functions; (c) motor function; and (d) sensory function as well as a GLASGOW COMA SCALE. Evaluation of these functions gives the nurse information about the person's ability to perform everyday activities such as thinking, remembering, seeing, eating, speaking, moving, smelling, feeling and hearing. A person with an acute and life-threatening alteration in neurological function is evaluated and monitored in four general areas: (a) level of consciousness; (b) sensory and motor function; (c) pupillary changes; and (d) vital signs and pattern of respiration.

neurologist (nyəˈroləjəst) a medical practitioner who specialises in neurology.

neurology (nyəˈroləjee) 1. the scientific study of the nervous system. 2. the branch of medicine concerned with diseases of the nervous system.

neuroma (nyəˈrohmə) a tumour consisting of nervous tissue.

neuromuscular (ˌnyoo·rohˈ-muskyələ) appertaining to nerves and muscles. *N. junction* the small gap between the end of the motor nerve and the motor endplate of the muscle fibre supplied. This gap is bridged by the release of acetylcholine whenever a nerve impulse arrives.

neuromyelitis (ˌnyoo·rohˌmieəˈ-lietəs) neuritis associated with MYELITIS. It is a condition akin to multiple sclerosis. *N. optica* a disease in which there is bilateral optic neuritis and PARAPLEGIA.

neurone (neuron) (ˈnyoo·rohn, ˈnyoo·ron) a nerve cell. *Lower motor n.* the anterior horn cell and its neurone which conveys impulses to the appropriate muscles. *Upper motor n.* that in which the cell is in the cerebral cortex and the fibres conduct impulses to associated cells in the spinal cord.

neuroparalysis (ˌnyoo·rohpəˈraləsəs) paralysis due to disease of a nerve or nerves.

neuropathy (nyəˈropəthee) a disease process of nerve degeneration and loss of function. *Alcoholic n.*

neuropathy due to thiamine deficiency in chronic alcoholism. *Diabetic n.* that associated with diabetes mellitus. *Entrapment n.* any of a group of neuropathies, e.g. carpal tunnel syndrome, due to mechanical pressure on a peripheral nerve; also known as nerve compression syndrome. *Ischaemic n.* that caused by a lack of blood supply. *Peripheral n.* occurs when nerves in the body's periphery are damaged.

neuroplasticity (ˌnyoorohplaˈ-stisətee) the capacity for nerve cells to regenerate and recover function.

neuroplasty (ˈnyoo·rohˌplastee) the surgical repair of a damaged nerve.

neuropsychiatry (ˌnyoorohˈsieˌkieətree) the medical specialty concerned with the effects on the mind and behaviour of organic disorders of the nervous system, combining both neurology and psychiatry.

neurorrhaphy (nyəˈro·rəfee) the operation of suturing a divided nerve.

neurosis (nyəˈrohsəs) now an outdated term for a group of mental health disorders in which symptoms are distressing to the person. Reality testing is intact, behaviour does not violate gross social norms and there is no apparent organic cause. *Anxiety n.* persistent anxiety and the accompanying symptoms of fear, rapid pulse, sweating, trembling, loss of appetite and insomnia. *Obsessive compulsive n.* one characterised by compulsions and obsessional rumination.

neurosurgery (ˌnyoo·rohˈsərjə·ree) that branch of surgery dealing with the brain, spinal cord and nerves.

neurosyphilis (ˌnyoo·rohˈsifələs) a manifestation of third stage syphilis in which the nervous system is involved. Symptoms of the disease may not occur for 20 years or so after the primary infection. The three most common forms are: (a) meningovascular syphilis, affecting the blood vessels to the meninges; (b) tabes dorsalis (*see* ATAXIA); and (c) general paralysis of the insane.

neurotic (nyəˈrotik) a loosely applied adjective denoting association with neurosis.

neurotmesis (ˌnyoo·rotˈmeesəs) degeneration of a nerve due to severance.

neurotoxic (ˌnyoo·rohˈtoksik) poisonous or destructive to nervous tissue.

neurotransmitter (ˌnyoo·rohtranz-ˈmitə, -trahnz-) a substance (e.g. noradrenaline, acetylcholine, dopamine) that is released from the axon terminal to produce activity in other nerves.

neurotripsy (ˈnyoo·rohˌtripsee) the surgical bruising or crushing of a nerve.

neurotropic (ˌnyoo·rohˈtropik) having an affinity for nerve tissue. *N. viruses* those that particularly attack the nervous system (such as measles, rabies, poliomyelitis, etc.).

neutral thermal environment (nyootrəl thərməl ˌənˈvierənmənt) an environment created by any method or apparatus to maintain the normal body temperature or minimise oxygen consumption and caloric expenditure, such as in an INCUBATOR or Isolette® for a premature, sick or low birth-weight infant.

neutropenia (ˌnyootrəˈpeeni·ə) a decrease in the number of neutrophils in the blood.

neutrophil (ˈnyootrəˌfil) a polymorphonuclear leucocyte that has a neutral reaction to acid and alkaline dyes.

nevus (ˈneevəs) *see* NAEVUS.

Newborn Screening Program (ˈnyoo ˌbawn ˈskreening ˈprohgram) an extension of the GUTHRIE TEST. In Australia, all babies are screened for PKU and HYPOTHYROIDISM. It may also include screening for cystic fibrosis and GALACTOSAEMIA.

next of kin (nekst ov kin) technically a person's closest living relative, whose name is often required as part of healthcare information. People should be asked whom they wish to nominate as their 'next of kin' or significant other in accordance with their own personal situation.

niacin (ˈnieəsən) NICOTINIC ACID.

nicotine (ˈnikəˌteen) a poisonous alkaloid in tobacco. *N. replacement therapy* preparations containing nicotine that are used in place of cigarettes to assist people to stop smoking. Preparations are available in a variety of forms, e.g. as patches, sublingual tablets, chewing gum or nasal spray; these therapies increase the chances of smokers quitting successfully. Some side effects may occur, e.g. nausea, headaches, palpitations and flu-like symptoms.

nicotinic acid (ˌnikəˈtinik ˈasəd) niacin. A water-soluble vitamin in the B complex. A deficiency of this vitamin causes PELLAGRA.

nidation (nieˈdayshən) implantation of the fertilised ovum in the uterus.

nidus (ˈniedəs) 1. a nest. 2. a place in which an organism finds conditions suitable for its growth and development. 3. the focus of an infection.

Niemann-Pick disease (ˌneemənˈpik diˈzeez) *Albert Niemann, German paediatrician, 1880–1921*; *Ludwig Pick, German physician, 1868–1944.* A group of rare inherited disorders in which there is lipoid storage abnormality and widespread deposition of lecithin in the tissues.

night blindness (niet ˈbliendnəs) nyctalopia; difficulty in seeing in the dark. This may be a congenital defect or may be caused by a vitamin A deficiency. Also occurs as a result of retinal degeneration.

nightmare (nietmair) a frightening or unpleasant dream that occurs during REM (rapid eye movement) sleep usually in the middle to later part of the night. The dreamer wakes completely, remembering the dream. Most common in young children; in adults may be a side effect of certain drugs, e.g. beta-blockers, or associated with a traumatic experience.

night sweat (ˈniet ˌswet) profuse perspiration during sleep, associated with an acute feverish illness or the menopause.

night terror (ˈniet ˌterə) an unpleasant experience in which the subject, usually a young child, screams while asleep and seems terrified. On waking, the individual is unable to remember the cause of the fear.

nihilism (ˈnieəˌlizəm) in psychiatry, a term used to describe feelings of not existing and of hopelessness, that all is lost or destroyed.

nil by mouth (NBM) (nil bie mowth) a patient care instruction advising that a patient is prohibited from ingesting food, beverages or medications, usually implemented prior to surgical anaesthesia, certain diagnostic procedures and when the patient is unable to tolerate oral foods or fluids for some reason.

nipple (ˈnipəl) the small conical projection at the tip of the breast, through which, in the female, milk may be withdrawn. *Accessory n.* a rudimentary nipple anywhere in a line from the breast to the groin. *Depressed n.* one that does not protrude. *N. shield* a shield fitted with a rubber teat which covers the AREOLA of a nursing mother when her nipple is sore or not sufficiently protractile for the baby to suck. *Retracted n.* one that is drawn inwards. It may be a sign of cancer of the breast.

Nissl granules (ˈnisəl ˈgranyəlz) *Franz Nissl, German neuropathologist, 1860–1919.* RNA-containing units found in the cytoplasm of cells. Probably associated with protein synthesis.

nit (nit) the egg of the head louse, attached to the hair near the scalp.

nitrate drugs (ˈnietrayt drugz) a group of coronary vasodilator drugs used to treat angina pectoris. These drugs provide rapid relief of symptoms and improve exercise tolerance. They may be given as tablets to be chewed or dissolved sublingually, as skin patches, gel or sublingual sprays.

nitrogen (ˈnietrəjən) *symbol* N. A gaseous element. Air is largely composed of nitrogen, and it is one of the essential constituents of all protein foods. *N. balance* the state of the body in regard to the rate of protein intake and protein utilisation. A negative nitrogen balance occurs when more protein is utilised by the body than is taken in. A positive nitrogen balance implies a net gain of protein in the body. Negative nitrogen balance can be caused by such factors as malnutrition, debilitating disease, blood loss and glucocorticoids. A positive balance can be caused by exercise, growth hormone and testosterone. *N. mustards* a group of toxic, blistering alkylating agents, including nitrogen mustard itself (mechlorethamine hydrochloride) and related compounds; some have been used as antineoplastics in certain forms of cancer.

nitrous oxide (ˈnietrəs oksied) N_2O; laughing gas. An inhalation anaesthetic ensuring a brief spell of unconsciousness.

NK cells (NKˌsels) *see* NATURAL KILLER CELLS.

NMBA *see* NURSING AND MIDWIFERY BOARD OF AUSTRALIA.

NNT *see* NUMBERS NEEDED TO TREAT.

nociassociation (ˌnohsee·əˌsohseeˈayshən) the discharge of nervous energy which occurs unconsciously in trauma, as in surgical shock. *See* ANOCI-ASSOCIATION.

noctambulation (ˌnoktambyəˈlayshən) sleep walking; SOMNAMBULISM.

nocturia (nokˈtyoo·ri·ə) the passing of urine at night, especially that associated with irritation of the bladder and urethra, or that associated with prostatic enlargement.

nocturnal (nokˈtərnˈl) referring to the night. *N. enuresis* bed wetting; incontinence of urine during sleep.

node (nohd) a swelling or protuberance. *Atrioventricular n.* the specialised tissue between the right atrium and the ventricle at the point where the coronary vein enters the atrium, from which is initiated the impulse of contraction down the atrioventricular bundle. *N. of Ranvier* a constriction occurring at intervals in a nerve fibre to enable the NEURILEMMA with its blood supply to reach and nourish the axon of the nerve. Also known as myelin sheath gaps. *Sinoatrial n.* known as the pacemaker of the heart. A group of specialised cells situated at the opening of the superior vena cava and the right atrium. These cells emit regular electric impulses which initiate and control the heartbeat.

nodule (ˈnodyool) a small swelling or protuberance.

no lift policy (noh lift polisee) a strategy developed to minimise the risks associated with manual handling of people. *See* MANUAL.

noma (ˈnohmə) an acute necrotising ulcerative process involving the mucous membranes of the mouth or genitalia. The condition is most commonly seen in severely malnourished, debilitated people, especially children with poor nutrition and hygiene. There is rapid spreading throughout the mouth, including teeth, jawbone, cheek, tongue, lips and nose, eventually leading to extensive necrosis and destruction of soft tissues and bones. Also known as CANCRUM ORIS or gangrenous STOMATITIS.

nominal (ˈnomənəl) the level of measurement that simply assigns data into categories that are mutually exclusive.

nomogram (ˈnoməˌgram, ˈnoh-) a graph with several scales arranged so that a ruler laid on the graph intersects the scales at related values of the variables; the values of any two variables can be used to find the values of the others.

non-accidental injury (NAI) (ˌnonaksəˈdentʼl injəree) injury inflicted upon children or infants by those looking after them, usually the parents. The injuries are usually physical (beating, burning, biting) but the term includes the giving of poisons and dangerous drugs, sexual abuse, starvation, neglect and any other form of physical assault.

non-compliance (ˌnonkəmˈplieəns) describes the decision made by a person not to comply with a drug regimen or other treatments, even though fully understanding the rationale for such therapy.

non compos mentis (non ˈkompəs ˈmentis) [L.] not of sound mind. Applied to people whose mental state is such that they are unable to manage their own affairs.

non-experimental research design (nonəkˌsperəˈmentʼl ˌreeˈsərch dəˈzien) research design in which an investigator observes a phenomenon without manipulating the independent variable(s).

non-invasive (non inˈvaysiv, -ziv) describes any medical procedure that does not penetrate the skin or organ of the body, e.g. CT screening, or blood pressure monitoring. The term may also be used to describe non-cancerous tumours that do not metastasise.

non-maleficence (ˌnonmaˈlefəsəns) the concept in the healthcare services of the duty to avoid harm to the interests of others.

non-shivering thermogenesis (nonˈshivəring ˌthərmohˈjenəsəs) the use of brown adipose tissue by the neonate to produce heat in times of cold stress. Brown fat is stored in the mediastinum, around the nape of the neck, between the scapulae and around the kidneys and suprarenal glands.

non-specific (ˌnonspəˈsifik) 1. not due to any single known cause. 2. not directed against a particular agent, but rather having a general effect. *N. urethritis* a common, sexually transmitted disease which may be due to a variety of agents, e.g. *Chlamydia trachomatis*, which causes 40% of cases. Also called non-gonococcal URETHRITIS.

non-steroidal anti-inflammatory drugs (NSAIDs) (non,stə'royd'l ,antee'inflamətree drugz) a group of drugs with analgesic, antipyretic and anti-inflammatory activity due to their ability to inhibit the synthesis of prostaglandins. It includes aspirin, phenylbutazone, indomethacin, tolmetin, ibuprofen and related drugs.

non-union (non'yoonyən) in a fracture, failure of the two pieces of bone to unite.

nonparametric statistics (,non,-parə'metrik ,stə'tistiks) statistics that are usually used when variables are measured at the nominal or ordinal level, because they do not estimate population parameters and involve less restrictive assumptions about the underlying distribution.

noradrenaline (,naw·rə'drenələn) *see* NOREPINEPHRINE.

norepinephrine (,nawr,epee'nefrən) a hormone present in extracts of the suprarenal medulla and at synapses in the peripheral sympathetic nervous system. It causes vasoconstriction and raises both the systolic and the diastolic blood pressures.

norm (nawm) a fixed standard or value against which values are measured.

normal ('nawməl) conforming to a standard; regular or usual. *N. distribution* in statistics, a symmetrical 'bell-shaped' distribution or curve that forms in the plotting of the scores. The most probable scores are concentrated around the mean or average with progressively less probable scores occurring further from the mean. *N. flora* bacteria which normally live on body tissues and have a beneficial effect. *N. saline* isotonic solution of sodium chloride. Physiological solution.

normoblast ('nawmoh,blast) a nucleated precursor red blood cell in bone marrow. *See* ERYTHROCYTE.

normochromic (,nawmoh'krohmik) normal in colour. Applied to the blood when the haemoglobin level is within normal limits.

normocyte ('nawmoh,siet) a red blood cell that is normal in size, shape and colour.

normoglycaemia (,nawmohglie-'seemi·ə) normal blood sugar level.

normotension (,nawmoh'tenshən) normal tone, tension or pressure. Usually used in relation to blood pressure.

norovirus (,nawroh'vierəs) common cause of vomiting and diarrhoea transmitted through faecal contamination of food and water. Norovirus infections are highly contagious and are a leading cause of gastroenteritis.

North American Nursing Diagnosis Association (NANDA) (,nawth a,merikan 'nərsing ,dieəg'nohsəs ə,sohsi'ayshən) professional organisation of registered nurses, formed in 1982. The purpose of NANDA is to promote patient safety by standardising evidence-based nursing diagnoses and to enable nurses to implement interventions with predictable outcomes.

Norton score ('nawtən skaw) a pressure sore risk assessment scale devised by Norton, McLaren and Exton Smith and used primarily in the care of older people. It has five health state components, each with a 4-point descending scale. Maximum points are 20 and the minimum 5; a 'score' of 14 or below indicates that the patient is at risk of developing pressure sores and needs 1–2-hourly changes of posture and the use of pressure-relieving devices. The system requires weekly application and whenever a change occurs in the person's condition and/or circumstances of care.

nose (nohz) the organ of smell and the airway for respiration.

nosocomial (ˌnohsə'kohmieəl) pertaining to or acquired in hospital. Now most commonly called healthcare-associated infection (HAI) as many of these occur at home or elsewhere in the community. *N. disease* for the patient a new disorder, not related to the original disease, that is caused or precipitated during hospitalisation.

nosocomial infection (ˌnohsə'kohmieəl in'fekshən) an infection acquired in hospital at least 72 hours after admission; also called HEALTHCARE-ASSOCIATED INFECTION. Contact-transmitted infection is the most important and frequent mode of transmission of nosocomial infections and may be either direct or indirect. Direct contact transmitted infections involve direct body-surface-to-body-surface contact, such as occurs in patient care activities, e.g. bathing a patient. Direct contact can also occur between two patients, with one serving as the source of infectious microorganisms, the other being a susceptible host. Indirect contact transmitted infections involve contact of a susceptible host with a contaminated intermediate object, usually inanimate (*see* FOMITES), e.g. contaminated instruments, needles, dressings or gloves that are not changed between patients. Unwashed, contaminated hands may also be a source of nosocomial infection.

nosology (ˌnoh'soləjee) the classification of disease into groups by criteria, based on (expert) agreement of the boundaries of the groups, e.g. by the DELPHI TECHNIQUE.

nostril ('nostrəl) one of the anterior orifices of the nose.

notifiable ('nohtəˌfieəbəl) applied to such diseases, incidents or occurrences that must by law be reported to the health authorities. These include measles, scarlet fever, typhus fever, typhoid fever, cholera, diphtheria, tuberculosis, dysentery and various forms of food poisoning.

notifiable conduct ('nohtəˌfieəbəl 'konˌdukt) under the HEALTH PRACTITIONER REGULATION NATIONAL LAW (the National Law), any registered health practitioner who has: i) practised the practitioner's profession while intoxicated by alcohol or drugs; or ii) engaged in sexual misconduct in connection with the practice of the practitioner's profession; or iii) placed the public at risk of substantial harm in the practitioner's practice of the profession because the practitioner has an impairment that detrimentally affects or is likely to detrimentally affect the person's capacity to practise the profession; or iv) placed the public at risk of harm because the practitioner has practised the profession in a way that constitutes a significant departure from accepted professional standards.

NPF *see* NURSE PRESCRIBERS' FORMULARY.

NSAIDs *see* NON-STEROIDAL ANTI-INFLAMMATORY DRUGS.

NSU non-specific URETHRITIS.

nucha (ˈnyookə) the nape of the neck.

nuchal (nyookəl) the back of the neck. *N. cord* an abnormal but common condition in which the umbilical cord is wrapped around the neck of the fetus in utero or of the child as it is being born. It is usually possible to slip the loop or loops of cord gently over the child's head. The condition occurs in more than 25% of deliveries, more often with long cords than with short cords. *N. displacement* a complication of breech labour, when an arm is displaced behind the child's neck. *N. scanning* ultrasound performed at 11–13 weeks' gestation to measure the thickness of the skin at the back of the fetal neck as an indication of possible DOWN SYNDROME.

nuclear (ˈnyookli ɔ) pertaining to a nucleus. *N. medicine* that branch of medicine concerned with the use of radionuclides in the diagnosis and treatment of disease.

nuclear family (nyookleeə faməlee) two people and their children living together in a household without members of the extended family, such as grandparents, aunts and uncles living with them, or in the same locality.

nuclear magnetic resonance (ˈnyookli·ə magˈnetik ˈrezənəns) a phenomenon exhibited by atomic nuclei having a magnetic moment, i.e. those nuclei that behave as if they are tiny bar magnets. In the absence of a magnetic field these magnets are arranged randomly, but when a strong magnetic field is applied they align with the field. These signals can be analysed and used for chemical analysis (NMR spectroscopy) or for imaging (magnetic resonance imaging).

nuclease (ˈnyookleeˌayz) an enzyme which breaks down nucleic acids.

nucleic acids (nyooˈklee·ik, -ˈklay-ˈasəds) DEOXYRIBONUCLEIC ACID (DNA) and RIBONUCLEIC ACID (RNA), both of which are found in cell nuclei; RNA is also found in the cytoplasm. They are composed of series of nucleotides.

nucleolus (ˌnyookleeˈohləs, nyoo-ˈkleeələs) a small dense body in the cell nucleus which contains ribonucleic acid. It disappears during MITOSIS.

nucleoprotein (ˌnyookleeoh-ˈprohteen) a compound of nucleic acid and protein.

nucleotide (ˈnyookleeəˌtied) a compound formed from pentose sugar, phosphoric acid and a nitrogen-containing base (a purine or a pyrimidine).

nucleotoxic (ˌnyookleeəˈtoksik) applied to drugs, toxins, viruses and other agents that are toxic to cell nuclei.

nucleus (ˈnyookli·əs) 1. the essential part of a cell governing nutrition and reproduction, its division being essential for the formation of new cells. 2. the positively charged centre portion of an atom. 3. a group of nerve cells in the central nervous system. *Caudate n.* and *lenticular n.* part of the basal ganglia. *N. pulposus* the jellylike centre of an intervertebral disc.

null hypothesis (nul ˌhicˈpothəsəs) a research concept indicating that there is no significant relationship between an independent variable and a dependent variable, and that the observed experimental results can therefore be attributed to chance alone.

nullipara (nu'lipə·rə) a woman who has never given birth to a child.

numbers needed to treat (NNT) (numbəs needəd too treet) a measure of clinical significance in medicine and pharmacology used to communicate the effectiveness of a healthcare intervention. It refers to the average number of patients who need to be treated with a specific intervention to prevent one additional bad outcome. It is used in pharmacology to make decisions between treatment options being based on the number of subjects receiving the medication before one subject has a positive outcome.

nurse (nərs) 1. a person who is qualified in the art and science of nursing and meets certain prescribed standards of education and clinical competence and, if practising in Australia, is registered with the Nursing and Midwifery Board of Australia (NMBA) (*see also* NURSING PRACTICE). 2. to provide services that are essential to or helpful in the promotion, maintenance and restoration of health and wellbeing. 3. to nourish at the breast (*see also* BREASTFEEDING). *Enrolled n. (EN)* a second-level nurse who has undertaken an approved program leading to registration as a Division 2 nurse and provides nursing care under the direction and supervision of a registered nurse. *Endorsed Enrolled n. (EEN)* an enrolled nurse who has completed further medication endorsement. *N. consultant* an experienced nurse educated to a Master's level, with advanced skills in a clinical area, e.g. mental health, neonatology, critical care, stroke services or dermatology. The role involves considerable patient contact. The nurse consultant will be expected to promote research and evaluation in practice, demonstrate leadership skills and participate in the education and development of staff in the clinical area. *N. practitioner* a nurse with specific preparation and development to function at an advanced level who works in the primary care setting or in an acute care setting, e.g. rural or remote areas, accident and emergency, drug and alcohol services, orthopaedic clinics and minor injuries departments. Nurse practitioners can offer a nurse-led service and patients have a choice of seeing the doctor or the nurse when they attend. In Australia, only registered nurses and registered midwives who have been authorised by the NMBA to practise as nurse practitioners and midwife practitioners may use the title 'nurse practitioner' and 'midwife practitioner'. *N. prescribing* registered nurses who have undertaken a specialist qualification and demonstrate prescribing competency may prescribe, and therefore are accountable for prescribing for patients from the NURSE PRESCRIBERS' FORMULARY. *N. working in a medical practice* qualified nurse who works with a general practitioner (GP), or a group of GPs in a health centre or surgery. *Primary n.* a named nurse who is responsible for the overall coordination of the patient's care. *Registered n.* in Australia, one who has completed a Bachelor of Nursing (previously a hospital Certificate in Nursing or a Diploma in Nursing) and is eligible for registration as a Division 1 nurse and whose name is on the register held by the NMBA of the particular state or territory.

nurse-initiated medication (nərs ə'nisheeaytəd medikayshən) medication that is approved by the healthcare facility to be administered by a registered nurse or accredited enrolled nurse or midwife without a medical practitioner's authorisation. Only unscheduled S2 and S3 medications may be administered by a nurse or midwife.

Nurse Prescribers' Formulary (NPF) (ners preskriebəs formyooləree) a formulary from which nurses who are appropriately qualified may prescribe for patients.

nursing ('nərsing) the profession of performing the functions of a NURSE. *N. assessment* the systematic collection and analysis of patient data pertaining to an individual's health status, abilities and preferences for care and treatment. The first step of the nursing process leading to a clinical nursing judgement. *See* ASSESSMENT. *N. audit* a systematic procedure for assessing the quality of nursing care rendered to a specific patient population. *N. care plan* devised by a nurse and based on a nursing assessment and nursing diagnosis for an individual patient. The plan has four essential components: (a) identification of the nursing care problems; (b) an outline of the means and methods of solving these; (c) a statement of the anticipated benefit to the patient; and (d) an account of the specific actions used to achieve the goals specified. *N. diagnosis* a statement of a health problem or of a potential health problem in the patient's/client's health status that a nurse is professionally competent to treat. *N. goal* the objective that the nurse hopes to achieve through nursing interventions and activities related to the patient's health status, needs and abilities, e.g. the development of self-care skills. *N. history* a written record providing data for assessing the nursing care needs of a patient. *N. models* a conceptual framework of nursing practice based on knowledge, ideas and beliefs. A model or theory of nursing that clarifies the meaning of nursing, provides criteria for policy and gives direction to team nursing, thereby obviating conflicts in approach and giving the framework for continuity of care. It identifies the nurse's role and highlights areas of practice where research is needed. *N. practice* the performance or compensation of any act in the observation, care and counsel of the ill, injured or infirm, or in the maintenance of health or prevention of illness of others, or in the supervision and teaching of other personnel, or in the administration of medications and treatments as prescribed by a doctor or dentist. This requires substantial specialised judgement and skill and is based on knowledge and application of the principles of biological, physical and social sciences. *N. process* a systematic approach to nursing care derived from many occupational groups. The system itself is not specific to nursing. It has been used as a framework for nursing care by American nurses and subsequently its principles have been adapted to the Australian culture and healthcare system by Australian nurses. It is an organised approach to the identification of a patient's nursing care problems and the use of nursing actions that effectively alleviate, minimise or prevent the problems being presented or from developing. *N. records* accurate record-keeping and careful documentation are essential to the delivery of nursing practice to a patient or client, whatever the setting, e.g. in general practice settings, the hospital setting, in aged care facilities or in the person's own home. The record provides an account of care planned or given to an individual person by a registered nurse or other caregivers under the direction of a registered nurse. Records should be made in writing with a black pen or in some other permanent form, e.g. directly into a computer. *Theories of n.* proposed explanations of the way in which nursing achieves its aims. They require a definition of the nurse's perception of the person's needs, the nurse's own role and the context in which nursing care is performed. An understanding of the relationship of these variables enables nursing care to be planned in such a way that the outcome may be predicted and set goals achieved.

Nursing and Midwifery Board of Australia (NMBA) (nərsing and midwifəree bawd ov ostrayleeə) this is a National Board that has established state and territory boards to support its work. The National Board sets policy and professional standards, while the state and territory boards will continue to make individual notification and registration decisions affecting individual nurses and midwives.

nutation (nyoo'tayshən) uncontrollable nodding of the head.

nutrient ('nyootri·ənt) food; any substance that nourishes. The six classes of nutrients are fats, carbohydrates, proteins, vitamins, minerals and water.

nutrition (nyoo'trishən) 1. the sum of the processes involved in taking in nutriments and assimilating and using them. 2. nutriment. Nutrition is particularly concerned with those properties of food that build sound bodies and promote health. Good nutrition means a balanced diet containing adequate amounts of the essential nutritional elements that the body must have to function normally. The essential ingredients of a balanced diet are proteins, vitamins, minerals, fats and carbohydrates. The body can manufacture sugars from fats and fats from sugars and proteins, depending on the need, but it cannot manufacture proteins from sugars and fats. *Enteral n.* the provision of nutrients in fluid form to the alimentary tract by mouth, nasogastric tube or via an opening into the tract such as through a GASTROSTOMY. *N. disease* one that is due to the continued absence of a necessary food factor. *Parenteral n.* a technique for meeting a person's nutritional needs by means of intravenous feedings; sometimes called HYPERALIMENTATION.

nutritional status (nyoo'trishən'l ˌstaytəs, ˌstat-) the condition of the body as a result of its receiving and using nutrients. Nutritional status may also be affected by biochemical individuality as well as environmental factors.

nyctalopia (ˌniktə'lohpi·ə) NIGHT BLINDNESS.

nymphomania (ˌnimfə'mayni·ə) excessive sexual desire in a woman.

nystagmus (ni'stagməs) an involuntary, rapid movement of the eyeball. It may be hereditary or result from disease of the semicircular canals or of the central nervous system. It can occur from visual defect or be associated with other muscle spasms.

Oo

O symbol for *oxygen*.

OAE *see* OTOACOUSTIC EMISSION.

obese (oh'bees) very overweight; corpulent.

obesity (oh'beesətee) corpulent; excessive development of fat throughout the body which impairs health and is the most common nutritional disorder worldwide. A body mass index (BMI) of over 30 and up to 39.9 BMI. Extreme or severe obesity defines someone with greater than 40 BMI. Waist circumference, waist–height ratio and waist–hip ratio are also used as indicators of the amount of fat in the abdomen. Obesity is linked to many conditions, such as cardiovascular disease, hypertension, sleep apnoea, Type 2 diabetes mellitus, stroke, arthritis and some cancers. *See* BODY MASS INDEX.

objective (əb'jektiv) 1. in microscopy, the lens nearest the object being looked at. 2. a purpose; a desired end result. 3. concerning matters outside oneself. *O. signs* signs that the observer notes, as distinct from symptoms of which the patient complains (subjective).

oblique (ə'bleek) slanting. *O. muscles* 1. a pair of muscles, the inferior and the superior, which turn the eye upwards and downwards, and inwards and outwards. 2. muscles found in the wall of the abdomen.

observation (obsərvayshən) the act or faculty of closely noticing and paying attention to someone or something. In nursing this is an active process whereby the nurse uses the senses for the purpose of collecting patient data for developing a nursing diagnosis or care plan.

observational study (obsərvayshənəl studee) a research methodology in which the researcher is a non-participant observer and records behaviour without influencing it.

obsession (əb'seshən) an idea which persistently recurs to an individual, although resisted and regarded as being senseless. A compulsive thought. *See* COMPULSION.

obsessive compulsive disorder (OCD) (obsesiv kompulsiv disawdə) a mental health condition characterised by obsessional thoughts and/or ideas associated often with compulsive acts which may interfere with daily living.

obstetrician (ˌobstə'trishən) one who is trained and specialises in OBSTETRICS.

obstetrics (ob'stetriks) the branch of medicine and surgery dealing with pregnancy, labour and the PUERPERIUM.

obstipation (obstə'payshən) intractable constipation.

obstruction (əb'strukshən) the act of blocking or clogging; the state of being clogged. *Intestinal o.* any hindrance to the passage of faeces.

obturator ('obtyəˌraytə) that which closes an opening. *O. foramen* the large hole in the hip bone, closed by fascia and muscle.

obtusion (ob'tyoozhən) weakening or blunting of normal sensations, a condition produced by certain diseases.

occipital (ok'sipət'l) relating to the occiput. *O. bone* the bone forming the back and part of the base of the skull.

occipitoanterior (ok,sipətoh·an'tiə·ri·ə) referring to the position of the fetal occiput when it is to the front of the maternal pelvis as it comes through the birth canal. The opposite of occipitoposterior.

occipitoposterior (ok,sipətoh·-po'stiə·ri·ə) referring to the position of the fetal occiput when it is to the back of the maternal pelvis as it comes through the birth canal. The opposite of occipitoanterior.

occiput ('oksi,puht) the back of the head.

occlusion (ə'kloozhən) closure, applied particularly to alignment of the teeth in the jaws. *Coronary o.* obstruction of the lumen of a coronary artery. *O. of the pupil* may be congenital or occur in IRIDOCYCLITIS or after injury. *Retinal artery o.* blockage of one of the small arteries that carry blood to the retina. *Retinal vein o.* blockage of one of the small veins that take blood away from the retina.

occult ('okult) hidden, concealed. *O. blood* blood excreted in the stools in such a small quantity as to require chemical tests to detect it.

occupational (okyə'payshənəl) relating to work and working conditions. *O. disease* one likely to occur among workers in certain trades. An industrial disease. *O. health nurse* provides immediate care to ill or injured workers in the workplace and follows up the return to work of the sick and injured. Develops accident prevention programs and promotes good health among the work force. Also has an educational role and a health and safety obligation. *O. health nursing* the branch of nursing that is concerned with the health of people in the workplace. *O. medicine* the branch of medicine concerned with people at work and the effects of work on health. Essentially a branch of preventative or environmental medicine. It is concerned with ensuring that health and safety in the workplace is maintained and legislation complied with. *O. therapist* identifies goals to help patients and service users improve independence by using techniques, changing the environment and equipment. *O. therapy* treatment by provision of support to people whose health problems limit their ability to do activities of daily living.

ocular ('okyələ) relating to the eye. *O. myopathy* a rare gradual bilateral loss of mobility of the eyes. *O. myositis* inflammation of the orbital muscles.

oculogyric (,okyəloh'jierik) causing movements of the eyeballs. *O. crisis* involuntary, violent movements of the eye, usually upwards.

oculomotor (,okyəloh'mohtə) relating to movements of the eye. *O. nerves* the third pair of cranial nerves, which control the eye muscles.

odontoid (oh'dontoyd) resembling a tooth. *O. process* a tooth-like projection from the axis vertebra upon which the head rotates.

odontoma (,odon'tohmə) a tumour of tooth structures.

oedema (ə'deemə) an excessive amount of fluid in the body tissues. If the finger is pressed on an affected part, the surface pits and slowly regains its original contour. *Angio-o.* characterised by the sudden appearance of urticaria which may involve the skin of the face, hands, feet or genitalia, and with swelling of the mucosal membrane of mouth and throat, oedema of the glottis may be fatal. The swelling may be due to an allergic reaction to food (most common), moulds, pollens or other allergens, infection or a reaction to an insect bite or sting. In many cases no identifiable cause can be found. *Cardiac o.* a manifestation of congestive heart failure due to increased venous and capillary pressures and often associated with renal sodium retention. *Dependent o.* oedema affecting most severely the lowermost parts of the body. *Famine o.* that due to protein deficiency. *Lymph o.* that due to blockage of the lymph vessels. *O. neonatorum* a disease of preterm and feeble infants resembling sclerema, marked by spreading oedema with cold, livid skin. *Pitting o.* oedema in which pressure leaves a persistent depression in the tissues. *Pulmonary o.* diffuse extravascular accumulation of fluid in the tissues and air spaces of the lung due to changes in hydrostatic forces in the capillaries or to increased capillary permeability.

Oedipus complex (ˈeedəpəs ˈkompleks) the suppressed sexual desire of a son for his mother, with hostility towards his father. It is a normal stage in the early development of the child but may become fixed if the child cannot solve the conflict during his early years or during adolescence. Named after a mythical Greek hero.

oesophageal (əˌsofəˈjeeəl) pertaining to the oesophagus. *O. atresia* a congenital abnormality in which the oesophagus is not continuous between the pharynx and the stomach. May be associated with a fistula into the trachea. *O. varices* varicose veins of the lower oesophagus secondary to portal hypertension.

oesophagitis (əˌsofəˈjietəs) inflammation of the oesophagus. *Reflux o.* caused by regurgitation of acid stomach contents through the cardiac sphincter.

oesophagojejunostomy (əˌsofəgohˌ-jejəˈnostəmee) an operation to create an anastomosis of the JEJUNUM with the oesophagus after a total gastrectomy.

oesophagus (əˈsofəgəs) the canal that extends from the pharynx to the stomach. It is about 23 cm long.

oestradiol (ˌeestrəˈdieol) the chief naturally occurring female sex hormone produced by the ovary. Prepared synthetically, it is used to treat menopausal conditions and AMENORRHOEA.

oestrogen (ˈeestrəjən, -trəˌjen) one of several steroid hormones, including oestradiol, all of which have similar functions. Although they are largely produced in the ovary, they can also be extracted from the placenta, the adrenal cortex and the testis. They control female sexual development.

ointment (ˈoyntmənt) an external application with a greasy base in which the remedy is incorporated.

olecranon (ohˈlekrəˌnon, ˌohliˈkraynən) the curved process of the ulna which forms the point of the elbow.

oleum (ˈohli·əm) [L.] oil.

olfactory (olˈfaktə·ree) relating to the sense of smell. *O. nerves* the first pair of cranial nerves; those of smell.

oligohydramnios (ˌoləgoh·hieˈdram-neeəs) a deficiency in the amount of AMNIOTIC fluid.

oligomenorrhoea (ˌoləgohˌmenəˈreeə) 1. a diminished flow at the menstrual period. 2. infrequent occurrence of menstruation.

oligospermia (ˌoləgohˈspərmi·ə) a diminished output of spermatozoa.

oliguria (ˌoləˈgyoo·ri·ə) a deficient secretion of urine.

olivary (ˈolivə·ree) shaped like an olive. *O. body* a mass of grey matter situated behind the anterior pyramid of the MEDULLA OBLONGATA.

ombudsman (ˈombədz·mən) a person appointed to receive complaints about unfair administration. The ombudsman investigates complaints about failures in the health service not resolved at a local level, and issues regular reports, but is not able to pass judgement on clinical matters.

omentectomy (ˌohmenˈtektəmee) the surgical removal of all or part of the OMENTUM.

omentopexy (ohˈmentəˌpeksee) the surgical fixation of the OMENTUM to some other tissue, usually the abdominal wall. *Cardio o.* attachment of the omentum to the heart to establish a collateral circulation following coronary occlusion.

omentum (ohˈmentəm) a fold of peritoneum joining the stomach to other abdominal organs. *Greater o.* the fold reflected from the greater curvature of the stomach and lying in front of the intestines. *Lesser o.* the fold reflected from the lesser curvature and attaching the stomach to the undersurface of the liver.

omnivorous (omˈnivərəs) eating food of both plant and animal origin.

omphalitis (ˌomfəˈlietəs) inflammation of the umbilicus.

omphalocele (ˈomfəlohˌseel) an umbilical hernia.

Onchocerca (ˈongkohˌsərkə) a genus of filarial worms found in tropical parts of Africa and America, which may give rise to skin and subcutaneous lesions and attack the eye.

onchocerciasis (ˌongkohsərˈkieəsəs) a tropical skin disease caused by infestation with *Onchocerca*.

oncogenesis (ˌongkohˈjenəsəs) the causation and formation of tumours.

oncogenic (ˌongkohˈjenik) giving rise to tumour formation.

oncology (ongˈkoləjee) the scientific study of tumours.

onychia (oˈniki·ə) inflammation of the matrix of a nail with suppuration which may cause the nail to fall off.

onychogryphosis (ˌoneekohgriˈfohsəs) enlargement of the nails with excessive ridging and curvature, most commonly affecting the older person.

onycholysis (ˌoneeˈkoləsəs) loosening or separation of a nail from its bed.

onychomycosis (ˌoneekohmieˈkohsəs) infection of the nails by a fungus.

oocyte (ˈoh·əˌsiet) the immature egg cell or ovum in the ovary.

oogenesis (ˌoh·əˈjenəsəs) the development and production of the ovum.

oophorectomy (ˌoh·əfəˈrektəmee) excision of an ovary; ovariectomy.

oophorocystectomy (ohˌofə·rohsəˈstektəmee) surgical removal of an ovarian cyst.

oophoron (ohˈofə·ron) an ovary.

oophoropexy (ohˈofə·rohˌpeksee) the surgical fixation of a displaced ovary to the pelvic wall.

oophorosalpingectomy (ohˌofə·rohˌsalpinˈjektəmee) removal of an ovary and its associated uterine tube.

opacity (ohˈpasitee) cloudiness, lack of transparency. Opacities occur in the lens of an eye when a cataract is forming. They also occur in the vitreous humour and appear as floating objects.

open-ended items (ˌohpən ˈendəd ietəmz) questions that the respondent may answer in their own words.

operant conditioning (ˈopə·rənt kənˈdishəning) a form of behaviour therapy in which a reward is given when the subject performs the action required. The reward serves to encourage repetition of the action.

operation (ˌopəˈrayshən) a surgical procedure in which instruments or hands are used by the operator on a part or organ of the body.

operational definition (ˌopəˈrayshənəl ˈdefiˈnishən) the measurements used to observe or measure a variable; delineates the procedures or operations required to measure a concept.

ophthalmia (ofˈthalmi·ə) severe inflammation of the eye or of the conjunctiva or deeper structures of the eye. Aso known as ophthalmitis. *O. neonatorum* any hyperacute purulent conjunctivitis which may be caused by the gonococcus, *Escherichia coli*, staphylococci or *Chlamydia trachomatis*, occurring within the first 28 days of life. *Sympathetic o.* granulomatous inflammation of the uveal tract of the uninjured eye following a wound involving the uveal tract of the other eye, resulting in bilateral granulomatous inflammation of the entire uveal tract. Also called sympathetic UVEITIS.

ophthalmologist (ˌofthalˈmoləjəst) a specialist in diseases of the eye.

ophthalmology (ˌofthalˈmoləjee) the study of the eye and its diseases.

ophthalmoscope (ofˈthalməˌskohp) an instrument fitted with a light and lenses by which the interior of the eye can be illuminated and examined.

ophthalmotomy (ˌofthalˈmotəmee) incision of the eyeball.

opiate (ˈohpeeət, ˈohpeeˌayt) any medicine containing opium.

opisthotonos (ˌohpəsˈthotənəs) a muscle spasm causing the back to be arched and the head retracted, with great rigidity of the muscles of the neck and back. This condition may be present in acute cases of meningitis, tetanus and strychnine poisoning.

opium (ˈohpi·əm) a drug derived from dried poppy juice and used as a narcotic. It produces deep sleep, slows the pulse and respiration, contracts the pupils and checks all secretions of the body except sweat. It is a highly addictive drug. Opium derivatives include acodeine, morphine and heroin.

opponens (oˈpohnənz) [L.] opposing. A term applied to certain muscles controlling the movements of the fingers. *O. pollicis* a muscle that adducts the thumb so that it and the little finger can be brought together.

opportunistic (ˌopətyooˈnistik) 1. taking advantage of immediate opportunities. 2. denoting a microorganism that does not ordinarily cause disease but becomes pathogenic under certain circumstances. 3. denoting a disease or infection caused by such an opportunistic pathogen.

opsonic index (opˌsonik ˈindeks) a measurement of the bactericidal power of the phagocytes in the blood of an individual.

opsonin (ˈopsənən) an antibody, present in the blood, which renders bacteria more easily destroyed by the phagocytes. Each kind of bacterium has its specific opsonin.

optic (ˈoptik) relating to vision. *O. atrophy* degeneration of the optic

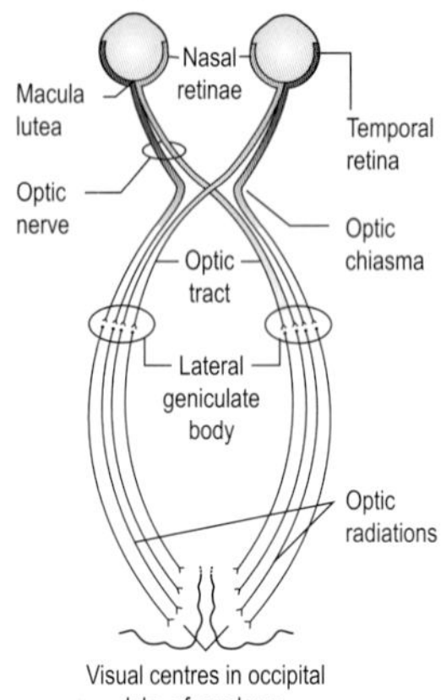

Optic chiasma.

nerve. *O. chiasma* the crossing of the fibres of the optic nerves at the base of the brain (*see* figure). *O. disc* the point where the optic nerve enters the eyeball. *O. foramen* the opening in the posterior part of the orbit through which pass the optic nerve and the ophthalmic artery. *O. nerve* a bundle of nerve fibres running from the optic chiasma in the brain to the optic disc on the eyeball.

optical (ˈoptikəl) pertaining to sight. *O. density* the refractive power of the transparent tissues through which light rays pass, changing the direction of the ray.

optician (opˈtishən) a professional trained in the detection of refractive errors and the dispensing of appropriate spectacles or contact lenses.

optimum (ˈoptəməm) the best and most favourable.

optometry (opˈtomətree) the assessing and measuring of visual acuity for the fitting of glasses or contact lenses to correct visual defects.

ora (ˈawra) [L.] a margin. *O. serrata* the jagged edge of the retina.

oral (ˈorəl) 1. pertaining to the mouth; taken through or applied in the mouth, as an oral medication or oral hygiene. 2. denoting that aspect of the teeth which faces the oral cavity or tongue. *O. contraceptive pill* a drug preparation taken orally containing one or more synthetic female hormones taken as part of the monthly cycle to prevent pregnancy. *O. hairy leucoplakia* an unusual form of leucoplakia that is seen only in human immunodeficiency virus (HIV) infected persons. It consists of fuzzy (hairy) patches on the tongue and, less frequently, elsewhere in the mouth. Hairy leucoplakia may be one of the first signs of HIV infection. *See* LEUCOPLAKIA. *O. rehydration therapy (ORT) see* REHYDRATION THERAPY. *O. syringe* a calibrated device with a plunger that is used to administer small doses of oral liquid medications to young children. The dose is drawn up into the syringe via the plunger and then squirted onto the inside of the cheek.

orbit (ˈawbət) 1. the bony cavity containing the eyeball. 2. the path of an object moving around another object.

orchidectomy (ˌawkəˈdektəmee) excision of a testicle. *Bilateral o.* the operation of castration.

orchidopexy (ˌawkədohˈpeksee) an operation to free an undescended testicle and place it in the scrotum.

orchiepididymitis (ˌawkeeˌepee-didəˈmietəs) inflammation of a testicle and its epididymis.

orchitis (aw'kietəs) inflammation of a testicle.

ordinal scale (awdənəl skayl) a measurement scale in which the data are arranged in order of size or magnitude but where there is no standard measure of difference between the data given.

orf (awf) a virus infection transmitted from sheep to humans. It may give rise to a boil-like lesion on the hands of meat handlers.

organ ('awgən) a part of the body designed to perform a particular function. *O. of Corti* a spiral structure situated in the inner ear. It contains the basilar membrane that converts sound waves into nerve impulses that are then transmitted to the brain via the cochlear nerve.

organelle (ˌawgə'nel) a structure within a cell that has specialised functions, e.g. nucleus, endoplasmic reticulum, mitochondrion, etc.

organic (aw'ganik) 1. pertaining to the organs. 2. pertaining to chemicals containing carbon. *O. disease* disease of an organ, accompanied by structural changes.

organism ('awgəˌnizəm) an individual living being, animal or vegetable.

orgasm ('awgazəm) the climax of sexual excitement.

orientation (ˌawreeən'tayshən) a sense of direction. 1. the ability of a person to estimate position in regard to time, place and persons. 2. the imparting of relevant information at the onset of a course or conference so that its content and objects may be understood. *Reality o.* the way in which older people who may be confused or mentally ill are assisted in keeping in touch with the world around them on a day-to-day basis. This may be achieved in a variety of ways, with large clocks, calendar boards, signs on doors and daily newspapers.

orifice ('o·rəfəs) any opening in the body.

origin ('o·rəjən) in anatomy: 1. the point of attachment of a muscle. 2. the point at which a nerve or a blood vessel branches from the main stem.

ornithosis (ˌawnə'thohsəs) a viral disease of birds, usually pigeons, that may be transmitted to humans in a form resembling BRONCHOPNEUMONIA.

orogenital (ˌaw·roh'jenət'l) pertaining to the mouth and external genitalia.

oropharynx (ˌaw·roh'faringks) the lower portion of the pharynx behind the mouth and above the oesophagus and larynx.

orphan (awfən) a child whose parents are dead. *O. drugs* those that have been found to be useful in the treatment of rare diseases but which are not commercially produced usually because of high costs involved in manufacture and minimal demand. *O. viruses* those that have been isolated in the laboratory but which do not appear to be associated with any particular disease.

orthodontics (ˌawthoh'dontiks) dentistry that deals with the prevention and correction of malocclusion and irregularities of the teeth.

orthodox sleep ('awthohˌdoks sleep) *see* SLEEP.

Orthomyxovirus ('awthohˌmiks-ohˌvierəs) RNA viruses belonging to the family of Orthomyxoviridae which cause influenza in humans and other mammals, e.g. birds and swine. *See* AVIAN INFLUENZA and SWINE INFLUENZA. These viruses originated in aquatic birds and crossed the species barrier (*see* zoonosis) about 10,000 years ago to infect humans.

orthopaedics (ˌawthəˈpeediks) the science dealing with deformities, injuries and diseases of the bones and joints.

orthopnoea (ˌawthopˈneeə) difficulty in breathing unless in an upright position, e.g. sitting up in bed.

orthoptics (awˈthoptiks) the practice of treating by non-surgical methods (usually eye exercises) abnormalities of vision such as STRABISMUS (squint).

orthosis (awˈthosəs) a supportive appliance that can be applied to or around the body in the care/treatment of physical impairment or disability.

orthostatic (ˌawthohˈstatik) pertaining to or caused by standing erect. *O. albuminuria see* ALBUMINURIA. *O. hypotension* low blood pressure occurring when a person stands up. Postural hypotension.

orthotic (awˈthotik) serving to protect or to restore or improve function.

orthotics (awˈthotiks) the use or application of an ORTHOSIS.

orthotist (ˈawthəˌtist) a person skilled in orthotics and practising its application in individual cases.

Ortolani's sign (ˌawtohˈlahneez sien) *Marino Ortolani, Italian orthopaedic surgeon, 1904–1983.* A test performed soon after birth to detect possible congenital dislocation of the hip. A 'click' is felt on reversing the movements of abduction and rotation of the hip while the child is lying with knees flexed.

os (ohs) [L.] 1. (*pl.* ora) any body orifice. 2. (*pl.* ora) the mouth. 3. (*pl.* ossa) a bone.

oscillation (ˌosəˈlayshən) 1. a backwards and forwards motion. 2. vibration.

oscilloscope (əˈsiləˌskohp) an apparatus using a cathode-ray tube to depict visibly data fed into it electronically, e.g. the way in which the heart is performing.

Osgood-Schlatter disease (ˈozgood ˈschlatə ˈdiˌzeez) *Robert Osgood, American orthopaedic surgeon 1873–1956; Carl Schlatter, Swiss physician 1864–1934.* Pain, swelling and tenderness in the knee in adolescents and young adults due to damage to the bone during growth spurt.

Osler's nodes (ˈohsləz nohdz) *Sir William Osler, Canadian physician, 1849–1919.* Small painful swellings which occur in or beneath the skin, especially of the extremities in subacute bacterial ENDOCARDITIS, caused by minute emboli. They usually disappear in 1–3 days.

osmolality (ˌozmohˈlalətee) the osmotic pressure of a solution expressed in osmoles or milliosmoles per kilogram of water.

osmolarity (ˌozmohˈlarətee) the osmotic pressure of a solution expressed in osmoles or milliosmoles per kilogram of the solution.

osmoreceptor (ˌozmohrəˈseptə) one of a group of specialised nerve cells which monitor the osmotic pressure of the blood and the extracellular fluid. Impulses from these receptors are relayed to the HYPOTHALAMUS.

osmosis (ozˈmohsəs, os-) the passage of fluid from a low concentration solution to one of a higher concentration through a semipermeable membrane.

osmotic (ozˈmotik) pertaining to osmosis. *O. pressure* the pressure exerted by large molecules in the blood, e.g. albumin and globulin proteins, which draws fluid into the bloodstream from the surrounding tissues. *O. diuretics* diuretics, e.g. mannitol, given intravenously to reduce elevated pressure in cerebral oedema or glaucoma, or to produce a diuresis in drug overdose.

osseous (ˈosi·əs) bony.

ossicle (ˈosikəl) a small bone. *Auditory o.* one of the three bones in the middle ear: the MALLEUS, INCUS and STAPES.

ossification (ˌosəfəˈkayshən) the process by which bone is developed; osteogenesis.

ostealgia (ˌostˈalji·ə) pain in a bone.

osteitis (ˌosteeˈietəs) inflammation of bone. *O. deformans see* Paget's disease. *O. fibrosa cystica* or *parathyroid o.* defects of ossification with fibrous tissue production leading to weakening and deformity. It affects children chiefly, and is associated with parathyroid tumour, removal of which checks it.

osteoarthritis (ˌosteeoh·ahˈthrietəs) often described as degenerative joint disease. *See* ARTHRITIS.

osteoarthrotomy (ˌosteeoh·ahˈ-throtəmee) surgical excision of the jointed end of a bone.

osteoblast (ˈosteeohˌblast) a cell that develops into an osteocyte and turns into bone.

osteochondritis (ˌosteeohkonˈdrie-təs) inflammation of bone and cartilage, particularly a degenerative disease of an EPIPHYSIS, causing pain and deformity. *O. of the tarsal scaphoid bone* Köhler's disease. *O. of the tibial tuberosity* Osgood–Schlatter disease.

osteochondroma (ˌosteeohkon-ˈdrohmə) a tumour consisting of both bone and cartilage.

osteoclasis (ˌosteeˈokləsəs) 1. the surgical fracture of bones to correct a deformity such as bowleg. 2. the restructuring of bone by osteoclasts during growth or the repair of damaged bone.

osteoclast (ˈosteeohˌklast) 1. a large cell that breaks down and absorbs bone and callus. 2. an instrument designed for surgical fracture of bone.

osteocyte (ˈosteeohˌsiet) a bone cell.

osteodystrophy (ˌosteeohˈdistrəfee) a metabolic disease of bone.

osteogenesis (ˌosteeohˈjenəsəs) the formation of bone. *O. imperfecta* a congenital disorder of the bones, which are very brittle and fracture easily. Fragilitas ossium.

osteoma (ˌosteeˈohmə) a benign tumour arising from bone.

osteomalacia (ˌosteeohməˈlayshi·ə) a disease characterised by painful softening of bones. Due to vitamin D deficiency.

osteomyelitis (ˌosteeohˌmieəˈlietəs) inflammation of bone, localised or generalised, due to a pyogenic infection. It may result in bone destruction, stiffening of joints and, in extreme cases occurring before the end of the growth period, in the shortening of a limb if the growth centre is destroyed. Acute osteomyelitis is caused by bacteria that enter the body through a wound, spread from an infection near the bone or come from a skin or throat infection. The infection usually affects the long bones of the arms and legs and causes acute pain and fever. It occurs most often in children and adolescents, particularly boys.

osteopath (ˈosteeohˌpath) one who practises OSTEOPATHY.

osteopathy (ˌosteeˈopəthee) a system of diagnosis and treatment of disease which involves massage, palpation and manipulation. Osteopathic treatment is aimed at freeing and loosening joints and re-establishing proper relationships of the spinal column, its component bones with the pelvis, and limb bones on the basis that many diseases are associated with disorders of the musculoskeletal system.

osteopenia (ˌosteeoh'peeni·ə) a condition where bone density is lower than normal but not low enough to be classified as OSTEOPOROSIS. Usually occurs when the rate of bone lysis exceeds the rate of bone matrix synthesis.

osteoperiostitis (ˌosteeohˌpereeoh-'stietəs) inflammation of bone and PERIOSTEUM.

osteopetrosis (ˌosteeohpə'trohsəs) (Albers–Schönberg disease). A rare congenital disease in which the bones become abnormally dense.

osteophyte ('osteeohˌfiet) a small outgrowth of bone, usually in a joint damaged by osteoarthritis.

osteoporosis (ˌosteeohpaw'rohsəs) a loss of bone density which may be idiopathic or secondary to other conditions. The disorder leads to thinning of the skeleton with inadequate calcium absorption into the bone and excessive bone reabsorption. The principal causes are lack of physical activity, lack of oestrogens or androgens and nutritional deficiency. Osteoporosis is associated with ageing in both men and women. Symptoms include pathological fractures and collapse of the vertebrae without compression of the spinal cord. Management involves minimising bone loss with vitamin D, dietary calcium and regular sustained exercise to build and maintain bone strength. Long-term hormone replacement therapy can prevent osteoporosis in postmenopausal women.

osteosarcoma (ˌosteeohsah'kohmə) an osteogenic sarcoma; a malignant bone tumour.

osteosclerosis (ˌosteeohsklə'rohsəs) an increase in density and a hardening of bone. *O. congenita* ACHONDROPLASIA. *O. fragilis* osteopetrosis.

osteotomy (ˌostee'otəmee) the cutting into or through a bone, sometimes performed to correct deformity. *O. of the hip* a method of treating osteoarthritis by cutting the bone and altering the line of weight-bearing.

ostium ('osti·əm) an opening or entrance. *Abdominal o.* the opening at the end of the uterine tube into the peritoneal cavity.

OTC drugs (OTC drugz) *see* OVER-THE-COUNTER DRUGS.

otoacoustic emission (OAE) (ˌohtohˌə'koostik ˌə'mishən) a computer linked hearing test used for screening infants in the first few weeks of life to ascertain hearing levels.

otic ('ohtik) relating to the ear.

otitis (oh'tietəs) inflammation of the ear. *Aviation o.* a symptom complex resulting from fluctuations between atmospheric pressure and air pressure in the middle ear; also called barotitis media. *Furuncular o.* the formation of FURUNCLES in the external ear. *O. externa* inflammation of the external ear. *O. interna*, *o. labyrinthica* LABYRINTHITIS. *O. media* inflammation of the middle ear, occurring most often in infants and young children and classified as serous, secretory and suppurative.

otolith ('otohˌlith) 1. a calculus in the middle ear. 2. one of a number of small calcareous concretions of the inner ear, at the base of the semicircular canals.

otomycosis (ˌohtohmie'kohsəs) a fungal infection of the auditory canal.

otorrhoea (ˌohtə'reeə) discharge from the ear, especially of pus.

otosclerosis (ˌohtohsklə'rohsəs) the formation of spongy bone in the labyrinth of the ear, causing the auditory ossicles to become fixed and less able to pass on vibrations when sound enters the ear. The cause of otosclerosis is still unknown. It may be hereditary or perhaps related to vitamin deficiency or OTITIS MEDIA. An early symptom is ringing in the ears with a progressive loss of hearing—conductive deafness.

otoscope ('ohtohˌskohp) an auriscope; an instrument for examining the ear.

ototoxic (ˌohtoh'toksik) anything that has a deleterious effect on the eighth cranial nerve or on the organs of hearing.

outbreak ('owtˌbrayk) an epidemic of an infectious disease limited to a localised increase in the incidence of the disease, e.g. in a village, town or institution. *See* EPIDEMIC.

outcome ('owtˌcum) a consequence or objective for a healthcare intervention, e.g. a personal goal. The implications are that the outcome is (a) measurable and (b) can be expected as a result of the planned intervention. *O. indicator* measurement of the success of a clinical treatment/intervention in terms of the impact on the health of the individual.

outlet ('owtlet) a means or route of exit or egress. *Pelvic o.* the inferior opening of the pelvis, literally that bounded by the ischial spines, lower border of the symphysis pubis and the sacrococcygeal joint.

out-of-body experience (owt ov bodee ˌek'spiereeənts) a sensation of leaving one's body and travelling through tunnels and lights onto another plane of experience. The condition has been attributed to anoxia of the brain following anaesthesia or severe illness.

outpatient ('owtˌpayshənt) a patient who has a medical consultation or receives treatment at a hospital but who does not require to stay overnight in a hospital bed.

output ('owtˌpuht) the yield or total of something produced by a system. *Cardiac o.* the effective volume of blood expelled by either ventricle of the heart per unit of time (usually volume per minute); it is equal to the stroke output multiplied by the number of beats per the time unit used in the computation. *Fluid o.* the amount of urine passed, usually measured in comparison to oral fluid intake.

outreach ('owtˌreech) healthcare services provided in an alternative setting, such as within a community setting, e.g. a specialised clinic held in a general practitioner's surgery or other public buildings enabling patients and/or clients to access care more conveniently and avoid long or difficult journeys.

ovarian (oh'vair·ri·ən) relating to an ovary. *O. cyst* a tumour of the ovary containing fluid.

ovariectomy (ˌohvə·ri'ektəmee) OOPHORECTOMY; excision of an ovary.

ovariotomy (ohˌvair·ree'otəmee) 1. surgical removal of an ovary. 2. excision of an ovarian tumour.

ovary ('ohvə·ree) one of a pair of glandular organs in the female pelvis. They produce ova which pass through the uterine tubes into the uterus, and steroid hormones which control the menstrual cycle.

over-the-counter drugs (ohvə thə kowntə drugz) abbreviated OTC drugs. Drugs that can be purchased from a pharmacy without a prescription from a doctor. The list of derestricted drugs available to the public is growing and includes corticosteroid ointments, antihistamines, aciclovir, ibuprofen and nicotine patches.

overbite (ˈohvəˌbiet) an overlapping of the lower teeth by the upper teeth.

overcompensation (ˌohvaˌkompən-ˈsayshən) a mental mechanism by which people try to assert themselves by aggressive behaviour or by talking or acting 'big' to compensate for a feeling of inadequacy.

overuse injury (ˈohvəˌyoos injəree) injury due to the repetitive movement of a joint or part of the body. *See* REPETITIVE STRAIN INJURY.

oviduct (ˈohviˌdukt, ˈovi-) a uterine tube.

ovulation (ˌovyəˈlayshən, ˌoh-) the process of rupture of the mature Graafian follicle when the ovum is shed from the ovary.

ovum (ˈohvəm) [L.] an egg. The reproductive cell of the female.

oxidisation (ˌoksədieˈzayshən) oxidation. The process by which combustion occurs and breaking up of matter takes place, e.g. oxidisation of carbohydrates gives carbon dioxide and water: $C_6H_{12}O_6 + 6O_2 = 6CO_2 + 6H_2O$. The opposite of reduction.

oximeter (okˈsimətə) a photoelectric cell used to determine the oxygen saturation of blood. *Ear o.* one attached to the ear by which the oxygen content of blood flowing through the ear can be measured.

oxygen (ˈoksəjən) *symbol* O. A colourless, odourless gas constituting one-fifth of the atmosphere. It is stored in cylinders at high pressure or as liquid oxygen. It is used medicinally to enrich the air when either respiration or circulation is impaired. *O. deficit* a physiological state that exists in cells during episodes of temporary oxygen shortage. *O. mask* a device used to administer supplemental oxygen. *O. saturation* the amount of oxygen bound to haemoglobin in the blood. *O. tent* a large plastic canopy that encloses the patient in a controlled environment; used for oxygen therapy, humidity therapy or aerosol therapy. Not widely used now, but still used for children with severe breathing difficulties. *O. therapy* supplementary oxygen administered for the purpose of relieving HYPOXAEMIA and preventing damage to the tissue cells as a result of oxygen lack. *O. toxicity* a condition of oxygen overdosage that can result in tissue damage, e.g. retinopathy in the neonate or bronchopulmonary dysplasia. Can also decrease the CO_2 drive to breathe. *O. transport* the mechanism by which oxygen is absorbed in the lungs by haemoglobin in circulating deoxygenated blood and carried to peripheral tissues (*see* figure, p. 351).

oxygenation (ˌoksəjəˈnayshən) saturation with oxygen; a process which occurs in the lungs to the haemoglobin of blood, which is saturated with oxygen to form OXYHAEMOGLOBIN.

oxygenator (ˈoksəjəˌnaytə) a machine through which the blood is passed to oxygenate it during open heart surgery.

oxyhaemoglobin (ˌokseeˌheemə-ˈglohbən) haemoglobin that has been oxygenated, as in arterial blood.

oxyntic (okˈsintik) acid forming. *O. cell* a parietal cell of the gastric

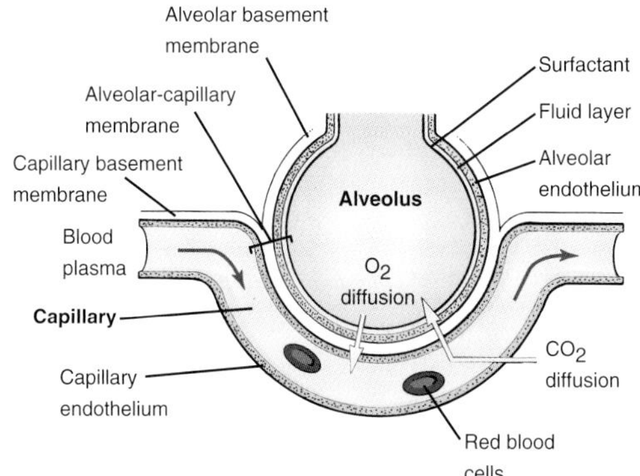

Oxygen transport.

glands which secretes hydrochloric acid.

oxytocic (ˌokseeˈtohsik) any drug that stimulates uterine contractions and may be used to hasten delivery.

oxytocin (ˌokseeˈtohsən) a pituitary hormone which stimulates uterine contractions and the ejection of milk. Synthetically prepared, it is used to induce labour and to control POSTPARTUM haemorrhage.

oxyuriasis (ˌokseeyəˈrieəsəs) infestation by threadworms of the genus *Enterobius*.

ozena (ohˈzeenə) a severe form of RHINITIS in which the mucous membrane of the nose atrophies. This is associated with a thick offensive nasal discharge that crusts and often results in severe halitosis.

ozone (ˈohzohn) an intensified form of oxygen containing three O atoms to the molecule (i.e. O_3), and often discharged by electrical machines, such as X-ray apparatus. In medicine it is employed as an antiseptic and oxidising agent. *O. sickness* sometimes experienced by jet travellers due to the levels of ozone in the aircraft.

Pp

Pa symbol for *pascal*.

pacemaker (ˈpaysˌmaykə) an object or substance that controls the rate at which a certain phenomenon occurs. The natural pacemaker of the heart is the sinoatrial NODE. *Electronic cardiac p.* an electrically operated mechanical device that stimulates the MYOCARDIUM to contract. It consists of an energy source, usually batteries, and electrical circuitry connected to an electrode, which is in direct contact with the myocardium. Pacemakers may be temporary or permanent. Temporary ones usually have an external energy source, whereas permanent ones have a subcutaneously implanted one. The rate at which the pacemaker delivers pulses may be either fixed or on demand. *Fixed* pacing means that pulses are delivered to the heart at a predetermined rate irrespective of any cardiac activity. A *demand* pacemaker is programmed to deliver pulses only in the absence of spontaneous cardiac activity. The need for replacement batteries is usually indicated when the rate of the pulse slows by five beats or more.

pachydermia (ˌpakeeˈdərmi·ə) an abnormal thickening of the skin. *P. laryngis* chronic hypertrophy of the vocal cords.

pachyonychia (ˌpakeeoˈniki·ə) abnormal thickening of the nails.

pacing (paysing) a series of techniques used by occupational therapists to assist people to perform tasks within their health limitations and to reduce adverse effects such as pain, joint stress and fatigue. Using a contractual arrangement with the person, the aim is to maximise performance and to meet personal objectives in achieving the desired task.

paediatrician (ˌpeedi·əˈtrishən) a medically qualified person specialising in childhood development and the diseases of children.

paediatrics (ˌpeediˈatriks) the branch of medicine dealing with the care and development of children and with the treatment of diseases that affect them.

paedophilia (ˌpeedəˈfili·ə) a sexual attraction towards children.

Paget's disease (ˈpajəts diˈzeez) *Sir James Paget, British surgeon, 1814–1899*. 1. a chronic disease of bone in which overactivity of the osteoblasts and osteoclasts leads to dense bone formation with areas of rarefaction. OSTEITIS deformans. 2. an inflammation of the nipple caused by cancer of the milk ducts of the breast.

pain (payn) a feeling of distress, suffering or agony, caused by stimulation of specialised nerve endings. Its purpose is chiefly protective; it acts as a warning that tissues are being damaged and induces the sufferer to remove or withdraw from the source. Pain is a subjective experience and one person's pain cannot be compared to another's experience. *Bearing-down p.*

pain accompanying uterine contractions during the second stage of labour. *False p.s* ineffective pains during pregnancy that resemble labour pains, but are not accompanied by cervical dilatation; also called false labour. *See also* BRAXTON HICKS CONTRACTIONS. *Gas p.s* pains caused by distension of the stomach or intestine by accumulations of air or other gases. *Hunger p.* pain coming on at the time of feeling hunger for a meal; a symptom of gastric disorder. *Intermenstrual p.* pain accompanying ovulation, occurring during the period between the menses, usually about midway. Also called mittelschmerz. *Labour p.s* the rhythmic pains of increasing severity and frequency due to contraction of the uterus at childbirth. *See also* LABOUR. *Lancinating p.* sharp, darting pain. *P. assessment* the measurement of a person's pain and its psychosocial and biological impact on the individual's personal

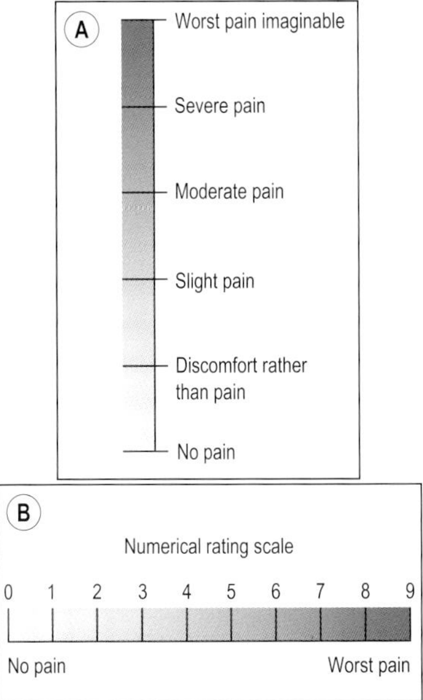

Visual analogue scale and numerical rating scale for pain assessment.

situation is especially difficult to assess where the person is unable to articulate their distress, e.g. children, infants and some adults. A number of assessment tools are available for use with children and adults; they are primarily longitudinal scales which list 'no pain' at one end to 'intense pain' at the other (*see* figure, p. 353). *Phantom p.* pain felt as if it were arising in an absent (amputated) limb. *See also* AMPUTATION. *Referred p.* pain in a part other than that in which the cause that produced it is situated. Referred pain usually originates in one of the visceral organs but is felt in the skin or sometimes in another area deep inside the body. Referred pain probably occurs because pain signals from the viscera travel along the same neural pathways used by pain signals from the skin. The person perceives the pain but interprets it as having originated in the skin rather than in a deep-seated visceral organ. *Rest p.* a continuous burning pain due to ischaemia of the lower leg, which begins or is aggravated after reclining and is relieved by sitting or standing.

painful arc syndrome (paynfuhl ark ˈsin͵drohm) a condition in which pain occurs when the arm is raised from the side between 45 and 160 degrees. The most usual cause is an inflamed tendon or bursa around the shoulder joint that is being squeezed between the scapula and humerus on movement. *See* FROZEN SHOULDER and *shoulder impingement syndrome*.

palate (ˈpalət) the roof of the mouth. *Artificial p.* a plate made to close a cleft palate. *Cleft p.* a congenital deformity where there is lack of fusion of the two bones forming the palate. *Hard p.* the bony part at the front. *Soft p.* a fold of mucous membrane that continues from the hard palate to the uvula.

palliative (ˈpali·ətiv) treatment that relieves, but does not cure, disease. *P. care* the active total care of patients whose disease no longer responds to curative treatment; should neither hasten nor postpone death. It pays equal attention to the physical, psychological, social and spiritual aspects of care of patients and those close to them.

pallor (ˈpalə) abnormal paleness of the skin.

palmar (ˈpalmə) relating to the palm of the hand. *Deep p. arches* the deep and superficial palmar arches are the chief arterial blood supply to the hand, formed by the junction of the ulnar and radial arteries. *P. fascia* the arrangement of tendons in the palm of the hand. *Superficial p. arches see* DEEP P. ARCHES above.

palpation (palˈpayshən) the examination of the organs by touch or pressure of the hand over the part.

palpebral (ˈpalpibrəl) referring to the eyelids. *P. ligaments* a band of ligaments which stretches from the junction of the upper and lower lid to the orbital bones, both medially and laterally.

palpitation (͵palpəˈtayshən) rapid and forceful contraction of the heart of which the person is conscious.

palsy (ˈpawlzee) a historical term for paralysis. *Bell's p.* paralysis of the facial muscles on one side, supplied by the seventh cranial nerve. *Crutch p.* paralysis due to pressure of a crutch on the radial nerve, and a cause of 'dropped wrist'. *Shaking p.* Parkinsonism; paralysis agitans.

panacea (͵panəˈseeə) a remedy for all diseases.

panarthritis (ˌpanahˈthrietəs) inflammation of all the joints or of all the structures of a joint.

pancreas (ˈpangkri·əs) an elongated, dual-purpose racemose gland about 15 cm long, lying behind the stomach, with its head in the curve of the duodenum and its tail in contact with the spleen (*see* figure). It secretes a digestive fluid (pancreatic juice) containing ferments which act on all classes of food. The fluid enters the duodenum by the pancreatic duct, which joins the common bile duct. The pancreas also secretes the hormones insulin and glucagon.

pancreatectomy (ˌpangkri·əˈtektəmee) surgical excision of the whole or a part of the pancreas.

pancreatin (ˈpangkri·ətən, panˈkreeə-) an extract from the pancreas containing the digestive enzymes. Used to treat deficiency, as in cystic fibrosis, and after pancreatectomy.

pancreatitis (ˌpangkri·əˈtietəs) inflammation of the pancreas. *Acute p.* a severe condition usually associated with alcohol misuse or biliary disease in which the person experiences sudden pain in the upper abdomen and back. The person often becomes severely shocked. *Chronic p.* chronic inflammation occurring after acute attacks. Pancreatic failure may lead to diabetes mellitus.

pancreozymin (ˌpangkreeohˈziemən) a hormone of the duodenal mucosa that stimulates the external secretory activity of the pancreas, especially its production of amylase.

pancytopenia (ˌpansietohˈpeeni·ə) a reduction in number of all types of blood cell due to failure of bone marrow formation.

pandemic (panˈdemik) an epidemic spreading over a wide area, sometimes all over the world.

panic (ˈpanik) an unreasoning and overwhelming fear or terror. It may occur in anxiety states and acute schizophrenia. *P. attack* a brief period of acute anxiety, distress and fear of dying or of losing one's reason. It may be recognised by the person that this experience is associated with specific situations,

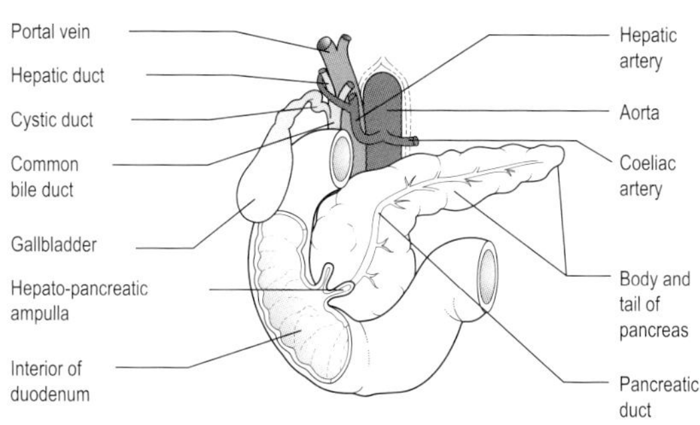

Pancreas.

e.g. being confined in a small space. Usually associated with other anxiety disorders or mental health problems. *P. disorder* a type of mental health disorder that is characterised by recurrent panic attacks of intense anxiety and distressing physical symptoms.

panniculitis (ˌpanˈikyooˌlietəs) inflammation of the fatty tissue under the skin, usually seen in women on the thighs and lower legs.

pannus (ˈpanəs) 1. in ophthalmology, pannus refers to an increased vascularity of the cornea leading to granulation tissue formation and impaired vision. Pannus may develop with contact lens wear, in trachoma after inflammation of the cornea or after chemical burns. 2. in rheumatoid arthritis, pannus tissue can form in the affected joint leading to loss of bone and cartilage.

panophthalmia (ˌpanofˈthalmi·ə) panophthalmitis; inflammation of all the tissues of the eyeball.

Papanicolaou test (ˌpapəˌnikəˈlayoo test) *Georgios Papanicolaou, Greek physician, anatomist and cytologist, 1883–1962.* A smear test to detect diseases of the uterine cervix and endometrium. Also called Pap test.

papilla (pəˈpilə) a small nipple-shaped protuberance. *Circumvallate p.* one surrounded by a ridge. A number are found at the back of the tongue arranged in a V-shape, and containing taste buds. *Filiform p.* one of the fine, slender filaments on the main part of the tongue which give it its velvety appearance. *Fungiform p.* a mushroom-shaped papilla of the tongue. *Optic p.* the optic disc, where the optic nerve leaves the eyeball. *Tactile p.* a projection on the true skin which contains nerve endings responsible for relaying sensations of pressure to the brain. A touch corpuscle.

papillitis (ˌpapiˈlietəs) 1. inflammation of the optic disc. 2. inflammation of a papilla.

papilloedema (ˌpapiləˈdeemə) oedema and hyperaemia of the optic disc, usually associated with increased intracranial pressure; also called choked disc.

papilloma (ˌpapəˈlohmə) a benign growth of epithelial tissue, e.g. a wart.

papillomatosis (ˌpapəˌlohməˈtoh-səs) the occurrence of multiple papillomas.

Papovavirus (pəˈpohvəˌvierəs) a family of DNA-producing viruses which cause tumours, usually benign, such as warts.

pappataci fever (pəpəˈtahˌchi ˈfeeˈvah) *see* PHLEBOTOMUS.

papule (ˈpapyool) a pimple, or small solid elevation of the skin.

papulopustular (ˌpapyəlohˈpustyəla) descriptive of skin eruptions of both papules and pustules.

papulosquamous (ˌpapyəlohˈ-skwayməs) descriptive of skin eruptions that are both papular and scaly. They include such conditions as lichen planus, pityriasis and psoriasis.

paracentesis (ˌparəsenˈteesəs) puncture of the wall of a cavity with a hollow needle in order to draw off excess fluid or to obtain diagnostic material.

paracusis (ˌparəˈkyoosəs) a disorder of hearing. *P. of Willis* an improvement in hearing when surrounded by noise.

paradigm (ˈparəˌdiem) an example or representative instance of a concept or theoretical approach.

paradoxical sleep (ˈparəˌdoksəˈkal sleep) rapid eye movement (REM) sleep. *See* SLEEP.

paraesthesia (ˌparəsˈtheezi·ə) an abnormal tingling sensation. ‘Pins and needles’.

Paragonimus (ˌparəˈgonimәs) a genus of trematode parasites. The flukes infest the lungs and are found mainly in tropical countries.

paralysis (pəˈraləsəs) loss or impairment of motor function in a part owing to a lesion of the neural or muscular mechanism; also, by analogy, impairment of sensory function (sensory paralysis). Paralysis is a symptom of a wide variety of physical and emotional disorders rather than a disease in itself. *P. agitans* Parkinsonism. *Bulbar p.* (*labio-glossopharyngeal p.*) paralysis due to changes in the motor centre of the medulla oblongata. It affects the muscles of the mouth, tongue and pharynx. *Facial p.* (*Bell's palsy*) paralysis that affects the muscles of the face and is due to injury or to inflammation of the facial nerve. *Flaccid p.* loss of tone and absence of reflexes in the paralysed muscles. *General p. of the insane* paralytic dementia occurring in the late stages of syphilis. *Infantile p.* the major form of POLIOMYELITIS. *Spastic p.* paralysis characterised by rigidity of affected muscles.

paralytic (ˌparəˈlitik) affected by or relating to paralysis. *P. ileus* obstruction of the ileum due to absence of peristalsis in a portion of the intestine.

paramedian (ˌparəˈmeedi·ən) situated on the side of the median line.

paramedic (ˌparəˈmedik) a person employed in the paramedical services, especially ambulance personnel qualified to provide pre-hospital procedures and care.

paramedical (ˌparəˈmedikəl) associated with the medical profession and the delivery of healthcare. The paramedical services include trained ambulance personnel, occupational and speech therapy, physiotherapy, radiography and social work.

parametritis (ˌparəməˈtrietəs) inflammation of the parametrium; pelvic CELLULITIS.

parametrium (ˌparəˈmeetri·əm) the connective tissue surrounding the uterus.

paramnesia (ˌparamˈneezi·ə) a defect of memory in which there is a false recollection. The person may fill in the forgotten period with imaginary events, which are often described in great detail.

paranoia (ˌparəˈnoyə) thinking and feeling of being under threat when there is no threat. Paranoid thoughts are delusions and may involve exaggerated suspicions or persecution that may be fully systematised in logical form, with the personality remaining fairly well preserved.

paranoid (ˈparəˌnoyd) resembling paranoia; refers to a condition that may occur in many forms of mental disease. Delusions of persecution are a marked feature. Associated with behaviour that denotes suspicion of others. *P. schizophrenia see* SCHIZOPHRENIA.

paraparesis (ˌparəpəˈreesəs) an incomplete paralysis affecting the lower limbs.

paraphimosis (ˌparəfieˈmohsəs) retraction of the prepuce behind the glans penis with inability to replace it, resulting in a painful constriction.

paraphrenia (ˌparəˈfreeniə) schizophrenia characterised by delusions (of persecution or grandeur or jealousy), but not accompanied by deterioration of the personality.

paraplegia (ˌparəˈpleeji·ə) paralysis of the lower extremities and lower trunk. All parts below the point of lesion in the spinal cord are affected. It may be of sudden onset from injury to the cord or may develop slowly as the result of disease.

parapraxia (parəpraksi·ə) describes minor aberrations of behaviour such as forgetfulness, the misplacing of things, verbal errors known also as 'Freudian slips' or 'senior moments' commonly associated with ageing.

paraprofessional (ˌparəprəˈfeshənəl) a person who is specially trained in a particular field or occupation to assist a professional.

parapsychology (ˌparəsieˈkoləjee) the branch of psychology dealing with psychical effects and experiences that appear to fall outside the scope of physical laws, e.g. telepathy and clairvoyance.

paraquat (ˈparəˌkwot) a poisonous compound used as a contact herbicide. Contact with concentrated solutions causes irritation of the skin, cracking and shedding of the nails, and delayed healing of cuts and wounds. After ingestion, renal and hepatic failure may develop, followed by pulmonary insufficiency and death.

parasite (ˈparəˌsiet) any animal or vegetable organism living on or within another, from which it derives its nourishment.

parasiticide (ˌparəˈsitəˌsied) a drug that kills parasites.

parasuicide (parəsooəsied) a suicidal action, such as self-mutilation or the taking of a drug overdose, which is motivated by a need to attract attention and seek help rather than commit suicide. Also known as deliberate self-harm (DSH).

parasympathetic nervous system (ˌparəˈsimpəthetik nərvəs sistəm) the craniosacral part of the autonomic nervous system.

parasympatholytic (ˌparəˈsimpətholitik) anticholinergic; an agent that opposes the effects of the parasympathetic nervous system.

parathormone (ˌparəˈthawmohn) the endocrine secretion of the parathyroid glands.

parathyroid gland (ˌparəˈthieroyd gland) one of four small endocrine glands, two of which are associated with each lobe of the thyroid gland, and sometimes embedded in it. The secretion from these has some control over calcium metabolism, and lack of it is a cause of tetany.

paratyphoid (ˌparəˈtiefoyd) a notifiable infection caused by *Salmonella* of all groups except *S. typhi.* The disease is usually milder and has a shorter incubation period, more abrupt onset and lower mortality rate than does typhoid. Clinically and pathologically, the two diseases cannot be distinguished. Also called paratyphoid fever.

paravertebral (parəvərtəbruhl) near or alongside the vertebral or spinal column. *P. block anaesthesia* induced by the infiltration of a local anaesthetic around the spinal nerve roots emerging from the intervertebral foramina. *P. injection* an injection of local anaesthetic into the sympathetic chain. May be used as a test in ischaemic limbs to ascertain if a SYMPATHECTOMY would be a useful treatment.

parenchyma (pəˈrengkəmə) the essential active cells of an organ, as distinguished from its vascular and connective tissue.

parent–infant relationship (pairənt infənt ˌreˈlayshənship) the unique relationship that develops between parents and their infant(s), sometimes referred to as 'bonding', which endures throughout life.

Promoted by early touching, fondling, speech with eye-to-eye contact and breastfeeding.

parenteral (pə'rentə·rəl) apart from the alimentary canal. Applied to the introduction into the body of drugs or fluids by routes other than the mouth or rectum, e.g. intravenously or subcutaneously. *P. nutrition see* NUTRITION.

paresis (pə'reesəs, 'parəsəs) partial paralysis.

parietal (pə'rieət'l) relating to the walls of any cavity. *P. bones* the two bones forming part of the roof and sides of the skull. *P. cells* the oxyntic cells in the gastric mucosa that secrete hydrochloric acid. *P. pleura* the pleura attached to the chest wall.

parity ('parətee) the classification of a woman with regard to the number of children that have been born live to her.

Parkinson's disease ('pahkənsənz di'zeez) *James Parkinson, British physician, 1755–1824.* Parkinsonism; paralysis agitans. A slowly progressive disease usually occurring in later life, characterised pathologically by degeneration within the nuclear masses of the extrapyramidal system, and clinically by mask-like facies (*see* Parkinson FACIES), a characteristic tremor of resting muscles, a slowing of voluntary movements, a festinating gait, peculiar posture and muscular weakness. When this symptom complex occurs secondarily to another disorder, the condition is called Parkinsonism.

paronychia (ˌparə'niki·ə) an abscess near the fingernail; a whitlow or felon. *P. tendinosa* a pyogenic infection that involves the tendon sheath.

parotid (pə'rotid) situated near the ear. *P. glands* two salivary glands, one in front of each ear.

parotitis (ˌparə'tietəs) inflammation of a parotid gland. Caused usually by ascending infection via its duct, when hygiene of the mouth is neglected or when the natural secretions are lessened, especially in severe illness or after operation. *Epidemic* p. mumps.

parous ('parəs) having borne one or more children.

paroxysm ('parokˌsizəm) 1. a sudden attack, worsening or recurrence of symptoms of a disease. 2. a spasm or seizure.

paroxysmal (ˌparok'sizməl) occurring in paroxysms. *P. cardiac dyspnoea* cardiac asthma. Recurrent attacks of DYSPNOEA associated with pulmonary oedema and left-sided heart failure. *P. tachycardia* recurrent attacks of rapid heartbeats that may occur without heart disease.

parrot disease (ˌparot di'zeez) *see* PSITTACOSIS.

particle ('pahtikəl) a minute piece of substance.

parturient (pah'tyoo·ri·ənt) giving birth; relating to childbirth.

parturition (ˌpahtyə'rishən) the act of giving birth.

parvovirus B19 (ˌpahro'vierəs 'bee nien'teen) *see* FIFTH DISEASE.

pascal (pa'skal, 'paskəl) *symbol* Pa. The SI unit of pressure.

passive ('pasiv) not active. *P. immunity see* IMMUNITY. *P. movements* in massage, manipulation by a physiotherapist without the help of the person. *P. smoking* inhaling tobacco smoke exhaled by others; associated with a significant risk of increase in lung cancer.

passivity (pa'sivətee) in psychiatry, a delusional feeling that a person is under some outside control and must therefore be inactive.

Pasteurella (ˌpahstəˈrelə) *Louis Pasteur, French chemist and bacteriologist, 1822–1895*. A genus of short Gram-negative bacilli.

pasteurisation (ˌpastə·rieˈzayshən, ˌpahstyə-) the process of heating foods to destroy disease-causing microorganisms, and to reduce the numbers of microorganisms responsible for fermentation and putrefaction. The pasteurisation process using moist heat is also used to disinfect medical instruments and other equipment.

Patau's syndrome (pəˈtowz ˈsinˌdrohm) a rare and serious genetic disorder caused by having an additional copy of chromosome 13. Also known as trisomy 13. Development is severely disrupted and in many cases leads to death in utero or shortly after birth.

patch test (pach test) a test of skin sensitivity in which a number of possible allergens are applied to the skin under a plaster. The causal agent of the allergy will produce an inflammation.

patella (pəˈtelə) the small, circular, sesamoid bone forming the kneecap.

patellar (pəˈtelə) belonging to the patella. *P. reflex* a knee jerk obtained by tapping the tendon below the patella.

patellectomy (ˌpatəˈlektəmee) excision of the patella.

patent (ˈpaytənt) open or unobstructed. *P. ductus arteriosus* failure of the ductus arteriosus to close, causing a shunt of blood from the aorta into the pulmonary artery and producing a continuous heart murmur.

paternity testing (ˌpəˈtərnətee testing) the use of blood samples to assist in establishing the paternity of a child. Blood taken from the suspected father, the child and sometimes the mother are tested to ascertain relationship via DNA.

pathogen (ˈpathəjən) a microorganism that can cause disease, e.g. *Clostridium tetani* causing tetanus.

pathogenicity (ˌpathəjəˈnisətee) the ability of a microorganism to cause disease.

pathognomonic (ˌpathəgnəˈmonik) specifically characteristic of a disease. A sign or symptom by which a pathological condition can positively be identified.

pathological (ˌpathəˈlojikəl) 1. pertaining to pathology. 2. causing or arising from disease. *P. fracture* a fracture occurring in diseased bone where there has been little or no external trauma.

pathology (pəˈtholəjee) the branch of medicine that deals with the essential nature of disease, especially of the structural and functional changes in tissues and organs of the body which cause or are caused by disease.

patient (ˈpayshənt) a person who is ill or is undergoing treatment for a health problem and/or is registered with a general practitioner. *P. advocate* a person who gives a voice to patients and their carers on health related matters. *P. allocation see* ALLOCATION. *P. pathway* the route followed by the patient into, through and out of health services and social care services. It can involve referral from primary care to hospital, visits to hospital departments and specialists, or a pathway through a clinical network. *P. representative*, a person who acts on behalf of an incapacitated patient.

patients' rights (ˈpayshənts riets) interests of patients in a range of standards and services. The *Australian Charter of Healthcare*

Rights (the Charter), for use in each Australian healthcare setting, identifies seven patient rights: the rights to access, safety, respect, partnership, information, privacy, redress and to give feedback. The Charter is not legislation; it does, however, express and incorporate a number of obligations health professionals owe patients under existing law, professional codes and employer policies.

Paul–Bunnell test (ˌpawlbəˈnel test) *John Paul, American physician, 1893–1971; Walls Bunnell, American physician, 1902–1966.* An agglutination test which, if positive, confirms the diagnosis of glandular fever.

Pavlov's method (ˈpavlovz ˈmethuhd) *Ivan Pavlov, Russian physiologist, 1849–1936.* A method for the study of the conditioned reflexes. Pavlov noticed that his experimental dogs salivated in anticipation of food when they heard a bell ring.

PDSA *see* PLAN, DO, STUDY, ACT.

peau d'orange (poh doˈronhzh) [Fr.] a dimpled appearance of the overlying skin. Blockage of the skin lymphatics causes dimpling of the hair follicle openings which resembles orange skin. Particularly associated with breast cancer.

pecten (ˈpektən) 1. the middle third of the anal canal. 2. a ridge on the pubic crest to which the inguinal ligament is attached.

pectoral (ˈpektə·rəl) relating to the chest. *P. muscles* two pairs of muscles, pectoralis major and pectoralis minor, which control the movements of the shoulder and upper arm.

pectus (ˈpektəs) the chest.

pedicle (ˈpedikəl) the stem or neck of a tumour. *P. graft* a tissue graft that is partially detached and inserted in its new position while temporarily still obtaining its blood supply from the original source.

pediculosis (pəˌdikyəˈlohsəs) the condition of being infested with lice.

Pediculus (pəˈdikyələs) a genus of lice. *P. humanus* a species that feeds on human blood and is an important vector of relapsing fever, typhus and trench fever. Subspecies are recognised: *P. humanus* var. *capitis* head louse found on the scalp hair, *P. humanus* var. *corporis* (body or clothes louse) and *P. pubis* the crab or pubic lice.

peduncle (pəˈdungkəl) a narrow part of a structure acting as a support. *Cerebellar p.* one of the collections of nerve fibres connecting the cerebellum with the medulla oblongata.

PEEP *see* POSITIVE END-EXPIRATORY PRESSURE.

peer (piə) a colleague usually of equal standing. *P. review* a basic component of quality assurance programs (*see* QUALITY) in which the results of health and/or nursing care given to a specific patient population are evaluated according to defined criteria established by the peers of the professionals delivering the care. Peer review is focused on the person and on the results of care given by a group of professionals rather than on individual professional practitioners. Peer review is also a feature of acceptance of journal submissions for publication. *P. support* the social support provided by one's peer group.

Pel–Ebstein syndrome (pel ˈebstien ˈsinˌdrohm) *Pieter Pel, Dutch physician, 1852–1919; Wilhelm Ebstein, German physician, 1836–1912.* A recurrent pyrexia, having a cycle of 15–21 days, which is a rare occurrence in people with Hodgkin's lymphoma.

pellagra (pəˈlagrə, -lay-) a syndrome caused by a diet seriously deficient in niacin (or by failure to convert tryptophan to niacin). Most persons with pellagra also suffer from deficiencies of vitamin B_2 (riboflavin) and other essential vitamins and minerals. The disease also occurs in persons suffering from alcoholism and drug addiction. Characterised by debility, digestive disorders, peripheral neuritis, ataxia, mental disturbance and erythema with exfoliation of the skin.

pelvic (ˈpelvik) pertaining to the pelvis. *P. exenteration* removal of all the pelvic organs. *P. floor exercises* a program of exercises to strengthen the muscles and tighten the ligaments at the base of the abdomen, which form the pelvic floor. *P. girdle* the ring of bone to which the lower limbs are jointed. It consists of the two hip bones and the sacrum and coccyx. *P. inflammatory disease (PID)* persistent infection of the internal reproductive organs of the female. If not treated it can result in infertility.

pelvimetry (pelˈvimətree) measurement of the pelvis.

pelvis (ˈpelvəs) a basin-shaped cavity. *Bony p.* the pelvic girdle formed of the hip bones and the sacrum and coccyx. *Contracted p.* narrowing of the diameter of the pelvis. It may be of the true conjugate or the diagonal. Effective antenatal care will recognise this condition, and caesarean section may be necessary. *False p.* the part formed by the concavity of the iliac bones above the iliopectineal line. *Renal p.* the dilatation of the ureter which, by enclosing the hilum, surrounds the pyramids of the kidney substance. *True p.* the basin-like cavity below the false pelvis, its upper limit being the pelvic brim.

pemphigoid (ˈpemfəˌgoyd) 1. resembling pemphigus. 2. a bullous disease of the older person with the blisters arising beneath the epidermis. The skin and the mucosa are affected, and, sometimes, the CONJUNCTIVA.

pemphigus (ˈpemfəgəs) a distinctive group of rare but serious diseases characterised by successive crops of large bullae ('water blisters'); the name is derived from the Greek word for blister, *pemphix*. Clusters of blisters usually appear first near the nose and mouth (sometimes inside them) and then gradually spread over the skin of the rest of the body. When the blisters burst, they leave round patches of raw and tender skin. Pemphigus is considered an autoimmune disorder.

pendulous (ˈpendyələs) hanging down. *P. abdomen* the hanging down of the abdomen over the pelvis, due to weakness and laxity of the abdominal muscles.

penicillin (ˌpenəˈsilən) an antibiotic cultured from certain moulds of the genus *Penicillium*. The drug is used in various forms to treat a wide variety of bacterial infections. It was first used therapeutically in 1941.

penicillinase (ˌpenəˈsiləˌnayz) an enzyme that inactivates penicillin. Many bacteria, particularly staphylococci, produce this enzyme.

Penicillium (ˌpenəˈsili·əm) a genus of mould-like fungi from some of which the penicillins are derived. Some species are pathogenic to humans.

penis (ˈpeenəs) the male organ of copulation and urination.

pentose (ˈpentohz, -s) a monosaccharide containing five carbon atoms in a molecule.

pepsin (ˈpepsən) an enzyme found in gastric juice. It partially digests proteins in an acid solution.

pepsinogen (pepˈsinəjən) the precursor of pepsin, activated by hydrochloric acid.

PEP *see* POST-EXPOSURE PROPHYLAXIS.

peptic (ˈpeptik) relating to pepsin or the action of the gastric juices in promoting digestion. *P. ulcer* an ulcer usually in the stomach or the duodenum caused by an erosion of the surface to expose the muscle wall by the stomach acid and digestive enzymes. It is often precipitated by *Helicobacter pylori* organisms.

peptide (ˈpeptied) any of a class of compounds of low molecular weight that yield two or more amino acids on hydrolysis. Peptides form the constituent parts of proteins.

peptone (ˈpeptohn) a substance produced by the action of pepsin on protein.

per os (per ohs) [L.] by the mouth.

percentile (pərˈsentiel) a term used in statistics to show how common some characteristic is. The line represents the percentage of the population who have this characteristic. The 90th percentile (or centile) for height means that 90% of the population will be no taller than the figure. The 50th percentile is the median or average.

percept; perception (ˈpərsept; pəˈsepshən) an awareness and understanding of an impression that has been presented to the senses. The mental process by which we perceive.

percussion (pəˈkushən) a method of diagnosis by tapping with the fingers or with a light hammer on any part the body. Information can thus be gained as to the condition of underlying organs.

percutaneous (ˌpərkyooˈtayni·əs) through the skin. *P. endoscopic gastrostomy (PEG)* a gastrostomy tube inserted endoscopically through the abdominal wall to allow feeding and the passage of drugs.

perforation (ˌpərfəˈrayshən) a hole or break in the containing walls or membranes of an organ or structure of the body. Perforation occurs when erosion, infection or other factors create a weak spot in the organ and internal pressure causes a rupture. It may also result from a deep penetrating wound.

performance indicators (PIs) (pəˈfawməns ˈindəˌkaytəs) quantifiable performance measurements. PIs evaluate the success of individuals or organisations against stated goals. This type of evaluation often leads to the identification of potential areas for improvement. Also known as key performance indicators (KPIs).

perfusion (pəˈfyoozhən) the passage of liquid through a tissue or an organ, particularly the passage of blood through the lung tissue.

perianal (ˌpereeˈayn'l) surrounding or located around the anus. *P. abscess* a small subcutaneous pocket of pus near the anal margin.

periarteritis (ˌpereeˌahtəˈrietəs) inflammation of the outer coat and surrounding tissues of an artery.

periarthritis (ˌpereeahˈthrietəs) inflammation of the tissues surrounding a joint.

pericarditis (ˌpereekahˈdietəs) inflammation of the pericardium. *Adhesive p.* the presence of adhesions between the two layers of pericardium owing to a thick fibrinous exudate. *Bacterial p.* inflammation of the pericardium due to bacterial infection. *Chronic constrictive p.* thickening and sometimes calcification of the pericardium, which inhibits the action of the heart. *Rheumatic p.* pericarditis due to rheumatic fever.

pericardium (ˌperee'kahdi·əm) the smooth membranous sac enveloping the heart, consisting of an outer fibrous and an inner serous coat. The sac contains a small amount of serous fluid.

perichondrium (ˌperee'kondri·əm) the membrane covering cartilaginous surfaces.

pericranium (ˌperee'krayni·əm) the periosteum of the cranial bones.

perilymph ('pereeˌlimf) the fluid that separates the bony and the membranous labyrinths of the ear.

perimeter (pə'rimətə) 1. the line marking the boundary of any area or geometrical figure; the circumference. 2. an instrument for measuring the field of vision.

perimetrium (ˌperee'meetri·əm) the peritoneal covering of the uterus.

perinatal (ˌperee'nayt'l) relating to the period from 20 weeks' gestation to the 28th day after birth. *P. mortality rate* the number of stillbirths plus deaths of babies under 7 days old per 1000 total births in any one year.

perinatologist (ˌpereenay'toləjəst) a medically qualified person specialising in perinatology.

perinatology (ˌpereenay'toləjee) the branch of medicine (obstetrics and paediatrics) dealing with the fetus and infant during the perinatal period.

perineal (ˌperee'neeəl) relating to the perineum.

perineum (ˌperee'neeəm) the tissues between the anus and external genitals. *Lacerated p.* a torn perineum, which may result from childbirth but is often forestalled by performing an episiotomy. Treatment is by suturing of the laceration.

period (ˌpiə·ree'əd) *see* MENSTRUATION.

periodic (ˌpiə·ree'odik) recurring at regular or irregular intervals. *P. apnoea of the newborn* occurring in the normal full-term infant, periodic episodes of rapid breathing followed by a brief period of apnoea, which is associated with rapid eye movements. *P. syndrome* recurrent head, limb or abdominal pains in children for which no organic cause can be found. It is often associated with migraine in adult life.

periodontitis (ˌperee·ədon'tietəs) inflammation of the periodontium.

periodontium (ˌperee·ə'donti·əm) the connective tissue between the teeth and their bony sockets.

perioperative (ˌperee'opə·rətiv) pertaining or relating to the period immediately before or after an operation as in perioperative care. Perioperative generally includes pre, intra- and post-operative phases.

periosteal (ˌperee'osti·əl) pertaining to or composed of periosteum. *P. elevator* an instrument for separating the periosteum from the bone.

periosteum (ˌperee'osti·əm) the fibrous membrane covering the surface of bone. It consists of two layers, the inner or osteogenetic layer, which is closely adherent and forms new cells (by which the bone grows in girth), and, in close contact with it, the fibrous layer richly supplied with blood vessels.

periostitis (ˌpereeoh'stietəs) inflammation of the periosteum, usually as a result of injury.

peripheral (pə'rifə·rəl) relating to the periphery. *P. arterial disease* a build-up of fatty deposits in the arteries restricting blood supply to leg muscles. *P. iridectomy* excision of a small piece of iris from its peripheral edge. *P. nervous system* those parts of the nervous system lying outside the central nervous system. *P. neuritis* inflammation of terminal nerves. *P. resistance* the resistance in the walls of the arterioles, which is a major factor in the control of blood pressure.

periphery (pə'rifə·ree) the outer surface or circumference.

peristalsis (ˌperee'stalsəs) a wave-like contraction preceded by a wave of dilatation that travels along the walls of a tubular organ, tending to press its contents onwards. It occurs in the muscle coat of the alimentary canal. *Reversed p.* a wave of contraction in the alimentary canal which passes *towards* the mouth. *Visible p.* a wave of contraction in the alimentary canal that is visible on the surface of the abdomen.

peritoneal (ˌperətə'neeəl) referring to the peritoneum. *P. cavity* the cavity between the parietal and the visceral peritoneum. *See also* ABDOMINAL CAVITY. *P. dialysis* a method of removing waste products from the blood by passing a cannula into the peritoneal cavity, running in a dialysing fluid and, after an interval, draining it off.

peritoneoscopy (ˌperətənee'oskəpee) visual examination of the peritoneum by means of a peritoneoscope.

peritoneum (ˌperətə'neeəm) the serous membrane lining the abdominal cavity and forming a covering for the abdominal organs. *Parietal p.* that which lines the abdominal cavity. *Visceral p.* the inner layer which closely covers the abdominal organs and includes the MESENTERIES.

peritonitis (ˌperətə'nietəs) inflammation of the peritoneum. This may be produced by inflammation of abdominal organs, by irritating substances from a perforated gallbladder or gastric ulcer, by rupture of a cyst or by irritation from blood, as in cases of internal bleeding. Less frequently, it may result from long-standing irritation caused by the presence in the abdomen of a foreign body, such as gunshot, or by chronic peritoneal dialysis.

peritonsillar (ˌperee'tonsələ) around the tonsil. *P. abscess* QUINSY.

perlèche (pər'lesh) [Fr.] inflammation with fissuring at the angles of the mouth; often due to vitamin B deficiency, poorly fitting dentures or thrush infection.

permeability (ˌpərmi·ə'bilətee) the degree to which a fluid can pass from one structure through a wall or membrane to another.

pernicious (pə'nishəs) highly destructive; fatal. *P. anaemia* an anaemia due to lack of absorption of vitamin B_{12} that is required for the formation of red blood cells.

perniosis (ˌpərnee'ohsəs) a condition resulting from persistent exposure to cold which produces vascular spasm in the superficial arterioles of the hands and feet, causing thrombosis and necrosis. Perniosis includes chilblains and RAYNAUD'S PHENOMENON (disease).

per oral (pər'ro·rəl) by the mouth.

perseveration (pərˌsevə'rayshən) the constant recurrence of an idea or the tendency to keep repeating the same words or actions.

persistent vegetative state (ˌpə'sistənt 'vejətətiv stayt) a long-term dependent state that may last for weeks, months or years. Caused by damage to the cerebral cortex of the brain that controls higher mental functions, while the brainstem controlling respiration and circulation remains undamaged. The individual appears awake but is totally dependent on others for all care and remains unresponsive.

persona (ˌpəˈsohnə) what one presents of one's self, to be perceived by others.

personal development plan (pərsən'l ˌdəˈveləpmənt plan) a planned process whereby an individual develops skills and knowledge that are beneficial to themselves and their career. This is part of a lifelong learning commitment for nurses and other health professionals.

personality (ˌpərsəˈnalətee) the sum total of heredity and inborn tendencies with influences from environment and education, which forms the mental make-up of a person and influences attitude to life. *Antisocial p. disorder (APD)* a personality disorder in which repetitive antisocial behaviour is associated with ego eccentricity, lack of guilt or anxiety, and imperviousness to punishment. Also called sociopathic (psychopathic) personality. *Double p., dual p.* multiple personality. *Multiple p.* a dissociative reaction in which an individual adopts two or more personalities alternatively, in none of which is there awareness of the experiences of the other(s). *Psychopathic p.* antisocial personality, sociopathic personality. *Schizoid p.* a personality disorder marked by timidness, self-consciousness, introversion, feelings of isolation and loneliness, and failure to form close interpersonal relationships; the individual is frequently ambitious, meticulous and a perfectionist.

perspiration (ˌpərspəˈrayshən) sweat or the act of sweating. *Insensible p.* water evaporation from the moist surfaces of the body such as the respiratory tract and skin, that is not due to the activity of the sweat glands. It occurs at a constant rate of about 500 mL/day. When treating dehydration this loss must be taken into account. *Sensible p.* sweat that is visible as droplets on the skin. Part of the mechanism for regulation of body temperature.

Perthes' disease (ˈpərtayz diˈzeez) *Georg Perthes, German surgeon, 1869–1927.* Osteochondritis of the head of the femur. PSEUDOCOXALGIA (Legg–Calvé–Perthes disease).

pertussis (pəˈtusəs) *see* WHOOPING COUGH.

perversion (pəˈvərshən) morbid diversion from a normal course. Any deviation from what is considered normal or natural. *Sexual p.* abnormal sexual desires and behaviour. A deviation.

pes (payz, peez) the foot or any foot-like structure. *P. cavus* a foot with an abnormally high arch. Claw foot. *P. malleus valgus* hammer toe. *P. planus* flat foot.

pessary (ˈpesə·ree) 1. a plastic or metal ring-shaped device which is inserted in the vagina to support a prolapsed uterus. 2. a medicated suppository inserted into the vagina for antiseptic or contraceptive purposes.

PET *see* POSITRON EMISSION TOMOGRAPHY.

petechia (pəˈteeki·ə) a small spot due to an effusion of blood under the skin, as in purpura.

petit mal (ˌpetee ˈmal) former name for a mild form of epilepsy common in children and characterised by a sudden and brief loss of consciousness. *See* EPILEPSY.

pétrissage (paytri'sahzh) [Fr.] a kneading action used in massage.

petrositis (,petroh'sietəs) inflammation of the petrous portion of the temporal bone, usually spread from a middle-ear infection.

Peyer's glands or patches ('pieəz glandz aw pachez) *Johann Peyer, Swiss anatomist, 1653–1712*. Small lymph nodules situated in the mucous membrane of the lower part of the small intestine.

Peyronie's disease ('payrəneez di'zeez) induration of the corpora cavernosa of the penis, producing a fibrous chordee leading to painful erection. Also known as induratio penis plastica (IPP).

pH a measure of the hydrogen ion concentration, and so the acidity or alkalinity of a solution. Expressed numerically 1 to 14; 7 is neutral, and below this is acid and above alkaline. *See* HYDROGEN ION CONCENTRATION.

phaeochromocytoma (,feeoh,krohmohsie'tohmə) a rare tumour of the adrenal medulla which gives rise to paroxysmal hypertension.

phage (fayj, fahzh) bacteriophage. A virus that lives on bacteria but is confined to a particular strain. *P.-typing* the identification of certain bacterial strains by determining the presence of strain-specific phages. Used in detecting the causative organisms of epidemics, especially food poisoning.

phagocyte ('fagə,siet) a blood cell that has the power of ingesting bacteria, protozoa and foreign bodies in the blood.

phagocytosis (,fagəsie'tohsəs) the engulfing and destruction of microorganisms and foreign bodies by phagocytes in the blood.

phalanges (fə'lanjeez) the bones of the fingers or toes.

phallus ('faləs) the penis.

phantasy ('fantəsee) *see* FANTASY.

phantom ('fantəm) 1. an image or impression not evoked by actual stimuli. 2. a model of the body or of a specific part thereof. 3. a device for simulating the in vivo interaction of radiation with tissues. *P. pain* pain felt as if it were arising in an absent (amputated) limb. Also known as phantom limb pain/experience. *P. pregnancy see* PSEUDOCYESIS. *P. tumour* a tumour-like swelling of the abdomen caused by contraction of the muscles or by localised gas.

Pharmaceutical Benefits Scheme (PBS) (,fahmə'syootikl bən'ifitz 'skeem) an Australian government program that provides subsidised prescription medication to residents of Australia.

pharmacist ('fahməsist) a person professionally qualified to prepare, dispense and provide clinical information on drugs or medications to health professionals and patients.

pharmacogenetics (,fahməkohjə'netiks) the study of genetically determined variations in drug metabolism and the response of the individual.

pharmacokinetics ('fahmakoh'kənetiks) the study of how drugs are processed within the body, including their absorption, distribution, metabolism and excretion.

pharmacology (,fahmə'koləjee) the science of the nature and preparation of drugs and particularly of their effects on the body.

pharmacopoeia (,fahməkə'pee·ə) an authoritative publication that gives the standard formulae and preparations of drugs used in a given country. *Australian p.* that authorised for use in Australia.

pharmacy (ˈfahməsee) 1. the activity or study of medicine preparations. 2. the art of preparing, compounding and dispensing medicines. 3. the place where drugs are stored and dispensed.

pharyngeal (ˌfarənˈjeeəl, fəˈrinji·əl) relating to the pharynx. *P. pouch* dilatation of the lower part of the pharynx.

pharyngitis (ˌfarənˈjietəs) inflammation of the pharynx.

pharyngolaryngeal (ˌfəˌring·goh-ˌlarənˈjeeəl) referring to both the pharynx and the larynx.

pharyngotympanic tube (fəˌring·gohˈtimpanik tyoob) the tube that joins the middle ear to the pharynx; the eustachian tube.

pharynx (ˈfaringks) the muscular tube, lined with mucous membrane, situated at the back of the mouth. It leads into the oesophagus, and also communicates with the nose through the posterior nares, with the ears through the pharyngotympanic (eustachian) tubes, and with the larynx. *See* LARYNGOPHARYNX, NASOPHARYNX and OROPHARYNX.

phenol (ˈfeenol) carbolic acid. A disinfectant derived from coal tar.

phenomenon (fəˈnomənən) 1. an objective sign or symptom. 2. a noteworthy occurrence.

phenomenology (fəˌnoməˈnoləjee) an approach in research, as the study of the lived experience of people or a way of thinking about what life experiences are like for people.

phenotype (ˈfeenohˌtiep) the characteristics of an individual that are due both to the environment and to genetic make-up.

phenylalanine (ˌfeenəlˈaləneen) an essential amino acid which cannot be properly metabolised in persons suffering from PHENYLKETONURIA.

phenylketonuria (PKU) (ˌfeenəlˌkee-təˈnyoo·ri·ə) a disease due to a defect in the metabolism of the amino acid phenylalanine. The condition is hereditary. It results from lack of an enzyme, phenylalanine hydroxylase, necessary for the conversion of phenylalanine into tyrosine. Thus, there is accumulation of phenylalanine in the blood, with eventual excretion of phenylpyruvic acid in the urine. If untreated, the condition results in learning difficulties and other abnormalities. The condition can be detected soon after birth, and screening of newborns for PKU is part of the newborn spot blood test at five days. Phenylalanine levels are assessed and treatment, if necessary, is with a diet low in phenylalanine. A special diet is usually recommended throughout life and especially during pregnancy as high phenylalanine levels in the mother's blood can damage the fetus.

phenylpyruvic acid (ˌfeenəlpieˈroovik ˈasəd) an abnormal constituent of the urine present in phenylketonuria.

pheromone (ferəmohn) a chemical substance with specific odour secreted externally by an organism and affecting the behaviour or physiology of members of the same species. These substances may be involved in the physiological communication within a species and provide an influence on sexual behaviour.

phimosis (fieˈmohsəs) constriction of the prepuce so that it cannot be drawn back over the glans penis. The usual treatment is circumcision.

phlebectomy (fləˈbektəmee) excision of a vein or a portion of a vein.

phlebitis (fləˈbietəs) inflammation of a vein, which tends to lead to the formation of a thrombus. The symptoms are pain and swelling, and redness along the course of the vein, which is felt later as a hard, tender cord.

phlebography (flə'bogrəfee) also known as venography 1. radiographic examination of a vein containing a contrast medium. 2. the graphic representation of the venous pulse.

phlebothrombosis (ˌflebohthrom'bohsəs) obstruction of a vein by a blood clot without local inflammation. It is usually in the deep veins of the calf of the leg, causing tenderness and swelling. The clot may break away and cause an embolism.

Phlebotomus (flə'botəməs) a genus of sandflies, the various species of which transmit LEISHMANIASIS in its many forms and also SANDFLY fever, which is also known as pappataci fever and three-day fever.

phlebotomy (fli'botəmee) the puncture of a vein for the withdrawal of blood. VENESECTION.

phlegm (flem) mucus secreted by the lining of the air passages.

phlegmasia alba dolens (fleg'mazia albə do'lenz) thrombophlebitis of the femoral vein resulting in pain, oedema and a white (alba) appearance of the leg. It may occur after childbirth, during a severe febrile illness or as a result of an underlying malignancy. Also called milk leg or white leg.

phlegmatic (fleg'matik) calm and unemotional.

phlycten ('fliktən) 1. a small blister caused by a burn. 2. a small vesicle containing lymph occurring in the conjunctiva or cornea of the eye. Often associated with tuberculosis.

phobia ('fohbi·ə) an irrational fear produced by a specific situation or object that the person attempts to avoid.

phocomelia (ˌfohkə'meeli·ə) a rare congenital deformity in which the long bones of the limbs are minimal or absent and the individual has stump-like limbs of various lengths. The drug thalidomide, used in the 1960s in early pregnancy, was associated with this deformity.

phonation (foh'nayshən) the art of uttering meaningful vocal sounds.

phonocardiogram (ˌfohnoh'kahdeeoˌgram) a record of the heart sounds made by a phonocardiograph.

phonocardiograph (ˌfohnoh'kahdeeəˌgrahf, -graf) an instrument that graphically records heart sounds and murmurs.

phonology (fə'noləjee) the study of speech sounds, their production and the relationship between sounds as elements of language.

phosphatase ('fosfəˌtayz) one of a group of enzymes involved in the metabolism of phosphate. *Alkaline p.* an enzyme formed by osteoblasts in the bones and by liver cells and excreted in the bile.

phosphate ('fosfayt) a salt or ester of phosphoric acid.

phospholipid (ˌfosfə'lipəd) a lipid of glycerol fats found in cells, especially those of the nervous system.

phosphorus ('fosfə·rəs) *symbol* P. An essential element in the diet. It is a major component of bone, is involved in almost all metabolic processes and also plays an important role in cell metabolism. It is obtained by the body from milk products, cereals, meat and fish. Its use by the body is controlled by vitamin D and calcium.

phosphorylase (fos'fo·rəˌlayz) an enzyme found in the liver and kidneys that catalyses the breakdown of glycogen into glucose 1-phosphate.

photocoagulation (ˌfohtohkohˌagyə'layshən) the use of a powerful light source to induce inflammation of the retina and CHOROIDS to treat retinal detachment.

photophobia (ˌfohtoh'fohbi·ə) intolerance of light. It can occur in many eye conditions including conjunctivitis, corneal ulceration, IRITIS and KERATITIS.

photophthalmia (ˌfohtof'thalmi·ə) inflammation of the eye due to over exposure to bright light, especially to ultraviolet light.

photopic (foh'topik, -'toh-) pertaining to bright light. *P. vision* vision in bright light when the cones of the retina provide the visual appreciation of colour and shape.

photopsia (foh'topsi·ə) a sensation of flashes of light sometimes occurring in the early stages of retinal detachment.

photosensitivity (ˌfohtohˌsensə'tivətee) an abnormal degree of sensitivity of the skin to sunlight.

phototherapy (ˌfohtoh'therəpee) treatment using fluorescent light containing a high output of blue light to reduce the amount of unconjugated BILIRUBIN in the skin of a jaundiced neonate.

phrenic ('frenik) 1. relating to the mind. 2. pertaining to the diaphragm. *P. avulsion* the surgical extraction of a part of the phrenic nerve. *P. nerve* one of a pair of nerves controlling the muscles of the diaphragm.

Phthirus pubis ('thirəs 'pyoobəs) the crab louse.

phthisis ('tiesəs) pulmonary tuberculosis. *P. bulbi* a shrinking of the eyeball following inflammation or injury.

physical ('fisikəl) in medicine, relating to the body as opposed to the mental processes. *P. abuse see* ABUSE. *P. disability* a term used when a physical disadvantage is due to impairment of physiological or anatomical structure or function. *P. examination* examination of the bodily state of a person by ordinary physical means, such as inspection, palpation, percussion and auscultation. *P. medicine* the treatment and rehabilitation of patients with physical disabilities. It includes physiotherapy and manipulation. *P. signs* those observed by inspection, percussion, etc.

physician (fə'zishən) a medically qualified person who practises medicine as opposed to surgery. *Community p.* a doctor who practises community medicine (*see* MEDICINE). *Consultant p.* senior doctor in overall charge of patients within a specialist medical field, and responsible for directing junior medical staff working for the same team. *Resident p.* a junior doctor, resident in hospital while on duty, acting under the orders of a consultant physician.

physiological (ˌfizi·ə'lojikəl) relating to physiology. Normal, as opposed to pathological. *P. jaundice see* JAUNDICE. *P. solutions* those of the same salt composition and same osmotic pressure as blood plasma.

physiology (ˌfizee'oləjee) the science of the functioning of living organisms.

physiotherapist (fizeeoh'therəpist) a healthcare professional concerned with function and movement as well as maximising mobility potential. They provide treatment for physical problems due to accident, illness or disability, and promote normal function and mobility, using skills of manipulation and electrotherapy with appropriate exercise programs as necessary. Physiotherapists are also involved in preventative healthcare and rehabilitation and committed to reviewing evidence that informs its practice and delivery.

physiotherapy (ˌfizeeohˈtherəpee) treatment and rehabilitation by natural forces, e.g. heat, light, electricity, massage, manipulation and remedial exercises.

physique (fəˈzeek) the structure of the body.

pia mater (ˌpieə ˈmahtə) [L.] the innermost membrane enveloping the brain and spinal cord, consisting of a network of small blood vessels connected by areolar tissue. This dips down into all the folds of the nerve substance.

pica (ˈpiekə) an unnatural craving for strange foods and for things not fit to be eaten. It may occur in pregnancy and sometimes in children with learning disabilities.

Pick's disease (ˈpiks diˈzeez) a progressive degenerative disease that causes irreversible destruction of brain cells.

Pickwickian syndrome (pikˈwiki·ən ˈsinˌdrohm) (*Pickwick Papers* by Charles Dickens). A condition in which people with extreme obesity fail to breathe rapidly enough or deeply enough, resulting in low blood oxygen levels and high blood carbon dioxide levels. Also known as obesity hypoventilation syndrome.

picornavirus (picˈkawnəˌvicrəs) a family of small RNA-containing viruses including ECHOVIRUSES and RHINOVIRUSES.

PICU paediatric intensive care unit. *See* INTENSIVE CARE UNIT.

PID *See* PELVIC INFLAMMATORY DISEASE; also prolapse of an intervertebral disc.

pie chart (ˈpie ˌchaht) a circular graph divided into sectors proportional to the magnitudes of the quantities represented.

pigeon breast (ˈpijən brest) a deformity in which the sternum is unduly prominent. *P. toed* walking with the toes of one foot or of both feet turned inwards.

pigment (ˈpigmənt) colouring matter. *Bile p.s* BILIRUBIN and biliverdin. *Blood p.* haemoglobin. *Melanotic p.* MELANIN.

pigmentation (ˌpigmenˈtayshən) the deposition of pigment in the tissues. In some conditions, e.g. jaundice or albinism, there is either an excess or a lack of pigmentation.

pile (piel) a HAEMORRHOID.

pill (pil) a rounded mass of one or more drugs, sometimes coated with sugar. Taken orally.

pilomotor (ˌpielohˈmohtə) capable of moving the hair. *P. nerves* sympathetic nerves that control muscles in the skin connected with hair follicles. Stimulation causes the hair to be erected and also the condition of goose-flesh of the skin.

pilonidal (ˌpieləˈnied'l) having a growth of hair. *P. cyst* a congenital infolding of hair-bearing skin over the coccyx. It may become infected and lead to sinus formation.

pilot study (ˈpielət ˈstuhdee) a small-scale version of a planned experiment or observation used initially to test the design of the larger study. A pilot study is helpful to see if any difficulties or problems arise in order that they can be clarified before embarking on the larger study, thus saving time and resources. A pilot study may also indicate possible extensions to the study or suggest restrictions of those aspects likely to be unhelpful.

pimple (ˈpimpəl) a small papule or pustule.

pineal (ˈpini·əl, ˈpie-) 1. pertaining to the pineal gland. Also known as the pineal body, a small endocrine gland in the vertebrate brain. 2. shaped like a pine cone.

pinguecula (pingˈgwekyələ) [L.] a small, benign, yellowish spot on the bulbar conjunctiva, seen usually in the older person. Caused by degeneration of the elastic tissue of the conjunctiva.

pinkeye (ˈpingkie) acute contagious conjunctivitis.

pinna (ˈpinə) the projecting part of the external ear; the auricle.

pinta (ˈpintə) a non-sexually transmitted skin infection caused by *Treponema carateum,* which is similar to the causative agent of syphilis. It is prevalent in the West Indies and Central America.

pinworm (ˈpinwərm) a threadworm; *Enterobius vermicularis*.

pituitary (pəˈtyooətree) an endocrine gland suspended from the base of the brain and protected by the SELLA TURCICA in the sphenoid bone. It consists of two lobes: (a) the anterior, which secretes a number of different hormones including adrenocorticotrophic hormone (ACTH), GONADOTROPHIN, thyroid-stimulating hormone (TSH) and prolactin; and (b) the posterior, which secretes oxytocin and vasopressin.

pityriasis (ˌpitəˈrieəsəs) a skin disease characterised by fine scaly desquamation. *P. alba* a condition common in children in which white scaly patches appear on the face. *P. capitis* dandruff. *P. rosea* an inflammatory form in which the affected areas are macular and ring-shaped. *P. versicolor* a common condition in which small patches of skin become scaly and discoloured.

PKU PHENYLKETONURIA.

placebo (pləˈseeboh) [L.] a substance given to a patient as medicine, or a procedure performed on a patient, that has no intrinsic therapeutic value and relieves symptoms or helps the patient in some way only because the patient believes or expects that it will. A placebo may be prescribed to satisfy a patient's psychological need for drug therapy and may also be given during controlled experiments. *P. effect* after the administration of a drug or treatment, a change (usually temporary) in a patient's physical or emotional condition following publicity or media interest in the drug or treatment. The placebo response is due more to the patient's expectations or to the expectations of the person giving the drug or treatment than to the result of any direct physiological or pharmacological substance response.

placenta (pləˈsentə) the afterbirth. A vascular structure inside the pregnant uterus supplying the fetus with nourishment through the connecting umbilical cord. The placenta develops at about the third month of pregnancy and is expelled after the birth of the child. *Battledore p.* one in which the cord is attached to the margin and not the centre. *P. praevia* one attached to the lower part of the uterine wall. It may cause severe antepartum haemorrhage. *See also* ABRUPTIO PLACENTAE.

plagiocephaly (ˌplayjeeohˈkefəlee, -ˈsef-) asymmetry of the head resulting from the irregular closing of the sutures.

plague (playg) an acute, febrile, infectious, highly fatal disease caused by the bacillus *Yersinia pestis.* A notifiable disease. Transmitted to humans by the bites of fleas that have derived the infection from diseased rats. *Bubonic p.* a type in which the lymph glands are infected and buboes form in the groins and armpits. Known in medieval times as 'The Black Death'. *Pneumonic p.* a type in which the infection attacks chiefly the lung tissues. A fatal form. *Septicaemic p.* a very severe and fatal form when the infection enters the bloodstream.

plan (plan) a detailed proposal for doing or achieving something.

plan, do, study, act (ˌplan ˌdoo ˈstudee ˈakt) a widely used method in service improvement methodology to test out small changes.

planes (playnz) used in the description of location and movement of parts of the body. Three planes are perpendicular to each other passing through the middle of the body. These are defined as follows: *sagittal*—vertical, front-to-back; *frontal*—vertical, side-to-side; *transverse*—horizontal (*see* figure, p. 374). *See* AXIS.

planned parenthood (pland pairənt-huhd) the practice of measures including contraception that limit the number and the spacing of pregnancies.

planning (planing) the stage of the nursing process in which the nurse and the patient together plan how to manage identified needs and problems and consider the measurable goals to achieve and produce an evidence-based, patient focused care plan. A forward date is also set for evaluation of whether or not the goals have been achieved.

plantar (ˌplantə) relating to the sole of the foot. *P. arch* the arch made by anastomosis of the plantar arteries. *P. fasciitis* heel pain usually caused when the plantar fascia becomes damaged and thickens. *P. flexion* bending of the toes downwards and so arching the foot. *P. reflex* contraction of the toes on stroking the sole of the foot. *P. wart* a common wart located on the sole of the foot. Plantar warts are epidermal tumours caused by a virus that may be picked up by going barefoot. Also called verruca plantaris.

plaque (plak, plahk) 1. a flat patch on the skin. 2. a deposit of food and bacteria on the enamel of teeth which may produce tartar and CARIES.

plasma (ˈplazmə) the fluid portion of the blood in which corpuscles are suspended. Plasma is to be distinguished from serum, which is plasma from which the fibrinogen has been separated in the process of clotting. *P. proteins* those present in the blood plasma: albumin, globulin and fibrinogen. *P. volume expander* a solution transfused instead of blood to increase the volume of fluid circulating in the blood vessels. Also called artificial plasma extender. *Reconstituted p.* dried plasma when again made liquid by addition of distilled water.

plasmapheresis (ˌplazməfəˈreesəs) a method of removing a portion of the plasma from circulation. VENESECTION is performed, the blood is allowed to settle, the plasma is removed and the red blood cells are returned to the circulation. Used in the treatment of those diseases caused by antibodies circulating in the patient's plasma.

plasmid deoxyribonucleic acid (plasmid DNA) (plazmid deeˌoksee-ˌriebohnyooˈklee·ik ˈasəd) present in the cytoplasm of some bacteria. This genetic material can be transferred during bacterial reproduction thus permitting the genes of antibiotic resistance to be passed on.

Sagittal plane
Frontal
(transverse)
axis
Transverse
plane
Sagittal axis
Frontal plane
Vertical axis

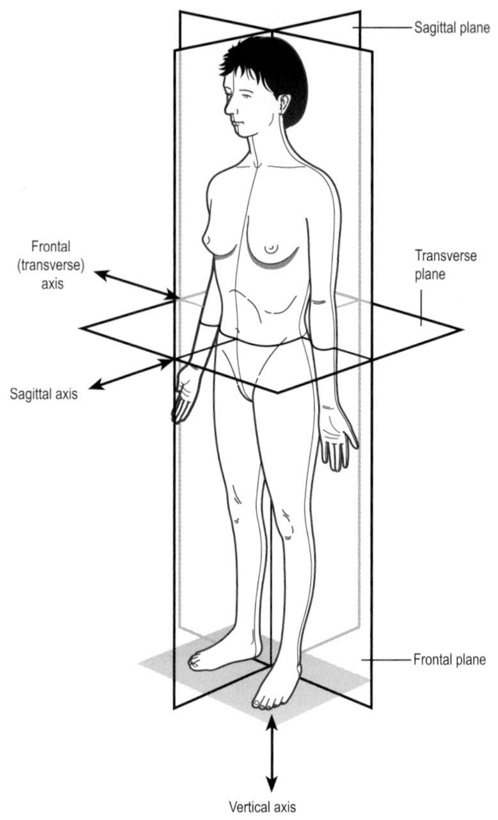

Planes.

plasmin (ˈplazmən) a fibrinolytic, found in blood plasma, which can dissolve fibrin clots.

plasminogen (plazˈminəjən) the inactive precursor of plasmin.

Plasmodium (plazˈmohdi·əm) a genus of protozoan parasites in the red blood cells of animals and humans. Human malaria is caused by four different species of *Plasmodium*: *P. falciparum*, *P. malariae*, *P. ovale* and *P. vivax*. Humans occasionally become infected with *Plasmodium* species that normally infect animals, such as *P. knowlesi*.

plaster (ˈplahstə, ˈplasta) 1. a mixture of materials that hardens; used for immobilising or making impressions of body parts. 2. an adhesive substance spread on fabric or other suitable backing material for application to the skin. Lightweight synthetic materials are now used to splint some fractures. Some synthetic materials are less pliable and cannot be moulded as effectively as plaster of Paris (POP) and occasionally cause allergy of the underlying skin. *Bohler's p.* plaster for Pott's fracture. A leg splint of plaster of Paris, in which is embedded an iron stirrup extending below the foot, which enables the patient to walk without putting weight on the joint. *Corn p.* an adhesive strip or patch impregnated with salicylic acid and applied to corns on the feet. *Frog p.* a plaster of Paris splint used to maintain the position after correction of the deformity due to congenital dislocation of the hip. *P. of Paris* calcium sulfate or gypsum which sets hard when water is added to it; it is used to form a plaster cast to immobilise a part, and in dentistry for making dental impressions.

plastic (ˈplastik) 1. constructive; tissue forming. 2. capable of being moulded; pliable. *P. surgery* the branch of surgery that deals with the repair and reconstruction of deformed or injured parts of the body, including their replacement, by tissue grafting or other means to restore function and appearance.

platelet (ˈplaytlət) a disc-shaped structure present in the blood and concerned in the process of clotting. A THROMBOCYTE.

play (play) an occupation for either children or adults which is voluntary and may be a spontaneous or an organised activity providing enjoyment, entertainment, amusement or a diversion. Play is important in childhood as a necessary part of psychological and physical development. *Normative p.* is by children that is spontaneous and child led, being pleasurable with no intrinsic goals. *P. group* a session of care and activities for preschool children. It can be organised by any interested person at home or in other premises, but it must be registered by the social services department. *P. specialist* a person who is qualified to use play constructively to help children come to terms with illness and hospitalisation. *P. therapist* one trained in the skills of play therapy. *P. therapy* a technique used in child psychotherapy in which play is used to reveal unconscious material. Play is the natural way in which children express and work through unconscious conflicts; thus play therapy is analogous to the technique of free association used in adult psychotherapy.

pleoptics (pleeˈoptiks) an orthoptic method of improving the sight in cases of STRABISMUS by stimulating the use of the macular part of the retina.

plethora (ˈplethə·rə) a general term denoting a red, florid complexion or, specifically, an excessive amount of blood.

plethysmography (ˌplethizˈmogrə-fee) the measurement of changes in the volume of organs or limbs due to alterations in blood pressure.

pleura (ˈploo·rə) the serous membrane lining the thorax and enveloping each lung. *Parietal p.* the layer that lines the chest wall. *Visceral p.* the inner layer which is in close contact with the lung.

pleurisy; pleuritis (ˈploo·rəsee; plooˈrietəs) inflammation of the pleura; it may be caused by infection, injury or tumour. It may be a complication of lung diseases, particularly of pneumonia, or sometimes of tuberculosis, lung abscess or influenza. The symptoms are cough, fever, chills, sharp, sticking pain that is worse on inspiration, and rapid shallow breathing. *Dry p., fibrinous p.* pleurisy in which the membrane is inflamed and roughened, but no fluid is formed. *P. with effusion* wet pleurisy. A type that is characterised by inflammation and exudation of serous fluid into the pleural cavity. *Purulent p.* empyema. The formation of pus in the pleural cavity. An operation for drainage is usually necessary. *Wet p.* pleurisy with effusion.

pleurodynia (ploorohdineeə) pain in the intercostal muscles, probably rheumatic in origin.

plexus (ˈpleksəs) a network of veins or nerves. *Auerbach's p.* the nerve ganglion situated between the longitudinal and circular muscle fibres of the intestine. The nerves are motor nerves. Also known as myenteric plexus. *Brachial p.* the network of nerves of the neck and axilla. *Choroid p.* a capillary network situated in the ventricles of the brain which forms the cerebrospinal fluid. *Coeliac p.* solar plexus. *Meissner's p.* the sensory nerve ganglion situated in the submucous layer of the intestinal wall. Also known as submucous plexus. *Rectal p.* the network of veins that surrounds the rectum and forms a direct communication between the systemic and portal circulations. *Solar p.* coeliac plexus. The network of nerves and ganglia at the back of the stomach, which supply the abdominal viscera.

plication (plieˈkayshən) the taking of tucks in a structure to shorten it; a folding to decrease the size of a structure or organ during a surgical procedure.

pluripotent stem cells (plooripohtənt stem sels) bone marrow cells that have the potential to develop into many other types of mature cells, e.g. erythrocytes, lymphocytes, granulocytes and thrombocytes.

pneumaturia (ˌnyoomәˈtyoo·ri·ә) the passing of flatus with the urine owing to a vesicointestinal fistula and air from the bowel entering the bladder.

pneumococcus (ˌnyoomohˈkokəs) the causative agent of a range of illnesses described as pneumococcal disease, e.g. pneumonia, septicaemia and meningitis. A Gram-positive, ovoid diplococcus, *Streptococcus pneumoniae*. Immunisation with pneumococcal vaccine helps prevent pneumococcal disease, and is recommended for babies, people aged 65 years and over, and those with certain medical conditions, e.g. diabetes, heart and lung conditions.

pneumoconiosis (ˌnyoomoh-ˌkohneeˈohsəs) an industrial disease of the lung due to inhalation of dust particles over a period of time.

See ANTHRACOSIS, ASBESTOSIS and SILICOSIS.

Pneumocystis (ˌnyoomoohˈsistəs) a genus of microorganisms of uncertain status but usually considered to be protozoans. *P. carinii* is an atypical fungus acquired by the airborne route which frequently causes pneumonia in people with human immunodeficiency virus (HIV) infection and in other immunosuppressed persons.

pneumodynamics (ˌnyoomohdieˈnamiks) the mechanics of respiration.

pneumoencephalography (ˌnyoomoh·enˌkefəˈlografee, -ˌsef-) *see* ENCEPHALOGRAPHY.

pneumogastric (ˌnyoomohˈgastrik) pertaining to lungs and stomach. *P. nerve* the 10th cranial nerve to the lungs, stomach, etc. The VAGUS nerve.

pneumomycosis (ˌnyoomohmieˈkohsəs) infection of the lung by microfungi, e.g. candidiasis or aspergillosis.

pneumonectomy (ˌnyoomәˈnektəmee) partial or total removal of a lung.

pneumonia (nyooˈmohni·ə) inflammation of the lung with consolidation and exudation. *Aspiration p.* an acute condition caused by the aspiration of infected material or acidic vomitus into the lungs. *Hypostatic p.* a form that occurs in weak, bedridden patients. *Lobar p.* an acute infectious disease caused by a pneumococcus and affecting whole lobes of either or both lungs. *Virus p.* inflammation of the lung occurring during some virus disease and secondary to it.

pneumonitis (ˌnyoomәˈnietəs) an imprecise term denoting any inflammatory condition of the lung.

pneumoperitoneum (ˌnyoomohˌperətəˈneeəm) the presence of air or gas in the peritoneal cavity, occurring pathologically or introduced intentionally for diagnostic or therapeutic purposes.

pneumoradiography (ˌnyoomohˌraydeeˈografee) radiographic examination of a cavity or part after air or a gas has been injected into it.

pneumotaxic (ˌnyoomohˈtaksik) regulating the rate of respiration. *P. centre* the centre in the pons that influences inspiratory effort during respiration.

pneumothorax (ˌnyoomohˈthor·raks) accumulation of air or gas in the pleural cavity, resulting in collapse of the lung on the affected side. The condition may occur spontaneously, as in the course of a pulmonary disease, or it may follow trauma to and perforation of the chest wall. *Spontaneous p.* sometimes occurs when there is an opening on the surface of the lung, allowing leakage of air from the bronchi into the pleural cavity. *Tension p.* is a particularly dangerous form of pneumothorax that occurs when air escapes into the pleural cavity from a bronchus but cannot regain entry into the bronchus. As a result, continuously increasing air pressure in the pleural cavity causes progressive collapse of the lung tissue.

podagra (pəˈdagrə) gout, particularly of the big toe.

podalic (pəˈdalik) relating to the feet. *P. version* a method of changing the lie of a fetus so that its feet will present.

podarthritis (ˌpodahˈthrietəs) inflammation of any of the joints of the foot.

podiatry (pəˈdieətree) chiropody. The examination, diagnosis, treatment and prevention of diseases and malfunction of the foot, lower limb and related structures. The main role of the podiatrist or chiropodist is to assess and treat abnormalities and diseases of the foot, and to give advice on proper care of the foot and the prevention of foot problems.

pointillage (ˌpwanhtiˈlahzh) [Fr.] a method of massage using the tips of the fingers.

poison (ˈpoyzən) any substance that, applied to the body externally or taken internally, can cause injury to any part or cause death.

poisoning (ˈpoyzəning) the morbid condition produced by a poison. The poison may be swallowed, inhaled (*see* CARBON MONOXIDE), injected by a stinging insect as in a BEE STING, or spilled or otherwise brought into contact with the skin.

polioencephalitis (ˌpohleeoh·enˌkefəˈlietəs, -ˌsef-) acute inflammation of the cortex of the brain.

poliomyelitis (ˌpohleeohˌmieəˈlietəs) an acute, notifiable, infectious viral disease that attacks the central nervous system, injuring or destroying the nerve cells that control the muscles and sometimes causing paralysis; also called polio. Paralysis most often affects the limbs but can involve any muscles, including those that control breathing and swallowing. Since the development and the use of vaccines against poliomyelitis, the disease has been virtually eliminated in wealthier countries, where vaccination rates are high, but is still common in many other parts of the world. (*See* Appendix 7.)

poliovirus (ˌpohleeohˈvierəs) a small RNA-containing virus which causes poliomyelitis.

pollinosis (ˌpoləˈnohsəs) hay fever; allergic rhinitis; an allergy caused by various kinds of pollen (also pollenosis).

pollution (pəˈlooshən) 1. the act of destroying the purity of or contaminating something. 2. contamination of the environment by poisons, radioactive substances, accidental chemical spillage, microorganisms or other wastes from industrial activity, vehicle exhausts or untreated sewage. Pollution into the environment has been linked at many levels as being injurious to good health. Air pollution causes respiratory problems while noise pollution has been linked to hearing loss, insomnia and poor concentration.

polyarteritis (ˌpoleeˌahtəˈrietəs) inflammatory changes in the walls of the small arteries.

polyarthralgia (ˌpoleeahˈthralji·ə) pain in several joints.

polyarthritis (ˌpoleeahˈthrietəs) inflammation of several joints at the same time, as seen in rheumatoid arthritis.

polycoria (ˌpoleeˈkor·ri·ə) a congenital abnormality in which there are one or more holes in the iris in addition to the pupil.

polycystic (ˌpoleeˈsistik) containing many cysts. *P. kidney disease* a hereditary disease in which there is massive enlargement of the kidney with the formation of many cysts. Severe bleeding into cysts can occur. End-stage renal disease can affect many members of one family. *P. ovary syndrome* STEIN–LEVENTHAL SYNDROME.

polycythaemia (ˌpoleesieˈtheemi·ə) an abnormal increase in the number of red cells in the blood. Erythrocythaemia. *P. vera* a rare disease in which there is a greatly increased production of red blood cells and also of leucocytes and platelets. The skin becomes flushed, with cyanosis, thrombosis and splenomegaly.

polydactylism (ˌpoleeˈdaktəˌlizəm) the condition of having more than the normal number of fingers or toes.

polydipsia (ˌpoleeˈdipsi·ə) abnormally excessive thirst. It may be a symptom of diabetes.

polyhydramnios (ˌpoleeˈhie·dramnee·os) *see* HYDRAMNIOS.

polymorphic light eruption (ˌpoleeˈmorfik ˈliet əˈrupshən) a common skin condition caused by exposure to sunlight.

polymorphonuclear (ˌpoleeˌmawfohˈnyookli·ə) 1. having nuclei of many different shapes. 2. a polymorphonuclear leucocyte.

polymorphous (ˌpoleeˈmawfəs) occurring in several or many different forms.

polymyalgia rheumatica (ˌpoleemieˌalji·ə rooˈmatikə) persistent aching pain in the muscles, often involving the shoulder or the pelvic girdle and spine. Associated with morning stiffness. More common in older people.

polymyositis (ˌpoleeˌmieohˈsietəs) a generalised inflammation of the muscles, with weakness and joint stiffness, particularly around the hips and shoulders.

polyneuritis (ˌpoleenyəˈrietəs) inflammation of many nerves at the same time.

polyneuropathy (ˌpoleenyəˈropəthee) a number of disease conditions of the nervous system.

polyopia (ˌpoleeˈohpi·ə) the perception of two or more images of the same object. Multiple vision.

polyp (ˈpolip) a pedunculated tumour of mucous membrane. A polypus.

polypharmacy (ˌpoleeˈfahməsee) 1. the administration of many drugs together. This increases the likelihood of side effects from drug interactions and of non-compliance by the patient. The taking of over-the-counter medications and the use of complementary therapies may enhance the problem. 2. the administration of excessive medication.

polyposis (ˌpoleeˈpohsəs) the presence of many polyps in an organ. *Familial adenomatous p.* a hereditary condition in which large numbers of polyps develop in the colon, which may become malignant.

polyuria (ˌpoleeˈyoo·ri·ə) an abnormally large output of urine due either to an excessive intake of liquid or to disease, often diabetes.

POMs *see* PRESCRIPTION-ONLY MEDICINES.

pompholyx (ˈpomfəliks) an intensely pruritic skin condition in which vesicles appear on the hands and feet, particularly on the palms and soles. Typically occurring in repeated, self-limiting attacks.

pons (ponz) a bridge of tissue connecting two parts of an organ. *P. varolii* the part of the brain that connects the cerebrum, cerebellum and MEDULLA OBLONGATA.

Pontiac fever (ˈponteeˌak ˈfeevə) an influenza-like illness with little or no pulmonary involvement, caused by *Legionella pneumophila*. It is not life-threatening, as is the pulmonary form known as Legionnaires' disease.

popliteal (ˌpopləˈteeəl, popˈliti·əl) relating to the posterior part of the knee joint. *P. cyst* fluid-filled cyst developing at the back of the knee. Also known as Baker's cyst.

poppers (popəz) a street name for nitrite inhalants generally, or amyl nitrite in particular, taken in substance misuse to achieve 'an elevated mood' or 'high'.

population (ˌpopyəˈlayshən) 1. the total number of persons inhabiting a given geographical area or location. 2. in statistics, the aggregate of individuals or items from which a sample for a study is drawn. 3. any group that is distinguished by a particular trait or situation.

pore (por) a minute circular opening on a surface. *Sweat p.* an opening of a sweat gland on the skin surface.

porphyria (paw'firi·ə) an inborn error in the metabolism of porphyrins, resulting in PORPHYRINURIA. Several types of porphyria are known depending on the affected gene. The manifestations of porphyria include gastrointestinal, neurological and psychological symptoms, cutaneous photosensitivity, pigmentation of the face (and later of the bones) and anaemia, with enlargement of the spleen.

porphyrin ('pawfərən) one of a number of pigments used in the production of the haem portion of haemoglobin.

porphyrinuria (ˌpawfərə'nyoo·ri·ə) the presence of an excess of porphyrin in the urine.

porta ('pawtə) an opening in an organ through which pass the main vessels.

portacaval (ˌpawtə'kahvəl) pertaining to the portal vein and the inferior vena cava. *P. anastomosis* the joining of the portal vein to the inferior VENA CAVA so that much of the blood bypasses the liver. It is used in the treatment of portal hypertension.

portage system ('pawtij ˌsistəm) a method of behaviour modification taught to family members to enable them to assist a child with special needs in development and acquiring skills for everyday living.

portfolio (pawtfohleeoh) a collection of competency evidence assembled by the practitioner/student, which demonstrates the owner's professional development. The portfolio may include such material as journals, marked assessments, evidence of reflective practice or other examples that document the acquisition of new skills, knowledge, understanding and achievements relevant to professional practice. *See* PROFILE.

port wine stain *see* NAEVUS FLAMMEUS.

position (pə'zishən) attitude or posture. *Dorsal p.* lying flat on the back. Also called supine position. *Dorsal recumbent p.* the person lies on the back with lower limbs flexed and rotated outwards; used in vaginal examination, application of obstetrical forceps and other procedures. *Fowler's p.* the person sits upright or leaning back slightly; legs can be straight or bent at the knees. *Genupectoral or knee–chest p.* resting on the knees and chest with arms crossed above the head. *Lateral p.* relating to lying on the left or right side. *Left lateral recumbent p.* the posture assumed by the person, lying on the left side with the right thigh and knee drawn up. Also called Sims' position or semi prone position. *Lithotomy p.* lying on the back with thighs raised and knees supported and held widely apart. *Orthopnoeic p.* a body position that enables a person to breathe comfortably; to achieve this the person assumes an upright or semivertical position by using pillows to support the head and chest, or sits upright in a chair. Used for people with orthopnoea (difficulty with breathing except in the upright position). *Prone p.* lying with the face down as opposed to the *supine p.,* which is lying with the face up. *Reverse Trendelenburg* *p.* a supine position with the person on a plane inclined with the head higher than the rest of the body and appropriate safety measures such as a footboard. *Right lateral recumbent p.* the posture assumed by the person, lying on the right side with the left thigh and knee drawn up. *Semi Fowler's p.* similar to Fowler's position but with the head less elevated. *Trendelenburg p.* a supine position in which the feet are higher (15–30 degrees) than the head.

positive (ˈpozətiv) having a value greater than zero; indicating existence or presence, as chromatin-positive or Wassermann-positive; characterised by affirmation or cooperation. The opposite of negative.

positive end-expiratory pressure (PEEP) (posətiv end ˌekˈspəraytəree preshə) in mechanical ventilation, a positive airway pressure maintained until the end of expiration. A PEEP higher than the critical closing pressure holds alveoli open until the end of expiration and can markedly improve the arterial PO_2 in patients with a lowered functional residual capacity (FRC), as in acute respiratory failure.

positron emission tomography (PET) (pozitron ˌəˈmishən ˌtəˈmogrəfee) a diagnostic imaging technique used in nuclear medicine based on the detection of positively charged particles with a short half-life known as positrons that are emitted by radioactive labelled substances introduced into the body. PET scanning produces three-dimensional images of the metabolic and chemical activity of tissues in the body, e.g. the brain.

posseting (ˈposəting) regurgitation of a small amount of milk by an infant immediately after a feed.

post-exposure prophylaxis (PEP) (pohst ekspohzhə profəlaksis) the administration of antibiotics, antiviral agents or active and/or passive vaccination following exposure to an infectious agent, e.g. antiretroviral drugs after exposure (usually occupationally, but may include sexual exposure) to human immunodeficiency virus (HIV).

post-traumatic stress disorder (PTSD) (pohst trawˈmatik stres disˈawdə) following the experience of a major incident, such as injury, rape or drowning, or other serious event, such as a natural disaster, warfare—the person may experience insomnia, acute anxiety, nightmares and 'flashbacks' resulting in depression, loss of concentration, apathy and guilt. This reaction may be immediate or delayed, and may last for a variable time. Support and counselling are needed and many people find antidepressants of the selective serotonin re-uptake inhibitor type are beneficial.

postconcussional syndrome (ˌpohst-kənˈkushən'l ˈsinˌdrohm) constant headaches with mental fatigue, difficulty in concentration and insomnia that may persist after head injury.

posterior (poˈstiə·ri·ə) behind a part. Dorsal. The opposite of anterior. *P. chamber* that part of the aqueous chamber that lies behind the iris, but in front of the lens.

postgastrectomy syndrome (pohst gaˈstrektəmee ˈsinˌdrohm) *see* DUMPING.

posthumous (ˈpostyəməs) occurring after death. *P. birth* one occurring after the death of the father, or by caesarean section after the death of the mother.

postmature (pohstməˈtyooə) a state in which the pregnancy is prolonged after the expected date of delivery. Due to many variables it is difficult to estimate, but may exist when a pregnancy has lasted 41–42 weeks from the last menstrual period.

postmenopausal (pohstmenəpawzəl) relating to or occurring in the period following the menopause. *See* MENOPAUSE. *P. bleeding* vaginal bleeding that happens at least 12 months after menstruation has ceased.

postmortem (pohst'mawtəm) [L.] after death. *P. examination* autopsy.

postnatal (pohst'nayt'l) after childbirth. *P. care* includes care of the mother for at least 6 weeks after delivery. *P. check* an examination of the mother preferably 6 weeks after childbirth: (a) regarding the mother's general health; and (b) to find out the state of the uterus, pelvic floor and vagina. *P. depression* a common problem affecting more than 1 in 10 women within a year of giving birth. It can also affect fathers. Symptoms include persistent low mood, difficulties in concentration and decision-making, loss of interest, lack of energy, feeling tired, disturbances of sleep and appetite and difficulty bonding. May occur shortly after delivery or up to a year later. Treatment includes psychological therapy, self-help, diet, exercise and maybe antidepressant drugs. *P. exercises* taught to the mother by the midwife or physiotherapist during the puerperium to strengthen the pelvic floor and abdominal muscles but also includes deep breathing and leg exercises as preventative measures against respiratory tract infection and deep vein thrombosis. *P. period* up to 6 weeks after the birth of the baby.

postpartum (pohst'pahtəm) occurring after labour. *P. psychosis* a rare but serious mental health condition occurring shortly after the birth of a baby where the mother has symptoms of hallucinations, delusions, manic mood and depression. Also known as puerperal psychosis.

postprandial (pohst'prandi·əl) occurring after a meal.

postural ('postyərəl) relating to a position or posture. *P. drainage* drainage of secretions from specific lobes or segments of the lung, aided by careful positioning of the patient. *P. psychosis* a rare but serious mental health condition occurring shortly after the birth of a baby where the mother has symptoms of hallucinations, delusions, manic mood and depression. Also known as puerperal psychosis.

potassium (pə'tasi·əm) *symbol* K. A metallic alkaline element which is a constituent of all plants and animals. Its salts are widely used in medicine.

Pott's disease (pots di'zeez) *Percivall Pott, British surgeon, 1714–1788.* Tuberculosis of the spine.

Pott's fracture (pots frakchə) a fracture-dislocation of the ankle, involving fracture of the lower end of the tibia, displacement of the talus and sometimes fracture of the medial malleolus.

pouch (powch) a pocket-like space or cavity. *Morison's p.* a fold of peritoneum below the liver also known as the hepatorenal pouch. *P. of Douglas* the lowest fold of the peritoneum between the uterus and rectum.

poultice ('pohltis) a soft, moist mass of about the consistency of cooked cereal, spread between layers of muslin, linen, gauze or towels and applied hot to a given area in order to create moist local heat or to counter irritation.

Poupart's ligament (ˈpoopahts ˈligəmənt) *François Poupart, French anatomist, 1661–1708.* The inguinal ligament. The tendinous lower border of the external oblique muscle of the abdominal wall, which passes from the anterior spine of the ilium to the os pubis.

poverty (povətee) the lack of sufficient material, economic and cultural resources to sustain an existence compatible with wellbeing. *Absolute p.* the situation of not having sufficient resources to maintain nutrition for good health or to provide shelter and living accommodation. *P. of speech* marked deficit in spontaneous speech; replies to questions are perfunctory, monosyllabic or unforthcoming. *P. trap* a situation whereby an increase in a person's income results in a loss of state benefits leaving them no better off. *Relative p.* where a person's living standards are below those of the community in which the person lives.

power calculation (powə kalkyoo-layshən) a measure of statistical power used in research. The likelihood of a study to produce statistically significant results.

powerlessness (ˈpowələsnəs) without power or ability leading to a feeling of being without influence on their personal situation. People may feel powerless in their dealings with health services and healthcare professionals.

practice (praktis) the exercise of a profession. *P. nurse* a member of the primary healthcare team who is a registered nurse employed by general practitioners to work within the practice setting, providing healthcare services to the population served by the practice. *General p.* the medical specialty concerned with the planning and provision of comprehensive primary health care on a continuing basis.

practitioner (prakˈtishənə) a person who practises a profession. *See* NURSE PRACTITIONER.

Prader-Willi syndrome (ˈpradah willee ˈsinˌdrohm) *Andrea Prader, Swiss paediatrician and endocrinologist, 1919–2001; Heinrich Willi, Swiss paediatrician, 1900–1971* a genetic disorder due to loss of function of specific genes. Symptoms include poor feeding in babies, weak muscles and delayed development. In childhood, there is constant hunger leading to obesity and type 2 diabetes, and mild to moderate learning disability.

pre-eclampsia (ˌpree·əˈklampsi·ə) a condition occurring in late pregnancy. The symptoms include proteinuria, hypertension and oedema.

preceptor (prəˈseptə) 1. a teacher, an instructor. 2. a registered nurse or midwife with experience in the relevant clinical field, who provides newly registered nurses or midwives with support and guidance in making the transition from student to registered nurse or midwife. Preceptors should be provided with specific preparation for their role.

preceptorship (preeˈseptəˌship) a period of support, given by a preceptor, of at least the first 4–12 months of registered practice for the newly registered nurse or midwife or for those returning to nursing after a break of more than 5 years.

precipitate (prəˈsipəˌtayt) a deposit of solid matter which was previously in solution.

precipitate labour (ˌprəˈsipətət laybə) unusually rapid labour with extremely quick delivery. There is danger to the mother of severe perineal lacerations, and to the child of intracranial trauma as a result of the rapid passage through the birth canal.

precocious (prəˈkohshəs) developed in advance of the norm, either mentally or physically or both.

precognition (ˌpreekogˈnishən) a direct perception of a future event which is beyond the reach of inference.

preconception (preekənˈsepshən) before pregnancy. Ensuring the mother is in optimum health before becoming pregnant.

precursor (preeˈkərsə) something that precedes. In biological processes, a substance from which another, usually more active or mature, substance is formed. In clinical medicine, a sign or symptom that heralds another.

prediabetes (preeˌdie·əˈbeetis, -teez) a state which precedes diabetes mellitus, in which the disease is not yet clinically manifested. In pregnancy, the diabetes may become evident, or the patient may remain well but give birth to an unusually large child. The condition can be detected by a fasting blood glucose or oral glucose tolerance test.

predisposition (ˌpreedispəˈzishən) susceptibility to a specific disease.

pregnancy (ˈpregnənsee) being with child; the condition from conception to expulsion of the fetus. The normal period is 280 days or 40 weeks counted from the first day of the last normal menstrual period. *Ectopic* or *extrauterine p.* pregnancy occurring outside the uterus, in the uterine tube (*tubal p.*) or very rarely in the abdominal cavity. *P. tests* tests used to demonstrate whether conception has occurred. These detect the human chorionic gonadotrophin (hCG) produced by the embryo from the days after the first missed period.

prejudice (ˈprejədəs) preconceived opinion, which can be used negatively or positively. *See* BIAS.

premature (ˌpreməˈtyooə) occurring before the anticipated time. *P. contraction* a form of cardiac irregularity in which the ventricle contracts before its anticipated time. *See* SYSTOLE. *P. ejaculation* emission of semen before or at the beginning of sexual intercourse. *P. infant* preterm infant. A child born before the 37th completed week of gestation.

premedication (ˌpreemedəˈkayshən) drugs given preoperatively in order to reduce fear and anxiety and to facilitate the induction and maintenance of, and recovery from, anaesthesia.

premenstrual (preeˈmenstrooəl) preceding menstruation. *P. endometrium* the hypertrophied and vascular mucous lining of the uterus immediately before the menstrual flow starts. *P. syndrome (PMS)* feelings of nervousness, depression, irritability, bloating, breast pain and loss of interest in sex experienced by some women in the days before their menstrual periods. Emotional and physical symptoms usually disappear with the onset of menstruation.

premolar teeth (preeˈmohlə teeth) a bicuspid tooth in front of the molars on each side of the upper and lower jaws. *See* DENTITION.

prenatal (preeˈnayt'l) preceding birth; antenatal. *P. care* care of the pregnant woman before delivery of the infant.

prepuce (ˈpreepyoos) foreskin; the loose fold of skin covering the glans penis.

presbyopia (ˌpresbeeˈohpi·ə) diminution of accommodation of the lens of the eye due to a loss of elasticity, occurring normally with ageing and usually resulting in hyperopia, or farsightedness.

prescription (prəˈskripshən) a formula written by a medically qualified doctor, or a specially qualified nurse, directing the pharmacist to supply the medication. Also contains instructions to the patient indicating how the medication is to be taken.

prescription-only medicines (POMs) (ˌprəˈskripshən ohnlee medsənz) drugs and medicines that are not available 'over the counter' and can only be obtained by prescription from the pharmacist.

presenile (preeˈseeniel) prematurely aged in mind and body. *See* DEMENTIA.

presentation (ˌprezənˈtayshən) in obstetrics, that portion of the fetus that appears in the centre of the neck of the uterus (*see* figure below).

pressure (ˈpreshə) stress or strain. The force exerted by one object upon another. *P. garment* often used

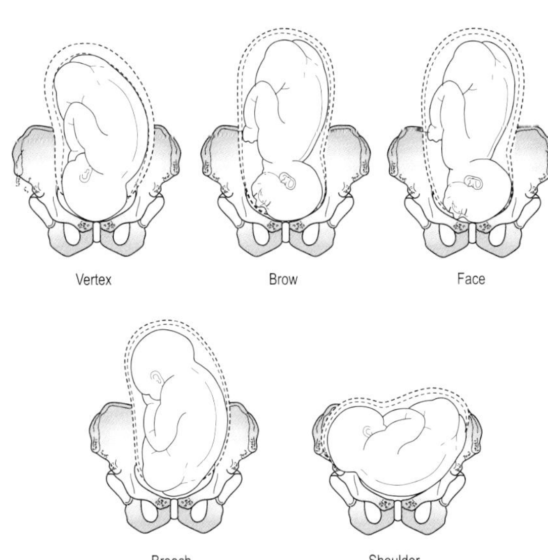

Fetal presentations.

in the treatment of burns and scalds to reduce scarring. Made of lycra (a strong, synthetic, slightly elastic fibre), the garment is worn by the patient to exert firm pressure on the affected area, e.g. to prevent keloid scarring following burns or scalds. *P. group* an organisation or charitable association that seeks to pressurise local and central government to advance the interests of that group. *P. point* the point at which an artery can be compressed against a bone in order to stop bleeding. *P. injury* a localised injury to the skin and/or underlying tissue usually over a bony prominence, as a result of pressure, shear and/or friction, or a combination of these factors; previously called a pressure ulcer, decubitus ulcer or bedsore. *P. injury risk areas* areas of the body where the tissues may be compressed between the bed and the underlying bone, especially the sacrum, greater trochanters and heels; the tissues become ischaemic (*see* figure, p. 387). *P. injury risk assessment scales* regular assessment of the patient's nutrition, general condition especially of the skin and pressure areas, is focal in the prevention of pressure ulcers. Pressure injury risk assessment scales are used to monitor and record data for the nursing care plan. *Braden scale* a pressure injury assessment scale mainly used in North America, similar to the Norton scale. *Norton scale* pressure injury risk assessment scale devised by Norton, McLaren and Exton Smith in the UK. Used primarily in the care of older people and reviewed on a weekly basis. It comprises five health state components, each with a four-point descending scale. Maximum points are 20 and the minimum 5; a 'score' of 14 and below indicates that the patient is at risk of developing pressure injuries and needs 1–2-hourly changes of posture and the use of pressure-relieving devices. *Waterlow scale* a comprehensive scale that recognises there are many factors influencing the development of pressure injuries. Waterlow's scale includes such factors as build (weight/height), mobility, sex, age, continence, appetite, the state of skin and other influencing factors such as medication, surgery and neurological deficits. *P. point* the point at which an artery can be compressed against a bone in order to stop bleeding (*see* figure, p. 387).

presystole (preeˈsistəlee) the period in the cardiac cycle just before systole.

preterm (ˈpreetərm) before term, i.e. before the 37th completed week of pregnancy. *P. infant* baby born before 37 weeks' gestation. The baby will be of low birth weight, but may also be small for gestational age. Gestational age is assessed using the Dubowitz score. Preterm infants are prone to respiratory distress syndrome, feeding problems due to immature sucking, swallowing and coughing reflexes, hypothermia, jaundice and infection. *P. labour* labour that occurs before 37 weeks' gestation. It may occur spontaneously as a result of changing hormone levels, an overstretched uterus or weak cervix or due to infection; the obstetrician may attempt to arrest labour by the administration of tocolytic drugs until conditions are more favourable for the baby to be born. Labour may be induced before term because of poor maternal or fetal health, and thus the extrauterine environment will be less hazardous for the infant.

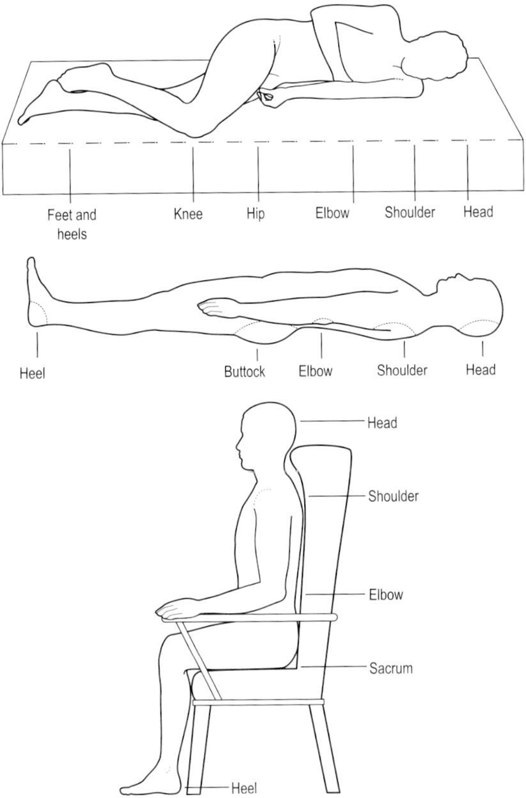

Pressure injury risk areas.

prevalence (ˈprevələns) the number of persons who have a specific disease or condition that are present in a defined population at one specific point in time. *See* INCIDENCE.

preventative (ˌprəˈventətiv) serving to avert the occurrence of; prophylactic.

priapism (ˈprieəˌpizəm) persistent erection of the penis, usually without sexual desire. It may be caused by local or spinal cord injury.

prickly heat (ˈpriklee heet) miliaria; heat rash. A skin eruption characterised by minute red spots with central vesicles.

primary (priemərее) first in order of time or importance.

primary care (ˌpriemərее ˈkair) the level of care in the HEALTHCARE SYSTEM that consists of initial care outside institutions. *P. healthcare* the care given to individuals in the community at the first point of contact with the primary healthcare team. First contact may be the general practitioner, a community nurse, paramedic or a community nurse.

primary nurse (ˌpriemərее ˈnərs) a nurse who is responsible for the planning, implementation and evaluation of nursing care for assigned patients and their families for the duration of the patients' stay in hospital. The primary nurse delegates to an associate nurse when off duty but the primary nurse remains responsible and accountable for the patient's nursing care.

primary nursing (ˌpriemərее ˈnərsing) a system for delivering nursing care that consists of four design elements: (a) allocation and acceptance of individual responsibility for decision-making to/by one individual; (b) individual assignment of daily care; (c) direct communication channels; and (d) one person responsible for the quality of care administered to patients on a unit 24 hours a day, 7 days a week.

primary source (priemərее saws) in a research study, the original source of data, e.g. manuscripts, documents or first-hand accounts. Primary sources are preferred over secondary sources because of the reduced potential for bias and distortion beyond the control of the researcher.

primigravida (ˌprieməˈgravidə) a woman who is pregnant for the first time.

primipara (ˌpriemiˈparə, prieˈmipərə) a woman who has given birth to her first child.

prion (prieon) tiny protein-based infectious agent similar to a virus. Prions transmit diseases, including CREUTZFELDT-JAKOB DISEASE in humans and BOVINE SPONGIFORM ENCEPHALOPATHY (BSE) in cattle. Prions do not contain nucleic acids and are difficult to destroy.

probability (ˌprobəˈbilətee) a statistical term meaning the likelihood of an association between variables being due to chance.

probiotics (ˌprohbieˈotiks) dietary supplements containing live microorganisms that may confer health benefits on the host.

problem-oriented record (ˌprobləmˌ ori·entəd ˈreˌkord) a multi-professional approach to patient care record-keeping that focuses on the patient's specific health problems and the structuring of a healthcare plan designed to cope with the identified problems.

process (ˈprohses) in anatomy, a prominence or outgrowth of any part.

procidentia (ˌprohsəˈdenshi·ə) complete prolapse of an organ, particularly the uterus so that the cervix extrudes through the vagina.

proctalgia (prokˈtalji·ə) pain in the rectum and anus; proctodynia.

proctitis (prokˈtietəs) inflammation of the rectum.

proctoscope (ˌproktohˈskohp) an instrument used to examine the rectum and the distal part of the colon. It is a short hollow tube that has a small light attached at the end.

proctosigmoiditis (ˌproktohˌsigmoyˈdietəs) inflammation of the rectum and sigmoid colon.

prodrome (ˈprohdrohm) a symptom that appears before the true diagnostic signs of a disease.

prodrug (ˈprohˌdrug) a compound that on administration must undergo chemical conversion by metabolic processes before becoming an active pharmacological agent, thus avoiding gastrointestinal side effects.

profession (prəˈfeshən) 1. an avowed, public declaration or statement of intention or purpose. 2. a calling or vocation requiring specialised knowledge, methods and skills, as well as preparation in an institution of higher learning in the scholarly, scientific and historical principles underlying such methods and skills. Members of a profession are committed to continuing study, to enlarging their body of knowledge, to placing service above personal gain and to providing practical services vital to human and social welfare. A profession functions autonomously and is committed to higher standards of achievement and conduct.

professional (prəˈfeshən'l) 1. pertaining to one's profession or occupation. 2. one who is a specialist in a particular field or occupation. *Allied health p.* a person with special training, and licensed when necessary, who works closely with other health professionals with responsibilities bearing on patient care. *P. disciplinary process* complaints against nurses from members of the public or an employer are reported to the statutory regulatory body (*see* P. SELF-REGULATION below). The professional conduct of the nurse is then investigated and judged by peers. The ultimate sanction is that the nurse is removed from the professional register. *P. organisation* an organisation formed to deal with issues of mutual concern for its members who share common goals and professional status (*see* PRESSURE GROUP). *P. self-regulation* the means whereby a profession monitors its own standards for quality and continuing professional and educational development. Each profession has its own professional regulatory body, e.g. Medical Board of Australia for medically qualified practitioners and the Nursing and Midwifery Board of Australia for nurses and midwives.

profile (ˈprohˌfiel) 1. a simple outline, as of the side view of the head or face; by extension, a graph representing quantitatively a set of characteristics determined by tests. 2. a record of achievements developed during a course of study, or subsequently. *See* PORTFOLIO.

progeny (ˈprojənee) issue. Descendants.

progeria (prohˈjeeri·ə) premature ageing, the signs of which appear in childhood.

progesterone (prohˈjestəˌrohn) a hormone of the corpus luteum which plays an important part in the regulation of the menstrual cycle and in pregnancy.

progestogen (prohˈjestəjən) one of a group of steroid hormones having an action similar to that of progesterone.

prognathism (ˈprognəˌthizəm) enlargement and protrusion of one or both jaws.

prognosis (progˈnohsəs) a forecast of the probable course and outcome of an attack of disease and the prospects of recovery, as indicated by the nature of the disease and the symptoms of the case.

progressive supranuclear palsy (proˈgressiv ˌsooprəˈnyookli·ə ˈpawlzee) a rare and progressive condition caused by damage to brain cells over time due to a build-up of the protein tau. Symptoms include problems with balance, movement, speech and swallowing.

projectile vomiting (prəˈjektieəl) *see* VOMITING.

projection (prəˈjekshən) in psychology, an unconscious process by which painful thoughts or impulses are made acceptable by transferring them on to another person or object in the environment.

prolactin (prohˈlaktən) a milk-producing hormone of the anterior lobe of the pituitary body which stimulates the mammary gland.

prolapse (ˈprohlaps) the downward displacement of an organ or part of one. *P. of the cord* expulsion of the umbilical cord before the fetus presents. *P. of an intervertebral disc* displacement of part of an intervertebral disc; 'slipped disc'; herniated disc. *P. of the iris* protrusion of a part of the iris through a wound in the cornea. *P. of the rectum* protrusion of the mucous membrane through the anal canal to the exterior. *P. of the uterus* descent of the cervix or of the whole uterus into the vagina owing to a weakening of its supporting ligaments.

proliferation (prəˌlifəˈrayshən) rapid multiplication of cells as may occur in a malignant growth and during wound healing.

prominence (ˈprominəns) in anatomy, a projection, usually on a bone.

pronation (prohˈnayshən) turning the palm of the hand downwards.

prone (prohn) lying face downwards. *See* SUPINE.

prophylactic (ˌprofəˈlaktik) 1. relating to prophylaxis. 2. a drug used to prevent a disease developing. *See* PREVENTATIVE.

prophylaxis (ˌprofəˈlaksəs) measures taken to prevent a disease.

proprietary name (prəˈprieətree naym) the name assigned to a drug or device by the manufacturer that first made it.

proprioception (ˌprohpreeohˈsepshən) the ability to sense stimuli originating from within the body, related to spatial position, motion and equilibrium. In humans, nerves within the body itself, as well as by the semicircular canals of the inner ear, detect these stimuli to make immediate and unconscious adjustments to the muscles to maintain balance.

proprioceptor (ˌprohpreeohˈseptə) one of the sensory end-organs that provide information about movements and position of the body. They occur chiefly in the muscles, tendons, joint capsules and labyrinth.

proptosis (propˈtohsəs) forward displacement of the eyeball; EXOPHTHALMOS.

prosopagnosia (ˌprosˈop·agˈnohs·iə) an inability to recognise faces.

prostaglandin (ˌprostəˈglandən) one of several hormone substances produced in many body tissues, including the brain, lungs, uterus and semen. They are active in many ways, having cardiac, gastric and respiratory effects and causing uterine contractions. They are sometimes used for the induction of abortion. Chemically they are fatty acids.

prostate (ˈprostayt) the gland surrounding the male urethra at its junction with the bladder; during ejaculation it produces a fluid which forms part of the semen. It often becomes enlarged after middle age and may require partial removal if it causes obstruction to the outflow of urine. *P. cancer* of unknown cause and one of the most common cancers in men, usually occurring in older men. Treatments include surgery, radiotherapy, chemotherapy and hormone therapy. *P. screening* routine examination and blood testing for prostate-specific antigen (PSA) in older men, as a means to detect cancer of the prostate at an early stage.

prostatectomy (ˌprostəˈtektəmee) surgical removal of the whole or a part of the prostate gland. *Retropubic p.* removal of the gland by incising the capsule of the prostate after making a suprapubic abdominal incision. *Transurethral p.* resection of the gland through the urethra using a resectoscope. *Transvesical p.* removal of the gland by incising the bladder after making a low abdominal incision.

prostatitis (ˌprostəˈtietəs) inflammation of the prostate gland.

prosthesis (prosˈtheesəs) [Gr.] 1. the replacement of an absent part by an artificial substitute. 2. an artificial substitute for a missing part.

prostration (proˈstrayshən) a condition of extreme exhaustion.

protease (ˈprohteeˌayz) a proteolytic enzyme in the digestive juices that causes the breakdown of protein.

protective isolation (prətektivˌiesəˈlayshən) a type of ISOLATION designed to prevent contact between potentially pathogenic microorganisms and uninfected persons who have seriously impaired resistance. Also called reverse isolation.

protein (ˈprohteen) one of a group of complex organic nitrogenous compounds formed from amino acids and occurring in every living cell of animal and vegetable tissue. *Bence Jones p.* an abnormal protein found in the urine of patients suffering from multiple myeloma. *First-class p.* one that provides the essential amino acids. Sources are meat, poultry, fish, cheese, eggs and milk. *P.-bound iodine* the iodine in the plasma that is combined with protein. Measurement of this is made when assessing thyroid function. *P.-losing enteropathy* a condition in which protein is lost from the lumen of the intestine. This causes hypoproteinaemia and oedema. *Second class p.* one that comes from a vegetable source (e.g. peas, beans and whole cereal) that cannot supply all the body's needs.

proteinuria (ˌprohtəˈnyoo·ri·ə) an excess of serum proteins in the urine.

proteolysis (ˌprohteeˈoləsəs) the processes by which proteins are reduced to an absorbable form by digestive enzymes in the stomach and intestines.

proteolytic (ˌprohteeohˈlitik) 1. pertaining to, characterised by or promoting proteolysis. 2. a proteolytic enzyme.

Proteus (ˈprohtee·əs) a genus of Gram-negative bacteria common in the intestines of humans and animals and in decaying matter. They are frequently to be found in secondary infections of wounds and in the urinary tract.

prothrombin (prohˈthrombən) a constituent of blood plasma; the precursor of THROMBIN, which is formed in the presence of calcium salts and THROMBOKINASE when blood is shed. *P. time* (PT) a test to measure the activity of clotting factors. Deficiency of any of these factors leads to a prolongation of clotting time. This test is widely used for the establishment and maintenance of anticoagulant therapy.

protocol (ˈprohtəkol) a term used by researchers to indicate the method or overall plan for procedures to be carried out in a particular study. Commonly used to indicate a specific program to be followed or with exclusion criteria for the study.

protoplasm (ˈprohtəˌplazəm) the essential chemical compound of which living cells are made.

prototype (ˈprohtəˌtiep) the original form from which all other forms are derived.

Protozoa (ˌprohtəˈzoh·ə) a phylum comprising the unicellular eukaryotic organisms; most are free-living but some lead commensalistic, mutualistic or parasitic existences. Pathogenic protozoa include *Entamoeba histolytica* (cause of amoebic dysentery) and *Plasmodium vivax* (cause of malaria). *See* METAZOA.

protuberance (prəˈtyoobə·rəns) in anatomy, a rounded projecting part.

proud flesh (prowd flesh) excessive granulation tissue in a wound or ulcer.

provider (prəˈviedə) in the health services, a person, group of people or organisation supplying a service.

provitamin (prohˈvitəmən, -ˈviet-) a precursor of a vitamin. *P. 'A'* carotene. *P. 'D'* ergosterol.

proxemics (ˌprokˈsemiks) the study of how the use of personal space and other spatial aspects affects human behaviour and interactions.

proximal (ˈproksəməl) in anatomy, nearest that point which is considered the centre of a system; the opposite to distal.

prurigo (prooˈriegoh) a chronic skin disease with an irritating papular eruption.

pruritus (ˈprooriˌtəs) great irritation of the skin. It may affect the whole surface of the body, as in certain skin diseases and nervous disorders, or it may be limited in area, especially involving the anus and vulva.

pseudoangina (ˌsyoodoh·anˈjienə) false angina. Pain experienced in the left side of the chest without clinical evidence of heart disease.

pseudoarthrosis (ˌsoodohˌahˈthroh-səs) a false joint formed when the two parts of a fractured bone have failed to unite together.

pseudocoxalgia (ˌsyoodohkokˈ-salji·ə) osteochondritis of the head of the femur. PERTHES' DISEASE.

pseudocyesis (ˌsyoodohsieˈeesəs) false pregnancy; development of all the signs of pregnancy without the presence of an embryo.

pseudogynaecomastia (ˌsyoodoh-ˌgienəkohˈmasti·ə) the deposition of adipose tissue in the male breast, which may give the appearance of enlarged mammary glands.

Pseudomonas (ˌsyoodohˈmohnəs) a genus of Gram-negative motile bacilli commonly found in decaying organic matter. *P. aeruginosa* found in pus from wounds ('blue pus') and also in urinary tract infections. Also called *P. pyocyanea*.

pseudomyopia (ˌsyoodohmieˈohpi·ə) spasm of the ciliary muscle causing the same focusing defect as in myopia.

psittacosis (ˌsitəˈkohsəs) a disease of parrots and budgerigars due to

Chlamydia psittaci, communicable to humans. The symptoms resemble paratyphoid fever with bronchopneumonia.

psoas (ˈsoh·əs) a long muscle originating from the lumbar spine and inserting into the lesser trochanter of the femur. It flexes the hip joint. *P. abscess* one that arises in the lumbar region and is due to spinal caries as a result of tuberculous infection.

psoriasis (səˈrieəsəs) a chronic, recurrent skin disease characterised by reddish marginated patches with profuse silvery scaling on extensor surfaces such as the knees and elbow but which may be more widespread and may be associated with arthritis of the joints. It is non-infectious and the cause is unknown. It tends to occur in families; about one-third of the cases are believed to be related to a hereditary factor. Psoriasis may present in different forms. The most common is discoid or plague psoriasis in adults. Guttate psoriasis occurs most commonly in children, consisting of small patches that may develop over a wide area of the body. Pustular psoriasis is characterised by small pustules.

psyche (ˈsiekee) the mind, both conscious and unconscious.

psychedelic (ˌsiekəˈdelik) mind altering; a term applied to hallucinatory or psychotomimetic drugs capable of profound effects on the nature of the perception and conscious experience. *See also* HALLUCINOGEN.

psychiatrist (sieˈkieətrəst) a medically qualified doctor who specialises in psychiatry.

psychiatry (sieˈkieətree) the branch of medicine that deals with the study, treatment and prevention of mental illness.

psychoanalysis (ˌsiekoh·əˈnaləsəs) 1. a method of investigating mental processes developed by Sigmund Freud which uses the techniques of free association, interpretation and dream analysis. 2. a system of theoretical psychology formulated by Freud, based on the recognition of unconscious mental processes such as resistance, repression and transference, and of the importance of infantile experience as a determinant of adult behaviour. 3. a method of psychotherapy based on the psychoanalytical method and psychoanalytical psychology.

psychoanalyst (ˌsiekohˈanələst) one who specialises in psychoanalysis.

psychodrama (ˌsiekohˈdrahmə) group PSYCHOTHERAPY in which patients dramatise their individual conflicting situations of daily life.

psychodynamics (ˌsiekohdieˈnamiks) the understanding and interpretation of psychiatric symptoms or abnormal behaviour in terms of unconscious mental mechanisms.

psychogenic (ˌsiekohˈjenik) originating in the mind. *P. illness* a disorder that has a psychological, as opposed to an organic, origin.

psychologist (sieˈkoləjəst) one who studies normal and abnormal mental processes, development and behaviour.

psychology (sieˈkoləjee) the study of the mind and mental processes.

psychometrics (ˌsiekohˈmetriks) the measurement of mental characteristics by means of a series of tests.

psychomotor (ˌsiekohˈmohtə) related to the motor effects of mental activity. The term is applied to those mental disorders that affect muscular activity.

psychoneurosis (ˌsiekohnyəˈrohsəs) a mental disorder characterised by an abnormal mental response to a normal stimulus. The psychoneuroses include anxiety states, depression, hysteria and obsessive–compulsive neurosis.

psychopath *see* PERSONALITY (antisocial).

psychopathic disorder (ˌsiekəˈpathik disawdə) a persistent disorder or disability of the mind (whether or not including significant impairment of intelligence) which results in abnormally aggressive or seriously irresponsible conduct on the part of the patient.

psychopathology (ˌsiekohpəˈtholəjee) the study of the causes and processes of mental disorders.

psychopharmacology (ˌsiekohˌfahməˈkoləjee) the study of drugs that have an action on the mind and how such action is produced.

psychoprophylaxis (ˌsiekohˌprofəˈlaksəs) 1. a psychological technique used to prevent emotional disturbances and mental health problems. 2. a technique involving breathing control and exercises used to relieve pain during childbirth.

psychosexual (ˌsiekohˈsekshooəl) relating to the mental aspects of sex. *P. development* the stages through which an individual passes from birth to full maturity, especially in regard to sexual urges, in the total development of the person.

psychosis (sieˈkohsəs) any major mental disorder of organic or emotional origin marked by derangement of the personality and loss of contact with reality, often with delusions, hallucinations or illusions. Psychoses are classified into different types, including: schizophrenia, bipolar disorder and organic brain syndrome.

psychosomatic (ˌsiekohsəˈmatik) relating to the mind and the body. *P. disorders* those illnesses in some individuals in which emotional factors (either causative or aggravating) have a profound influence, including ANOREXIA NERVOSA and asthma respectively.

psychotherapy (ˌsiekohˈtherəpee) any of a number of related techniques for treating mental illness by psychological methods. These techniques are similar in that they all rely mainly on establishing communication between the therapist and the patient as a means of understanding and modifying the patient's behaviour. On occasion, drugs may be used, but only in order to make this communication easier.

psychotropic (ˌsiekohˈtrohfik) pertaining to drugs that have an effect on the psyche. These include antidepressants, stimulants, sedatives and tranquillisers.

ptosis (ˈtohsəs) 1. drooping of the upper eyelid due to paralysis of the third cranial nerve. It may be congenital or acquired. 2. prolapse of an organ.

ptyalin (ˈtieələn) an enzyme (amylase) in saliva which metabolises starches.

puberty (ˈpyoobətee) the period during which secondary sexual characteristics develop and the reproductive organs become functional. Generally between the 12th and 17th years.

pubes (ˈpyoobeez) pubic hair or the area on which it grows.

pubic (ˈpyoobik) pertaining to the pubis.

pubis (ˈpyoobəs) the anterior part of a hip bone. The left and right pubic bones meet at the front of the pelvis at the pubic symphysis.

public domain (publik dohmayn) intellectual property, e.g. published documents, programs or files, usually from government sources and other organisations, that have been released for unconditional access and use by the public.

public health (ˈpublik helth) the area of healthcare that is concerned with promoting and protecting health and wellbeing, preventing ill health and prolonging life through organised efforts in the population. To achieve these goals various methods are used, including health surveillance, monitoring and analysis of data, assessment of evidence and interventions, the identification of significant trends, the development of policy and strategy, the investigation of outbreaks of disease and of any risk to health, health protection, health improvement and public health intelligence. *P. h. nursing* a field of nursing that is concerned with the health needs of the community. Public health nurses may work with families in the home, community groups, in schools, at the workplace, in government agencies, in rural and remote areas and at major health facilities. Also called community health nursing.

pudendal block (pyooˈdendʼl blok) a form of local analgesia induced by injecting a solution of 0.5% or 1% lignocaine around the pudendal nerve. Used mainly for EPISIOTOMY and forceps delivery.

pudendum (pyooˈdendəm) the external genitalia, especially those of a woman.

puerperal (pyooərˈperəl) pertaining to childbirth. *P. fever* or *sepsis* infection of the genital tract following childbirth.

puerperium (ˌpyooəˈperi·əm) a period of about 6 weeks following childbirth when the reproductive organs are returning to their normal state.

Pulex (ˈpyooleks) a genus of fleas. *P. irritans* those parasitic on humans. The type that infests rats may transmit plague to humans.

pulmonary (ˈpulməˌnə·ree, ˈpuhl-) pertaining to or affecting the lungs. *P. embolism* obstruction of the pulmonary artery or one of its branches by an embolus. *P. function test* a procedure for determining the capacity of the lungs to move gas in and out of the lungs and to exchange oxygen and carbon dioxide efficiently. The results are compared with predicted values which adjust for gender, age, height and race. *P. hypertension* an increase of blood pressure in the lungs, usually as a result of disease of the lung. *P. oedema* an excess of fluid in the lungs. *P. stenosis* a narrowing of the passage between the right ventricle of the heart and the pulmonary artery. The condition is frequently congenital. *P. tuberculosis see* TUBERCULOSIS. *P. valve* the valve at the point where the pulmonary artery leaves the heart.

pulp (pulp) any soft, juicy animal or vegetable tissue. *P. cavity* the centre of a tooth containing blood tissue and nerves. *Splenic p.* the reddish-brown tissue of the spleen.

pulsation (pulˈsayshən) a beating or throbbing.

pulse (puls) the local rhythmic expansion of an artery, which can be felt with the finger, corresponding to each contraction of the left ventricle of the heart. It may be felt in any artery sufficiently near the surface of the body, which passes over a bone, and the normal adult resting rate is 60–100 beats/min. In childhood it is more rapid, varying from 130 in infants to 80 in older children. *Alternating p.* alternate strong

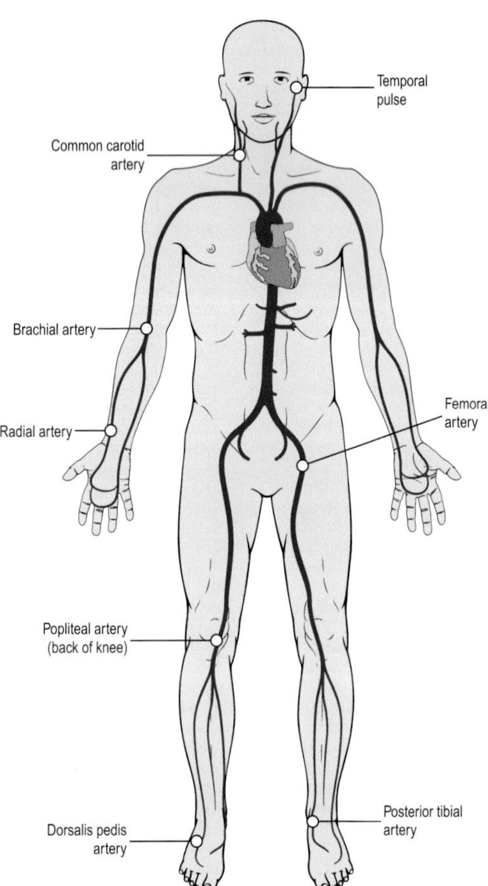

Pulse points.

and weak beats; pulsus alternans. *Paradoxical p.* pulsus paradoxus; the pulse rate slows on inspiration and quickens on expiration. It may occur in constrictive pericarditis. *P. deficit* a sign of atrial fibrillation; the pulse rate is slower than the apex beat. *P. oximetry* a non-invasive method for measuring haemoglobin oxygen saturation in the body using a sensor from an oximeter that is attached, usually to a finger but may be elsewhere, e.g. nose, finger or ear lobe. *P. point* one of the sites on the surface of the body where arterial pulsations can be easily palpated. The most commonly used pulse point is over the radial artery at the wrist (*see* figure p. 396). *Running p.* there is little distinction between the beats. It occurs in haemorrhage. *Thready p.* thin and almost imperceptible pressure. *Venous p.* that felt in a vein; it is usually taken in the right jugular vein.

pulseless disease (ˈpulsləs diˈzeez) progressive obliteration of the vessels arising from the aortic arch leading to loss of the pulse in both arms and carotids and to symptoms associated with ischaemia of the brain, eyes, face and arms. Also known as Takayasu's disease.

punctate (ˈpungktayt) dotted. *P. erythema* a rash of very fine spots.

punctum (ˈpungktəm) a point or small spot. *P. lacrimalis* one of the two openings of the lacrimal ducts at the inner CANTHUS of the eye.

puncture (ˈpungkchə) 1. the act of piercing with a sharp object. 2. the wound so produced. *Cisternal p.* the withdrawal of fluid from the cisterna magna. *Lumbar p.* the removal of cerebrospinal fluid by puncture between the third and fourth lumbar vertebrae. *Sternal p.* the withdrawal of bone marrow from the manubrium of the sternum. *Ventricular p.* the withdrawal of cerebrospinal fluid from a cerebral ventricle.

pupil (ˈpyoopəl) the circular aperture in the centre of the iris through which light passes into the eye. *Argyll Robertson p.* absence of response to light but not to accommodation; characteristic of neurosyphilis of the central nervous system and diabetic neuropathy. *Artificial p.* one made by cutting a piece out of the iris when the centre part of the cornea or the lens is opaque. *Fixed p.* one that fails to respond to light or convergence. *Multiple p.* two or more openings of the iris. *Tonic p.* one that reacts slowly to light or to convergence or both.

pupillary (pyooˈpilə·ree) referring to the pupil.

purgative (ˈpərgətiv) a laxative, an aperient drug. Purgatives may be: (a) irritants like cascara, senna, rhubarb and castor oil; (b) lubricants like liquid paraffin; or (c) mechanical agents that increase bulk, such as bran and agar preparations.

purine (ˈpyoo·reen) a heterocyclic compound that is the nucleus of the purine bases such as adenine and guanine, which occur in DNA and RNA. *See* PYRIMIDINE.

purpura (ˈpərpyərə) a condition characterised by extravasation of blood in the skin and mucous membranes, causing purple spots and patches. There are two general types of purpura: (a) primary or idiopathic (usually autoimmune) thrombocytopenic purpura, in which the cause is unknown; and (b) secondary or symptomatic thrombocytopenic purpura, which may be associated with exposure to drugs or other chemical agents, systemic diseases (such as systemic lupus erythematosus), diseases affecting the bone marrow (such as leukaemia) and infections (such as septicaemia viral infections and allergic reactions). *Allergic p., anaphylactic p.* Schönlein–Henoch purpura; also called Henoch–Schönlein. *Idiopathic thrombocytopenic p.* (ITP) an acquired thrombocytopenia which may be acute or chronic in its course. Acute ITP is common in young children. The disorder is usually self-limiting and rarely fatal. Chronic ITP is more insidious in onset, and is more common in young adult women. *P. senilis* dark purplish–red ecchymoses occurring on the forearms and backs of the hands in the older person; the platelet count is normal. *Schönlein–Henoch p.* non-thrombocytopenic purpura of unknown cause, most often seen in children; associated with various clinical symptoms, such as urticaria and erythema, arthropathy and arthritis, gastrointestinal symptoms and renal involvement. *Steroid p.* purpura secondary to prolonged use of steroids. The platelet count is normal, the basic defect being the loss of supporting connective tissue. *Thrombocytopenic p.* purpura associated with a decrease in the number of platelets in the blood.

purulent (ˈpyoo·rələnt) containing or resembling pus.

pus (pus) a thick, yellow semi-liquid substance consisting of dead leucocytes and bacteria, debris of cells and tissue fluids. It results from inflammation caused by invading bacteria, mainly *Staphylococcus aureus* and *Streptococcus haemolyticus*, which have destroyed the phagocytes and set up local suppuration. *Blue p.* that produced by infection with *Pseudomonas pyocyanea*.

pustule (ˈpustyool) a small pimple or elevation of the skin containing pus. *Malignant p. see* ANTHRAX.

putative (ˈpyootətiv) supposed, reputed. *P. father* the man believed to be the father of an illegitimate child.

putrefaction (ˌpyootrəˈfakshən) decomposition of animal or vegetable matter under the influence of microorganisms, usually accompanied by an offensive odour due to gas formation.

P value (pee ˈvalyoo) the symbol used to denote the probability of test results occurring by chance.

pyaemia (pieˈeemi·ə) a condition resulting from the circulation of pyogenic microorganisms from some focus of infection. Multiple abscesses occur, the development of which causes rigor and high fever. *Portal p.* PYLEPHLEBITIS.

pyarthrosis (ˌpieahˈthrohsəs) suppuration in a joint.

pyelography (ˌpieəˈlogrəfee) *see* UROGRAPHY.

pyelolithotomy (ˌpieəlohliˈthotəmee) the surgical removal of a stone from the renal pelvis.

pyelonephritis (ˌpieəlohnəˈfrietəs) inflammation of the renal pelvis and renal substance characterised by fever, acute loin pain and increased frequency of micturition, with the presence of pus and albumin in the urine.

pyeloplasty (ˈpieəlohˌplastee) a surgical reconstruction of the renal pelvis.

pylephlebitis (ˌpieləfləˈbietəs) inflammation of the portal vein which gives rise to severe symptoms of septicaemia or PYAEMIA.

pyloric (pie'lo·rik) relating to the PYLORUS. *P. stenosis* stricture of the pyloric orifice. It may be: (a) hypertrophic when there is thickening of normal tissue; this is congenital and occurs in infants from 4–7 weeks old, usually males and first babies; (b) cicatricial, when there is ulceration or a malignant growth near the pylorus.

pyloromyotomy (pie,lo·rohmie'otə-mee) Ramstedt's operation; an incision of the pylorus performed to relieve congenital pyloric stenosis.

pyloroplasty (pie'lo·roh,plastee) a surgical procedure performed on the PYLORUS to enlarge the outlet. A longitudinal incision is made and it is resutured transversely (*see* figure). The procedure is undertaken if conservative treatment with medication is ineffective.

pylorospasm (pie,lo·roh'spazəm) forceful muscle contraction of the pylorus which delays emptying of the stomach and causes vomiting.

pylorus (pie'law·rəs) the opening into the duodenum at the lower end of the stomach. It is surrounded by a circular muscle, the *pyloric sphincter*, which contracts to close the opening.

pyoderma (,pieoh'dərmə) any purulent skin disease, e.g. impetigo.

pyogenic (,pieoh'jenik) producing pus.

pyorrhoea (pieə'reeə) a discharge of pus. *P. alveolaris* pus in the sockets of the teeth; suppurative periodontitis.

pyramidal (pə'ramid'l) of pyramid shape. *P. cells* cortical cells shaped like a pyramid from which originate nerve impulses to voluntary muscle.

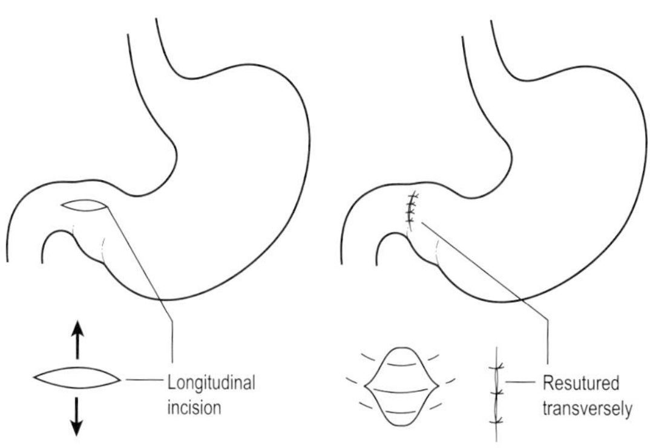

Pyloroplasty.

P. tract the nerve fibres that transmit impulses from pyramidal cells through the cerebral cortex to the spinal cord.

pyrexia (pieˈreksi·ə) fever; a rise of body temperature to any point between 37 and 40°C; above this is hyperpyrexia.

pyridoxine (ˌpirəˈdokseen) vitamin B_6. This vitamin is concerned with protein metabolism and blood formation. It is found in many types of food and deficiency is rare.

pyrimidine (pieˈrimiˌdeen) a nitrogen-containing organic compound. Thymine and cytosine are essential constituents of DNA, and uracil and cytosine of RNA. *See* PURINE.

pyrogen (ˈpierohˌjen) a substance that can produce fever.

pyromania (ˌpierohˈmayni·ə) an irresistible desire to set things on fire.

pyrosis (pieˈrohsəs) heartburn; a symptom of indigestion marked by a burning sensation in the stomach and oesophagus, with eructation of acid fluid.

pyuria (pieˈyoo·ri·ə) the presence of pus in the urine; more than three leucocytes per high-power field on microscopic examination.

Qq

QALY *see* QUALITY ADJUSTED LIFE YEAR.

Q fever (ˈkyoo ˌfeeva) an acute infectious disease of cattle which is transmitted to humans, usually by infected milk. It is caused by a RICKETTSIA, *Coxiella burnetii*, and has symptoms resembling pneumonia.

qi energy (chee enərjee) in Chinese medicine, the energy believed to be present in all living things. Qi energy is considered to flow through 12 meridian channels in the body, mainly connected to the internal organs, and considered essential to good health and wellbeing. This concept is used in a variety of complementary therapies, e.g. reflexology and acupuncture. Complementary therapy practitioners consider that any disturbance or blockage to the flow of qi energy results in illness or bodily and mental disturbance but that with manipulation, e.g. through acupuncture, the qi flow can be increased. Also called chi, prana and aura.

QRS complex (kyoo ah·r es ˈkompleks) a group of waves depicted on an electrocardiogram; also called the QRS wave. It actually consists of three distinct waves created by the passage of the cardiac electrical impulse through the ventricles and occurs at the beginning of each contraction of the ventricles (*see* figure on page 155). In a normal ELECTROCARDIOGRAM, the R wave is the most prominent of the three; the Q and S waves may be extremely weak, and are sometimes absent.

quadriceps (ˈkwodrəˌseps) four-headed. *Q. femoris muscle* the principal extensor muscle of the thigh.

quadriplegia (ˌkwodrəˈpleeji·ə) paralysis in which all four limbs are affected; tetraplegia.

quadruplets (ˌkwoˈdrooplәts) four children born at the same labour. Once very rare, but now more common with the use of fertility drugs.

qualitative research (ˌkwolətətiv ˈreeˌsərch) *see* RESEARCH.

quality (ˈkwolətee) 1. a distinguishing characteristic, property or attribute. 2. a degree or standard of excellence. *Q. adjusted life year (QALY)* a measure which assesses variations in the quality of life for the person resulting from an intervention, in relation to cost and length of life. Used for measuring the clinical and cost effectiveness of interventions. *Q. assurance* in the healthcare field, a pledge to the public by those within the various health disciplines that they will work towards the goal of an optimal achievable degree of excellence that is measured and evaluated in the services rendered to every person. *Q. indicator* a defined, measurable variable used to monitor the quality or appropriateness of an important aspect of care. Indicators may be activities, events, occurrences or outcomes. *Q. of life* a measure of the optimum energy or force that endows a person with the power to cope successfully with the full range of challenges encountered in everyday life. The term applies to all individuals, regardless of illness or handicap.

quantitative research (ˈkwontitətiv ˌreeˈsərch) *see* RESEARCH.

quarantine (ˈkwo·rənˌteen) the period of isolation of an infectious or suspected case to prevent the spread of disease. For contacts, this is the longest incubation period known for the specific disease.

quartan (ˈkwawtən) 1. recurring in 4-day cycles (i.e. by inclusive reckoning, every third day). 2. a variety of intermittent fever of which the paroxysms recur on every third day (*see* MALARIA).

quasi-experiment (ˌkwahzee əkˈ-sperəmənt) research design in which the researcher initiates an experimental treatment but some character of a true experiment is lacking.

Queensland tick typhus (ˈkweens-ˌland tik ˈtiefəs) an infection caused by *Rickettsia australis,* occurring in Australia, transmitted by ticks.

quickening (ˈkwikəning) the first perceptible fetal movement felt by the mother, usually between the fourth and fifth months of pregnancy.

quiescent (kweeˈesənt) inactive or at rest. Descriptive of a time when the symptoms of a disease are not evident.

quinsy (ˈkwinzee) a peritonsillar abscess; acute inflammation of the tonsil and surrounding cellular tissue with suppuration.

quintuplets (ˌkwinˈtyooplәts) five children born at the same labour.

quotidian (kwoˈtidi·ən) recurring every day. *Q. fever* a variety of malaria in which the fever recurs daily.

quotient (ˈkwohshənt) a number obtained by dividing one number by another. *Intelligence q. (IQ)* the degree of intelligence, estimated by dividing the mental age, reckoned from standard tests, by the age in years. *Respiratory q.* the ratio between the carbon dioxide expired and the oxygen inspired during a specified time.

qwerty (kwərtee) the standard typewriter keyboard layout that is also used for computers, with some additions.

Rr

Ra symbol for *radium*.

rabid (ˈrabid) infected with rabies.

rabies (ˈraybeez) an acute notifiable infectious disease of the central nervous system of animals, especially dogs, foxes, wolves and bats. The virus is found in the saliva of infected animals and is usually transmitted by a bite. Symptoms include fever, muscle spasms and intense excitement, followed by convulsions and paralysis, and death usually occurs. Vaccines are available.

race (rays) a term formerly used to describe a group of people sharing the same culture, language, values and beliefs. The preferred terms are now ethnic group or ethnicity.

racemose (ˈrasəˌmohz) grape-like. *R. gland* a compound gland composed of a number of small sacs, e.g. the salivary gland.

racism (raysism) the belief that races are inherently different from one another. A belief that is usually associated with the view that one race has an intrinsic superiority over others, leading to stereotyping, prejudice and discrimination. Also called racialism.

radiant (ˈraydi·ənt) emitting rays.

radiation (ˌraydeeˈayshən) the emanation of energy in the form of electromagnetic waves, including gamma rays, X-rays, infrared and ultraviolet rays and visible light rays. Radiation may cause damage to living tissues, e.g. in sunburn. *Ionising r*. a form of radiation that destabilises an atom to produce highly reactive ions, e.g. X-rays, gamma rays and particle radiation. When used therapeutically ionising radiation needs careful control and monitoring as it can cause tissue damage. *R. dosimetry* the method used to calculate the amount of radiation received by an individual. Also called radiation monitoring. *R. pneumonitis* inflammatory changes in the alveoli and interstitial tissue caused by radiation and which may lead to fibrosis. *R. sickness* a toxic reaction of the body to radiation. Any or all of the following may be present: anorexia, nausea, vomiting and diarrhoea.

radical (ˈradikəl) dealing with the root or cause of a disease. *R. cure* one which cures by complete removal of the cause.

radioactivity (ˌraydeeoh·akˈtivətee) disintegration of certain elements to ones of lower atomic weight with the emission of alpha and beta particles and gamma rays. *Induced r.* that brought about by bombarding the nuclei of certain elements with neutrons.

radiobiology (ˌraydeeohbieˈoləjee) the branch of medical science that studies the effect of radiation on live animal and human tissues.

radiodermatitis (ˌraydeeohˌdərmə-ˈtietəs) a late skin complication of radiotherapy in which there is atrophy, scarring, pigmentation and TELANGIECTASES of the skin.

radiograph (ˈraydeeohˌgrahf, -ˌgraf) the picture obtained, on specially sensitised film, by passing X-rays through the body.

radiographer (ˌraydeeˈogrəfə) a professional healthcare worker handling the radiological equipment in a diagnostic X-ray department (diagnostic radiographer) or in a radiotherapy department (therapy radiographer).

radiography (ˌraydeeˈogrəfee) the making of film records (radiographs) of internal structures of the body by exposure of film sensitised to X-rays or gamma rays. *Body-section r.* a special technique to show in detail images and structures lying in a predetermined plane of tissue, while blurring or eliminating detail in images in other planes; various mechanisms and methods for such radiography have been given various names, e.g. laminography, tomography, etc. *Double-contrast r.* a technique for revealing an abnormality of the intestinal mucosa; it involves injection and evacuation of a barium enema followed by inflation of the intestine with air under light pressure. *Neutron r.* that in which a narrow beam of neutrons from a nuclear reactor is passed through tissues; especially useful in visualising bony tissue. *Serial r.* the making of several exposures of a particular area at arbitrary intervals.

radioisotope (ˌraydeeohˈiesəˌtohp) an isotope of an element that emits radioactivity. These isotopes can occur naturally or be produced artificially by bombardment with neutrons.

radiologist (ˌraydeeˈoləjəst) a medically qualified doctor who specialises in the science of radiology.

radiology (ˌraydeeˈoləjee) the science of radiation. Using X-rays and other allied imaging techniques in the diagnosis and treatment of disease.

radiomimetic (ˌraydeeohmiˈmetik) producing effects similar to those of ionising radiations.

radionuclide (ˌraydeeohˈnyooklied) a radioactive substance which is inherently unstable. It is used in both radiodiagnosis and in radiotherapy.

radioscopy (ˌraydeeˈoskəpee) the examination of X-ray images on a fluorescent screen.

radiosensitive (ˌraydeeohˈsensətiv) pertaining to those structures that respond readily to radiotherapy.

radiotherapist (ˌraydeeohˈtherəpəst) a medically qualified doctor specialising in radiotherapy.

radiotherapy (ˌradeeohˈtherəpee) a method of treating disease and eradicating tumour cells aiming to deliver a therapeutic dose of radiation while preserving normal tissue function and structure.

radium (ˈraydi·əm) *symbol* Ra. A radioactive element obtained from uranium ores which gives off emanations of great radioactive power. Used in the treatment of some malignant diseases.

raised intracranial pressure (RIP) (rayzd intəˈkrayˌneel preshə) may be associated with a variety of conditions, e.g. haemorrhage, oedema, brain tumour, head injury or disturbance to the flow of cerebrospinal fluid.

rale (rahl) an abnormal rattling sound, heard on auscultation of the chest during respiration when there is fluid in the bronchi.

Ramsay Hunt syndrome (ˈramsee ˈhunt ˈsinˌdrohm) *James Ramsay Hunt, American neurologist, 1872–1937*. A complication of shingles involving peripheral facial nerve palsy accompanied by an erythematous vesicular rash on the ear (zoster oticus) or in the mouth.

Ramstedt's operation (ˈramshtets ˌopəˈrayshən) *Conrad Ramstedt, German surgeon, 1867–1963.* A pyloroplasty for congenital stricture of the PYLORUS in which the fibres of the sphincter muscle are divided, leaving the mucous lining intact.

randomised controlled trial (RCT) (randomiesəd ˌkənˈtrohld trieəl) a study in which experimental and control groups are randomly selected for research. There are also a number of other synonyms for this term, such as randomised clinical trial, controlled clinical trial and true experiment. *See* CONTROLLED TRIAL.

random sample (ˈrandəm ˈsahmpəl, -ˈsampəl) sample from a population obtained by ensuring that each member of that population has an equal chance of being selected. The sample selected should then demonstrate the same profile as the parent population.

range (raynj) a measure of variability; the difference between the highest and lowest scores in a set of sample data.

ranula (ˈranyələ) a retention cyst usually under the tongue when blockage occurs in a submaxillary or sublingual duct, or in a mucous gland.

rape (rayp) sexual assault or abuse; criminal forcible sexual intercourse (i.e. penetration) without the consent of the adult or child. Many cases are not reported because of feelings of shame, guilt, embarrassment or fear. Rape can occur between men, but it is most usually associated with victims who are female.

raphe (ˈrayfee) a seam or ridge of tissue indicating the junction of two parts.

rapport (raˈpaw) in psychiatry, a satisfactory relationship based upon respect, understanding and mutuality between two persons, either the doctor and the patient, or the nurse and the patient, or the patient with any significant other.

rarefaction (ˌrair·rəˈfakshən) the process of becoming less dense, e.g. in bone disease.

rash (rash) a superficial eruption on the skin, frequently characteristic of some specific fever.

Rashkind catheter (ˈrashkint ˈkathətə) a balloon catheter used to increase the size of the atrial septal defect in children who have transposition of the great vessels.

rate (rayt) the speed or frequency with which an event or circumstance occurs per unit of time, population or other standard of comparison. *Basal metabolic r. (BMR)* an expression of the rate at which oxygen is utilised in a fasting subject at complete rest as a percentage of a value established as normal for such a subject. *Birth r.* the number of live births in a population in a specified period of time (crude birth rate), for the female population (refined birth rate), or for the female population of childbearing age (true birth rate), usually expressed per year per 1000 of the estimated mid-year population. *Death r.* the number of deaths per stated number of persons (1000, 10,000 or 100,000) in a certain region in a certain time (crude death rate). The death rate calculated with allowances made for age and sex distribution in the population is termed the standardised death rate. Also called *mortality r. Glomerular filtration r.* an expression of the quantity of glomerular filtrate formed each minute in the nephrons of both kidneys, calculated by measuring the clearance of specific substances, e.g. insulin or creatinine.

ratio (ˈrayˌsheeoh) an expression of the quantity of one substance or entity in relation to that of another; the relationship between two quantities expressed as the quotient of one divided by the other or the highest level of measurement that possesses the characteristics of categorising, ordering and ranking, and also has an absolute or natural zero that has empirical meaning. *Lecithin–sphingomyelin r.* the ratio of lecithin to sphingomyelin in AMNIOTIC FLUID.

rationalisation (ˌrashənəlieˈzayshən) in psychiatry, the mental process by which individuals explain their behaviour, giving reasons that are advantageous to themselves or are socially acceptable. It may be a conscious or an unconscious act.

Rauwolfia (rawˈwuhlfi·ə, row-) a genus of tropical trees and shrubs. The dried root of *R. serpentina* is sometimes used as an antihypertensive and sedative, e.g. reserpine.

Raynaud's phenomenon (disease) (ˈraynohz fəˈnomənən (diˈzeez)) *Maurice Raynaud, French physician, 1834–1881.* Raynaud's phenomenon is characterised by episodic digital ischaemia producing pallor or cyanosis of the fingers or toes, provoked by stimuli such as emotion, cold, trauma, hormones and drugs. Treatment includes keeping the hands and feet as warm as possible. Vasodilator drugs may be helpful in severe cases.

RBC red blood cell (erythrocyte).

RCT *see* RANDOMISED CONTROLLED TRIAL.

RDS respiratory distress syndrome (infants). *See* RESPIRATORY.

re-education (ˌree·edyəˈkayshən) the rehabilitation through education and training of people with physical disabilities or those with learning difficulties to enable them to develop their potential.

reaction (reeˈakshən) counteraction; a response to the application of a stimulus. *R. time* the interval between the stimulus and the response.

reactive (reeˈaktiv) in psychiatry, used to describe a mental condition brought about by adverse external circumstances. *R. arthritis* formerly known as Reiter's syndrome. A rare type of arthritis that causes inflammation of the urinary tract, eyes, skin and mucous membrane and joints; usually following an infection. *R. depression* one that arises in this way and is not endogenous.

reagent (reeˈayjənt) a substance employed to produce a chemical reaction.

reality (reeˈalətee) agreed as an absolute by members of the same culture as the total of all things related to perception, meaning and behaviour. Not imaginary, fictitious or pretended. *R. orientation see* ORIENTATION.

real-time scanner (reel tiem skanə) 1. an ultrasound scanner that gives a moving visual display. 2. Antiviral software which continuously scans files for viruses each time the computer accesses them.

rebound (rəˈbownd) sudden contraction of a muscle after a period of relaxation.

rebreathing bag (reeˈbreething bag) a flexible bag (attached to a mask) which is squeezed to pump anaesthetic gases during surgery or for oxygen during resuscitation into the lungs.

recall (rəˈkawl, ˈreekawl) to bring back to consciousness.

receptor (rə'septə) 1. a sensory nerve ending that receives stimuli for transmission through the sensory nervous system. 2. a molecule on the surface or within a cell that recognises and binds with specific molecules, producing some effect in the cell.

recessive (rə'sesiv) tending to recede; the opposite to dominant. *R. gene* a gene that will produce its characteristics only when present in a HOMOZYGOUS state; both parents need to possess the particular gene, and there is a 1 in 4 chance of a child inheriting it homozygously.

recipient (rə'sipi·ənt) one who receives, as with a blood transfusion, or a tissue or organ graft. *Universal r.* a person thought to be able to receive blood of any 'type' without agglutination of the donor cells.

Recklinghausen's disease ('rekling,howzənz di'zeez) *see* NEUROFIBROMATOSIS.

recombinant (,ree'kombinant) 1. a new cell or individual that results from genetic recombination. 2. pertaining or relating to such cells or individuals. *R. DNA technology* the process of taking a gene from one organism and inserting it into the DNA of another. Also called gene splitting.

recommended daily allowance (RDA) (rekə'mended daylee əlowanz) a standard for the daily intake of individual nutrients and calories for groups of people.

recommended international non-proprietary name (rekə'mended inter,nashənəl nonprə'prieətree naym) a system whereby all drugs have a recommended non-proprietary name that is used internationally.

reconstituted family (ree'kən stuhtyooted faməlee) *see* FAMILY (BLENDED).

record ('re,kord) 1. a piece of evidence or information relating to the subject of the record, e.g. a change that has occurred or an account of an incident. 2. a document preserving the written account. 3. the state of being set down of information; individual personal details for preservation in writing or some other permanent form.

recrudescence (,reekroo'desəns) renewed aggravation of symptoms after an interval of abatement.

rectal ('rekt'l) relating to the rectum. *R. examination* inspection by insertion of a glove-covered finger or with the aid of a PROCTOSCOPE. *R. varices* haemorrhoids.

rectocele ('rektoh,seel) hernia or prolapse of the rectum, usually caused by overstretching of the vaginal wall at childbirth. Proctocele.

rectopexy ('rektoh,peksee) the operation for fixation of a prolapsed rectum.

rectosigmoid (,rektoh'sigmoyd) the junction of the pelvic colon with the rectum.

rectovaginal (,rektohvə'jienəl) concerning the rectum and vagina.

rectovesical (,rektoh'vesikəl) concerning the rectum and bladder.

rectum ('rektəm) the lower end of the large intestine from the sigmoid flexure to the anus.

recumbent (ree'kumbənt) lying down in the dorsal position.

recuperation (ree,koopə'rayshən) convalescence; recovery of health and strength. *See* REHABILITATION.

recurrent (ree'kurənt) liable to recur.

redback spider (redbak spiedə) *Latrodectus hasseltii*, a species of spider found in Australasia from the Latrodectus family of spiders found worldwide.

redback spider antivenom (redbak spiedə anteevenəm) a refined

F(ab)^2 portion of IgG which binds to venom fractions, neutralising venom activity and promoting clearance. May be administered by IV or IM route.

Redivac® drainage tube (ˈrediˌvak ˈdraynij tyoob) a proprietary closed suction drainage system used mainly postoperatively for abdominal wounds.

reduction (reeˈdukshən, rə-) 1. the correction of a fracture, dislocation or hernia. 2. the removal of oxygen or the addition of hydrogen to a substance or, more generally, the gain of electrons; the opposite of oxidation. *Closed r.* the manipulative reduction of a fracture without incision. *Open r.* reduction of a fracture after incision into the fracture site.

referred pain (rəˈfərd payn) pain which occurs at a distance from the place of origin due to the sensory nerves entering the spinal cord at the same level. For example, the phrenic nerve supplying the diaphragm enters the spinal cord in the cervical region, as do the nerves from the shoulder, and so an abscess on the diaphragm may cause pain in the shoulder. *See* SYNALGIA.

reflection (rəˈflekshən) 1. a turning or bending back, as in the folds produced when a membrane passes over the surface of an organ and then passes back to the body wall that it lines. 2. in nursing and healthcare practice, conscious and systematic thinking about one's actions; the review, analysis and evaluation of those situations that have occurred, usually after but maybe during an event. An active process by which the practitioner learns from situations with a view to improving future practice.

reflective practice (rəflektiv praktis) an active process by which the healthcare professional is able to review, analyse and evaluate events or situations. This conscious monitoring process can be based on any conceptual model, and may use supervision of peers in the process. The aim is to facilitate and enhance professional practice.

reflex (ˈreefleks) reflected or thrown back. *Accommodation r.* the alteration in the shape of the lens according to the distance of the image viewed. *Conditioned r.* that which is not natural but is developed by association and frequent repetition until it appears natural. *Corneal r.* the automatic reaction of closing the eyelids after exertion of light pressure on the cornea. This is a test for unconsciousness, which is absolute when there is no response. Also known as the blink reflex. *Deep r.* a muscle reflex elicited by tapping the tendon or bone of attachment. *Gag r.* the reflex action that occurs when the back of the throat is stimulated. *Light r.* alteration of the size of the pupil in response to exposure to light. *R. action* an involuntary action following immediately upon some stimulus, e.g. the knee jerk or the withdrawal of a limb from a pinprick. *R. arc* the sensory and motor neurones, together with the connector neurone, which carry out a reflex action (*see* figure, p. 409). *R. zone therapy* a system of complementary therapy, similar to reflexology, in which it is believed that the body is divided into 10 longitudinal and three transverse zones, with corresponding divisions in the feet. Reflex zone therapy can be used to identify areas of disorder or disease in the body and a sophisticated grip technique is used to massage

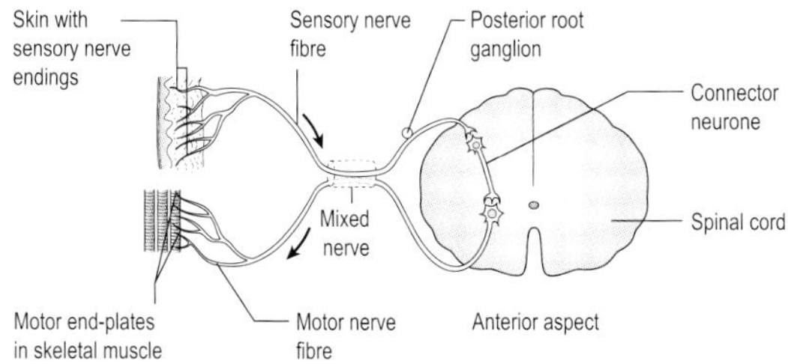

Reflex arc.

the feet and to treat the problem. The therapy may also be performed on the hands, which correspond closely to the feet, the tongue, the face and the back.

reflexology (ˌreefleksˈoləjee) a technique for treating certain disorders by deep massaging to the soles of the feet or palms of the hands, using principles similar to those of acupuncture.

reflux (ˈreefluks) a backward flow; regurgitation.

refraction (rəˈfrakshən) 1. the bending or deviation of rays of light as they pass obliquely through one transparent medium and penetrate another of different density. 2. in ophthalmology, the testing of the eyes to ascertain the amount and variety of refractive error that may be present in each of them.

refractory (rəˈfraktə·ree) not yielding to, or resistant to, treatment; resistant. *R. period* the period immediately after some activity during which a nerve or muscle is unable to react to a fresh impulse.

regeneration (rəˌjenəˈrayshən, ree-) renewal, as in new growth of tissue in its specific form after injury.

regimen (ˈrejimən) a regulated system, program or schedule such as diet, therapy or exercise intended to promote health or achieve another beneficial effect for a person's wellbeing. Regimen is used in preference to the word regime, which usually refers to a political system or structure.

register (ˈrejəstə) an epidemiological term meaning an index or file of all cases with a particular disease or condition in a defined population.

registered nurse (ˈrejəstərd nərs) *see* NURSE.

registrar (ˈrejəˌstrah) 1. an official keeper of records. 2. a doctor training to be a specialist.

regression (rəˈgreshən) 1. a return to a previous state of health. 2. in psychiatry, a tendency to return to primitive or child-like modes of behaviour. Some degree of regression frequently accompanies physical illness and hospitalisation. People who have a mental illness may exhibit regression to an extreme degree, reverting to infantile behaviour (atavistic regression).

regulatory bodies (ˌregyooˈlaytə·ree bodeez) organisations responsible for defining and monitoring preparation and practice of a specific professional group, e.g. Australian Health Practitioner Regulatory Agency; *see* AHPRA.

regurgitation (rəˌgurjəˈtayshən) backward flow, e.g. of food from the stomach into the mouth. Fluids regurgitate through the nose in paralysis, affecting the soft palate. *Aortic r.* backward flow of blood into the left ventricle when the aortic valve is incompetent. *Mitral r.* mitral incompetence. *See* MITRAL.

rehabilitation (ˌreehəˌbiləˈtayshən) (rehab) re-education, particularly where an individual has been ill or injured, to enable them to become capable of useful activity. *R. centre* one that provides services (such as physical, occupational and speech therapy), vocational training and programs designed to facilitate recovery and restore functional ability after illness or surgery.

rehydration therapy (reehiedrayshən therəpee) the treatment of dehydration by administering fluid and salts by mouth (oral rehydration) or by intravenous infusion. *See* FLUID BALANCE.

reinforcement (ˌree·ənˈfawsmənt) the increasing of force or strength. In behavioural science, the process of presenting a reinforcing stimulus to strengthen a response. *See* CONDITIONING. A positive reinforcer is a stimulus that is added to the environment immediately after the desired response. It serves to strengthen the response, i.e. to increase the likelihood of its occurring again. Examples of a positive reinforcer are food, money, a special privilege or some other reward that is satisfying to the subject.

Reiter's syndrome (ˈrietərz ˈsinˌdrohm) *Hans Reiter, German bacteriologist, 1881–1969.* Former name for REACTIVE ARTHRITIS.

rejection (rəˈjekshən) 1. in immunology, the formation of antibodies by the host against transplanted tissue, with eventual destruction of the transplanted tissue. 2. in psychosocial terms, the denial of acceptance or affection, or the exclusion of another person.

relapse (rəˈlaps, ˈreeˌlaps) the return of a disease after an interval of convalescence.

relapsing fever (rəˈlapsing ˈfeevə) one of a group of similar notifiable infectious diseases transmitted to humans by the bites of ticks. Marked by alternating periods of normal temperature and periods of fever relapse. The diseases in the group are caused by several different species of SPIROCHAETES belonging to the genus *Borrelia*.

relaxant (rəˈlaksənt) a drug or other agent that brings about muscle relaxation or relieves tension.

relaxation (reeˌlakˈsayshən) a lessening of tension, which may be observed when muscles slacken after they have contracted; it is characterised by feelings of peace and calmness. *R. therapy* classes in which people are taught breathing and other exercises to use for the relief of pain, stress and tension. Used as part of the preparation for childbirth.

relaxin (rəˈlaksən) a hormone that is produced by the CORPUS LUTEUM of the ovary; it softens the cervix and loosens the pelvic ligaments to aid the birth of the baby.

releasing factor (rəˈleesing ˈfaktə) a substance (hormone) produced in the HYPOTHALAMUS which causes the anterior pituitary gland to release other hormones.

reliability (rə,lieə'bilətee) the quality of being trustworthy or dependable. In research the consistency or constancy of a measuring instrument. *Interrater r.* the consistency of observations between two or more observers, often expressed as a percentage of agreement between observers or a coefficient of agreement that takes into account the element of chance. This is usually used with the direct observation method. *R. coefficient* a number between 0 and 1 that expresses the relationship between the error variance, true variance and the observed score. A 0 correlation indicates no relationship. The closer to 1 the coefficient is, the more reliable the tool. *Test–retest r.* administration of the same instrument twice to the same subjects under the same conditions within a prescribed time interval, with a comparison of the paired scores to determine the stability of the measure.

REM (rem) rapid eye movement, a phase of SLEEP associated with dreaming and characterised by rapid movements of the eyes. Paradoxical sleep.

reminiscence therapy (remə'nisəns 'therəpee) measures to stimulate long-term elderly patients with memorabilia, films and songs meaningful to their generation. Used in conjunction with or as a prelude to reality orientation therapy. *See* ORIENTATION.

remission (rə'mishən) subsidence of the signs and symptoms of a disease for a long time.

remittent (rə'mitənt) decreasing at intervals. *R. fever* one in which a partial fall in the temperature occurs daily.

remotivation (rə,mohtə'vayshən) in psychiatry, a group therapy technique administered by the nursing staff in a psychiatric unit, which is used to stimulate the communication skills and an interest in the environment of long-term, withdrawn patients.

renal ('reenəl) relating to the kidney. *R. calculus* stone in the kidney. *R. clearance tests* laboratory tests that determine the ability of the kidney to remove certain substances from the blood. *R. dialysis* the application of the principles of dialysis for treatment of renal failure (*see* below). *See also* HAEMODIALYSIS and PERITONEAL DIALYSIS. *R. failure* inability of the kidney to maintain normal function. It may be *acute* or *chronic*. Acute renal failure is a sudden, severe interruption of kidney function. It is normally the complication of another disorder and is reversible. Chronic renal failure is a progressive loss of kidney function. In its early stage, renal function can remain adequate but the GLOMERULAR FILTRATION RATE (GFR) is depressed and plasma chemistry begins to show abnormalities as waste products accumulate. In the later stage, known as end-stage renal disease (ESRD), the GFR deteriorates and when URAEMIA becomes evident and the person becomes symptomatic, dialysis is started or the person receives a transplant. *R. threshold* the level of the blood glucose beyond which it is excreted in the urine; normally 10 mmol/L (180 mg/100 mL). *R. transplant* transfer of a healthy kidney from a donor into the body of someone with serious kidney disease. *R. tubule* the thin tubular part of a nephron. A uriniferous tubule.

renin (ˈreenən) a proteolytic enzyme released into the bloodstream when the kidneys are ischaemic. It causes vasoconstriction and increases the blood pressure.

rennin (ˈrenən) an enzyme present in gastric juice that curdles milk.

reorganisation (reeˌawgənieˈzayshən) healing by formation of new tissue identical to the tissue that was injured or destroyed.

reovirus (ˌreeohˈvierəs) any of a group of RNA viruses isolated from healthy children, children with febrile and afebrile upper respiratory disease or children with some forms of diarrhoea.

repetitive strain injury (rəˈpetətiv strayn injəree) (RSI) a soft-tissue disorder produced by repetitive use of muscle, especially if the muscle activity involves an awkward or uncomfortable position of the body. Particularly affects keyboard operators, musicians, packers and machine operators.

replication (ˌrepləˈkayshən) 1. the turning back of a tissue on itself. 2. the process by which DNA duplicates itself when the cell divides.

replogle tube (riˈplohgəl tyoob) a double-lumen aspiration catheter attached to low-pressure suction apparatus.

repolarisation (ˌreepohlə·rieˈzayshən) the process by which the cell is restored to its resting potential.

representative sample (ˌreprəˈzentətiv ˈsahmpəl) a sample whose key characteristics closely approximate those of the population.

repression (rəˈpreshən) 1. the act of restraining, inhibiting or suppressing. 2. in psychiatry, a defence mechanism whereby a person unconsciously banishes unacceptable ideas, feelings or impulses from consciousness. A person using repression to obtain relief from mental conflict is unaware that he or she is 'forgetting' unpleasant situations as a way of avoiding them (motivated forgetting).

reproductive system (ˌreeprəˈduktiv sistəm) all those parts of the male and female bodies associated with the production of children.

research (ˌˈreeˌsərch) the systematic, logical and empirical inquiry into the possible relationships among particular phenomena to produce verifiable knowledge. *Applied r.* tests the practical limits of descriptive theories but does not examine the efficacy of actions taken by practitioners. *Basic r.* theoretical or pure research that generates, tests and expands theories that explain or predict phenomena. *Qualitative r.* the study of research questions about human experiences. It is often conducted in natural settings, and uses data that are words or text rather than numerical in order to describe the experiences that are being studied. *Quantitative r.* the process of testing relationships, differences and cause and effect interactions among and between variables. These processes are tested against hypotheses and/or research questions. *R. design* the plan or blueprint for conduct of a study. *R. question* a key preliminary step wherein the foundation for a study is developed from the research problem, thus resulting in the research hypothesis/question.

resection (reeˈsekshən) surgical removal of a part. *Submucous r.* removal of part of a deflected nasal septum from beneath a flap of mucous membrane which is then replaced. *Transurethral r.* a method of removing portions of an enlarged prostate gland via the urethra.

resectoscope (ree'sektə,skohp) a telescopic instrument by which pieces of tissue can also be removed. Used for transurethral PROSTATECTOMY.

reservoir ('rezə,vwah) 1. a storage place or cavity. 2. the host or environment in which an organism lives and from which it is able to infect susceptible individuals, e.g. hands, skin, nose and bowel.

residential care (,rezə'denshəl kair) the provision of care for frail, older people in a variety of settings, e.g. local authority residential homes for the older person or private residential homes.

residual (rə'zidyooəl) remaining. *R. air, r. volume* the amount of air remaining in the lungs after breathing out fully. *R. urine* urine remaining in the bladder after voiding; seen with bladder outlet obstruction and disorders affecting nerves controlling bladder function.

resistance (rə'zistəns) the degree of opposition to a force. 1. in electricity, the opposition made by a non-conducting substance to the passage of a current. 2. in psychology, the opposition, stemming from the unconscious, to repressed ideas being brought to consciousness. *Drug r.* the ability of a microorganism to withstand the effects of a drug that are lethal to most members of its species. *Peripheral r.* that offered to the passage of blood through small vessels and capillaries. *R. to infection* the natural power of the body to withstand the toxins of disease.

resolution (,rezə'looshən) 1. in medicine, the process of returning to normal. 2. the disappearance of inflammation without the formation of pus.

resonance ('rezənəns) in medicine, the reverberating sound obtained on percussion over a cavity or hollow organ, such as the lung.

respiration (,respə'rayshən) the gaseous interchange between the tissue cells and the atmosphere. *Artificial r.* the production of respiratory movements by external effort. *External r.* breathing, which comprises inspiration (when the external intercostal muscles and the diaphragm contract and air is drawn into the lungs) and expiration (when the air is breathed out). *Intermittent positive pressure r. (IPPR)* respiration produced by a ventilator. *Internal* or *tissue r.* the interchange of gases that occurs between tissues and blood through the walls of capillaries. *Laboured r.* that which is difficult and distressed. *Stertorous r.* snorting; a noisy breathing. *See* CHEYNE–STOKES RESPIRATION.

respirator ('respə,raytə) an apparatus to qualify the air breathed through it, or a device for giving artificial respiration or to assist pulmonary ventilation (*see also* VENTILATOR).

respiratory (rə'spirətree) pertaining to respiration. *Acute r. distress syndrome (ARDS)* a group of signs and symptoms resulting in acute respiratory failure; characterised clinically by TACHYPNOEA, DYSPNOEA, TACHYCARDIA, CYANOSIS and low PaO_2 that persists even with oxygen therapy. *R. acidosis* reduced alveolar ventilation resulting in raised arterial PCO_2 and carbonic acid. *R. alkalosis* an abnormal condition characterised by raised blood pH and decreased arterial PCO_2.

R. arrest cessation of breathing. *R. distress syndrome of newborn (NRDS), idiopathic r. distress syndrome, infant r. distress syndrome (IRDS)* a condition occurring in preterm infants, full-term infants of diabetic mothers, and infants delivered by caesarean section, and associated with pulmonary immaturity and inability to produce sufficient lung surfactant. Also called hyaline membrane disease. *R. failure* a life-threatening condition in which respiratory function is inadequate to maintain the body's need for oxygen supply and carbon dioxide removal while at rest; also called acute ventilatory failure. *See* TYPE I and TYPE II RESPIRATORY FAILURE. *R. insufficiency* a condition in which respiratory function is inadequate to meet the body's needs when increased physical activity places extra demands on it. *R. quotient* the ratio of the volume of expired carbon dioxide to the volume of oxygen absorbed by the lungs per unit of time. *R. shock* circulatory SHOCK due to interference with the flow of blood through the great vessels and chambers of the heart, causing pooling of blood in the veins and abdominal organs and a resultant vascular collapse. The condition sometimes occurs as a result of increased intrathoracic pressure in patients who are being maintained on a mechanical ventilator. *R. syncytial virus* a virus isolated from children with bronchopneumonia and bronchitis, characteristically causing severe respiratory infection in very young children but less severe infections as the children grow older. *R. therapy* the technical specialty concerned with the treatment, management and care of people with respiratory problems including administration of medical gases.

respite care (ˈrespət kair) temporary care provided for those with disabilities or serious and terminal conditions to allow relief for family and other carers. Provision may be on a daily or longer-term basis and in a variety of settings, e.g. in a hospice, residential aged care facility, hostel or in the family home. *See* HOSPICE.

restless legs syndrome (restləs legz ˈsinˌdrohm) characterised by weakness and coldness in the lower limbs, with an unpleasant feeling of a creeping tingling sensation firstly in the lower limbs but possibly extending to the thighs, arms and hands. Symptoms most commonly occur in people in bed at night, or sometimes in those sitting in chairs for prolonged periods during the day. Occurs primarily in the older person. The cause is unknown but it may be due to a vascular disorder. *See also* WILLIS-EKBOM DISEASE.

resuscitation (rəˌsusəˈtayshən) restoration to life or consciousness of one apparently dead, or whose respirations have ceased. *Cardiopulmonary r.* an emergency technique used in cardiac arrest to re-establish heart and lung function until more advanced life support is available. (*See* Appendix 6.)

retching (ˈreching) strong, involuntary effort to vomit.

retention (rəˈtenshən) holding back. *R. cyst see* CYST. *R. defect* a defect of memory. Inability to retain material in the mind so that it can be recalled when required. *R. of urine* inability to pass urine from the bladder which may be due to obstruction or be of neurological origin.

reticular (rə'tikyələ) resembling a network. *R. formation* areas in the brainstem from which nerve fibres extend to the cerebral cortex.

reticulocyte (rə'tikyəloh,siet) a red blood cell that is not fully mature. It retains strands of nuclear material.

reticulocytosis (rə,tikyəlohsie'toh-sis) the presence of an increased number of immature red cells in the blood, indicating overactivity of the bone marrow.

reticuloendothelial system (rə,tikyəloh,endə'theeli·əl sistəm) a collection of endothelial cells in the liver, spleen, bone marrow and lymph glands that produce large mononuclear cells or MACROPHAGES. They are phagocytic, destroy red blood cells and have the power of making some antibodies.

retina ('retənə) the innermost coat of the eyeball, formed of nerve cells and fibres from which the optic nerve leaves the eyeball and passes to the visual area of the cerebrum. The impression of the image is focused upon it.

retinal ('retənəl) relating to the retina. *R. detachment* partial detachment of the retina from the underlying choroid layer, resulting in loss of vision. It may result from several causes, including trauma or the presence of a tumour, or from high myopia. *R. migraine* an eye condition with brief spells of blindness or flashing lights, usually in one eye. The episodes are frightening but generally harmless. Also known as ocular migraine.

retinitis (,retə'nietəs) inflammation of the retina. *R. pigmentosa* a group of diseases, frequently hereditary, marked by progressive loss of retinal function, especially associated with contraction of the visual field and impairment of vision. The disorder often follows a slow course over a period of many years, but there is considerable variation in the progression of the disease.

retinoblastoma (,retənohbla'stohmə) a rare malignant tumour arising from retinal cells. Occurs in infancy and may be hereditary. Treatment includes cryotherapy, laser treatment, irradiation and chemotherapy, but ENUCLEATION may be required.

retinol (retənohl) a light-absorbing molecule obtained from vitamin A. *See* RHODOPSIN.

retinopathy (,retə'nopəthee) any non-inflammatory disease of the retina. *R. of prematurity* previously known as retrolental fibroplasia. Scarring and retinal detachment in babies who have received oxygen therapy due to prematurity. *R. pigmentosa* a group of diseases, frequently hereditary, marked by progressive loss of retinal function, especially associated with contraction of the visual field and impairment of vision. The disorder often follows a slow course over a period of many years, but there is considerable variation in the progression of the disease. *Diabetic r.* a complication of diabetes. Retinal haemorrhages occur, resulting in permanent visual damage, and retinal detachment may follow. Photocoagulation of damaged retinal blood vessels by a laser beam may be performed to prevent haemorrhage from the vessels. *Hypertensive r.* retinal change occurring as a result of high blood pressure.

retinoscope (ˈretinəˌskohp) an instrument which illuminates the retina and is used to detect and measure refractive errors. Retinoscopy.

retrobulbar (ˌretrohˈbulbə) pertaining to the back of the eyeball. *R. neuritis* dimness of vision due to inflammation of the optic nerve.

retroflexion (ˌretrohˈflekshən) a bending back, particularly of the uterus when it is bent backwards at an acute angle, the cervix being in its normal position. *See* RETROVERSION.

retrograde (ˈretrəˌgrayd) going backwards. *R. amnesia* forgetfulness of events occurring immediately before an illness or injury. *R. urography* radiographic examination of the kidney after the introduction of a radio-opaque substance into the renal pelvis through the urethra.

retrolental fibroplasia (ˌretrohˈlent'l ˌfiebrohˈplayzi·ə) a fibrous condition of the anterior vitreous body which develops when a premature infant is exposed to high concentrations of oxygen. Both eyes are affected, seriously interfering with vision and leading to retinal detachment. Early treatment with a freezing probe (cryopexy) can prevent retinal detachment.

retroperitoneal (ˌretrohˌperətəˈneeəl) behind the peritoneum.

retropharyngeal (ˌretrohfəˈrinji·əl, -ˌfarənˈjeeəl) behind the pharynx.

retropubic (ˌretrohˈpyoobik) behind the pubic bone.

retrospection (ˌretrohˈspekshən) looking back, especially into the past.

retrospective (ˌretrohˈspektiv) looking back on or dealing with past events. *R. study* a non-experimental research design that begins with the phenomenon of interest (dependent variable) in the present and examines the relationship to another variable (independent variable) in the past, e.g. discharged patients' records, to discover causal factors relevant to outcomes.

retrosternal (ˌretrohˈstərnəl) behind the sternum.

retroversion (ˌretrohˈvərshən) a lifting backwards, particularly of the uterus when the whole organ is tilted backwards. *See* RETROFLEXION.

retrovirus (ˈretrohˌvierəs) a group of viruses belonging to the family Retroviridae, principally infecting and frequently causing diseases in animals, but also including viruses that infect and cause disease in humans, e.g. HUMAN IMMUNODEFICIENCY VIRUS (HIV) and human T-cell leukaemia/lymphoma/lymphotropic virus type I (HTLV-I).

Rett syndrome (ˈret ˈsinˌdrohm) *Andreas Rett, Austrian neurologist, 1924–1997.* A rare genetic disorder affecting brain development resulting in severe physical and learning disabilities caused by a mutation in the MECP2 gene.

Reverdin's graft (ˈrevərdahnz grahft) *Jaques-Louis Reverdin, Swiss surgeon, 1842–1929.* A form of skin graft in which pieces of skin are placed as islands over the area.

Reye's syndrome (riez ˈsinˌdrohm) *Douglas Reye, Australian pathologist, 1912–1977.* An acute, potentially fatal illness that may follow a virus occurring in children, in which there is fatty degeneration of the liver and the brain and raised intracranial pressure, accompanied by vomiting, convulsions and coma. The cause of Reye's syndrome is unknown, but administration of salicylates in children under the age of 16 years is not recommended unless advised by a doctor. This follows evidence that aspirin may be a contributory factor in the development of Reye's syndrome.

rhabdomyosarcoma (ˌrabdohˌmieohsahˈkohmə) a rare malignant growth of striated muscle. It grows rapidly and metastasises early.

rhagades (ˈragəˌdeez) cracks or fissures in the skin, especially those round the mouth.

Rhesus factor (ˈreesəs ˈfaktə) *see* RH FACTOR.

rheumatism (ˈroomə‚tizəm) any of a variety of disorders marked by inflammation, degeneration or metabolic derangement of the connective tissue structures, especially the joints and related structures, and attended by pain, stiffness or limitation of motion. *Acute r.* or *rheumatic fever* an acute fever associated with previous streptococcal infection and occurring most commonly in children. The onset is usually sudden, with pain, swelling and stiffness in one or more joints. There is fever, sweating and TACHYCARDIA, and CARDITIS is present in most cases. Sometimes the symptoms are minor and ignored. This disease is the most common cause of MITRAL STENOSIS because scar tissue results from the inflammation.

rheumatoid (ˈroomə‚toyd) resembling rheumatism. *R. arthritis see* ARTHRITIS.

rheumatology (ˌroomәˈtoləjee) the branch of medicine dealing with disorders of the joints, muscles, tendons and ligaments.

Rh factor (ahˈaych ˈfakˌtə) the red blood cells of most humans carry a group of genetically determined antigens and are said to be Rh-positive (Rh^+). Those who do not are said to be Rh-negative (Rh^-). This is of importance as a cause of anaemia and jaundice in a newborn when the infant is Rh^+ and the mother Rh^-. The result of this incompatibility (isoimmunisation) is the formation of an antibody which causes excessive HAEMOLYSIS in the child's blood. *See* ANTI-D GAMMA GLOBULIN.

rhinitis (rieˈnietəs) inflammation of the mucous membrane of the nose.

rhinoplasty (ˈrienohˌplastee) a plastic operation on the nose; repairing a part of or forming an entirely new nose.

rhinorrhoea (ˌrienəˈreeə) an abnormal discharge of mucus from the nose.

rhinoscopy (rieˈnoskəpee) examination of the interior of the nose. *Anterior r.* examination through the nostrils with the aid of a speculum. *Posterior r.* examination through the nasopharynx by means of a rhinoscope.

rhinovirus (ˈrienohˌvierəs) one of a genus of small RNA-containing viruses that cause respiratory diseases, including the common cold.

Rhipicephalus (ˌriepiˈkefələs, -ˈsef-) a genus of ticks that can transmit the *RICKETTSIAE* which cause typhus and relapsing fever.

rhodopsin (rohˈdopsən) the visual purple of the retina, the formation of which is dependent upon vitamin A in the diet.

rhomboid (ˈromboyd) any one of two pairs of muscles in the upper back which control the shoulder blades.

rhonchus (ˈrongkəs) a wheezing sound produced in the bronchial tubes which is caused by partial obstruction and can be heard on auscultation.

rhythm (ˈrithəm) a regular recurring action. *Cardiac r.* the smooth action of the heart when systole is followed by diastole. *R. method* a contraceptive technique in which intercourse is limited to the 'safe period' (avoiding the 2–3 days immediately before and after ovulation).

rib (rib) any one of the 12 pairs of long, flat curved bones of the thorax, each united by cartilage to the spinal vertebrae at the back. *Cervical r.* a short extra rib, often bilateral. Pressure on this may cause impairment of nerve or vascular function. *See* SCALENUS SYNDROME. *False r.s* the last five pairs, the upper three of which are attached by cartilage to each other. *Floating r.s* the last two pairs connected only to the vertebrae. *True r.s* the seven pairs attached directly to the sternum.

riboflavin (ˌrieboh'flayvən) a chemical factor in the vitamin B complex.

ribonuclease (ˌrieboh'nyookleeˌayz) an enzyme from the pancreas which is responsible for the breakdown of nucleic acid.

ribonucleic acid (RNA) (ˌriebohnyoo'-klee·ik, -'klay- 'asəd) a complex chemical found in the cytoplasm of animal cells and concerned with protein synthesis. *RNA viruses* viruses which contain ribonucleic acid as their genetic material.

ribosome (ˌriebə'sohm) an RNA- and protein-containing particle which is the site of protein synthesis in the cell.

rickets ('rikəts) a condition of infancy and childhood caused by deficiency of vitamin D which leads to altered calcium and phosphorus metabolism and consequent disturbance of ossification of bone, resulting in deformity such as bowing of the legs. Since the action of sunlight on the skin produces vitamin D in the human body, rickets often occurs in parts of the world where the winter is especially long, and where smoke and fog constantly intercept the sun. *Adult r.* osteomalacia; a rickets-like disease affecting adults. *Fetal r.* ACHONDROPLASIA. *Late r.* OSTEOMALACIA, that occurring in older children. *Vitamin D resistant r.* an hereditary condition almost indistinguishable from ordinary rickets clinically but resistant to unusually large doses of vitamin D; it is also known as X-linked dominant hypophosphataemic rickets.

Rickettsia (ri'ketsi·ə) a genus of microorganisms which are parasitic in lice and similar insects. The bite of the host is thus the means of transmitting the organisms, some of which are responsible for the typhus group of fevers.

rigidity ('rijiditee) sustained muscle tension causing the affected part to be stiff and inflexible; may be due to stress, injury or neurological disease.

rigor ('rigə) an attack of intense shivering, occurring when heat regulation is disturbed. The temperature rises rapidly and may either stay elevated or fall rapidly as profuse sweating occurs. *R. mortis* stiffening of the body which occurs soon after death.

Ringer's solution ('ringəz ˌsə'looshən) *Sidney Ringer, British physiologist, 1835–1910.* A physiological solution of saline to which small amounts of calcium and potassium salts have been added. Used to replace fluids and electrolytes intravenously.

ringworm ('ringˌwərm) tinea. A contagious skin disease characterised by circular patches, pinkish in colour, with a desquamating surface, and due to a parasitic fungus.

Rinne's test (ˈrinəz test) *Heinrich Rinne, German biologist, 1819–1868.* A test for deafness in which the degree of conductivity through bone is tested by holding a vibrating tuning fork alternately in front of the ear and over the mastoid bone.

risk (risk) hazard, or chance of developing a disease or of complications during or after treatment. This may arise because of inherent problems with the treatment itself (e.g. drug side effects) or because of the frailty of the person. *Relative r.* the likelihood of developing a disease after a given exposure; in epidemiological terms, calculated as incidence rate of disease in an exposed group divided by incidence rate in the non-exposed group. *R. assessment* 1. a study of a person by a healthcare professional in which the details of the person's health record are considered together with other relevant factors to assess the likelihood of the development of a particular disease, or, if the disease is already present, the probability of exacerbation or remission. 2. an assessment of a situation or activity for risks with a view to prevention of any damaging effects upon health, e.g. procedures and environment related to moving and handling. *R. factor* a factor which, when added to others, increases the likelihood of a disease or complication (e.g. smoking and obesity are risk factors for the development of coronary artery disease). *R. management* use of a structured approach to reduce identifiable risks in the health services before problems occur in order to protect the interests of patients and staff by improving the quality of care, reducing costs and potential litigation.

risus (ˈriesəs) laughter. *R. sardonicus* a peculiar grin caused by muscle spasm around the mouth; seen in tetanus and in strychnine poisoning.

rite of passage (riet ov pasəj) the cultural ceremonies and rituals that may accompany the changes in status that occur in the course of a person's life, e.g. 18th birthday parties or bar mitzvah. These ceremonies serve to draw attention to changes in status and social identity and also to the management of the social tensions that such changes may involve.

RNA (ar en ay) *see* RIBONUCLEIC ACID.

Rocky Mountain spotted fever (rokee ˈmowntən spotəd ˌfeeva) a tick-borne infection caused by a *RICKETTSIA*, common in the US, with rash, fever, muscle pain and often an enlarged liver. The disease lasts about 3 weeks.

rod (rod) a straight, thin structure. *Retinal r.* one of the two types of light-sensitive end organ of the retina, which contain RHODOPSIN and are responsible for night vision.

role (rohl) a pattern of behaviour developed in response to the demands or expectations of others; the pattern of responses to the persons with whom an individual interacts in a particular situation. *R. play* an educational technique used in teaching interpersonal, communication and practice skills. Students are given roles (or parts) and asked to act these roles out. Some members of the group may be given observational tasks related to the exercise. At the end of the session, there is an opportunity for the group to evaluate the exercise. This technique may also be used therapeutically, usually in the psychiatric setting. *Sick r.* the role played by people who have defined themselves as ill. Adoption of the sick role changes the behavioural expectations of others towards the sick person, who is exempted from normal social responsibilities and is not held responsible for the condition. The person is obliged to 'want to get well' and to seek competent medical help.

Romberg's sign (ˈrombərgz sien) *Moritz Romberg, German physician, 1795–1873.* Inability to stand erect with the feet close together without swaying if the eyes are closed. A sign of TABES DORSALIS and other diseases of the posterior columns.

rooting reflex (rooting reefleks) a reflex which may be elicited in the newborn by stroking the cheek or side of the mouth and in response babies will turn to the side stimulated and open their mouth ready to suckle.

Rorschach test (ˈrorshahk test) *Hermann Rorschach, Swiss psychiatrist, 1884–1922.* A personality trait test that consists of 10 ink-blot designs, some in colours and some in black and white.

rosacea (rohˈzayshi·ə) *see* ACNE ROSACEA.

roseola (rohˈzeeohlə) 1. a rose-coloured rash. 2. roseola infantum. *R. infantum* a common acute viral disease that usually occurs in children under 24 months old; it attacks suddenly but disappears in a few days, leaving no permanent marks. *Syphilitic r.* an eruption of rose-coloured spots in early secondary syphilis.

Ross River virus (ˈros ˌrivə ˈvierəs) Australian epidemic polyarthritis virus. An acute febrile illness characterised by fever and arthritic pain in the joints, often accompanied by a rash; caused by a virus infection spread by mosquitoes.

Roth's spots (rohts spotz) *Moritz Roth, Swiss physician, 1839–1914.* Small white spots seen in the retina early in the course of sub-acute bacterial ENDOCARDITIS.

roughage (ˈrufij) coarse vegetable fibres and cellulose that give bulk to the diet and stimulate peristalsis.

rouleau (ˈrooloh) a rounded formation found in blood, caused by red cells piling on each other.

roundworm (ˈrowndwərm) any of various types of parasitic nematode worm, somewhat resembling the common earthworm, which sometimes invade the human intestinal tract and multiply there. Very common among them is the pinworm or threadworm.

Rovsing's sign (ˈrohvsingz sien) *Niels Rovsing, Danish surgeon, 1868–1927.* A test for acute appendicitis in which pressure in the left iliac fossa causes pain in the right iliac fossa.

RSI *see* REPETITIVE STRAIN INJURY.

rubefacient (ˌroobəˈfayshənt) an agent causing redness of the skin.

rubella (rooˈbelə) German measles; an acute, notifiable virus infection of short duration, characterised by PYREXIA, enlarged cervical lymph glands and a transient rash. The greatest risk from this disease is to the offspring of mothers who contract it during the early weeks of pregnancy. The child may be born with cataract, heart defects, deafness, or have other congenital defects including brain damage. When a woman is exposed to rubella during the first 20 weeks of pregnancy, a sample of saliva or blood should be taken to test for immunity to rubella. If this shows immunity and if there is no infection, reassurance can be given to continue the pregnancy. The second serum should be taken 4 weeks later, if the first shows no immunity. If this shows evidence of infection further investigation of the baby will be undertaken to check for any sign of problems in the baby to enable informed choice, should termination of the pregnancy be considered. Rubella vaccination is given, in conjunction with immunisation against mumps and measles (MMR), when an infant is approximately 12 months old with a second booster before the start of school.

rumination (ˌroomə'nayshən) 1. recurring thoughts. 2. voluntary regurgitation of food, which is then chewed and swallowed again. *Obsessional r.* thoughts which persistently recur against the person's will.

rupture ('rupchə) 1. tearing or bursting of a part, as in rupture of an aneurysm; of the membranes during labour; or of a tubal pregnancy. 2. a term commonly applied to refer to a hernia.

R wave (R wayv) *see* QRS COMPLEX.

Ryle's tube ('rieəlz tyoob) *John Ryle, British physician, 1889–1950.* A thin tube with a weighted end, introduced via the nose into the stomach. It may be used for the withdrawal of gastric contents or for the administration of fluids.

Ss

Sabin vaccine (ˈsaybin vakˈseen) *Albert Sabin, American biologist, 1906–1993.* A live oral attenuated polio-virus vaccine active against poliomyelitis.

saccharide (ˈsakəˌried) one of a series of carbohydrates, including the sugars.

saccule (ˈsakyool) a small sac, particularly the smaller of the two sacs within the membranous labyrinth of the ear.

sacral (ˈsaykrəl) relating to the sacrum.

sacroiliac (ˌsaykrohˈili·ak) relating to the sacrum and the ilium.

sacrum (ˈsaykrəm) a triangular bone composed of five united vertebrae situated between the lowest lumbar vertebra and the coccyx. It forms the back of the pelvis.

sadism (ˈsaydizem) a form of sexual perversion in which the individual takes pleasure in inflicting mental and physical pain on others.

SADS *see* SEASONAL AFFECTIVE DISORDER SYNDROME.

Safe Motherhood Initiative (sayf ˈmuhthəˌhuhd iˈnishəˌtiv) the World Health Organisation (WHO) campaign to reduce worldwide maternal mortality and morbidity with the implementation of simple, appropriate and cost-effective strategies to enable mothers to have access to high-quality, affordable care during pregnancy and childbirth. The campaign also seeks to improve the health, nutrition and the general wellbeing of girls and women of reproductive age and to the reduction of any long-term sequelae of childbirth which often result in lifelong disabilities.

safe sex (sayf seks) preventative measures to reduce the risk of sexually transmitted infections, e.g. maintaining a monogamous sexual relationship and using a condom. Known risks of infections by human immunodeficiency virus and other organisms transmitted through sexual contact can be reduced by safe sex practices.

sagittal (ˈsajət'l) arrow-shaped. *S. suture* the junction of the PARIETAL bones.

salicylate (səˈlisəˌlayt) a salt of salicylic acid. *Methyl s.* the active ingredient in ointments and lotions for joint pains and sprains. *Sodium s.* a drug that acts as a non-steroidal anti-inflammatory drug (NSAID) and reduces PYREXIA and relieves pain.

saline (ˈsaylien, -een) a solution of sodium chloride and water. *Hypertonic s.* a greater than normal strength. *Hypotonic s.* a lower than normal strength. *Normal* or *physiological s.* a 0.9% solution which is isotonic with blood.

saliva (səˈlievə) the secretion of the salivary glands. When food is taken, saliva moistens and partially digests carbohydrates by the action of its enzyme, PTYALIN amylase.

salivary (səˈlievə·ree, ˈsaləvə·ree) relating to saliva. *S. calculus* a small stone (calculi) which has formed in the salivary duct. The calculi can block the flow of saliva causing swelling and pain. *S. fistula* an abnormal opening on the skin of the face leading into a salivary duct or gland. *S. glands* the parotid, submaxillary and sublingual glands.

salivation (ˌsalə'vayshən) 1. the process of salivating. 2. excessive salivation which may lead to soreness of mouth and gums. Ptyalism.

Salk vaccine (sawlk 'vakseen) *Jonas Salk, American virologist, 1914–1995.* The first poliomyelitis vaccine of killed viruses, given by injection. *See* VACCINE.

Salmonella (ˌsalmə'nelə) any of the genus of Gram-negative, non-sporing, rod-like bacteria that are parasites of the intestinal tract of humans and animals. *S. typhi* and *S. paratyphi* are exclusively human pathogens which cause typhoid and paratyphoid fevers.

Salmonellosis (ˌsalmənə'lohsəs) infection with the genus *Salmonella*, usually caused by the ingestion of food containing salmonellae or their products. The organisms can be found in raw meats, raw poultry, eggs and dairy products; they multiply rapidly at temperatures between 7°C and 46°C. Symptoms of salmonellosis include violent diarrhoea attended by abdominal cramps, nausea and vomiting, and fever. It is rarely fatal and can be prevented by adequate cooking.

salpingectomy (ˌsalpin'jektəmee) excision of one or both of the uterine tubes.

salpingitis (ˌsalpin'jietəs) 1. inflammation of the uterine tubes. 2. inflammation of the PHARYNGOTYMPANIC (eustachian) TUBES. Eustachitis. *Acute s.* most often a bilateral ascending infection due to a streptococcus, a gonococcus or chlamydia trachomatis. *Chronic s.* a less acute form that may be blood-borne.

salpingo-oophorectomy (salˌping-gohoh·əfə'rektəmee) removal of a uterine tube and its ovary.

salpingography (ˌsalping'gogrəfee) radiographic examination of the uterine tubes after injection of a radio-opaque substance to determine their patency.

salpingostomy (ˌsalping'gostəmee) the making of a surgical opening in a uterine tube near the uterus to restore patency.

salpinx ('salpingks) a tube. Applied to the uterine or PHARYNGOTYMPANIC (eustachian) TUBES.

salt (solt, sawlt) 1. sodium chloride, common salt, used in solution as a cleansing lotion, a stimulating bath or for infusion into the blood, etc. 2. any compound of an acid with an alkali or base. 3. a saline purgative such as Epsom salts. *S. depletion* a loss of salt from the body due to sweating or persistent diarrhoea or vomiting. Common in hot climates when it may be prevented by the taking of salt tablets. *Smelling s.s* aromatic ammonium carbonate. A restorative in fainting.

sample ('sahmpəl) 1. a selection of individuals made for research purposes from a larger population and intended to reflect that population in all significant aspects. 2. a small part of anything intended as representative of the whole, e.g. blood specimen. *Convenience s.* a non-probability sampling strategy that uses the most readily accessible persons or objects as subjects in a study. *Non-probability s.* a procedure in which elements are chosen by non-random methods. *Probability sampling* a procedure that uses some form of random selection when the sample units are chosen. *Purposive s.* a non-probability sampling strategy in which the researcher selects subjects who are considered to be typical of the population. *Quota s.* a non-probability sampling strategy that identifies the strata of the population and proportionately represents the strata in the sample. *Snowball effect s.* a strategy used for locating samples that are difficult to locate. It uses social network and the fact that friends tend to have characteristics in common; subjects who meet the eligibility criteria are asked for assistance in getting in touch with others who meet the same criteria. *Systematic s.* a probability sampling strategy that involves the selection of subjects randomly drawn from a population list at fixed intervals.

sandfly (ˈsandˌflie) a very small fly of the genus *Phlebotomus*, common in tropical climates and the vector of most types of LEISHMANIASIS. *S. fever* a fever transmitted by the bites of sandflies and common in Mediterranean countries. Similar to DENGUE and sometimes known as 3-day fever, pappataci fever or phlebotomus fever.

sanguineous (sangˈgwini·əs) pertaining to or containing blood.

saphenous (səˈfeenəs) relating to the saphena veins that carry blood from the foot upwards.

sapphism (ˈsafizəm) female homosexuality; lesbianism.

sarcoid (ˈsahkoyd) 1. tuberculoid; characterised by non-caseating epithelioid cell tubercles. 2. pertaining to or resembling SARCOIDOSIS. 3. sarcoidosis.

sarcoidosis (ˌsahkoyˈdohsəs) a chronic, progressive, generalised disease resembling tuberculosis which may affect any part of the body but most frequently involves the lymph nodes, liver, spleen, lungs, skin, eyes and small bones of the hands and feet.

sarcoma (sahˈkohmə) a malignant tumour developed from connective tissue cells and their stroma. *Ewing s.* a rare type of cancer affecting bones or tissues around bones. Mostly seen in young people and more common in males. *Kaposi's s.* one principally involving the skin, although visceral lesions may be present; it usually begins on the distal parts of the extremities, most often on the toes or feet, as reddish-blue or brownish soft nodules and tumours. It is viral in origin and is frequently associated with AIDS. *Melanotic s.* a highly malignant type pigmented with melanin. *Round-celled s.* a rare highly malignant growth composed of a primitive type of cell.

sarcomatosis (ˌsahkohməˈtohsəs) multiple sarcomatous growths in various parts of the body.

Sarcoptes (sahˈkopteez) a genus of mites. *S. scabiei* the cause of scabies.

SARS (sahz) *see* SEVERE ACUTE RESPIRATORY SYNDROME.

sartorius (sahˈtor·ri·əs) a long muscle of the thigh which flexes both the thigh and the lower leg.

saturation (ˌsatyəˈrayshən) 1. a condition in which a solution contains as much solute as can remain dissolved. 2. a measure of the degree to which oxygen is bound to haemoglobin, expressed as a percentage of the possible limit.

3. (in research) a point in which no new or relevant information emerges. The researcher looks for this point because no new data need be collected.

satyriasis (ˌsatəˈrieəsəs) abnormally excessive sexual appetite in men.

scab (skab) the crust on a superficial wound consisting of dried blood, pus, etc.

scabies (ˈskaybeez) 'the itch'; a parasitic skin disease caused by the itch mite (*Acarus sarcoptes scabiei*), the female of which burrows beneath the skin and deposits eggs at intervals. It is intensely irritating and the rash is aggravated by scratching. The sites affected are chiefly between the fingers and toes, the axillae and groins. Acquired by close direct contact and highly contagious. All members of the family should be treated with topical applications containing either permethrin or malathion to the whole body (except for the head). Two applications 1 week apart are required.

scald (ˈskawld) a burn caused by hot liquid or vapour.

scale (skayl) 1. a scheme or instrument by which something can be measured. A pair of scales is a balance for measuring weight. 2. a self-report inventory that provides a set of response symbols for each item. A rating or score is assigned to each response. 3. compact layers of dead epithelial tissue shed from the skin. 4. to scrape deposits of tartar from the teeth.

scalenus (skəˈleenəs) one of four muscles which move the neck to either side and raise the first and second ribs during inspiration. *S. syndrome* symptoms of pain and tenderness in the shoulder with sensory loss and wasting of the medial aspect of the arm. It may be caused by pressure on the brachial plexus, by spasm of the scalenus anterior muscle or by a cervical rib.

scalp (skalp) the hairy skin that covers the cranium. *S. vein needle* a thin-gauge needle designed for use in the veins of the scalp or other small veins, especially in infants and children. Also called butterfly needle.

scalpel (ˈskalpəl) a small, pointed surgical knife with a convex edge to the blade.

scan (skan) an image produced using a moving detector or a sweeping beam of radiation, as in scintiscanning, B-mode ultrasonography, scanography or computed tomography.

scanning (ˈskaning) 1. visual examination of an area. 2. a speech disorder that may be present in cerebellar disease. The syllables are inappropriately separated from each other and are evenly stressed, with rhythmically occurring pauses between them.

scaphoid (ˈskayfoyd) boat-shaped. *S. bone* a boat-shaped bone of the wrist which articulates with the radius and with the trapezium and the trapezoid bones.

scapula (ˈskapyəla) the large, flat, triangular bone forming the shoulderblade.

scar (skah) the mark left after a wound has healed with the formation of connective tissue.

scarlet fever (ˈskahlət ˈfeevə) scarlatina; an acute, notifiable, rare, infectious disease of childhood with an incubation period of 2–4 days. It is caused by a group A beta-haemolytic streptococcus. There is sore throat, high fever and a punctate rash. It is readily treated by antibiotics, and the complications of NEPHRITIS and middle ear infection are less common.

scattergram (ˈskatəˌgram) used in research and statistics, where two variables are represented by a single plot against an x and y axis.

Schilling test (ˈshiling test) *Robert Schilling, American haematologist, 1919–2014*. A test used to confirm the diagnosis of PERNICIOUS ANAEMIA by estimating the absorption of ingested radioactive vitamin B_{12}.

Schistosoma (ˌshistəˈsohmə) a genus of minute blood flukes, some of which are parasitic in humans. *S. haematobium* a species that infests the urinary bladder; widely found in Africa and the Middle East, especially in Egypt. *S. japonicum* and *S. mansoni* species that infest the large intestine. They are found respectively in China, Japan and the Philippines, and in Africa, the West Indies and tropical America.

schistosomiasis (ˌshistəsohˈmieəsəs) a parasitic infection of the intestinal or urinary tract by *Schistosoma*. The parasite enters the skin from contaminated water and causes diarrhoea, HAEMATURIA and anaemia. The secondary hosts are freshwater snails. Bilharziasis.

schizoid personality disorder (SPD) (ˈskitsoyd ˌpərsəˈnalətee ˈdisˈawdah) a personality disorder that is marked by introspection, self-consciousness, solitariness and a failure in affection towards others. SPD is not the same as schizophrenia or schizotypal disorder.

schizophrenia (ˌskitsəˈfreeni·ə) is a chronic, severe and disabling brain disorder characterised by mental deterioration from a previous level of functioning and characteristic disturbances of multiple psychological processes, including delusions, false beliefs, loosening of associations, poverty of the content of speech, auditory hallucinations, inappropriate affect, disturbed sense of self and withdrawal from the external world. Antipsychotic medication is the mainstay of treatment together with psychotherapy, vocational and social rehabilitation, as well as community mental health support to prevent relapse. Family counselling is also supportive. *Paranoid s.* predominance of delusions of a persecutory nature. *S. nursing assessment* used by mental health nurses to assess all family members including the person as a means of identifying the main issues for care and treatment. *Simple s.* a progressive deterioration of the person's efficiency with increasing social withdrawal.

Schlemm's canal (shlemz kəˈnal) *Friedrich Schlemm, German anatomist, 1795–1858*. A venous channel at the junction of the cornea and sclera for the draining of aqueous humour. Also known as scleral venous sinus.

Schönlein-Henoch purpura or syndrome (ˌshərnlien ˈhenok ˈpərpyərə aw ˈsinˌdrohm) *Johann Schönlein, German physician, 1793–1864; Eduard Henoch, German paediatrician, 1820–1910. See* PURPURA.

school health service (skool helth ˈservəs) the provision of medical and dental inspection and treatment, immunisation and health programs in schools.

school nurse (skool nərs) a registered nurse who has undertaken further education to specialise in the healthcare of school-age children.

Responsibilities include carrying out health assessments, health promotion, advice and education, monitoring growth and development, screening and caring for those with special educational needs.

sciatica (sie'atikə) pain down the back of the leg in the area supplied by the sciatic nerve. It is usually caused by pressure on the nerve roots by a protrusion of an intervertebral disc.

scintillography (sin'tilogrəfee) the visual recording of the distribution of radioactivity in an organ after injection of a small dose of a radioactive substance specifically taken up by that organ.

sclera ('skliə·rə) the fibrous coat of the eyeball, the white of the eye, which covers the posterior part and in front becomes the cornea.

scleroderma (ˌskliə·roh'dərmə) a disease marked by progressive hardening of the skin in patches or diffusely, with rigidity of the underlying tissues. It is often a chronic condition. *See* RAYNAUD'S PHENOMENON.

sclerosis (sklə'rohsəs) the hardening of any part from an overgrowth of fibrous and connective tissue, often due to chronic inflammation. *Multiple s. (MS)* an autoimmune disease of unknown cause affecting the myelin which insulates nerves. It is a long-term condition which results in a wide range of symptoms. It usually begins in young adults and continues throughout life with periods of exacerbation and remission. Also known as disseminated sclerosis.

sclerotherapy (ˌskleroh'therəpee) treatment of oesophageal varices, varicose veins and haemorrhoids by the injection of sclerosing solutions to produce fibrosis.

sclerotic (sklə'rotik) 1. hard; indurated; affected by sclerosis. 2. pertaining to the sclera of the eye. *S. coat* the tough membrane forming the outer covering of the eyeball, except in front of the iris where it becomes the clear horny cornea.

sclerotomy (sklə'rotəmee) incision of the sclerotic coat, usually for the removal of a foreign body or for the relief of GLAUCOMA.

scoliosis (ˌskohli'ohsəs) lateral curvature of the spine (*see* figure). *See* LORDOSIS and KYPHOSIS.

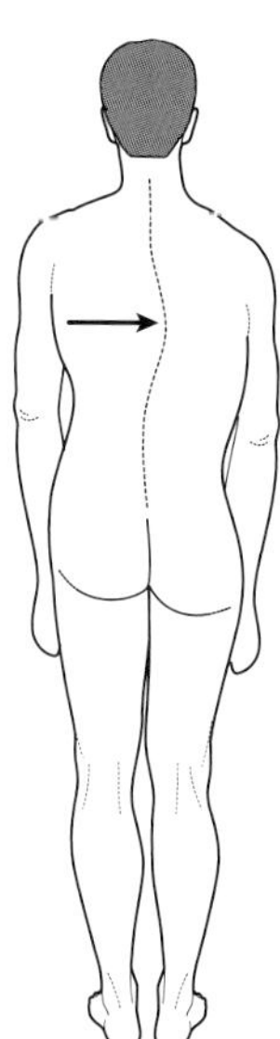

Scoliosis.

scotoma (skoh'tohmə) a blind or depressed area in the field of vision due to some lesion of the retina. It is also found in GLAUCOMA and in detachment of the retina.

screening ('skreening) the carrying out of a test on a large number of people to identify those that have a particular disease for which treatment may be available. Screening tests include: testing of neonates for disorders which benefit from early diagnosis and treatment, e.g. cystic fibrosis; breast screening with mammography, testing for faecal occult blood, blood pressure measurement, blood tests and ultrasound examination in pregnancy, testing for prostate specific antigen and abdominal aortic aneurysm in men.

scrotum ('skrohtəm) the pouch of skin and soft tissues containing the testicles.

scurf (skərf) dandruff.

scurvy ('skərvee) hypoascorbemia; a rare deficiency disease caused by lack of vitamin C (which is found in raw fruits and vegetables). Clinical features of scurvy include fatigue, oozing of blood from the gums and bruising. The condition rapidly improves with adequate diet.

seasonal affective disorder syndrome (SADS) (ˌseezənəl əˌfektiv ˌdis'awdə sinˌdrohm) a condition in which the person notices a change in mood or feelings according to the season of the year and hence the amount of exposure to (sun) light.

sebaceous (sə'bayshəs) fatty, or pertaining to the SEBUM. *S. cyst see* CYST. *S. glands* are found in the skin, communicating with the hair follicles and secreting sebum.

seborrhoea (ˌsebə'reeə) a disease of the sebaceous glands marked by an excessive secretion of sebum which collects on the skin in oily scales.

sebum ('seebəm) the fatty secretion of the sebaceous glands.

secondary ('sekəndree) second in order of time or importance. *S. deposits see* METASTASIS. *S. intention* wound healing as the edges of the wound unite after formation of granular tissue. *See* HEALING.

secretin (sə'kreetən) the hormone originating in the duodenum which, in the presence of bile salts, is absorbed into the bloodstream and stimulates the secretion of pancreatic juice.

secretion (sə'kreeshən) a substance formed or concentrated in a gland and passed into the alimentary tract, the blood or to the exterior. The secretions of the endocrine glands include various hormones and are important in the overall regulation of body processes.

sedation (sə'dayshən) the allaying of irritability or the relief of pain or mental distress, and the promotion of sleep, particularly by drugs.

sedative ('sedətiv) a drug or agent that lessens excitement and relieves tension. Sedative drugs are used to induce sleep.

sedentary ('sedəntree) pertaining to sitting; physically inactive.

sedimentation (ˌsedəmen'tayshən) the deposit of solid particles at the bottom of a liquid. *Erythrocyte s. rate (ESR) see* ERYTHROCYTE.

segregation (ˌsegrə'gayshən) 1. put or come apart from the rest. 2. the separation during meiosis of allelic genes as the chromosomes migrate towards opposite poles of the cell.

seizure ('seezhə) a sudden involuntary contraction of a group of muscles. Also known as a fit, caused by a disturbance in the electrical activity of the brain. *Absence s.* seizure lasting around 15 seconds manifested by a brief period of staring and a lapse in awareness.

selective mutism (sə'lektiv ˌmu'tizəm) a severe anxiety disorder where a person is unable to speak in certain situations.

self (self) 1. a term used to denote an animal's own antigenic constituents, in contrast to 'not-self', denoting foreign antigenic constituents. 2. the complete being of an individual, comprising both physical and psychological characteristics and including both conscious and unconscious components.

self-actualisation (selfˌakshooəlie'-zayshən) a level of psychological development in which innate potential is realised to the full, allowing transcendence of the environment. *See* MASLOW'S HIERARCHY OF NEEDS.

self-care (self'kair) the personal care carried out by the person, e.g. bathing, personal grooming, eating and toilet hygiene. May be with assistance or instruction from a healthcare worker. The aim of rehabilitative care is to maximise self-care and personal independence.

self-catheterisation (selfˌ-kə'theetərieˌzayshen) men, women and older children may be taught to pass a fine catheter into the urinary bladder to evacuate urine as required.

self-disclosure (selfˌdis'klohz·iə) the process by which one person lets their inner being, thoughts and emotions be known to another. It is important for psychological growth in the individual and group psychotherapy, both for the therapist and for the person in the group.

self-esteem (selfˌə'steem) a person's evaluation of their own worth as an individual.

self-examination of testes (ˌselfˌegzamə'nayshən ov testees) *see* TESTICULAR SELF-EXAMINATION.

self-harm (ˌself hahm) deliberate damage to one's own body. Over half of people who die by suicide have a history of self-harm; however, the intention is more often to punish themselves, express their distress or relieve unbearable tension. Self-harm may sometimes be linked to anxiety and depression. Most often occurs in young adults and is more common in women. Also referred to as self-injury or self-mutilation.

self-image (self'imij) an individual's concept of their own personality and abilities based on their own ideas and perceptions.

self-limited (self'limətəd) descriptive of a condition affecting health and wellbeing that runs a definite course regardless of external factors or influences, e.g. the common cold.

self-retaining catheter (ˌself re'tayning 'kathətə) *see* CATHETER.

sella turcica (ˌselə 'tərsika) a depression in the sphenoid body which protects the pituitary gland.

semen ('seemən) the secretion of seminal fluid from the prostate gland and spermatozoa from the testicles which is ejaculated from the penis during sexual intercourse. Seminal fluid.

semicircular (ˌsemee'sərkyələ) formed in a half-circle. *S. canals* part of the labyrinth of the internal ear consisting of three canals in the form of arches which contain fluid and are connected with the cerebellum by their nerve supply. Impressions of change of position of the body are registered in these canals by oscillation of the fluid, and are conveyed by the nerves to the CEREBELLUM.

semicomatose (ˌsemeeˈkohmatohs, -tohz) in a condition of unconsciousness from which the person may be roused. *See* COMA.

semilunar (ˌsemeeˈloonə) shaped like a half-moon. *S. cartilages* two crescent-shaped cartilages in the knee joint. *S. valve* either of two valves at the junction of the pulmonary artery and aorta, respectively, with the heart.

seminoma (ˌsemeeˈnohmə) a malignant tumour of the testis that is highly radiosensitive.

semipermeable (ˌsemeeˈpərmi·əbəl) of a membrane, permitting the passage of some molecules and hindering that of others.

semiprone (ˌsemeeˈprohn) partly prone. Applied to a position in which the person is lying face down but the knees are turned to one side.

senescence (səˈnesəns) the process of growing old.

Sengstaken-Blakemore tube (ˌsengzˈtaykən ˈblaykmor tyoob) *Robert Sengstaken, American neurosurgeon, 1923–1978*; *Arthur Blakemore, American surgeon, 1879–1970*. A compression tube used in the treatment of bleeding oesophageal varices.

senile (ˈseeniel) related to the involutional changes associated with old age or the ageing process. *S. dementia* deterioration of mental activity in the older person associated with an impaired blood supply to the brain.

sensation (senˈsayshən) a feeling resulting from impulses sent to the brain by the sensory nerves.

sense (sens) the faculty by which conditions and properties of things are perceived, e.g. hunger or pain. *S. organ* one that receives a sensory stimulus, for instance the eyes and ears. *Special s.* any one of the faculties of sight, hearing, touch, smell, taste and muscle sense, through which the consciousness receives impressions from the environment.

sensible (ˈsensəbəl) 1. capable of being perceived. 2. sensitive. *S. perspiration* that obvious on the skin as moisture.

sensitisation (ˌsensətieˈzayshən) 1. the process of rendering susceptible. 2. an increase in the body's response to a certain stimulus, as in the development of an allergy. *Protein s.* the condition occurring in an individual when a foreign protein is absorbed into the body, e.g. shellfish causing URTICARIA when eaten. *See* DESENSITISATION.

sensory (ˈsensə·ree) relating to sensation. *S. cortex* that part of the cerebral cortex to which information is relayed by the sensory nerves. *S. deprivation* the effecting of a major reduction of sensory information received by the body. This is damaging to the person's ability to function normally, which is dependent upon constant stimulation. *S. nerve* an afferent nerve conveying impressions from the peripheral nerve endings to the brain or spinal cord. *S. overload* exposure to bright lights, constant loud music and noise that may result in distress, confusion and headaches. May occur in intensive care units.

sentiment (ˈsentəmənt) an emotion directed towards some object or person. Sentiments are acquired and profoundly influence a person's actions.

sentinel event (ˈsentənəl eeˈvent) any unanticipated and wholly preventable event in a healthcare setting resulting in death or serious harm to a patient or patients, not related to the natural course of the patient's illness.

separation anxiety disorder (ˌsepəˈrayˌshen ˌangˈzie·əˌtee dəˈsawdə) developmentally, young children experience feelings of distress at separation from home, parents or carers to whom they have formed an attachment. If hospitalised at this time without a 'live-in' parent or carer, the child may regress to a former stage of development, with food refusal and incontinence. Separation anxiety usually diminishes by the age of 3 or 4 years but occasionally may occur in older children, resulting in nightmares, complaints of somatic symptoms (e.g. headaches, nausea or vomiting) and refusal to attend school. May be associated with depression.

sepsis (ˈsepsəs) an infection of the body by pus-forming bacteria. *Focal s.* a local focus of infection which produces general symptoms. *Oral s.* infection of the mouth which causes general ill health by absorption of toxins. *Puerperal s.* infection of the uterus occurring after labour.

septic (ˈseptik) referring to or produced by sepsis. *S. arthritis* inflammation of a joint due to bacterial infection, most commonly affecting the knees or hips. *S. shock* a life-threatening condition in which there is tissue damage and a severe fall in blood pressure as a result of septicaemia. TOXIC SHOCK SYNDROME is one type of septic shock.

septicaemia (ˌseptəˈseemi·ə) the presence in the blood of large numbers of bacteria and their toxins. The symptoms are a rapid rise of temperature (which is later intermittent), rigors, sweating and all the signs of acute fever.

septum (ˈseptəm) a division or partition. *Atrial s., atrioventricular s., ventricular s.* the partitions dividing the various cavities of the heart. *Nasal s.* the structure made of bone and cartilage which separates the nasal cavities.

sequela (səˈkweelə) a pathological condition occurring after a disease and resulting from it.

sequestrum (səˈkwestrəm) a piece of dead bone. Inflammation in bone leads to THROMBOSIS of blood vessels, resulting in necrosis of the affected part, which separates from the living structure.

serological (ˌsiə·rəˈlojikəl) relating to serum. *S. tests* those that are dependent on the formation of antibodies in the blood as a response to specific organisms or proteins.

serology (siəˈroləjee) the scientific study of serum.

serosa (səˈrohsə) a serous membrane. It consists of two layers: the visceral (in close contact with the organ) and the parietal (lining the cavity).

serotonin (ˌsiə·rohˈtohnən, ˌserə-) an amine present in blood platelets, the intestine and the central nervous system, which acts as a vasoconstrictor. It is derived from the amino acid tryptophan and is inactivated by monoamine oxidase.

serotype (ˈsairohˌtiep) the type of organism identified by the kinds of antigens present in the cell. Used to classify microorganisms.

serous (ˈsiə·rəs) related to serum. *S. effusion* an effusion of serous exudate.

serum (ˈsiə·rəm) the clear, fluid residue of blood from which the corpuscles and fibrin have been removed. *S. hepatitis* jaundice caused by hepatitis B virus, usually after a blood transfusion or an inoculation with contaminated material. *S. sickness* an allergic reaction usually 8–10 days after a serum injection. It may manifest as an irritating urticaria, pyrexia and painful joints. It readily responds to adrenaline and antihistaminic drugs. *See* ANAPHYLAXIS.

serum glutamic oxaloacetic transaminase (SGOT) (ˈsiərəm ˌglooˈtamik ˌoksaləˈseetik ˌtranzˈamənayz (es jee oh tee)) an enzyme excreted by damaged heart muscle. A raised serum level occurs in MYOCARDIAL INFARCTION.

serum glutamic pyruvic transaminase (SGPT) (ˈsiərəm ˌglooˈtamik ˌpieˈroovik ˌtranzˈamənayz (es jee pee tee)) an enzyme excreted by the parenchymal cells of the liver. There is a raised blood level in infectious hepatitis.

severe acute respiratory syndrome (SARS) (səˌviər əˌkyoot rəˈspirə-tree ˌsindrohm; sahz) a serious acute respiratory illness caused by the SARS coronavirus known as SARS Co-V. The WHO monitors countries throughout the world for outbreaks—there have been none since 2004. Infected persons develop high fever (> 38°C) and cough and/or dyspnoea followed by rapidly progressive respiratory compromise. Infected persons may also experience chills, muscle aches, headache and loss of appetite. The SARS virus is highly contagious and is predominantly transmitted by droplets or by direct and indirect contact. Shedding of the virus in faeces and urine also occurs. Mortality rates vary depending on age and underlying medical conditions. Treatment is symptomatic and intensive respiratory support including mechanical ventilation may be required.

sex (seks) 1. either of the two divisions of organic organisms described respectively as male and female. 2. to discover the sex of an organism. *S. chromosome* a chromosome that determines sex. Women have two X chromosomes and men have one X chromosome and one Y chromosome. *S. hormone* a steroid hormone produced by the ovaries or the testes and controlling sexual development. *S.-limited* pertaining to a characteristic found in only one sex. *S.-linked* pertaining to a characteristic that is transmitted by genes that are located on the sex chromosomes, e.g. HAEMOPHILIA.

sexism (ˈseksˌəsm) a belief that one sex is superior to the other and the superior sex has endowments, rights, prerogatives and status greater than those of the inferior sex. Often results in discrimination in all areas of life and acts as a limiting factor in educational, professional and psychological development.

sexual (ˈseksyooəl) pertaining to sex. *S. abuse see* ABUSE. *S. development* the biological and psychosocial changes that lead to sexual maturity. *S. deviation* aberrant sexual activity; expression of the sexual instinct in practices which are socially prohibited or unacceptable, or biologically undesirable. *S. intercourse see* COITUS.

sexuality (ˌseksyooˈalətee) 1. the characteristic quality of the male and female reproductive elements.

2. the constitution of an individual in relation to sexual attitudes and behaviour.

sexually transmitted infection (STI) (ˈseksyooəlee tranzˈmitəd inˈfekshən (es tee ie)) an infection transmitted either by means of sexual intercourse between heterosexual or homosexual individuals, or by intimate contact with the genitals, mouth and/or rectum. STIs include syphilis, gonorrhoea, human immunodeficiency virus (HIV) infection, acquired immunodeficiency syndrome (AIDS), chlamydial infection, genital herpes, non-specific urethritis, trichomoniasis, genital lice, scabies, genital warts, hepatitis B infection and yaws. 'Sexually transmitted infection' is now the preferred term for what was formerly known as sexually transmitted disease (STD) and venereal disease (VD).

SGA *see* SMALL FOR GESTATIONAL AGE.

SGOT *see* SERUM GLUTAMIC OXALOACETIC TRANSAMINASE.

SGPT *see* SERUM GLUTAMIC PYRUVIC TRANSAMINASE.

shaken baby syndrome (shaykən ˈbaybee ˈsindrohm) the presence of unexplained fractures in the long bones, together with evidence of a subdural haematoma (bleeding under the membrane surrounding the brain), retinal bleed and brain swelling in a baby. These injuries are caused by the violent shaking of the baby resulting in vomiting, convulsions, irritability, coma and death. *See* ABUSE.

shared care (shaird kair) the coordinated care of people across the primary and secondary healthcare interface. In obstetrics, a term used to describe antenatal care carried out by a midwife, an obstetrician and/or a general practitioner. *S. c. protocols* consensus protocols for the clinical management of people across the interface of primary and secondary healthcare.

sharps (shahps) any needles, scalpels or other articles that could cause wounds or punctures to personnel handling them. *See also* NEEDLESTICK INJURY.

shearing force (ˈshiəˌring faws) a strain produced by pressure in the structure of a substance so that each layer slides over the next. In the body this may occur when any part is on a gradient; the deeper tissues slide towards the lower gradient and the skin remains with the supporting contact, e.g. sheets on a bed or on a chair. In the presence of moisture this friction is exacerbated and the deeper tissues become ischaemic. *See* PRESSURE INJURY.

sheath (sheeth) 1. an enveloping tubular structure or part. 2. a condom worn on the erect penis during sexual intercourse to trap seminal fluid, preventing the transmission of human immunodeficiency virus (HIV) and other viruses and also reducing the risk of pregnancy.

shiatsu (sheeˈatsoo) a form of manipulation in which the practitioner uses the thumbs, fingers and palms of the hands, knees, forearms, elbows and feet to apply pressure to the client's body in order to promote and maintain health.

Shigella (shiˈgelə) a genus of Gram-negative, rod-like bacteria. Some species cause bacillary dysentery. *S. flexneri* and *S. shigae* are common in Asia, *S. dysenteriae* in the USA and *S. sonnei* in Western Europe.

shin (shin) the bony front of the leg below the knee. The tibia.

shingles (ˈshing·gəlz) *see* HERPES ZOSTER.

Shirodkar's operation (shiˈrodkəz ˌopəˈrayshən) *Vithal Nagesh Shirodkar, Indian obstetrician, 1900–1971.* A cervical cerclage procedure to prevent abortion resulting from cervical incompetence. The internal os is closed by means of a purse-string suture, which is removed shortly before term, or earlier if labour should begin.

shock (shok) a condition produced by severe illness or trauma in which there is a sudden fall in blood pressure. This leads to lack of oxygen in the tissues and greater permeability of the capillary walls, so increasing the degree of shock by greater loss of fluid. The person has a cold, moist skin, a feeble pulse and a low blood pressure, and is distressed, thirsty and restless. *Allergic* or *anaphylactic s.* shock produced by the injection of a protein to which the person is sensitive. *Cardiogenic s.* shock as a result of an acute heart condition such as MYOCARDIAL INFARCTION. *Hypovolaemic s.* shock resulting from a reduction in the volume of blood in the circulation after haemorrhage or severe burns. *Neurogenic s.* shock due to nervous or emotional factors. *Septic s. see* SEPTIC. *Shell s.* a form of POST-TRAUMATIC STRESS DISORDER, first described in World War 2 and caused by the stresses of warfare (*see* POST-TRAUMATIC STRESS DISORDER). *Toxic s. see* TOXIC.

short-sightedness (ˌshawtˈsietədnəs) *see* MYOPIA.

shoulder (ˈshohldə) the junction of the clavicle and the scapula where the arm joins the body. *S. impingement syndrome* a common cause of shoulder pain affecting the rotator cuff tendon. *Frozen s.* also known as adhesive capsulitis. Pain and stiffness in the shoulder caused by inflammation and thickening of the capsule.

show (shoh) the blood-stained discharge that occurs at the onset of labour.

shunt (shunt) a diversion, particularly of blood, due to a congenital defect, disease or surgery.

sialolith (ˈsieəlohˌlith) a salivary calculus.

sibling (ˈsibling) one of a family of children having the same parents. Applied in psychology to one of two or more children of the same parent or substitute parent figure. *S. rivalry* jealousy, compounded of love and hate of one child for his or her sibling.

sickle-cell disease (SCD) (ˈsikəl sel diˈzeez) a group of inherited red blood cell disorders. People with SCD have abnormal haemoglobin, called haemoglobin S or sickle haemoglobin in the red blood cells. *See also* ANAEMIA.

side effect (sied əˈfekt) a result other than the one for which the drug or agent used is being given. Some side effects are predictable, e.g. hair loss with cytotoxic therapy, but others are unpredictable, e.g. skin eruptions or anaphylactic shock.

siderosis (ˌsidəˈrohsəs) 1. chronic inflammation of the lung due to inhalation of particles of iron. 2. excess iron in the blood. 3. the deposit of iron in the tissues.

SIDS (sidz) *see* SUDDEN INFANT DEATH SYNDROME.

sigmoid (ˈsigmoyd) shaped like the Greek letter sigma, Σ. *S. colon* or *s. flexure* that part of the colon in the left iliac fossa just above the rectum.

sigmoidoscope (sigˈmoydəˌskohp) an instrument by which the interior of the rectum and sigmoid colon can be seen.

sign (sien) 1. any objective evidence of disease or dysfunction. 2. an observable physical phenomenon so frequently associated with a given condition as to be considered indicative of its presence. *S. language* hand and body language used by deaf people to communicate with others. *Vital s.s* the signs of life, namely pulse, respiration and temperature. Although not strictly a vital sign, blood pressure can also be included.

significant other (ˌsigˈnifəkənt uthə) a person designated by the person as the person who should be consulted in the event of an emergency or to contact when making arrangements for discharge.

silicosis (ˌsiləˈkohsəs) fibrosis of the lung due to the inhalation of silica dust particles. It occurs in miners, stone masons and quarry workers.

Sims' position (simz pəˈzishən) *James Sims, American gynaecologist, 1813–1883*. A semiprone position. *See* POSITION.

singultus (ˌsingˈguhltəs) hiccups.

sinoatrial (ˌsienohˈaytri·əl) situated between the SINUS venosus and the atrium of the heart. *S. node* the pacemaker of the heart. *See* NODE.

sinus (ˈsienəs) 1. a cavity in a bone. 2. a venous channel, especially within the cranium. 3. an unhealed passage leading from an abscess or internal lesion to the surface. *Cavernous s.* a venous sinus of the DURA MATER which lies along the body of the sphenoid bone. *Coronary s.* the vein that returns the blood from the heart muscle into the right atrium. *Ethmoidal s.* air spaces in the ethmoid bone. *Frontal s.* air spaces in the frontal bone. *S. arrhythmia see* ARRHYTHMIA. *S. thrombosis* clotting of blood in a cranial venous channel. In the lateral sinus it is a complication of MASTOIDITIS. *Sphenoidal s.* air spaces in the sphenoid bone.

sinusitis (ˌsienooˈsietəs) inflammation of the lining of a sinus, especially applied to the bony cavities of the face.

sitz bath (ˌsits bahth) a bath in which only the rectal and perineal areas are immersed in water or saline solution.

SI units (es ie yoonətz) [Fr. Système International d'Unités] the international units of physical amounts. Examples of these units are the mass of a kilogram, and the length in a metre.

six sigma (siks ˈsigmə) a set of tools and techniques for improvement of processes.

skeleton (ˈskelətən) the bony framework of the body, supporting and protecting the organs and soft tissues.

skewed distribution (skyood ˌdistrəˈbyooshən) in statistics, the degree to which the distribution is asymmetric around the mean. The normal distribution is symmetric, thus having a zero skewness.

skill mix (skil miks) the ratio of staff employed in an area of healthcare activity, whether qualified, trained or untrained, representing the availability of skills possessed by these staff.

skin (skin) the outer protective covering of the body. It consists of an outer layer, the epidermis or cuticle, and an inner layer, the dermis or corium, which is known as 'true skin'. *S. grafting* transplantation of pieces of healthy skin to an area where loss of surface tissue has occurred. *S. patch* a drug-impregnated adhesive patch which is applied to the skin. The drug is slowly absorbed, allowing its level in the blood to be maintained over a given period of time. *S. tags* small, soft, skin-coloured growths that hang from the skin resembling a wart. *S. test* application of a substance to the skin, or intradermal injection of a substance, to permit observation of the body's reaction to it. *S. to s. contact see* KANGAROO CARE.

skinfold callipers (skinfohld 'kaləpəz) the instrument used to measure the breadth of a fold of skin, usually on the posterior aspect of the upper arm or over the lower ribs of the chest.

skinfold thickness (skinfohld thiknəs) the measurement of the amount of subcutaneous fat, obtained by inserting a fold of skin into the jaws of a calliper. Indirectly measures an individual's body fat against predetermined standard tables.

skull (skul) the bony framework of the head consisting of the cranium and facial bones.

slapped cheek syndrome (slap'd cheek 'sindrohm) also known as fifth disease. A viral infection most commonly seen in children, resulting in a bright red rash on the cheeks. It will usually clear up in 1–3 weeks.

sleep (sleep) a period of rest for the body and mind during which volition and consciousness are in partial or complete abeyance and the bodily functions partially suspended. It occurs in a 24-hour biological rhythm. Sleep occurs in cycles which have two distinct phases. Each phase lasts approximately 60–90 minutes: orthodox or non-rapid eye movement sleep (NREM), and paradoxical or rapid eye movement sleep (REM). Sleeping requirements vary, with each individual averaging between 4 and 10 hours in a 24-hour period. The purpose of sleep is unknown but sleep deprivation is harmful. *S. walking see* SOMNAMBULISM.

sleep apnoea (sleep 'apni·ə) *see* APNOEA.

sleeping sickness ('sleeping 'siknəs) TRYPANOSOMIASIS; a tropical fever occurring in parts of Africa and caused by a protozoal parasite (*Trypanosoma*), which is conveyed by the tsetse fly.

sleep studies (sleep 'studees) electrodiagnostic tests to diagnose obstructive sleep apnoea (OSA), and performed in a sleep laboratory where the person is monitored by electrocardiogram, pulse oximetry, electroencephalogram and electromyography. Also known as polysomnography.

slide sheet (slied sheet) a strong and lightweight slippery nylon sheet, approximately 1 m by 1.5 m or larger, used for turning or moving people in bed. Two surfaces of the slide sheet are placed under the person and the carer(s) slide the top surface over the lower surface. Also called slip sheet or turning sheet.

sling (sling) a bandage or device used to support an injured part of the body; especially a forearm.

slipped disc (slipt disk) a prolapsed intervertebral disc which causes pressure on the spinal nerves. It may be very painful.

slit lamp (slit lamp) an instrument that provides a three-dimensional view of the eye. Used in ophthalmology for examining the external, surface and internal segments of the eye, including the eyelid(s), lashes, conjunctiva, cornea, anterior chamber, pupil, iris, anterior vitreous and retina. A second hand-held lens is also used to examine the retina. *See* BIOMICROSCOPY.

slough (sluf) dead tissue caused by injury or inflammation. It separates from the healthy tissue and is ultimately washed away by exuded serum, leaving a granulating surface.

slow (sloh) taking a long time before acting or showing signs of activity. *S.-acting drugs* those that are absorbed in the small intestine and have a sustained release over a period of time. Many of these drugs are now incorporated into skin patches. *S. viruses* those infective agents that produce infection after a latent period in the body which may last weeks to months. *See* PRION.

small for gestational age (SGA) (smawl faw ˌjəˈstayˌshənəl ayj) term for a baby who is smaller or lighter in weight than expected for its gestational age. There is some variance in definition, from inclusion of babies below the 10th percentile to only those below the 5th percentile.

smallpox (ˈsmawlˌpoks) once a highly infectious viral disease, associated with high mortality. Eradicated from the world in 1980. Smallpox vaccination is no longer required for travellers to any part of the world.

smear (smiə) a specimen for microscopic examination that has been prepared by spreading a thin film of the material across a glass slide.

smegma (ˈsmegmə) the secretion of sebaceous glands of the clitoris and prepuce.

smell (smel) one of the five senses. Airborne particles are deposited and dissolved in the mucous membrane lining the nose, stimulating the endings of the olfactory nerve. The nose is able to distinguish a wide range of odours.

smoking (ˈsmohking) the act of drawing into the mouth and puffing out the smoke of tobacco contained in a cigarette, cigar or pipe. A close relationship between smoking and lung cancer, heart disease and bronchitis and chronic obstructive airway disease has been established. Smoking is also harmful in pregnancy because the inhaled carbon monoxide reduces oxygen transportation in the body and the nicotine causes vasoconstriction of the arterioles. *Anti-s. initiatives* a range of programs aimed at smoking cessation, e.g. slogans such as 'smoking kills' and nicotine replacement therapy. *Passive s.* the involuntary inhalation of tobacco smoke by people who do not smoke. Passive smoking has been shown to increase the risks of chest infections, coronary disease and tobacco-induced cancers in adults. The infants of mothers who smoke are likely to suffer from fetal growth restriction, and development may be delayed. Children exposed to passive smoking are prone to develop ear and chest infections and asthma. Smoking in the workplace and other public environments, e.g. restaurants, shops, planes and buses, is regarded as an environmental health hazard and is banned in Australia and many other countries.

snake (snayk) a limbless reptile; a serpent. The bites of many snakes are poisonous to humans. *S. bite* a wound resulting from penetration of the flesh by the fangs or teeth of a snake. Bites from snakes known to be non-venomous are treated as puncture wounds; those produced by an unidentified or poisonous snake require immediate attention. Management includes immobilising the bitten area, keeping the person still and prompt transportation to an emergency department. *S. venom antitoxin* antivenin; a serum made from animals, usually horses, which have been immunised against the venom of a specific type of snake.

Snellen's test types (ˈsnelənz test tiepz) *Herman Snellen, Dutch ophthalmologist, 1834–1908.* Square-shaped letters on a chart used for sight testing.

snow (snoh) frozen water vapour. *Carbon dioxide s.* solid CO_2 which is used as a refrigerant; 'dry ice'. *S. blindness* photophobia due to the glare of snow also known as photokeratitis.

snowball sampling (snohbawl ˈsampling) a method of obtaining participants for a study by soliciting names of potential participants from those already in the study.

snuffles (ˈsnufəlz) a chronic discharge from the nose occurring in children as a result of infection of the nasal mucous membrane.

social (ˌsohshəl) in healthcare, the prefix 'social' denotes a role, function or description to do with society, its peoples and its organisation. *S. anxiety disorder* fear of social situations. *S. class* a category arising from the division of society into economic or occupational groupings. *S. media* online and mobile tools that people use to share opinions, information, experiences, images and video or audio clips. It includes websites and applications used for social networking. *S. norms* socially accepted patterns of behaviour within a community or population. *S. worker* a professional trained in the treatment of individual and social problems of people and their families.

socialisation (ˌsohshəlieˈzayshən) the process by which society integrates the individual, and the individual learns to behave in socially acceptable ways.

sociology (ˌsohseeˈoləjee) the scientific study of the development of human social relationships and organisation, i.e. interpersonal and intergroup behaviour as distinct from the behaviour of an individual.

sociopath (ˈsohseeohˌpath) a person with an antisocial personality, morally irresponsible and seeking instant gratification; a psychopath.

sodium (ˈsohdi·əm) *symbol* Na. A metallic alkaline element widely distributed in nature and forming an important constituent of animal tissue. *S. aminosalicylate* an anti-tuberculous drug used in conjunction with other drugs in an established regimen of management. *S. bicarbonate* an antacid widely used to treat digestive disorders, especially flatulence. Repeated use can cause ALKALOSIS. *S. chloride* common salt. Its presence in the diet is necessary to health. *S. citrate* compound used to prevent clotting of blood during blood transfusions. *S. cromoglycate* a drug used as an inhalant in the treatment of asthma. *S. fluoride* a salt used in the fluoridation of water and also in toothpastes to prevent the formation of caries. *S. hypochlorite* a compound with germicidal properties used in solution to disinfect utensils, and diluted as a topical antibacterial agent in many environmental situations. *S. potassium pump* a protein that transports sodium and potassium ions across cell membranes against their concentration gradients. Sodium is normally moved from the inside of the cell, where its concentration is low, to the extracellular fluid, where its concentration is much higher. Potassium is moved in the opposite direction (*see* figure). *S. salicylate* an antipyretic and analgesic drug which acts as a non-steroidal anti-inflammatory (NSAID).

soft tissue mobilisation (soft tisyoo ˌmobəlie'zayshən) *see* MASSAGE.

software ('soft ˌwair) computer data and programs containing instructions that detail how to use a specific computer facility.

solar keratoses ('sohlə' ˌkerə'tohsəz) rough patches of skin caused by damage from repeated exposure to the sun.

solar plexus ('sohlə pleksəs) coeliac plexus. A network of sympathetic nerve ganglia in the abdomen; the nerve supply to abdominal organs below the diaphragm.

solution (sə'looshən) a liquid in which one or more substances have been dissolved.

solvent ('solvənt) a liquid that dissolves or has power to dissolve. *S. abuse* breathing in fumes from

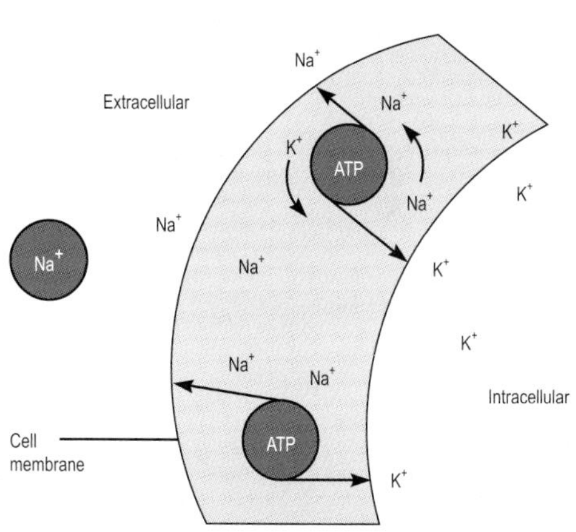

Sodium-potassium pump.

substances such as glue and other volatiles in order to feel high.

soma (ˈsohmə) the body tissue as distinct from the germ cells.

somatic (səˈmatik) relating to the body wall as distinct from the viscera.

somnambulism (somˈnambyəˌlizəm) walking and carrying out other complex activities during a state of sleep.

Somogyi effect (sohˈmohgee əˈfekt) *Michael Somogyi, American biochemist, 1883–1971*. A rebound phenomenon occurring in DIABETES MELLITUS. Overtreatment with insulin induces HYPOGLYCAEMIA, resulting in rebound HYPERGLYCAEMIA and KETOSIS.

Sonne dysentery (sonh ˈdisənˌtree) *Carl Sonne, Danish bacteriologist, 1882–1948*. Bacillary dysentery which is common in the UK. The symptoms are diarrhoea, vomiting and abdominal pain. The causative agent is *Shigella sonnei.*

sonogram (ˈsonəgram) a record or display obtained by ultrasonic scanning. *See* ULTRASONOGRAPHY.

sonography (səˈnogrəfee) *see* ULTRASONOGRAPHY.

sorbitol (ˈsawbəˌtol) a sweetening agent which is converted into sugar in the body, although it is slowly absorbed from the intestine. It is used in some diabetic foods and in intravenous feeding.

sordes (ˈsawdeez) brown crusts which form on the teeth and lips of unconscious patients, or those suffering from acute or prolonged fevers.

sore (saw) a general term for any ulcer or open skin lesion. *Cold s.* herpes simplex. *Hard s.* a syphilitic chancre. *Pressure s. See* PRESSURE INJURY. *Soft s.* a chancroid ulcer. *S. throat* inflammation of the larynx or pharynx, including tonsillitis.

souffle (ˈsoofəl) a blowing sound heard on auscultation. *Uterine s.* a sound due to the blood passing through the uterine arteries of the mother, particularly over the placental site. It is synchronous with the maternal pulse.

soya bean (soyə been) a legume that contains high-quality protein and little starch. *S. milk* historically used as a milk substitute for babies who could not tolerate constituents of breast or cow's milk. Other substitutes are now available and used instead.

Spansule® (ˈspanˌsyool) trade name for a delayed release form of capsule.

spasm (ˈspazəm) a sudden involuntary muscle contraction. *Carpopedal s.* spasm of the hands and feet. A sign of tetany. *Clonic s.* alternate muscle rigidity and relaxation. *Habit s.* a tic. *Nictitating s.* spasmodic twitching of the eyelid. *Tetanic s.* violent muscle spasms, including OPISTHOTONOS. *Tonic s.* a sustained muscle rigidity.

spastic (ˈspastik) 1. caused by spasm; convulsive. 2. term with negative connotations for one affected by spasticity *S. colon* irritable bowel syndrome. *S. paralysis* paralysis associated with lesions of the upper motor neuron, as in cerebral vascular accidents, and characterised by increased muscle tone and rigidity.

spasticity (spaˈstisətee) marked rigidity of muscles.

spatial (ˈspayshəl) pertaining to space.

spatula (ˈspatyələ) 1. a flexible, blunt blade used for spreading ointment. 2. a rigid blade-shaped instrument used, for example, for depressing the tongue in throat examination.

special needs (ˈspeshəl needz) a term generally used to describe the educational or learning needs of a child or adult with a learning disability. The expression may also be used in a wider context to describe the special educational needs of any child, e.g. one who is musically gifted.

specific (spəˈsifik) 1. relating to a species. 2. a remedy that has a distinct curative influence on a particular disease. 3. related to a unit mass of a substance. *S. gravity* the density of fluid compared with that of an equal volume of water.

specimen (ˈspesəmən) a sample or part taken to show the nature of the whole, e.g. for chemical testing or microscopic survey.

specular reflection (ˈspekyələ ˌrəˈflekshən) reflecting as from a surface. A term used in ultrasound to describe an interface which gives a strong reflection or echo, e.g. the fetal skull or bony prominence.

spectacles (ˈspektəkəlz) a frame containing lenses worn in front of the eyes to correct errors of vision or to protect from glare.

spectrometer (spekˈtromətə) an instrument for measuring the strength and wavelengths of visible or invisible electromagnetic radiations.

speech (speech) the act of communicating by sounds by means of a linguistic code. *Clipped s.* speech in which the words are cut short. *Explosive s.* loud, sudden utterances; a sign of mental disorder. *Incoherent s.* disconnected utterances made when the sequence of thought is disturbed, as in delirium. *Oesophageal s.* speech produced after LARYNGECTOMY by swallowing air and using it to vibrate within the oesophagus against the closed cricopharyngeal sphincter. *S. pathologist* a professional trained to identify, assess and rehabilitate persons with speech or language disorders, learning difficulties and feeding difficulties. *Scanning s.* speech in which the syllables are inappropriately separated from each other and are evenly stressed. Characteristic of cerebellar damage. *Staccato s.* speech in which each syllable is separately pronounced; characteristic of multiple sclerosis.

sperm (spərm) 1. a spermatozoon. 2. the semen. *S. count* a method of determining the concentration of spermatozoa in a semen sample. *S. donation* seminal fluid provided by donors for the fertilisation of women whose partners are sterile.

spermatocele (ˈspərmətohˌseel) a cystic swelling in the EPIDIDYMIS containing semen.

spermatozoon (ˌspərmətohˈzoh·ən) a mature male germ cell consisting of a flat-shaped head, a short middle part and a long tail. There are 300–500 billion spermatozoa in a normal ejaculate.

spermicide (ˈspərməˌsied) any agent that will destroy SPERMATOZOA.

SPF *see* SUN PROTECTION FACTOR.

sphenoid (ˈsfeenoyd) wedge-shaped. *S. bone* the central part of the base of the skull.

spherocytosis (ˌsfiə·rohsieˈtohsəs) the presence in the blood of erythrocytes that are more nearly spherical than biconcave; characteristic of ACHOLURIC jaundice. It may also be hereditary.

sphincter (ˈsfingktə) a ring-shaped muscle, contraction of which closes a natural orifice.

sphygmomanometer (ˌsfigmohməˈnomətə) an instrument for directly measuring the arterial blood pressure.

spica (ˈspiekə) a bandage or plaster cast applied to a joint, e.g. shoulder spica, to hold it in the required position.

spigot (ˈspigət) a small plastic peg or bung to close the opening of a tube.

spina (ˈspienə) spine; a slender, thorn-like projection that occurs on many bones. *S. bifida* a congenital defect of non-union of one or more vertebral arches, allowing protrusion of the meninges and possibly their contents. The condition can be detected during pregnancy by ultrasonography, or by testing the blood of the mother or the amniotic fluid for the presence of increased levels of alpha-fetoprotein. Associated with this condition is a folate deficiency in the diet of women of childbearing age who should be encouraged to take sufficient amounts in their diet. *See* MENINGOCELE and MENINGOMYELOCELE.

spinal (ˈspienəl) relating to the spine. *S. anaesthesia see* ANAESTHESIA. *S. canal* the hollow in the spine formed by the neural arches of the vertebrae. It contains the spinal cord, meninges and cerebrospinal fluid. *S. caries* disease of the vertebrae, usually tuberculous. *See* POTT'S DISEASE. *S. column* the backbone; the vertebral column. *S. cord see* CORD. *S. cord compression* an abnormal and often serious condition resulting from pressure on the spinal cord. Causes include spinal fracture, vertebral dislocation, tumour, haemorrhage and oedema associated with contusion. *S. curvature* abnormal curving of the spine. If associated with caries, it is known as Pott's disease. *See* KYPHOSIS, LORDOSIS and SCOLIOSIS. *S. jacket* a moulded support for the spine, used to provide stabilisation to treat a number of spinal conditions including scoliosis. *S. muscular atrophy* a serious progressive genetic disorder causing muscle weakness. *S. nerves* the 31 pairs of nerves which leave the spinal cord at regular intervals throughout its length. They pass out in pairs, one on either side between each of the vertebrae, and are distributed to the periphery. *S. puncture* lumbar or cisternal puncture.

spine (spien) 1. the backbone or vertebral column consisting of 33 vertebrae, separated by fibro-cartilaginous discs and enclosing the spinal cord. 2. a sharp process of bone.

spinnbarkeit (ˈspinbahˌkiet) [Ger.] a thread of mucus secreted by the cervix uteri; used to determine ovulation.

spirochaete (ˈspieraˌkeet) one of a group of microorganisms in the form of a spiral, some of which are found in impure fresh or salt water. The group includes the species *Treponema*, *Borrelia* and *Leptospira*.

spirograph (ˈspieraˌgrahf, -ˌgraf) an instrument for registering respiratory movements.

spirometer (spieˈromətə, spiˈrom-) an instrument for measuring the air capacity of the lungs.

Spitz-Holter valve (ˌspits ˈholtəˌvalv) *Eugene Spitz, American engineer, 1919–2006*; *John Holter, American engineer, 1916–2003*. A device used in the treatment of HYDROCEPHALUS to drain the cerebrospinal fluid from the ventricles into the superior vena cava or the right atrium.

splanchnic (ˈsplangknik) pertaining to the viscera. *S. nerves* sympathetic nerves to the viscera.

spleen (spleen) a large, vascular, gland-like but ductless organ, coloured a reddish-purple and situated in the left HYPOCHONDRIUM under the border of the stomach. It manufactures lymphocytes and breaks down red blood corpuscles.

splenectomy (spləˈnektəmee) excision of the spleen.

splenomegaly (ˌspleenohˈmegəlee) enlargement of the spleen.

splint (splint) an appliance used to support or immobilise a part while healing takes place, or to correct or prevent deformity.

spondylitis (ˌspondəˈlietəs) inflammation of the vertebrae. *Ankylosing s.* a rheumatic disease, chiefly of young males, in which there is abnormal ossification with pain and rigidity of the intervertebral, hip and sacroiliac joints.

spondylolisthesis (ˌspondə-lohlisˈtheesəs) a sliding forwards or displacement of one vertebra over another, usually the fifth lumbar over the sacrum, causing symptoms such as low back pain as a result of pressure on the nerve roots.

spondylosis (ˌspondəˈlohsəs) ANKYLOSIS of the vertebral joints, usually caused by a degenerative disease of the intervertebral discs such as OSTEOARTHRITIS.

spontaneous (sponˈtayni·əs) occurring without apparent cause. Applied to certain types of fracture and to recovery from a disease without any specific treatment.

sporadic (spoˈradik) pertaining to isolated cases of a disease that occurs in various and scattered places (compare endemic and epidemic).

spore (spaw) 1. a reproductive stage of some of the lowest forms of vegetable life, e.g. moulds. 2. a protective state which some bacteria are able to assume in adverse conditions such as lack of moisture, food or heat. In this form, the organism can remain alive but inert for years.

sporulation (ˌsporuhˈlayshən) the formation of spores by bacteria, e.g. Clostridia or Bacilli.

spotted fever (ˈspotəd ˈfeevə) a febrile disease characterised by a skin eruption, such as Rocky Mountain spotted fever, and other infections due to tick-borne rickettsiae.

sprain (sprayn) wrenching of a joint, producing laceration of the capsule or stretching of the ligaments with consequent swelling which is due to effusion of fluid into the affected part.

spreadsheet (ˈspredˌsheet) a computer program that aligns data in tables, rows and columns.

sprue (sproo) a disease of malabsorption in the intestine which may be tropical or non-tropical in form. There is STEATORRHOEA, DIARRHOEA, GLOSSITIS and ANAEMIA.

SPSS *see* STATISTICAL PACKAGE FOR THE SOCIAL SCIENCES.

sputum (ˈspyootəm) material expelled from the air passages through the mouth. It consists chiefly of mucus and saliva, but in diseased conditions of the air passages it may be purulent, blood-stained and frothy, and may contain many bacteria. It must always be regarded as highly infectious. *Rusty s.* that in which altered blood permeates the mucus. Characteristic of acute lobar pneumonia.

squamous (ˈskwayməs) scaly. *S. bone* the thin part of the temporal bone which articulates with the parietal and frontal bones. *S. cell carcinoma* a malignancy of the squamous cells of the bronchus. *S. epithelium* epithelium composed of flat and scale-like cells.

squint (skwint) *see* STRABISMUS.

staging (ˈstayjing) 1. the determination of distinct phases or periods in the course of a disease. 2. the classification of neoplasms according to the extent of the tumour. *TNM s.* staging of tumours according to three basic components: primary tumour (T), regional nodes (N) and metastasis (M). Subscripts are used to denote size and degree of involvement; e.g. 0 indicates undetectable and 1, 2, 3 and 4 indicate a progressive increase in size or involvement.

stammering (ˈstamə·ring) stuttering; a speech disorder in which the utterance is broken by hesitation and repetition or prolongation of words and syllables.

standard deviation (ˌstandədˌdee-veeyˈayshən) (Σ) in statistics, a measure of the dispersion of a random variable: the square root of the average squared deviation from the mean. For data that have a normal distribution, about 68% of the data points fall within one standard deviation from the mean and about 95% fall within two standard deviations.

standard error of the mean (ˈstandəd erə əv thə meen) in statistics, the standard deviation of a theoretical distribution of sample means. It indicates the average error in the estimation of the population mean.

standards (ˈstandədz) statements of the levels of service or care related to specific topics which staff agree to provide. Often accompanied by a description of the structure (staff, equipment, etc.) and process needed to attain specified observable outcomes. *S. of care* a measure by which a professional's conduct is compared, comprises a list of those acts that a prudent professional practitioner would have carried out (or not performed) in similar circumstances within healthcare.

standard precautions (ˈstandəd prəˈcawshənz) work practices that are applied to everyone and are required to achieve a basic level of infection control in healthcare settings; they are recommended for the management and care of all people regardless of their diagnosis or presumed infection status. Implementing standard precautions has the potential to reduce the risk of transmission of infectious agents from person to person, even in high risk situations. Standard precautions consist of: hand hygiene, before and after every episode of patient contact; the use of personal protective equipment; the safe use and disposal of sharps; routine environmental cleaning; reprocessing of reusable medical equipment and instruments; respiratory hygiene and cough etiquette; aseptic non-touch technique; waste management; and appropriate handling of linen. Standard precautions should be used in the handling of: blood (including dried blood); all other body substances, secretions and excretions (excluding sweat), regardless of whether they contain visible blood; non-intact skin;

and mucous membranes. (*See* Appendix 10.)

stapedectomy (ˌstaypiˈdektəmee) removal of the STAPES and insertion of a vein graft or other device to re-establish conduction of sound waves in OTOSCLEROSIS.

stapediolysis (stəˌpeedeeˈoləsəs) an operation in which the foot piece of the stapes is mobilised to aid conduction in deafness from otosclerosis.

stapes (ˈstaypeez) the stirrup-shaped bone of the middle ear. The stapes transmits sound vibrations from the incus to the internal ear.

Staphylococcus (ˌstafəlohˈkokəs) a genus of Gram-positive non-mobile bacteria which under the microscope appear grouped together in small masses like bunches of grapes. They are normally present on the skin and mucous membranes. *S. pyogenes* (or *S. aureus*) is a common cause of boils, carbuncles and abscesses.

staphyloma (ˌstafəˈlohmə) a protrusion of the cornea or the sclerotic coat of the eyeball as the result of inflammation or a wound.

starch (stahch) carbohydrates are stored as starch in many plants. Starch consists of linked glucose units in two forms, amylose and amylopectin, providing a valuable source of energy and fibre in the diet.

startle reflex (ˈstahtlˈreefleks) *see* MORO REFLEX.

stasis (ˈstaysəs) the stagnation or stoppage of the flow of a fluid. *Intestinal s.* sluggish movement of faeces through the bowel owing to partial obstruction or to impairment of the action of the intestinal muscles also known as gastrointestinal hypomobility or ileus. *Venous s.* congestion of blood in the veins.

Statistical Package for the Social Sciences (SPSS) (ˌstəˈtistikəl pakij faw thə ˌsohshəl ˈsieənsəs) a statistical computer program used in research to analyse numerical data from large samples.

statistical significance (ˌstəˈtistikəl ˌsigˈnifəkəns) in research, a conclusion that the results achieved have little probability of occurring by chance alone.

statistics (ˌstəˈtistiks) 1. numerical facts pertaining to a particular subject or body of objects. 2. the science dealing with the collection, tabulation and analysis of numerical facts.

status (ˈstaytəs, ˈstat-) condition. *S. asthmaticus* a severe and prolonged attack of asthma. *S. epilepticus* a serious condition in which there is rapid succession of epileptic fits. *S. lymphaticus* a condition in which all lymphatic tissues are hypertrophied, also known as lymphatism.

STD sexually transmitted disease. *See* SEXUALLY TRANSMITTED INFECTION.

steapsin (steeˈapsən) the fat-splitting enzyme (lipase) of the pancreatic juice.

steatoma (stiəˈtohma) 1. a sebaceous cyst. 2. a LIPOMA; a fatty tumour.

steatorrhoea (ˌstiətəˈreeə) the presence of an excess of fat in the stools owning to malabsorption of fat by the intestines.

Stein–Leventhal syndrome (shtien ˈlevənˌthawl ˈsindrohm) *Irving Stein, American gynaecologist, 1887–1976; Michael Leventhal, American gynaecologist, 1901–1971.* Condition affecting females in which obesity, hirsutism and sterility are associated with polycystic ovaries and menstrual irregularities. Polycystic ovary syndrome (PCOS).

Steinmann pin (ˈstienmən pin) *Fritz Steinmann, Swiss surgeon, 1872–1932.* A fine metal rod passed through a bone by which extension is applied to overcome muscle contraction in certain fractures. *See* KIRSCHNER WIRE.

stellate (ˈstelayt) star-shaped. *S. fracture* a radiating fracture of the patella. *S. ganglion* the inferior cervical ganglion. A star-shaped collection of nerve cells at the base of the neck.

stem cell (ˈstem sel) an undifferentiated cell which is capable of giving rise to infinitely more cells of the same type, and from which certain other kinds of cell arise by differentiation. *S.c. transplant* replacement or damaged blood cells caused by conditions such as leukaemia and lymphoma. An allogeneic transplant involves transplanting cells from a healthy compatible donor. An autologous stem cell transplants involves taking and later replacing cells from the host after any damaged or diseased cells have been removed.

stenosis (stəˈnohsəs) abnormal narrowing or contraction of a channel or opening. *Aortic s.* narrowing of the opening of the aortic valve due to scar tissue formation as the result of inflammation. *Mitral s.* narrowing of the orifice of the mitral valve, usually following rheumatic fever. *Pulmonary s.* a congenital narrowing of the opening from the right ventricle of the heart into the pulmonary artery. *Pyloric s.* narrowing of the pyloric orifice of the stomach due to scar tissue, new growth or congenital hypertrophy.

stent (stent) a tube of metal or plastic placed inside a canal, duct or artery to prevent or counteract a disease-induced, localised flow constriction, thus keeping the passageway open.

stercobilin (ˌstərkohˈbielən) a brown-orange pigment derived from bile and present in faeces.

stereognosis (ˌstereeogˈnohsəs, ˌstiə-) the ability to visualise the shape of an object by touch alone.

stereotype (ˈstairi·əˌtiep) an oversimplified generalisation about a group or class of people which is often then applied to an individual. May form a basis for discrimination and prejudice.

stereotypy (ˈstereeohˌtiepee, ˈstiə-) repetitive actions carried out or maintained for long periods in a monotonous fashion.

Steri-Strips® (ˈsteri ˌstrips) proprietary skin closure strips which are placed across a wound. A final strip is placed on either side parallel to the wound.

sterile (ˈsteriel) 1. aseptic; free from microorganisms. 2. infertile; incapable of producing young.

sterility (stəˈrilətee) 1. the state of being free from microorganisms. 2. the inability of a woman to become pregnant, or of a man to produce potent SPERMATOZOA.

sterilisation (ˌsterəlieˈzayshən) 1. rendering dressings, instruments, etc. aseptic by destroying or removing all microbial life. 2. rendering incapable of reproduction by any means.

steriliser (ˈsterəˌliezə) an apparatus in which objects can be sterilised. *See* AUTOCLAVE.

sternal angle of Louis (stərnəl angəl ov looəs) *Antoine Louis, French surgeon, 1723–1792.* The sternal angle between the manubrium and the body of the sternum. Also called angle of Louis.

sternotomy (stər'notəmee) the operation in which the sternum is cut through to enable the heart to be reached.

sternum ('stərnəm) the breastbone; the flat narrow bone in the centre of the anterior wall of the thorax.

steroid ('steroyd, 'stiə-) one of a group of hormones chemically related to cholesterol. They include oestrogen, androgen, progesterone and the corticosteroids. They may be naturally occurring or synthetic.

sterol ('sterol, 'stiə·rol) one of a group of steroid alcohols which includes cholesterol and ergosterol.

stertorous ('stərtə·rəs) snore-like; applied to a snoring sound produced in breathing during sleep or in coma.

stethoscope ('stethə,skohp) the instrument used for listening to internal body sounds, especially from the heart and lung. It consists of a hollow tube, one end of which is placed over the part to be examined and the other at the ear of the examiner.

Stevens-Johnson syndrome (,steevənz 'jonsən 'sin,drohm) *Albert Stevens, American paediatrician, 1884–1945*; *Frank Johnson, American paediatrician, 1894–1934*. A severe form of ERYTHEMA multiforme in which the lesions may involve the oral and anogenital mucosa, eyes and viscera, associated with such constitutional symptoms as malaise, headache, fever, ARTHRALGIA and conjunctivitis.

STI *see* SEXUALLY TRANSMITTED INFECTION.

stigma ('stigmə) any mark characteristic of a condition or defect, or of a disease. May also be applied to any physical or social quality of a person that is perceived by others as a negative attribute.

stillbirth ('stil,bərth) a baby born after the 24th week of pregnancy and who has not, at any time after being completely expelled from its mother, breathed or shown any sign of life.

Still's disease (stilz di'zeez) *Sir George Still, British paediatrician, 1868–1941. See* JUVENILE RHEUMATOID ARTHRITIS.

stimulant ('stimyələnt) an agent that causes increased energy or functional activity of any organ.

stimulus ('stimyələs) *pl.* stimuli [L.] Any agent, act or influence that produces functional or trophic reaction in a receptor or an irritable tissue. *Conditioned s.* a neutral object or event that is psychologically related to a naturally stimulating object or event and which causes a CONDITIONED RESPONSE (*see also* CONDITIONING). *Discriminative s.* a stimulus associated with reinforcement which exerts control over a particular form of behaviour; the subject discriminates between closely related stimuli and responds positively only in the presence of that stimulus. *Eliciting s.* any stimulus, conditioned or unconditioned, that elicits a response. *Structured s.* a well organised and unambiguous stimulus, the perception of which is influenced to a greater extent by the characteristics of the stimulus than by those of the perceiver. *Threshold s.* a stimulus that is just strong enough to elicit a response. *Unconditioned s.* any stimulus that is capable of eliciting an unconditioned response (*see also* CONDITIONING). *Unstructured s.* an unclear or ambiguous stimulus, the perception of which is influenced to a greater extent by the characteristics of the perceiver than by those of the stimulus.

stitch (stich) 1. a popular term used to describe a sudden sharp pain usually due to spasm of the diaphragm. 2. a suture. *S. abscess* pus from a formation where a stitch has been inserted.

Stokes-Adams syndrome (ˌstohks ˈadəmz ˈsinˌdrohm) *William Stokes, Irish surgeon, 1804–1878*; *Robert Adams, Irish physician, 1791–1875.* Attacks of SYNCOPE or fainting due to cerebral anaemia in some cases of complete heart block. The heart stops temporarily but breathing continues. The syndrome is treated by using an artificial pacemaker.

stoma (ˈstohmə) *pl.* stomata. 1. a mouth or mouth-like opening. 2. an artificial opening in the skin surface leading into one of the tubes forming the alimentary canal. *See* COLOSTOMY and ILEOSTOMY.

stomach (ˈstumək) the dilated portion of the alimentary canal between the oesophagus and the duodenum, just below the diaphragm. *Bilocular* or *hourglass s.* one divided into two parts by a constriction. *S. pH electrode* apparatus used to measure gastric contents in situ. *S. pump* a pump that removes the contents of the stomach by suction. *See* GASTRIC *lavage*.

stomatitis (ˌstohməˈtietəs) inflammation of the mouth, either simple or with ulceration caused by a vitamin deficiency, or by a bacterial or fungal infection. *Angular s.* cracking at the corners of the mouth usually due to riboflavin deficiency. *Aphthous s.* that characterised by small, white, painful ulcers on the mucous membrane. *Ulcerative s.* painful shallow ulcers on the tongue, cheeks and lips; a severe type that may produce serious constitutional effects.

stone (stohn) a CALCULUS.

stool (stool) a motion or discharge from the bowels. *Fatty s.* that which contains undigested fat. *Hunger s.* stool passed by underfed infants: frequent, small and green. *Ricewater s.* the water stool containing small white flakes seen in cholera. *Tarry s.* a black tarry stool due to the presence of blood from a peptic ulcer or oesophageal varices; MELAENA.

strabismus (strəˈbizməs) squint; HETEROTROPIA. A deviation of the eye from its normal direction. It is called convergent when the eye turns in towards the nose, and divergent when it turns outwards. *Concomitant s.* a squint in which the angle of deviation stays constant.

strabotomy (strəˈbotəmee) the division of ocular muscles in the treatment of STRABISMUS.

strain (strayn) 1. overuse or stretching of a part, e.g. a muscle or tendon. 2. a group of microorganisms within a species. 3. to pass a liquid through a filter.

strangulated (ˈstrang·gyəˌlaytəd) compressed or constricted so that the circulation of the blood is arrested. *S. hernia see* HERNIA.

strangulation (ˌstrang·gyəˈlayshən) 1. choking caused by compression of the air passages. 2. arrested circulation to a part, which will result in GANGRENE.

strangury (ˈstrang·gyəˌree) a painful, frequent desire to micturate, but in which only a few drops of urine are passed with difficulty.

stratified (ˈstratəˌfied) arranged in layers. *S. tissue* a covering tissue in which the cells are arranged in layers. The germinating cells are the lowest and, as surface cells are shed, there is continual replacement.

stratum (ˈstrahtəm, ˈstray-) a layer; applied to structures such as the skin and mucous membranes. *S. corneum* the outer, horny layer of the epidermis.

Streptococcus (ˌstreptəˈkokəs) a genus of Gram-positive spherical bacteria occurring in chains or pairs. Divided into various groups. The first group includes the beta-haemolytic human and animal pathogens; the second and third include alpha-haemolytic parasitic forms occurring as normal flora in the body; and the fourth is made up of saprophytic forms. *S. mutans* implicated in dental caries. *S. pneumoniae* pneumococcus, the most common cause of lobar pneumonia; also causes serious forms of meningitis, septicaemia, empyema and peritonitis. *S. pyogenes* beta-haemolytic, toxigenic, pyogenic streptococci causing many conditions, including pharyngitis, erysipelas and cellulitis, scarlet fever, rheumatic fever, necrotising fasciitis, and toxic shock syndrome and acute GLOMERULONEPHRITIS.

streptokinase (ˌstreptəˈkinayz) an enzyme derived from a streptococcal culture and used to liquefy clotted blood and pus.

Streptomyces (ˌstreptohˈmieseez) a genus of soil bacteria from which some antibiotics are derived.

stress (stres) any factor, mental or physical, the pressure of which can adversely affect the functioning of the body. *S. disorders* those resulting from an individual's inability to withstand stress. *S. fracture* one that occurs as a result of repetitive jarring of a bone, e.g. metatarsal bones in the foot associated with long-distance running and walking. *S. incontinence* incontinence, usually of urine, when the intra-abdominal pressure is raised, such as in coughing, sneezing or laughing. *S. ulcer* an acute peptic ulcer, which may be multiple and develop after severe burns, major injuries and occur sometimes during serious illness. The cause is unknown.

stressor (ˈstresə) any life event or change that causes a person stress and which in some circumstances may precipitate distress or deterioration in mental health. These factors may be physical, physiological or psychosocial, e.g. pain and hunger, loss of job, bereavement, divorce.

stria (ˈstrieə) *pl.* striae. A line or stripe. *Striae gravidarum* the lines that appear on the abdomen of pregnant women. They are red in first pregnancy but white subsequently, and are due to stretching and rupture of the elastic fibres. Stretch marks.

striated (strieˈaytəd) striped. *S. muscle* voluntary muscle. *See* MUSCLE.

stricture (ˈstrikchə) a narrowing or local contraction of a canal. It may be caused by muscle spasm, new growth or scar tissue formation after inflammation.

stridor (ˈstriedaw) a harsh, vibrating, shrill sound, produced during respiration when there is partial obstruction of the larynx or trachea.

stroke (strohk) a term to describe the sudden onset of symptoms that occurs when the blood supply to part of the brain is cut off, affecting movement, sensation, speech and vision. There may be paralysis and loss of sensation down one side of the body or one side of the face.

Stroke may be ischaemic, where the blood supply is stopped due to a blood clot, or haemorrhage, where a weakened blood vessel supplying the brain bursts. *See* CEREBROVASCULAR *accident*. *Heat s.* a HYPERPYREXIA accompanied by cerebral symptoms. It may occur in someone newly arrived in a very hot climate.

stroma (ˈstrohmə) the connective tissue forming the ground substance, framework or matrix of an organ, as opposed to the functioning part or PARENCHYMA.

Strongyloides (stronjəˈloydeez) a genus of nematode worms, one of which, *S. stercoralis*, is common in tropical countries and causes diarrhoea and intestinal ulcers.

strontium (ˈstronti·əm) *symbol* Sr. A metallic element. Isotopes of strontium are used in bone scanning to detect abnormalities. *S.-90* a radioactive isotope used in radiotherapy in the treatment of bone malignancies.

structuralism (ˈstrukchərəlizəm) in psychology, the view that the important influences on people's lives are the basic content of consciousness including intellect, feelings, memory and behaviour. Structuralist approaches in anthropology and sociology are concerned with the social structures within which people function.

Stryker frame (ˈstriekə fraym) an apparatus specially designed for care of patients with injuries of the spinal cord or paralysis. It is constructed of pipe and canvas and is designed so that one nurse can turn the patient without difficulty.

study skills (ˈstudee skilz) a set of techniques, strategies and behaviour patterns which form a structured approach to learning.

stupor (ˈstyoopə) a state of semi-unconsciousness occurring in the course of many varieties of mental illness in which the person does not move or speak, and usually only responds to noxious stimuli.

Sturge-Weber syndrome (ˌstərj ˈwebə ˈsinˌdrohm) *William Sturge, British physician, 1850–1919; Frederick Weber, British physician, 1863–1962*. A rare congenital abnormality in which there is a port wine stain on the face with an ANGIOMA of the meninges on the same side. Common symptoms are epilepsy, HEMIPLEGIA and associated learning difficulties. Also known as encephalotrigeminal angiomatosis.

stuttering (ˈstutə·ring) *see* STAMMERING.

stye (stie) *see* HORDEOLUM.

stylet (ˈstielət) a wire or rod for keeping clear the lumen of catheters, cannulae and hollow needles.

styloid (ˈstieloyd) like a pen. *S. process* a long pointed spine, particularly one projecting from the temporal bone. Also processes on the ulna and radius.

styptic (ˈstiptik) an astringent which, applied locally, arrests haemorrhage.

subacute (ˌsubəˈkyoot) moderately acute. Applied to a disease that progresses moderately rapidly, but does not become ACUTE.

subarachnoid (ˌsubəˈraknoyd) below the arachnoid. *S. haemorrhage* bleeding into the subarachnoid space from a vessel in the brain. Commonly, due to a rupture of a cerebral aneurysm or to trauma. Blood is present in the cerebrospinal fluid. *S. space* between the arachnoid and pia mater of the brain and spinal cord and containing cerebrospinal fluid.

subclavian (subˈklayvi·ən) beneath the clavicle. *S. artery* the main vessel of supply to the neck and arms.

subclinical (subˈklinikəl) without clinical manifestations; said of the early stages or a very mild form of a disease.

subconscious (subˈkonshəs) 1. not conscious, yet able to be recalled to consciousness. 2. in psychoanalysis, the part of the mind that retains memories which cannot, without much effort, be recalled to mind.

subculture (ˈsubˌkulchə) a subgroup that diverges from the dominant culture in a society but may retain some of its customs and values, while rejecting others.

subcutaneous (ˌsubkyooˈtayni·əs) beneath the skin. *S. injection* one given hypodermically.

subdural (subˈdyoo·rəl) below the DURA MATER. *S. haematoma* a blood clot between the arachnoid and dura mater. It may be acute or arise slowly from a minor injury.

subinvolution (ˌsubinvəˈlooshən) incomplete or delayed return of the uterus to its pregravid size during the PUERPERIUM, usually as the result of retained products of conception and infection.

subjective (səbˈjektiv) related to the individual. *S. symptoms* those of which the person is aware by sensory stimulation, but which cannot easily be seen by others. *See also* OBJECTIVE.

sublimate (ˈsubləˌmayt) a substance obtained by sublimation.

sublimation (ˌsubləˈmayshən) 1. the vaporisation of a solid and its condensation into a solid deposit. 2. in psychoanalysis, a redirecting of energy at an unconscious level. The transference into socially acceptable channels of tendencies that cannot be expressed. An important aspect of maturity.

subliminal (subˈlimənəl) below the threshold of perception.

sublingual (subˈling·gwəl) beneath the tongue. *S. glands* two small salivary glands in the floor of the mouth.

subluxation (ˌsublukˈsayshən) partial dislocation of a joint.

submaxillary (ˌsubmakˈsilə·ree) beneath the lower jaw. *S. glands* two salivary glands situated under the lower jaw.

submucous (subˈmyookəs) beneath mucous membrane. *S. resection* an operation to correct a deflected nasal septum.

subnormal (subˈnawməl) below normal.

subphrenic (subˈfrenik) beneath the diaphragm. *S. abscess* one that develops below the diaphragm usually after peritonitis or from postoperative infection.

substitution (ˌsubstəˈtyooshən) the act of putting one thing in place of another.

substrate (ˈsubstrayt) a substance on which an enzyme acts.

succus (ˈsukəs) a juice. *S. gastricus* gastric juice.

succussion (suˈkushən) a method of determining when free fluid is present in a cavity in the body. A sound of splashing is heard when the person moves or is deliberately moved.

sucrose (ˈsookrohz, -ohs) a disaccharide obtained from cane or beet sugar.

suction (ˈsukshən) 1. the process of sucking. 2. the removal of gas or fluid from a cavity or other container by means of reduced pressure. *Post-tussive s.* a sucking noise heard in the lungs just after a cough.

sudamen (soo'daymən) a small white vesicle formed in the sweat glands after prolonged sweating.

sudden infant death syndrome (SIDS) (sudən 'infənt deth 'sin,drohm) the sudden and unexpected death of an apparently healthy infant, typically occurring in the first 6 months and not explained by postmortem studies. Called cot death because often the infant is found dead in the cot and dies while asleep. The prone position, respiratory illness and infection, tobacco smoke and overheating have been found to be risk factors. Parents and carers are advised to put their babies to sleep on their backs at the foot of the cot to prevent them from wriggling under the bed clothes, not to overheat the room, not to smoke in the same room and to seek advice from a health professional if the baby seems unwell.

sudor ('syoodaw) sweat; perspiration.

sudorific (,syoodə'rifik) 1. pertaining to an agent or condition such as heat or emotional tension that causes or stimulates sweating. *S. agent* a substance that stimulates the sweat glands, e.g. cholinergic drugs. Also called diaphoretic.

suffocation (,sufə'kayshən) asphyxiation; a cessation of breathing caused by occlusion of the air passages, leading to unconsciousness and ultimately to death.

suffusion (sə'fyoozhən) a process of diffusion or overspreading, as in flushing of the skin; blushing.

sugar ('shuhgə) a group of sweet carbohydrates classified chemically as monosaccharides or disaccharides. The following are included: *beet s.* obtained from sugar beet; *cane s.* obtained from sugar cane; *fructose* fruit sugar; *grape s.* dextrose, glucose; *milk s.* lactose. *Muscle s.* INOSITOL; a sugar-like compound found in animal tissue, particularly in muscle, and also in many plant tissues.

suggestibility (sə,jestə'bilətee) inclination to act on the suggestions of others.

suggestion (sə'jeschən) a tool of psychotherapy in which an idea is presented to, and accepted by, a person. *Posthypnotic s.* one implanted in a person under hypnosis which lasts after return to a normal condition.

suicide ('sooə,sied) the intentional taking of one's own life. Legally, a death suspected of being due to violence that is self-inflicted is not termed a suicide unless the victim leaves positive evidence of the intention to commit suicide, or the method of death is such that a verdict of suicide is inevitable. Attitudes to suicide are culturally determined and vary from one group to another. Depression is the commonest cause of suicide and severely depressed people are always at risk.

sulcus ('sulkəs) a furrow or fissure; applied especially to those of the brain.

sunburn ('sun,bərn) a dermatitis due to exposure to the sun's rays causing burning and redness.

sun protection factor (SPF) (sun ,prə'tekshən 'fak,tə, es pee ef) a system of evaluating the effectiveness of various formulations for protecting the skin from ultraviolet radiation. Sunscreens are rated from 1 to 50+ in accordance with the Australian and New Zealand

Standard for Sunscreens. The SPF number is derived from the time or dose required to produce minimal reddening of skin, divided into time or dose required to produce the same degree of reddening with the product applied.

sunstroke (ˈsun͵strohk) a profound disturbance of the body's heat-regulating mechanism caused by prolonged exposure to excessive heat from the sun. Persons over 40 and those in poor health are most susceptible to it. *See* STROKE.

superego (͵soopəˈreegoh) that part of the personality that is concerned with moral standards and ideals that are derived unconsciously from parents, teachers and environment, and influence a person's whole mental make-up, acting as a control on impulses of the ego.

superfecundation (͵soopə͵fekən-ˈdayshən, -͵fee-) the fertilisation of two or more ova produced during the same menstrual cycle by SPERMATOZOA from separate coital acts.

superfetation (͵soopəfeeˈtayshən) the fertilisation of a second ovum when pregnancy has already started, producing two fetuses of different maturity.

superior (sooˈpiə·ri·ə) above; the upper of two parts.

supernumerary (͵soopəˈnyoomə͵rəree) 1. present in excess of the normal or required number; extra, as in supernumerary digit. 2. students and new staff placed in clinical areas for orientation and/or for supervised practice who are not included in the staffing numbers.

supine (ˈsoopien) 1. lying on the back, with the face upwards. 2. the turning of the palm of the hand upwards. *See* PRONE.

suppository (səˈpozətree) a medicated solid substance prepared for insertion into the rectum or vagina which will dissolve at body temperature.

suppression (səˈpreshən) 1. complete cessation of a secretion. 2. in psychology, conscious inhibition as distinct from repression, which is unconscious. *S. of urine* no secretion of urine by the kidneys.

suppuration (͵supyəˈrayshən) the formation of pus.

supracondylar (͵sooprəˈkondələ) above the condyles. *S. fracture* one above the lower end of the humerus or femur.

supraorbital (͵sooprəˈawbət'l) above the orbit of the eye.

suprapubic (͵sooprəˈpyoobik) above the pubic bones. *S. cystotomy* surgical incision of the urinary bladder just above the pubic bones.

suprarenal (͵sooprəˈreenəl) above the kidney. *S. gland* adrenal gland; one of a pair of triangular endocrine glands situated on the upper surface of the kidneys. *See* ADRENAL.

supraventricular tachycardia (SVT) (͵sooprəˈ venˈtrikyələ ͵takeeˈkahdi·ə) abnormally fast heartbeat of over 100 beats per minute not connected with exercise.

surface tension (ˈserfəs ˈtenshən) the tendency of a liquid to minimise the area of its surface by contracting. This property causes liquids to rise in a capillary tube, affects the exchange of gases in the alveoli and alters the ability of various liquids to wet another surface.

surfactant (sərˈfaktənt) a surface active agent; a mixture of phospholipids that is secreted into the pulmonary alveoli and reduces the surface tension of pulmonary fluids, thus contributing to the elastic properties of pulmonary tissue. Surfactant can be instilled via a tracheal catheter as treatment for respiratory distress syndrome. *See also* RESPIRATORY DISTRESS SYNDROME OF NEWBORN.

surgeon (ˈsərjən) a medical practitioner who specialises in surgery.

surgery (ˈsərjə·ree) the branch of medicine that treats disease by operative measures.

surrogate (ˈsurəgət) a real or imaginary substitute for a person or object in someone's life. *S. mother* a woman who carries a child for another (the commissioning parent) with the intention that the child be handed over after birth for adoption.

surveillance (sərˈvayləns) the monitoring, recording, analysing and reporting of the occurrence of infectious outbreaks of disease, e.g. hospital-acquired infections, bacterial bloodstream infections and wound infection following orthopaedic surgery. The process can be applied to other incidences, e.g. the cases of notifiable disease in a population.

survey (ˈsərˌvay) the systematic collection of information, not forming part of a scientific epidemiological study.

survivor (ˈsəˈvieˌvə) 1. a person who continues to live despite nearly dying. 2. A person who is able to continue living their life successfully despite experiencing difficulties. *S. guilt* the condition of feeling guilty after surviving a tragedy in which others were harmed or died. In some cases, the person may believe the tragedy occurred because they did something bad; in others, the person may feel they did not do enough to avert the tragedy. Also called survivor's guilt, survival guilt or survivor syndrome.

susceptibility (səˌseptəˈbilətee) lack of resistance to infection. The opposite to immunity.

suspensory (səˈspensə·ree) supporting a part. *S. bandage* one applied to support a part of the body, particularly the scrotum or the lower jaw. *S. ligament* a ligament that supports or suspends an organ, e.g. that of the lens of the eye.

suture (ˈsoochə) 1. a stitch or series of stitches used to close a wound (*see* figure, p. 455). 2. the jagged line of junction of the bones of the cranium. *Atraumatic s.* a suture fused to the needle to obtain a single thickness through each puncture of the needle. *Cerclage s.* encircling with a ring or loop of non-absorbable suture to keep an incompetent cervix closed to prevent miscarriage. Cervical cerclage, *see* SHIRODKAR'S PROCEDURE. *Continuous s.* a form of oversewing with one length of suture. *Coronal s.* the junction between the frontal and parietal bones. *Everting s.* a type of mattress stitch that turns the edges outwards to give a closer approximation. *Fascial s.* a strip of fascia taken from the person and used to form a suture. *Interrupted s.* a series of separate sutures. *Lambdoid s.* the junction between the parietal and occipital bones. *Mattress s.* one in which each suture is taken twice through the wound, giving a loop one side and a knot the other. *Purse-string s.* a circular continuous suture round a small wound or appendix stump. *Sagittal s.* the junction between the two occipital bones. *Subcuticular s.* a continuous suture placed just below the skin. *Tension s.* or *relaxation s.* one taking a large bite and relieving the tension on the true stitch line.

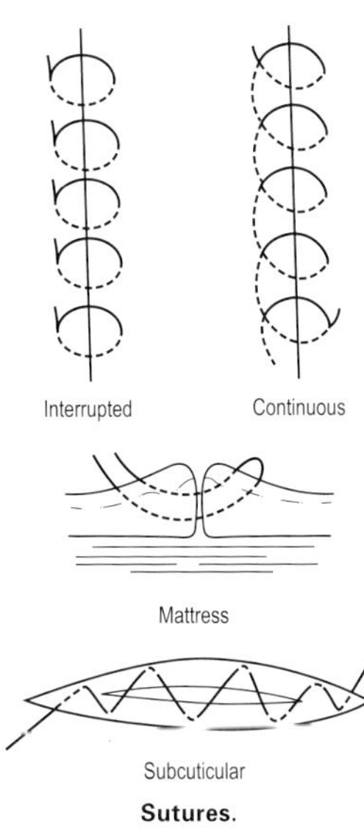

Sutures.

swab (swob) 1. a small piece of cotton wool or gauze. 2. in pathology, a dressed sterile stick used in taking bacteriological specimens.

swallowing (ˈswoloh·ing) the taking in of a substance through the mouth and pharynx and into the oesophagus. It is a combination of a voluntary act and a series of reflex actions. Once begun, the process operates automatically. Also called deglutition.

sweat (swet) perspiration; a clear watery fluid secreted by the sweat glands. *S. glands* coiled tubular glands situated in the dermis with long ducts to the skin surface.

swine influenza (swien ˌinflooˈenzə) a highly contagious respiratory disease of pigs caused by infection with the swine fever influenza virus. A/H1N1pdm09 virus (shortened to H1N1). Infected swine can infect and cause symptomatic disease in humans with fever of sudden onset, cough or shortness of breath associated with headache, tiredness, aching muscles, sneezing and runny nose. The virus was first identified in 2009. The regular flu vaccine protects against H1N1. *See* INFLUENZA, AVIAN INFLUENZA and ORTHOMYXOVIRUS.

sycosis (sieˈkohsəs) a pustular inflammation of the hair follicles, usually of the beard and moustache.

Sydenham's chorea (ˈsidənəmz koˈreeə) *Thomas Sydenham, British physician, 1624–1689.* A disorder of the central nervous system closely linked with rheumatic fever; also called chorea minor or historically St Vitus's dance. The condition, usually self-limited, is characterised by purposeless, irregular movements of the voluntary muscles that cannot be controlled by the person.

symbiosis (ˌsimbieˈohsəs) in parasitology, an intimate association between two different organisms for the mutual benefit of both.

symblepharon (simˈblefə·rən) adhesion of an eyelid to the eyeball.

symbolism (ˈsimbəˌlizəm) in psychology, an abnormal mental condition in which events or objects are interpreted as symbols of the person's own thoughts. In psychiatry, the re-entry into consciousness of repressed material in an acceptable form.

sympathectomy (ˌsimpəˈthektəmee) division of autonomic nerve fibres which control specific involuntary muscles. An operation performed for many conditions, among them RAYNAUD'S PHENOMENON and focal hyperhidrosis.

sympathetic (ˌsimpəˈthetik) 1. exhibiting sympathy. *S. ophthalmia* inflammation leading to loss of sight in the opposite eye after a perforating injury in the ciliary region. 2. relating to the autonomic nervous system. *S. nervous system* one of the two divisions of the autonomic nervous system. It supplies involuntary muscle and glands; it stimulates the ductless glands and the circulatory and respiratory systems but inhibits the digestive system. *S. ophthalmia* inflammation leading to loss of sight in the opposite eye after a perforating injury in the ciliary region.

sympathomimetic (ˌsimpəthəˈmimetik) pertaining to drugs that produce effects similar to those caused by a stimulation of the sympathetic nervous system.

symphysis (ˈsimfisəs) a cartilaginous joint along the line of union of two bones. *S. pubis* the cartilaginous junction of the two pubic bones.

symptom (ˈsimptəm) any indication of disease perceived by the person. *Cardinal s.s* 1. symptoms of greatest significance to the doctor, establishing the identity of the illness. 2. the symptoms shown in the temperature, pulse and respiration. *Dissociation s.* anaesthesia to pain and to heat and cold, without impairment of tactile sensibility. *Objective s.* one perceptible to others than the person, such as pallor, rapid pulse or respiration, restlessness, etc. *Presenting s.* the symptom or group of symptoms about which the person complains or from which relief is sought. *Subjective s.* one perceptible only to the person, as pain, pruritus, vertigo, etc. *Withdrawal s.s* symptoms that follow sudden abstinence from a drug on which a person is dependent.

symptomatology (ˌsimptəməˈtolәjee) 1. the study of the symptoms of a disease. 2. the symptoms of a particular disease taken together.

synalgia (siˈnalji·ə) pain felt in one part of the body but caused by inflammation of or injury to another part. Referred pain.

synapse (ˈsienaps) the junction between the termination of an axon and the dendrites of another nerve cell. Chemical transmitters pass the impulse across the space.

syncope (ˈsingkəpee) a simple faint or temporary loss of consciousness due to cerebral ischaemia, often caused by dilatation of the peripheral blood vessels and a sudden fall in blood pressure.

syndactyly (sinˈdaktəˌlee) a congenital abnormality characterised by the fusion of the fingers or toes.

syndactylism (sinˈdaktəˌlizəm) possessing webbed fingers or toes. A condition in which two or more fingers or toes are joined together.

syndrome (ˈsindrohm) a group of signs or symptoms typical of a distinctive disease which frequently occur together and form a distinctive clinical picture.

synergist (ˈsinəjəst, siˈnər-) 1. a muscle that works in conjunction with another muscle. 2. a drug that works in combination with another drug, the two drugs having a greater effect when taken together than when taken separately.

synovectomy (ˌsienohˈvektəmee, ˌsi-) excision of a diseased synovial membrane to restore joint movement.

synovial fluid (sie'nohvi·əl, si- 'flooəd) the fluid that surrounds a joint and is secreted by the synovial membrane. It is a thick, colourless, lubricating substance.

synovial membrane (sie'nohvi·əl 'membrayn, si-) a serous membrane lining the articular capsule of a movable joint and terminating at the edge of the articular cartilage.

synovitis (ˌsienə'vietəs) inflammation of a synovial membrane usually with an effusion of fluid within the joint.

synthesis ('sinthəsəs) the building up of a more complex structure from simple components. This may apply to drugs or to plant or animal tissues.

syphilis ('sifələs) a sexually transmitted infection caused by the spirochaete *Treponema pallidum*. The initial sign is the appearance of a painless sore, appearing on the genitals, anus, rectum, lips, throat or fingers, which heals within a few weeks. A rash then ensues, which may be transient, recurrent or last for months. Other symptoms include lymphadenopathy, malaise, headaches, fever and fatigue. Following the symptomatic phase, the disease becomes latent for a few years or sometimes indefinitely. For untreated cases the disease progresses to the development of gummatous lesions involving the cardiovascular and neurological systems. Syphilis can be vertically transmitted from mother to fetus from 9 weeks of gestation, causing miscarriage, stillbirth, neonatal death and long-term morbidity. Practising safer sex can help to prevent syphilis infection. People with syphilis are infectious in the early stages but not in the latent and final stages. By law, syphilis is a notifiable disease in Australia and New Zealand and most other developed countries, such as the United States.

syringe (si'rinj) an instrument for injecting fluids or for aspirating or irrigating body cavities. It consists of a hollow tube with a tight-fitting piston. A hollow needle or a thin tube can be fitted to the end. *S. driver* a small battery-operated pump used to give medication continually.

syringomyelia (siˌring·gohmie'eeli·ə) the formation of cavities filled with fluid inside the spinal cord. Impairment of muscle function and sensation result at the level of and below the lesion. Painless injury may be the first symptom. It is a progressive disease.

syringomyelitis (siˌring·gohˌmieə'-lietəs) inflammation of the spinal cord, as the result of which cavities are formed in it.

syringomyelocele (siˌring·goh'mieə-lohˌseel) a type of SPINA BIFIDA in which the protruded sac of fluid communicates with the central canal of the spinal cord.

system (sistəm) 1. a collection or assemblage of parts that, unified, make a whole. 2. a set of computer programs and hardware that work together for a specific purpose. *Health service s.* a multi-faceted organisation of people, institutions and resources that provide government funding and private health insurance to meet the health needs of the Australian population. *Health service area s.* a geographic region designated under the various states and territories, covering such factors as geographic features, political boundaries, population and health resources, for the effective planning and development of health services. *S. overload* an inability to cope with messages and expectations from a number of sources within a given timeframe.

systematic (ˈsistəˌmatik) describing a process that is carried out according to a method or a system. *S. review* a methodical approach to literature reviews that reduces random error and bias. This requires a review of clinical literature in a particular field that has set explicit tests for whether research is valuable enough to be included in an overview of the area. This is often combined with a statistical meta-analysis of clinical trial results. *S. sampling* a type of sampling in which a convenient number is chosen, e.g. every 10th or fourth member of the population is selected into the sample.

Système International d'Unités *see* SI UNITS.

systemic (siˈstemik) pertaining to or affecting the body as a whole. *S. circulation* circulation of the blood throughout the whole body, other than the pulmonary circulation. *S. lupus erythematosus (SLE) See* LUPUS, SCLEROSIS.

systole (ˈsistəlee) the period of contraction of the heart. *See* DIASTOLE. *Atrial s.* the contraction of the heart by which the blood is pumped from the atria into the ventricles. *Extra s.* a premature contraction of the atrium or ventricle, without alteration of the fundamental rhythm of the pacemaker. *Ventricular s.* the contraction of the heart by which the blood is pumped into the aorta and pulmonary artery.

systolic (siˈstolik) relating to a systole. *S. murmur* an abnormal sound produced during systole in heart infections. *S. pressure* the highest pressure of the blood reached during systole.

Tt

T symbol for *thymine*.

T-cell (ˈtee ˌsel) a lymphocyte which is derived from the thymus and is responsible for cell-mediated immunity. *T. cytotoxic cells* (also known as T-killer cells) T-cells that are activated by circulating T-helper cells in the blood and lymphatic systems, and which recognise body cells displaying antigens to which they have become sensitised, targeting those which are viral or bacterially infected, triggering cell-mediated immunity. *T. helper cells* T-cells that activate B lymphocytes to release antibodies and T-killer cells to destroy cells that have a specific antigenic profile. *T. receptor* cells, formerly known as suppressor cells, T-cells keep the immune response at an appropriate level and also stop or slow down the activity of B lymphocytes and other T-cells once the immune response has dealt with the antigen.

TAB (typhoid-paratyphoid A and B vaccine) (tee ay bee ˈtieˌfoydˌ parəˈtieˌfoyd ay ənd bee ˈvakseen) a sterile suspension of the killed salmonellae causing these diseases. Used as a preventive, it provides an active immunity.

tabes (ˈtaybeez) a wasting away. *T. dorsalis* or *locomotor ataxia see* ATAXIA.

tablet (tablət) a small solid dosage form of a medication. Compressed or moulded during manufacture and may be of almost any size, shape weight and colour. *T. computer* a mobile computer integrated into a flat screen and operated by touching the screen.

taboo (ˌtəˈboo) any ritual prohibition of certain activities, e.g. incest in many societies, or the open discussion of death and dying.

tachycardia (ˌtakeeˈkahdi·ə) abnormally rapid action of the heart and consequent increase in pulse rate. *See* BRADYCARDIA. *Paroxysmal t.* spasmodic increase in cardiac contractions of sudden onset lasting a variable time from a few seconds to hours.

tachyphasia (tachyphrasia) (ˌtakee-ˈfayzi·ə; ˌtakeeˈfrayzi·ə) extreme volubility of speech. It may be a sign of mental disorder.

tachyphrenia (ˌtakeeˈfreeni·ə) hyperactivity of the mental processes.

tachypnoea (ˌtakipˈneeə) rapid, shallow respirations; a reflex response to stimulation of the vagus nerve endings in the pulmonary vessels.

tactile (ˈtaktiel) relating to the sense of touch.

Taenia (ˈteeniə) a genus of tapeworms. *T. saginata* the beef tapeworm. The most common type of tapeworm found in the human intestine. *T. solium* the pork tapeworm. Can also be parasitic in humans, causing CYSTICERCOSIS. *See* TAPEWORM.

taeniasis (teeˈnieəsəs) an infestation with tapeworms.

TAF 1. toxoid-antitoxin floccules. A vaccine used for diphtheria immunisation. *See* TOXOID. 2. tumour angiogenesis factor.

tai chi (ˌtieˈchee) a system of postures, linked by elegant and graceful movement, originating in China, promoting general health and wellbeing.

Takayasu arteritis (takay-ahsoo ˌahtəˈrietəs) a rare type of vasculitis that mainly affects the aorta of young women.

Takotsubo cardiomyopathy (tako-tsooboh ˌkahdeeohmieˈopəthee) also known as acute stress cardiomyopathy. Temporary and reversible symptoms of chest pain and breathlessness after significant emotional or physical stress.

talipes (ˈtaləpeez) clubfoot. A deformity caused by a congenital or acquired contraction of the muscles or tendons of the foot (*see* figure). *T. calcaneus* the heel alone touches the ground on standing. *T. equinus* the toes touch the ground but not the heel. *T. valgus* the inner edge of the foot only is in contact with the ground. *T. varus* the person walks on the outer edge of the foot.

talus (ˈtayləs) the astragalus or ankle bone.

tampon (ˈtampon) a plug of absorbent material inserted in the vagina, the nose or other orifice to restrain haemorrhage or absorb secretion.

tamponade (ˈtampəˌnayd) the surgical use of tampons. *Cardiac t.* impairment of heart action by haemorrhage or effusion into the pericardium; may be due to a stab wound or follow surgery.

tantrum (ˈtantrəm) an outburst of ill temper. *Temper t.* a behaviour disorder of childhood. A display of bad temper in which the child performs uncontrolled actions in a state of emotional stress.

tapeworm (ˈtaypˌwərm) any of a group of cestode flatworms including the *Taenia* genus which are parasitic in the intestines of humans and many animals. The adult consists of a round head with suckers or hooklets for attachment (scolex). From this, numerous segments (proglottids) arise, each of which produces ova capable of independent existence for a considerable length of time. Treatment is by ANTHELMINTIC drugs.

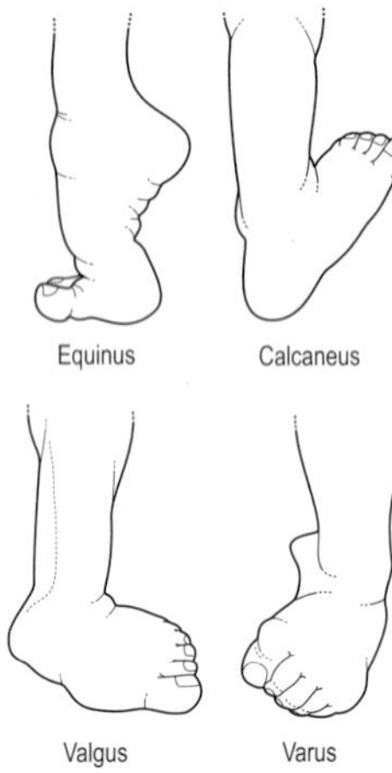

Talipes.

tapotement (ˌtapohtˈmonh) [Fr.] a tapping movement used in massage.

tapping *see* PARACENTESIS.

target cells (ˈtahgət selz) abnormal flat red blood cells seen in liver and spleen disease and in the haemoglobinopathies. The haemoglobin is distributed as a small inner mass with a pale outer ring.

tarsal (ˈtahsəl) relating to a tarsus. *T. bones* the seven small bones of the ankle and instep. *T. cyst* MEIBOMIAN CYST; CHALAZION.

T. glands meibomian glands of the eyelids. *T. plates* small cartilages in the upper and lower eyelids.

tarsalgia (tahˈsalji·ə) pain in the foot, usually associated with flattening of the arch.

tarsorrhaphy (tahˈso·rəfee) a rarely performed procedure involving partial stitching of the eyelids together to protect the cornea or to allow healing of an abrasion.

tartar (ˈtahtə) a hard incrustation deposited on the teeth and on dentures.

task allocation (ˈtahsk ˌaləkayˌshən) a method of organising care whereby each specific type of care is carried out by a separate nominated nurse or healthcare assistant, e.g. for the same patient, one nurse records the blood pressure and another nurse gives the prescribed medications.

taste (tayst) the sense by which it is possible to identify what is eaten and drunk. Taste receptors (buds) lie on the tongue and give the sensations of sweet, sour, salt and bitter.

tattoo (taˈtoo) a permanent discolouration of the skin due to a foreign pigment.

tattooing (ˌtaˈtoo·ing) the deliberate (usually for decorative purposes) or accidental, perhaps as a result of an explosion, insertion of coloured material into the deeper layers of the skin.

taxis (ˈtaksəs) manipulation by manual pressure of displaced organs or long bones to restore any part to its normal position. It can be used to reduce a hernia or a dislocation.

taxonomy (takˈsonəmee) the theory and practice of the classification into ordered categories of animals, plants and concepts.

Tay-Sachs disease (tay zahks diˈzeez) *Waren Tay, English ophthalmologist, 1843–1927; Bernard Sachs, American neurologist, 1858–1944.* A rare and usually fatal genetic disorder that causes progressive damage to the nervous system usually within the first 6 months of life, caused by a mutated HEXA gene.

TB *see* TUBERCULOSIS.

TBI *see* TOTAL BODY IRRADIATION.

TCA tricyclic antidepressants. *See* ANTIDEPRESSANT.

team nursing (ˈteem ˌnərsing) a method of organising care based on the allocation of each nurse to a team that cares for a group of patients.

tears (tiəz) the watery, slightly alkaline and saline secretion of the lacrimal glands that moistens the conjunctiva. Tears contain lysozyme, a bactericidal enzyme. *Artificial t.* preparations used to supplement tear production in people with dryness of the cornea and conjunctiva caused by a deficiency in tear production or altered tear film composition or dry eye associated with autoimmune disorder, e.g. rheumatoid arthritis, or to relieve irritation.

teat (teet) 1. a nipple of the breast. 2. a manufactured nipple used on infants' feeding bottles.

technetium (tekˈneeshi·əm) *symbol* Tc. A metallic element. *Radioactive t.* an isotope (^{99m}Tc) used in a number of diagnostic tests. As it has a short half-life (6 hours), a high dose may be given for scanning organs, but the person receives only a low radiation dose.

teeth (teeth) *see* DENTITION.

tegument (ˈtegyəmənt) the skin.

telangiectasis (təˌlanjeeˈektəsəs) a group of dilated capillary blood vessels, web-like or radiating in form.

telangioma (təˌlanjeeˈohmə) a tumour of the blood capillaries.

telemedicine (ˈtelee͵medsən) the use of communication systems (such as electronic networks and visual display units) to provide remote diagnosis, advice, treatment and monitoring. Used widely in primary, acute care rural and remote settings.

telepathy (təˈlepəthee) the transmission of thought without any normal means of communication between two persons.

telereceptor (͵teleerəˈseptə) a sensory nerve ending which can respond to distant stimuli. Those of the eyes, ears and nose are examples. Teleceptor.

telophase (ˈteloh͵fayz) the last stage in the division of cells when the chromosomes have been reconstituted in the nuclei at either end of the cell and the cell cytoplasm divides to form two new cells.

temperament (ˈtempərəmənt) a person's nature; the habitual and emotional attitude, as distinct from mood, which is temporary.

temperature (ˈtemprəchə) the degree of heat of a substance or body as measured by a thermometer. *Normal t.* the normal temperature of the human body is 37°C, with a slight decrease in the early morning and a slight increase at night. It indicates the balance between heat production and heat loss.

template (ˈtemplayt, templət) a mould or pattern. In radiotherapy, a map of the area of the patient requiring treatment and of those areas to be protected from radiation.

temple (ˈtempəl) the region on either side of the head above the zygomatic arch.

temporal (ˈtempə·rəl) pertaining to the side of the head. *T. arteritis* giant cell arteritis. A chronic inflammatory condition of the carotid arterial system, occurring usually in older people. There is persistent headache, and partial or total blindness may result. *T. bone* one of a pair of bones on either side of the skull and containing the organ of hearing. *T. lobe* the part of the cerebrum below the lateral SULCUS.

temporomandibular (͵tempə·rohmanˈdibyələ) relating to the temporal bone and the mandible. *T. joint* the hinge of the lower jaw. *T. joint syndrome* painful dysfunction of the temporomandibular joint, marked by a clicking or grinding sensation in the joint; commonly caused by malocclusion of the teeth.

tenacious (təˈnayshəs) thick and viscid, as applied to sputum or other body fluids.

tendinitis (͵tendəˈnietəs) inflammation of a tendon and its attachments.

tendon (ˈtendən) a band of fibrous tissue forming the termination of a muscle and attaching it to a bone. *Achilles t.* that inserted into the CALCANEUM. *T. grafting* an operation which repairs a defect in one tendon by a graft from another. *T. insertion* the point of attachment of a muscle to a bone which it moves. *T. reflex* the muscular contraction produced on percussing a tendon.

tenesmus (təˈnezməs) a painful, ineffectual straining to empty the bowel or bladder.

tennis elbow (ˈtenəs ˈelboh) a painful disorder which affects the extensor muscles of the forearm at their attachment to the external EPICONDYLE.

tenorrhaphy (teˈno·rəfee) the suturing together of the ends of a divided tendon.

tenosynovitis (͵tenoh͵sienəˈvietəs) inflammation of a tendon sheath.

TENS *see* TRANSCUTANEOUS ELECTRICAL NERVE STIMULATION.

tension (ˈtenshən) the act of stretching or the state of being stretched. *Arterial t.* the pressure of blood on the vessel wall during cardiac contraction. *Intraocular t.* the pressure of the contents of the eye on its walls, measured by a tonometer. *Intravenous t.* the pressure of blood within the veins. *Surface t.* tension or resistance which acts to preserve the integrity of a surface, particularly the surface of a liquid.

tensor (ˈtensə, -saw) a muscle that stretches a part.

teratogen (ˌtəˈratəjən) an agent or influence that causes physical defects in the developing embryo.

teratoma (ˌterəˈtohmə) a solid tumour containing tissues similar to those of a dermoid cyst. Found most often in the ovaries and testes. Many of these tumours are malignant.

term (tərm) the end of pregnancy, normally calculated as 280 days or 40 weeks from the date of the last normal menstrual period but considered to be any time after the 37th week of pregnancy.

termination of pregnancy (TOP) (ˈtərmənˌayshən əv ˈpregˌnənsee) abortion that is induced, legally or illegally.

tertiary (ˈtərshə·ree) third. *T. care* care and treatment that is given in a regional hospital providing specialist care, e.g. cardiac surgery, intensive, neonatal, oncological services. *T. prevention* prevention of ill health, mitigating the effects of illness and disease that have already occurred.

test (test) 1. an examination or trial. 2. analysis of the composition of a substance by the use of chemical reagents, and/or to determine the presence or absence of a substance.

testicle (ˈtestikəl) a testis; one of the two glands in the scrotum which produce SPERMATOZOA. *Undescended t.* a condition in which the organ remains in the pelvis or inguinal canal.

testicular self-examination (tesˈtikyələ ˌselfˌegzaməˈnayshən) should be performed regularly once a month for the detection of early tumours of the testis which are highly curable if detected at an early stage. Self-examination should take place after a warm bath or shower, which relaxes the scrotal skin. It is performed as follows: standing in front of a mirror, look for any swelling. One testicle may appear larger than the other or hang lower; this is usually perfectly normal. Examine each testicle with both hands and gently roll each testicle between the fingers and thumb. A small lump is felt for and, if found, almost always occurs in only one testis and is usually painless. A cordlike structure found on the top and back of each testicle should be found and examined for any swelling (*see* figure, p. 464). *T. torsion* severe twisting of the spermatic cord.

testis (ˈtestəs) a testicle.

testosterone (tesˈtostəˌrohn) the hormone produced by the testes which stimulates the development of sex characteristics. It can now be made synthetically and is used medicinally in cases of failure of sex function and as a palliative treatment in some cases of advanced metastatic breast cancer in females.

tetanus (ˈtetənəs) an acute disease of the nervous system caused by the contamination of wounds by the spores of a soil bacterium, *Clostridium tetani.* Muscle stiffness around the site of the wound occurs,

Testicular self-examination

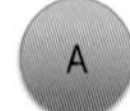

Make sure your scrotum is warm and relaxed. This can be achieved during or after showering or after a bath.

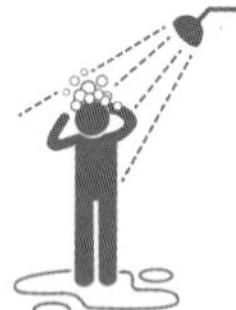

B

Firmly but gently roll one testicle between the fingers and thumbs of both hands checking for lumps, swelling or pain.

Become familiar with the structure of the epididymis by feeling along the underside of the testicle. It feels like tightly curled tubes.

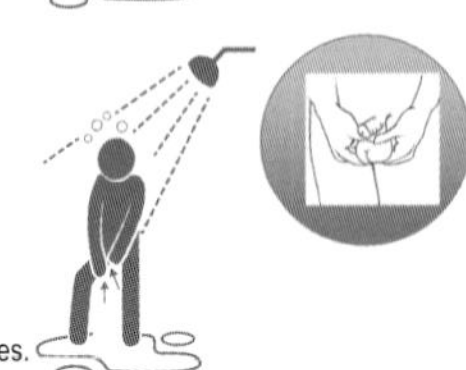

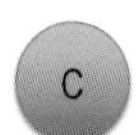

Repeat on the other testicle.

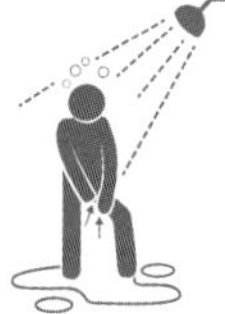

Symptoms of testicular cancer include a lump or a painless swelling in the testicle.
Other testicular changes to look/feel for include:

- a feeling of heaviness in the scrotum
- any changes in the feel, size or shape of the testicle
- feelings of unevenness or enlargement of the testicle
- any pain or ache in the lower abdomen, the testicle or scrotum
- any back pain
- a collection of fluid in the scrotum
- enlargement or tenderness of the breast tissue (due to hormones created by cancer cells).

There is no routine screening test for testicular cancer; therefore it is important to take note of any changes or anything unusual in the testicle and report the findings to your general practitioner (GP). Undertaking regular testicular self-examination lets men know what is normal for each testicle. If changes are detected, they need to be reported to their GP without delay. For more information on how to be testicular aware, visit the Cancer Council Australia website or relevant organisations related to the country of your practice.

Testicular self-examination.

followed by rigidity of face and neck muscles—hence 'lockjaw'. All muscles are then affected and OPISTHOTONOS may occur. *T. immunoglobulin* also known as tetanus antitoxin and tetanus immune globulin (TIG) a serum that gives a short-term passive immunity and may be used for immediate treatment of a case of tetanus. Also *T. vaccine* or *toxoid* will give an active immunity.

tetany (ˈtetənee) an increased excitability of the nerves due to a lack of available calcium, accompanied by painful muscle spasm of the hands and feet (carpopedal spasm). The cause may be HYPOPARATHYROIDISM or ALKALOSIS owing to excessive vomiting or hyperventilation.

tetralogy (teˈtraləjee) a series of four. *T. of Fallot see* FALLOT'S TETRALOGY. (*See* figure below.)

tetraplegia (ˌtetrəˈpleeji·ə) also known as quadriplegia. Paralysis of all four limbs.

thalamus (ˈthaləməs) a mass of nerve cells at the base of the cerebrum. Most sensory impulses from the body pass to this area and are transmitted to the cortex.

thalassaemia (ˌthaləˈseemi·ə) a group of inherited haemolytic

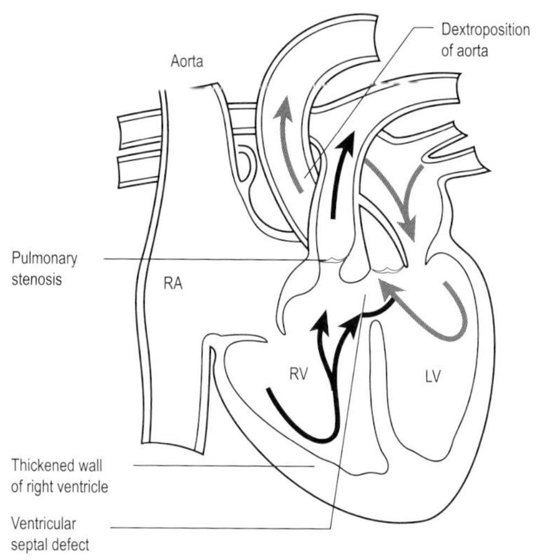

Tetralogy of Fallot.

anaemias where there is interference with the synthesis of haemoglobin resulting in anaemia. Several types are recognised, according to the symptoms. Thalassaemia is prevalent in the Mediterranean, Middle East and South-East Asian regions, and occurs in families from these regions as the disease is genetically inherited. The only possible cure is a stem cell or bone marrow transplant, but this carries significant risks so is not often performed. Genetic counselling is advised for the parents or other close relatives of a child with thalassaemia and also for any person with thalassaemia trait.

thalassotherapy (thəˌlasohˈtherəpee) treatment involving sea bathing, sea products or a sea voyage.

thanatology (ˌthanəˈtoləjee) 1. the study of death and dying. 2. the forensic study of the causes of death.

theca (ˈtheekə) a sheath, such as the covering of a tendon. *T. folliculi* the covering of a Graafian follicle. *T. vertebralis* the membranes enclosing the spinal cord; the DURA MATER.

thenar (ˈtheenə) 1. the palm of the hand. 2. the fleshy part at the base of the thumb.

theory (ˌthiəree) a set of interrelated concepts, definitions and propositions that present a systematic view of phenomena for the purpose of explaining and making predictions about those phenomena.

therapeutic (ˌtherəˈpyootik) pertaining to therapeutics or treatment of disease; curative. *T. abortion see* ABORTION. *T. community* any treatment setting (usually psychiatric) which provides a living–learning situation through group processes emphasising social, environmental and personal interactions and which encourages the individual to learn socially from these processes. *T. drug monitoring (TDM)* some drugs require that blood levels are maintained within a certain range (often called a therapeutic window) to avoid inefficacy as a result of low blood levels and producing side effects for the person as a result of levels in the blood being too high. To do this blood levels of the drug concerned need to be measured at appropriate intervals and medication regimens altered as necessary. *T. index* the margin of difference between the desired and safe effect that a drug dose achieves and the dose that is known to produce toxic effects. This measure varies between people, who all process drugs differently, but it does alert the prescriber to the margins of safety in the use of a particular drug. *T. touch* techniques that are used to facilitate healing and wellbeing of a person based on the concept that the body is an energy field and that this field can be influenced from outside itself. Body energies can be transferred to and through the hands of a therapist who has been trained to assume the role of healer. *See* MASSAGE. *T. use of self* the ability of the caregiver such as a nurse to use therapy, experimental knowledge, self-awareness and the ability to explore and use personal impact on others. *T. window* range of blood levels in the use of certain drugs. *See TDM* above.

therapeutics (ˌtherəˈpyootiks) the science and art of healing and the treatment of disease.

therapy (ˈtherəpee) the treatment of disease.

thermal (ˈthərməl) relating to heat.

thermocautery (ˌthərmohˈkawtə·ree) the deliberate destruction of tissue by means of heat. *See* CAUTERY.

thermography (ˌthərˈmogrəfee) a method of measuring the amount of heat produced by different areas of the body using infrared photography. Used as a diagnostic aid in the detection of breast tumours and the assessment of rheumatic joints; also used in the study of pain.

thermolysis (thərˈmoləsəs) the loss of body heat by radiation, by excretion and by the evaporation of sweat.

thermometer (thəˈmomətə) an instrument for measuring temperature. *Clinical t.* one used to measure the body temperature.

thermoreceptor (ˌthərmohrəˈseptə) a nerve ending that responds to heat and cold.

thermoregulation (ˈthərmohˌregyooˌlayshən) the normal regulation of body temperature by the maintenance of the balance between heat production and heat loss.

thermotherapy (ˌthərmohˈtherəpee) the treatment of disease by application of heat.

thiamine (ˈthieəˌmeen) vitamin B_1, or aneurine. An essential vitamin involved in carbohydrate metabolism. A deficiency causes beriberi. The source is liver and unrefined cereals.

Thiersch skin graft (tiərsh skin grahft) *Karl Thiersch, German surgeon, 1822–1895.* The transplantation of areas of partial thickness skin. *See* GRAFT.

thirst (thərst) an uncomfortable sensation of dryness of the mouth and throat with a desire for oral fluids. *Abnormal t.* POLYDIPSIA.

Thomas splint (ˈtomas splint) *Hugh Thomas, British orthopaedic surgeon, 1834–1891.* A splint consisting of an oval metal ring that fits over the lower limb. Attached to the ring are two round metal rods which are bent into a W shape at the lower end. Used to immobilise fractures of the leg during transportation and for use with traction as it supports the limb and moves the weight from the knee joint to the pelvis.

thoracic (thawˈrasik) relating to the thorax. *T. duct* the large lymphatic vessel situated in the thorax along the spine. It opens into the left subclavian vein.

thoracocentesis (ˌthaw·rəkohsenˈteesəs) puncture of the wall of the thorax to allow aspiration of pleural fluid.

thoracoscopy (ˌthaw·rəˈkoskəpee) examination of the pleural cavity by means of an endoscopic instrument.

thoracotomy (ˌthaw·rəˈkotəmee) a surgical incision into the thorax.

thorax (ˈthaw·raks) the chest; a cavity containing the heart, lungs, bronchi and oesophagus. It is bounded by the diaphragm, the sternum, the thoracic vertebrae and the ribs. *Barrel-shaped t.* a development in chronic obstructive pulmonary disease, such as EMPHYSEMA, when the chest is malformed like a barrel.

threadworm (ˈthredˌwərm) a species of roundworm, *Enterobius vermicularis*, parasitic in the large intestine, particularly of children.

threonine (ˈthreeəˌneen) one of the essential amino acids.

thrill (thril) a tremor discerned by palpation.

throat (throht) 1. the anterior surface of the neck. 2. the pharynx. *Clergyman's sore t.* LARYNGITIS. *Sore t.* PHARYNGITIS.

thrombectomy (thromˈbektəmee) surgical excision of a clot from a vein or an artery.

thrombin (ˈthrombən) an enzyme that converts fibrinogen to fibrin during the later stages of blood clotting.

thromboangiitis (ˌthrombohˌanjeeˈ-ietəs) inflammation of blood vessels with clot formation. *T. obliterans* inflammation of the arteries, usually of the legs of young males, causing intermittent claudication and gangrene. Buerger's disease.

thrombocyte (ˈthrombohˌsiet) a disc-shaped blood platelet that is essential for the clotting of shed blood.

thrombocytopenia (ˌthrombohˌsie-tohˈpeeni·ə) a reduction in the number of platelets in the blood; bleeding may occur. Destruction of platelets can be caused by infections, certain drugs, transfusion-related purpuras, idiopathic thrombocytopenic PURPURA and disseminated intravascular coagulation.

thrombocytosis (ˌthrombohsieˈtoh-səs) an increase in the number of platelets in the blood.

thromboembolism (ˈthrombohˌ-embəlizm) a clot or embolism, which has become detached from a thrombus formed in another site that is carried in the blood flow to obstruct a blood vessel elsewhere in the body.

thromboendarterectomy (ˌthrom-bohˌendahtəˈrektəmee) surgical removal of a clot from an artery together with a portion of the lining of the artery.

thromboendarteritis (ˌthromboh-ˌendahtəˈrietəs) inflammation of the lining of an artery with clot formation as a result.

thrombokinase (ˌthrombohˈkienayz) THROMBOPLASTIN; a lipid-containing protein activated by blood platelets and injured tissues which is capable of activating prothrombin to form thrombin, which, combined with fibrinogen, forms a clot.

thrombolysis (thromˈboləsəs) the disintegration or dissolving of a clot by the infusion of an enzyme such as streptokinase into the blood.

thrombophilia (ˌthrombohˈfiliə) increased tendency for blood to clot.

thrombophlebitis (ˌthromboh-fləˈbietəs) the formation of a clot, associated with inflammation of the lining of a vein.

thromboplastin (ˌthrombohˈplastən) *see* THROMBOKINASE.

thrombosis (thromˈbohsəs) the formation of a thrombus. *Cavernous sinus t.* thrombosis of the cavernous sinus, usually the result of infection of the face, when the veins in the sinus are affected via ophthalmic vessels. *Cerebral t.* the occlusion of a cerebral artery, the most common cause of cerebral infarction (a 'stroke'). *Coronary t.* the occlusion of a coronary vessel, by which the heart muscle is deprived of blood, causing myocardial ischaemia and often leading to MYOCARDIAL INFARCTION (a heart attack). *See* DEEP VENOUS THROMBOSIS. *Lateral sinus t.* a rare complication of a middle ear infection when the lateral sinus of the DURA MATER is infected and there is clot formation.

thrombus (ˈthrombəs) a stationary blood clot caused by coagulation of the blood in the heart or in an artery or a vein.

thrush (thrush) an infection of the mucous membranes, most commonly of the skin, mouth and vagina, by a fungus, *Candida albicans*. *See* CANDIDIASIS.

thymectomy (thieˈmektəmee) surgical removal of the thymus.

thymine (ˈthiemeen) one of the pyrimidine bases found in DNA.

thymoma (thieˈmohmə) a tumour that originates in thymus tissue.

thymus (ˈthieməs) a gland-like structure situated in the upper thorax and neck. Present in early life, it reaches its maximum development during puberty and continues to play an immunological role throughout life, even though its function declines with age.

thyroglossal (ˌthieroh'glosəl) relating to the thyroid and the tongue. *T. cyst see* CYST.

thyroid ('thieroyd) 1. shaped like a shield. 2. pertaining to the thyroid gland. *T. cartilage* the largest cartilage of the larynx. It forms the 'Adam's apple' in the front of the throat. *T. gland* a ductless gland consisting of two lobes situated in front and on either side of the trachea. It secretes the hormones thyroxine and triiodothyronine which are concerned with regulating the metabolic rate. *Overactive T. see* THYROTOXICOSIS. *T.-stimulating hormone (TSH)* thyrotrophin; a hormone produced by the anterior pituitary gland which controls the activity of the thyroid gland.

thyroidectomy (ˌthieroy'dektəmee) partial or complete removal of the thyroid gland. *Underactive T.* hypothyroidism. The thyroid gland does not produce sufficient hormones, resulting in a range of symptoms, including weight gain, tiredness and depression.

thyroiditis (ˌthieroy'dietəs) inflammation of the thyroid. Acute thyroiditis, usually due to a virus infection, is characterised by sore throat, fever and painful enlargement of the gland. *Hashimoto's t.* also known as chronic lymphocytic thyroiditis, is a progressive autoimmune disease of the thyroid gland with degeneration of its epithelial elements and replacement by lymphoid and fibrous tissue.

thyroparathyroidectomy (ˌthierohˌ-parəˌthieroy'dektəmee) surgical removal of the thyroid and parathyroid glands.

thyrotoxicosis (ˌthierohˌtoksə'-kohsəs) hyperthyroidism. The symptoms arise when there is overactivity of the thyroid gland. The metabolism is speeded up and there is enlargement of the gland and EXOPHTHALMOS.

thyrotrophin (ˌthieroh'trohfən) *see* THYROID-STIMULATING HORMONE.

thyroxine (thie'rokseen) one of the two hormones secreted by the thyroid gland. It is used in the treatment of HYPOTHYROIDISM.

TIA *see* TRANSIENT ISCHAEMIC ATTACK.

tibia ('tibi·ə) the shin bone; the larger of the two bones of the leg, extending from knee to ankle.

tic (tik) a spasmodic twitching of certain muscles, usually of the face, neck or shoulder. *T. douloureux* paroxysmal trigeminal neuralgia.

tick (tik) a bloodsucking parasite which can transmit the organisms of various diseases.

tidal volume ('tied'l 'volyoom) the amount of gas passing into and out of the lungs in each respiratory cycle.

tincture ('tingk·chə) a medical substance dissolved in alcohol.

tinea ('tini·ə) a group of skin infections caused by a variety of fungi and named after the area of the body affected, thus: *T. barbae*, the beard; *T. capitis*, the head; *T. circinata* or *T. corporis*, the body; *T. cruris*, the groin; and *T. pedis*, the feet. *See* RINGWORM.

tinnitus (ti'nietəs, 'tinətəs) a ringing, buzzing or roaring sound in the ears.

tissue ('tisyoo, 'tishoo) a group or layer of similarly specialised cells that together perform certain special functions.

titration (tie'trayshən) determination of a given component in solution by addition of a liquid reagent of known strength until a given endpoint, e.g. change in colour, is reached, indicating that the component has been consumed by reaction with the reagent.

TLC *see* TOTAL LUNG CAPACITY.

tobacco (tə'bakoh) the dried leaves of the plant *Nicotiana tabacum*, containing the drug nicotine, which may be smoked, chewed or inhaled. All these activities are potentially dangerous to health. Cigarette smoking in particular is responsible for an increase in cancer of the lung and mouth and bronchitis. Smoking increases the likelihood of chronic obstructive pulmonary disease, including emphysema and coronary artery disease. It is also harmful during pregnancy, leading to smaller and less healthy babies. *T. withdrawal syndrome* a change in mood or behaviour associated with the stopping of or reduction in cigarette smoking.

tocography (to'kogrəfee) the measurement of alterations in the intrauterine pressure during labour.

tocopherol (to'kofə·rol) vitamin E, present in wheatgerm, green leaves and milk.

token economy program (ˌtohkən ə'konəmee 'prohgram) a behavioural approach to modifying troublesome behaviours and restoring lost self-help behaviours by the systematic rewarding of desired behaviour through giving tokens which may be exchanged for goods or privileges.

tolerance ('tolə·rəns) the ability to endure without effect or injury. *Drug t.* decrease of susceptibility to the effects of a drug due to its continued administration. *Exercise t.* test to determine how much oxygen a person's myocardium requires during exercise. The results indicate the person's capacity for exercise and in the estimation of the extent of coronary disease. *Immunological t.* or immune tolerance is a specific non-reactivity of lymphoid tissues to a particular antigen capable, under other conditions, of inducing immunity.

tomography (tə'mogrəfee) body section radiography in which X-rays or ultrasound waves are used to produce an image of a layer of tissue at any depth.

tone (tohn) 1. the normal degree of tension, e.g. in a muscle. 2. a particular quality of sound.

tongue (tung) a muscular organ attached to the floor of the mouth and concerned in taste, mastication, swallowing and speech. It is covered by a mucous membrane from which project numerous PAPILLAE. *T. tie* also known as ankyloglossia is where a strip of skin connecting the tongue and floor of the mouth in a baby is shorter than usual.

tonic ('tonik) 1. a term popularly applied to any drug supposed to brace or tone up the body or any particular part or organ. 2. possessing tone in a state of contraction, e.g. muscles. *T. spasm* a prolonged contraction of one or several muscles, as seen in epilepsy, for example. *See* CLONIC.

tonography (to'nogrəfee) the measurement made by an electric tonometer recording the intraocular pressure and so, indirectly, the drainage of aqueous humour from the eye.

tonsil ('tonsəl) a mass of lymphoid tissue, particularly one of two small, almond-shaped bodies, situated one on each side between the pillars of the FAUCES. It is covered by mucous membrane and its surface is pitted with follicles. *Pharyngeal t.* the lymphadenoid tissue of the pharynx between the pharyngotympanic tubes. Adenoids. *T. test* a small sample of tonsil obtained in suspected cases of CREUTZFELDT-JAKOB DISEASE (CJD) for the identification of the prion found in new variant CJD, a spongiform encephalopathy.

tonsillectomy (ˌtonsəˈlektəmee) excision of one or both tonsils.

tonsillitis (ˌtonsəlˈietəs) inflammation of the tonsils, usually due to a viral infection.

tonus (ˈtohnəs) the normal state of partial contraction of the muscles.

tooth (tooth) a structure in the mouth designed for the mastication of food. Each is composed of a crown, neck and root with one or more fangs. The main bulk is of dentine enclosing a central pulp; the crown is covered with a hard white substance called enamel. *See* DENTITION.

TOP *see* TERMINATION OF PREGNANCY.

tophus (ˈtohfəs) a small, hard, chalky deposit of sodium urate in the skin and cartilage, occurring in gout and sometimes appearing on the auricle of the ear.

topical (ˈtopikəl) relating to a particular spot; local. *T. lotion* one for local or external application.

topography (təˈpografee, toh-) the study of the surface of the body in relation to the underlying structures.

torpor (ˈtawpə) a sluggish condition in which response to stimuli is absent or very slow.

torsion (ˈtawshən) twisting: (a) of an artery to arrest haemorrhage; (b) of the pedicle of a cyst which produces venous congestion in the cyst and consequent gangrene (a possible complication of ovarian cyst).

torso (ˈtawsoh) the body, excluding the head and the limbs; the trunk.

torticollis (ˌtawtəˈkoləs) wryneck, a contracted state of the cervical muscles producing torsion of the neck. The deformity may be congenital or hysterical, or secondary to pressure on the accessory nerve, to inflammation of glands in the neck or to muscle spasm.

total (ˈtohtəl) complete, the whole number or amount. *T. body irradiation (TBI)* the complete exposure of the person's body to radiotherapy, used in the treatment of some cancers and prior to bone marrow transplantation. *T. burn surface area (TBSA)* a formula for predicting outcomes after a burn injury: (age 1 TBSA) 5 percentage chance of surviving. *See* LUND AND BROWDER CHART. *T. lung capacity (TLC)* the volume of air held in the lungs following deep inspiration. *T. parenteral nutrition (TPN)* the supplying of all essential nutrients to a person via the intravenous route. *T. quality management (TQM)* a largely superseded approach to management based on the idea that quality of service depends on the active involvement of all members of staff in achieving and maintaining high standards of care throughout an organisation.

touch (tuch) 1. the ability to feel objects and to distinguish their various characteristics; the tactile sense. 2. the ability to perceive pressure when it is applied on the skin. 3. to palpate or examine with the hands different parts of the body.

Tourette's syndrome (tooretz ˈsindrohm) *George Gilles de la Tourette, French physician, 1857–1904.* An inherited neurological disorder which starts in childhood.

Characterised by repetitive grimaces and tics, involuntary barks, grunts, shouting and other noises may appear as the disease progresses. Some sufferers may also use obscene language (coprolalia). Also known as Gilles de la Tourette's syndrome. Causes are unknown although there may be a genetic cause in some cases.

tourniquet (ˈtooənəˌkay, ˈtawnə-) a constrictive band applied to a limb to arrest arterial haemorrhage. Now used to obstruct the venous return from a limb and so facilitate the withdrawal of blood from a vein.

toxaemia (tokˈseemi·ə) poisoning of the blood by the absorption of bacterial toxins. *T. of pregnancy* a condition affecting pregnant women and characterised by ALBUMINURIA, hypertension and oedema, with the possibility of pre-eclampsia and ECLAMPSIA developing.

toxic (ˈtoksik) 1. poisonous, relating to a poison. 2. caused by a toxin. *T. shock syndrome* a severe illness characterised by high fever of sudden onset, vomiting, diarrhoea and, in severe cases, death. A sunburn-like rash with peeling of the skin occurs. The syndrome affects almost exclusively menstruating women using tampons, although a few women who do not use tampons and a few males have been affected. It is thought to be caused by infection with *Staphylococcus aureus*.

toxicity (tokˈsisətee) the degree of virulence of a poison.

toxicology (ˌtoksəˈkoləjee) the science dealing with poisons.

toxidrome (ˌtoksəˈdrohm) a collection of signs and symptoms that indicate poisoning by a certain drug.

toxin (ˈtoksən) any poisonous compound, usually referring to that produced by bacteria.

Toxocara (ˌtoksohˈkah·rə) a genus of nematode worms, parasitic in the intestines of dogs and cats, which may also infest humans, especially children. The spleen, liver and lungs are most often affected but the parasite may also infest the retina, causing inflammation and granulation.

toxoid (ˈtoksoyd) a toxin which has been deprived of some of its harmful properties, but is still capable of producing immunity and may be used in a vaccine.

Toxoplasma (ˌtoksohˈplazmə) a genus of protozoa which infests birds and animals and may be transmitted from them to humans.

toxoplasmosis (ˌtoksohplazˈmohsəs) a disease due to *Toxoplasma gondii* carried by cats, birds and other animals and in contaminated soil. The congenital form may result in miscarriage or stillbirth of the infant. The disease may also cause enlarged liver and spleen, blindness, brain defects and death. The acquired infection is often asymptomatic but may result in pneumonia, skin rashes and NEPHRITIS. Can cause severe multisystem disease in immunocompromised people.

TPN (tee pee en) *see* TOTAL PARENTERAL NUTRITION.

trabecula (trəˈbekyələ) a dividing band or septum extending from the capsule of an organ into its interior and holding the functioning cells in position.

trabeculectomy (trəˌbekyəˈlektəmee) an operation to lower the intraocular pressure in glaucoma that cannot be controlled by medication.

trace element (trays ˈeləmənt) an element that is essential in the diet, for the normal functioning of the body, but is required only in minute amounts, e.g. zinc, manganese, fluorine.

tracer (ˈtraysə) a means by which something may be followed, as: (a) a mechanical device by which the outline or movements of an object can be graphically recorded; or (b) a material by which the progress of a compound through the body may be observed, e.g. a radioactive isotope tracer.

trachea (trəˈkeeə, ˈtraki·ə) the windpipe: a cartilaginous tube lined with ciliated mucous membrane extending from the lower part of the larynx to the commencement of the bronchi.

tracheitis (ˌtrakeeˈietəs) inflammation of the trachea causing pain in the chest, with coughing.

tracheobronchitis (ˌtrakeeohbrongˈkietəs) acute infection of the trachea and bronchi due to viruses or bacteria.

tracheostomy (ˌtrakeeˈostəmee) a surgical opening into the third and fourth cartilage rings of the trachea. *T. tubes* those used to maintain an airway after tracheotomy, either permanently or until the normal use of the air passages is regained.

tracheotomy (ˌtrakeeˈotəmee) surgical incision of the trachea. *Inferior* or *low t.* that in which the opening is made below the thyroid isthmus. *Superior* or *high t.* that in which the opening is made above the thyroid isthmus.

trachoma (trəˈkohmə) a chronic infectious disease of the conjunctiva and cornea, producing photophobia, pain and lacrimation, caused by an organism once thought to be a virus but now classified as a strain of the bacterium *Chlamydia trachomatis*. Trachoma is more prevalent in Africa and Asia than in other parts of the world.

traction (ˈtrakshən) 1. the exertion of a pulling force, such as that applied to a fractured bone or dislocated joint or to relieve muscle spasm to maintain proper position and facilitate healing. 2. in obstetrics, that along the axis of the pelvis to assist in delivery of a fetal part, or the placenta and membranes. *Hamilton-Russell t.* a form of continuous traction that is generated by weights and pulleys to immobilise, position and align the lower extremities in the treatment of fractures of the femurs, hip and knee contractures. Also known as Russell's traction. *Head t.* traction exerted on the head in the treatment of cervical injury. *Skeletal t.* a method of keeping the fractured ends of bone in position by traction on the bone. A metal pin or wire is passed through the distal fragment or adjacent bone to overcome muscle contraction.

trait (trayt) an inherited or developed physical or mental characteristic.

trance (trans) a condition of semiconsciousness of hysterical, cataleptic or hypnotic origin. It is not due to organic disease.

tranquilliser (ˈtrangkwəˌliezə) a drug which allays anxiety, relieves tension and has a calming effect on the patient.

transactional analysis (tranˈzakshənəl, trahn- əˈnaləsəs) a theory of personality structure and a psychotherapeutic method. The human personality is viewed as consisting of three ego states: the parent, the adult and the child. The aim is to allow the adult ego to take control over the child and parent egos.

transaminase (tranˈzaməˌnayz) one of a group of enzymes which catalyse the transfer of an amine group from one amino acid into another. Transaminases include *glutamic oxalacetic t. (GOT)* and *glutamic pyruvic t. (GPT)*.

transcendental meditation (ˌtransən-ˌdent'l ˌmedəˈtayshən, ˌtrahn-) a technique for attaining a state of physical relaxation and psychological calm by the regular practice of a relaxation procedure which entails the repetition of a mantra. Has been successfully used by some people to reduce hypertension.

transcultural nursing (tranzˈkul-chərəl ˈnərsing) being aware of the person's cultural health beliefs and values and incorporating these into the agreed care plan with the patient.

transcutaneous blood gas monitors (tranzˌkyooˈtaynee·əs blud gas ˈmonətəz) the application to the skin of a probe which is heated to a temperature of 44°C and enables measurements of PO_2 and PCO_2 to be made. Accuracy depends on the quality of the peripheral circulation thus transcutaneous blood gas monitoring is usually used in conjunction with intermittent arterial sampling.

transcutaneous electrical nerve stimulation (TENS) (tranz-ˌkyooˈtaynee·əs əˈlektrikəl nərv ˈstimyəˈlayshən, tenz) a method of treating persistent pain by passing small electrical currents into the spinal cord or sensory nerves by means of electrodes applied to the skin. TENS is non-invasive and non-addictive, with no known side effects.

transdermal (ˌtranzˈdərm'l) through the skin. *T. patch* a medicated adhesive patch that is placed onto the skin to deliver a specific dose of medication through the skin and into the bloodstream. The main advantage of the transdermal patch is that it provides a controlled release of the medication into the person. The main disadvantage is that only drugs whose molecules are small enough to penetrate the skin can be delivered by this method.

transference (ˈtransfə·rəns, transˈfər·rəns, ˈtrahns-) in psychiatry, the unconscious transfer by the person onto the psychiatrist of feelings that are appropriate to other people significant to the person.

transferrin (ˌtranzˈfairən) a glycoprotein that acts as a carrier for iron in the bloodstream.

transfusion (transˈfyoozhən) the introduction of whole blood or a blood component into a vein, performed in cases of severe loss of blood, shock, septicaemia, etc. It is used to supply actual volume of blood or to introduce constituents, such as clotting factors or antibodies, that are deficient in the person. *Direct t.* the transfer of blood directly from a donor to a recipient. *Exchange* or *replacement t.* the removal of most or all of the recipient's blood and its replacement with fresh blood. Used with infants suffering from ERYTHROBLASTOSIS. *See* RH FACTOR. *Feto-maternal t.* from fetus to mother via the placenta; transplacental transfusion (TPT). *Replacement t.* exchange transfusion.

transgender (transˈjendə) people who have a gender identity or gender expression that differs from their assigned sex.

transient ischaemic attack (TIA) (ˈtranzeeˌənt isˈkeemik əˈtak) an episode of cerebrovascular insufficiency usually associated with partial occlusion of the cerebral artery by an atherosclerotic plaque or an embolus.

transillumination (ˌtranzəˌlooməˈnayshən, ˌtrahnz-) the illumination of a translucent body structure by a strong light as an aid to diagnosis, particularly of tumours of the retina and of abnormalities in the ethmoidal and frontal sinuses.

translocation (ˌtranzlohˈkayshən, ˌtrahnz-) in morphology, the transfer of a segment of a chromosome to a different site on the same chromosome or to a different chromosome. It may be a cause of congenital abnormality.

translucent (tranzˈloosənt, trahnz-) allowing light rays to pass through indistinctly.

transmigration (ˌtranzmieˈgrayshən, ˌtrahnz-) a movement from one place to another, as in the passage of blood cells through the walls of the capillaries; DIAPEDESIS. *External t.* the passage of an ovum from an ovary to the uterine tube on the opposite side. *Internal t.* the movement of an ovum from one uterine tube to the other through the uterus.

transmission-based precautions (ˌtranzˈmishən baysʼd prəˈcawshənz) precautions designed to be applied to people known or suspected to be infected with pathogens that are highly transmissible or epidemiologically important, and for which additional measures beyond STANDARD PRECAUTIONS are needed to interrupt transmission in hospital. There are three types of transmission-based precaution: airborne, droplet and contact precautions. They may be combined for diseases that have multiple routes of transmission. When employed either singly or in combination, they are used in addition to standard precautions. (*See* Appendix 10.)

transplacental (ˌtranspləˈsentʼl, ˌtrahns-) across the placenta. Movement may be from mother to fetus, or vice versa. *T. infection* may affect the unborn child.

transplant (ˈtransplant, ˈtrahnsplahnt) 1. an organ or tissue taken from the body and grafted into another area of the same individual or another individual. 2. to transfer tissue from one part to another or from one individual to another.

transplantation (ˌtransplanˈtayshən, ˌtrahnsplahn-) the transfer of living organs from one part of the body to another (autotransplant) or from one individual to another (allograft). Transplantation is often called grafting, although the term 'grafting' is more commonly used to refer to the transfer of skin.

transposition (ˌtranzpəˈzishən, ˌtrahnz-) 1. displacement of any of the viscera to the opposite side of the body. 2. the operation which partially removes a piece of tissue from one part of the body to another, the complete severance being delayed until it has become established in its new position. *T. of the great vessels* a congenital abnormality of the heart in which the positions of the pulmonary artery and aorta are reversed.

transsexualism (tranzˈsekshooəˌlizəm, trahnz) people who experience gender identity that is inconsistent with their assigned sex.

transudate (ˈtransyəˌdayt, ˈtrahn-) any fluid that passes through a membrane.

transverse (transˈvərs, trahnz-) crosswise. *T. presentation* position of the fetus whereby it lies across the pelvis, which position must be corrected before normal birth can take place.

transvestite (tranz'vestiet) a person who experiences a habitual and strongly persistent desire to dress and act in a style transitionally associated with a member of the opposite sex ('cross-dressing'). The majority are male and have no desire to physically change sex.

trapezius (trə'peezi·əs) the large triangular muscle of the upper back and shoulder.

trauma ('trawmə) 1. physical injury caused by violent or disruptive action or by the introduction into the body of a toxic substance. 2. psychological injury resulting from severe emotional shock. *Birth t.* an injury to the infant sustained during the process of being born.

treatment ('treetmənt) the mode of dealing with a person or disease. *Active t.* that in which specific medical or surgical treatment is undertaken. *Conservative t.* that which aims at preserving and restoring injured parts by natural means, e.g. rest, fluid replacement, etc., as opposed to radical or surgical methods. *Empirical t.* treatment based on observation of symptoms and not on science. *Palliative t.* that which relieves distressing symptoms but does not cure the disease. *Prophylactic t.* that which aims at the prevention of disease.

Trematoda (ˌtremə'tohdə, ˌtree-) a class of fluke worms, some of which are parasitic in humans. Many of them have freshwater snails as secondary hosts.

tremor ('tremə) an involuntary, muscular quivering which may be due to fatigue, emotion or disease. Tremor, first of one hand and later affecting the other limbs, is the first symptom of PARKINSON'S DISEASE. *Intention t.* one that occurs on attempting a movement, as in disseminated SCLEROSIS.

Trendelenburg's position (tren'-delənˌbərgz pə'zishən) *Friedrich Trendelenburg, German surgeon, 1844–1924. See* POSITION.

Trendelenburg's sign (ˌtren'delənˌ-bərgz sien) a test of the stability of the hip. The person stands on the affected leg and flexes the other knee and hip. If there is dislocation, the pelvis is lower on the side of the flexed leg, which is the reverse of normal.

Treponema (ˌtrepə'neemə) a genus of spirochaetes. Anaerobic bacteria, they are motile, spiral and parasitic in humans and animals. *T. careatum* the causative agent of PINTA. *T. p. pallidum* the causative agent of syphilis. *T. p. immobilisation test* a serological test for syphilis. *T. p. pertenue* the causative agent of YAWS (framboesia).

tri-iodothyronine (trieˌieədoh-'thierəˌneen) a hormone produced by the thyroid gland together with thyroxine.

triage (tree'ahzh) [Fr.] 1. to choose, classify or sort. 2. a process by which a person is assessed upon arrival to determine the urgency of the problem, and to designate appropriate healthcare resources to care for the identified problem. *T. nurse* a registered nurse with specialist skills and knowledge who carries out the assessment and classification of casualties according to the type and severity of their injuries in order to assign them for treatment in the accident and emergency department.

triangulation (trieˌang·gyə'layshən) the expansion of research methods in a single study or multiple studies to enhance diversity, enrich understanding and accomplish specific goals.

triceps (ˈtrieseps) having three heads. *T. muscle* that situated on the back of the upper arm, which extends the forearm.

trichiasis (triˈkieəsis) 1. a condition of ingrowing hairs about an orifice, or ingrowing eyelashes. 2. the appearance of hair-like filaments in the urine.

trichinosis (ˌtrikəˈnohsəs) a disease caused by eating undercooked pork containing a parasite, *Trichinella spiralis*. This becomes deposited in muscle and causes stiffness and painful swelling. There may also be nausea, diarrhoea and fever. Trichiniasis.

trichology (triˈkoləjee) the study of hair.

Trichomonas (ˌtrikohˈmohnəs) a genus of flagellate protozoa that are parasitic to humans. *T. hominis* infests the bowel and may cause dysentery. *T. tenax* infests the mouth and may be present in cases of PYORRHOEA. *T. vaginalis* is commonly present in the vagina and may cause LEUCORRHOEA and VAGINITIS.

trichomoniasis (ˌtrikohməˈnieəsəs) infestation with a parasite of the genus *Trichomonas*.

Trichophyton (ˌtrikohˈfietən) a genus of fungi that affect the skin, nails and hair.

trichophytosis (ˌtrikohfieˈtohsəs) infection of the skin, nails or hair with one of the genus *Trichophyton*. *See* TINEA.

trichosis (triˈkohsəs) any abnormal growth of hair.

trichuriasis (ˌtrikyəˈrieəsəs) infestation by the whipworm.

Trichuris (triˈkyoo·rəs) a genus of nematode worms which may infest the colon and cause diarrhoea. A whipworm.

tricuspid (trieˈkuspəd) having three flaps or cusps. *T. valve* that at the opening between the right atrium and the right ventricle of the heart.

trifocal (trieˈfohkəl) pertaining to a spectacle lens that has three foci: one for distant vision, one for intermediate vision and one for near vision.

trigeminal (trieˈjeminəl) divided into three. *T. nerves* the fifth pair of cranial nerves, each of which is divided into three main branches and supplies one side of the face. *T. neuralgia* pain in the face which is confined to branches of the trigeminal nerve; tic douloureux.

trigeminy (trieˈjemənee) the type of pulse in which there are three beats and then a missed beat; a regular irregularity. Pulsus trigeminus.

trigger (ˈtrigə) a substance, object or agent that initiates or stimulates an action.

trigger finger (ˈtrigə ˌfing·gə) a stenosing of the tendon sheath at the metacarpophalangeal joint, allowing flexion of the finger but not extension without assistance when it 'clicks' into position.

triglyceride (trieˈglisəˌried) 'human fat', an ester of glycerol and three fatty acids.

trigone (ˈtriegohn) a triangular area. *T. of the bladder* the triangular space on the floor of the bladder, between the ureteric openings and the urethral orifice.

trimester (trieˈmestə) a period of 3 months. *First t. of pregnancy* the first 3 months, during which rapid development is taking place.

trimethylaminuria (trieˈmethəˌlam·ənooriə) a rare genetic disorder that causes a strong body odour due to the inability to process trimethylamine. Also known as fish odour syndrome.

triplets (ˈtripləɪz) three children carried in the uterus at once and born at one labour. The incidence was formerly about 1 in 6400 births; now, as a result of treatment of infertility, it is more common.

triple vaccine (ˈtrip'l ˈvakseen) a combined dose of diphtheria, tetanus and pertussis immunisation.

triplopia (triˈplohpi·ə) a condition in which three images of an object are seen at the same time.

trismus (ˈtrizməs) lockjaw; a tonic spasm of the muscles of the jaw.

trisomy (ˈtriesəmee) the presence of an extra chromosome in each cell in addition to the normal paired set of 46. The cause of several chromosome disorders including DOWN SYNDROME and KLINEFELTER'S SYNDROME.

trocar (ˈtrohkah) a sharp pointed surgical instrument used with a cannula to pierce the skin and the wall of a cavity or canal in the body to aspirate fluids, to instil a medication or to guide the placement of a soft catheter.

trochanter (trohˈkantə) either of two bony prominences below the neck of the femur. *Greater t.* that on the outer side forming the bony prominence of the hip. *Lesser t.* that on the inner side at the neck of the femur.

trochlea (ˈtrokli·ə) any pulley-shaped structure, but particularly the fibrocartilage near the inner angular process of the frontal bone, through which passes the tendon of the superior oblique muscle of the eye.

trophoblast (ˈtrofəˌblast) the layer of cells surrounding the blastocyst at the time of, and responsible for, implantation.

tropia (ˈtrohpi·ə) a manifest deviation of the eye, one that is present when both eyes are open.

tropical (ˈtropikəl) relating to the areas within 23.5° north and south of the equator, termed the tropics. *T. medicine* that concerned with diseases that are more prevalent in hot climates.

tropism (ˈtrohpizəm) an affinity or attraction of one cell to another.

troponin (troˈponin) a complex of globular muscle proteins that is integral to muscle contraction. Found in skeletal and cardiac muscle but not smooth muscle. Useful as a diagnostic marker for various cardiac disorders, specifically is a marker for myocardial infarction or heart muscle death.

Trousseau's sign (ˈtroosohz sien) *Armand Trousseau, French physician, 1801–1867.* 1. spontaneous peripheral venous thrombosis. 2. a sign of tetany in which carpal spasm can be elicited by compressing the upper arm and causing ischaemia to the nerves distally.

truncus (ˈtrungkəs) a trunk; the main part of the body, or a part of it, from which other parts spring. *T. arteriosus* the arterial trunk connected to the fetal heart which develops into the aortic and pulmonary arteries.

Trypanosoma (ˌtripənohˈsohmə) a genus of protozoan parasites which pass some of their life cycle in the blood of vertebrates, including humans. *T. gambiense* and *T. rhodesiense* are transmitted by the bite of the tsetse fly and are the cause of sleeping sickness.

trypanosomiasis (ˌtripənohsəˈmieə-səs) a disease caused by infestation with *Trypanosoma*. Sleeping sickness.

trypsin (ˈtripsən) a digestive enzyme that converts protein into amino acids.

trypsinogen (tripˈsinəjən) the precursor of trypsin. It is secreted in the pancreatic juice and activated by the enterokinase of the intestinal juices into trypsin.

tryptophan (ˈtriptəˌfan) one of the essential amino acids.

tsetse fly (ˈtetsee, ˈtse- ˌflie) a fly of the genus *Glossina* which transmits the parasite *Trypanosoma* to humans, causing TRYPANOSOMIASIS.

TSH *see* THYROID-STIMULATING HORMONE.

***t* statistic** (ˈtee stəˈtistik) commonly used in nursing research; it tests whether two group means are more different than would be expected by chance. Groups can be related or independent.

tsutsugamushi disease (ˌtsootsoo-gəˈmooshee diˈzeez) scrub typhus which occurs in Japan and is transmitted by the bite of a mite. *See also* TYPHUS.

tubal (ˈtyoobəl) relating to a tube. *T. ligation* tying of the fallopian tubes as method of female sterilisation. *T. pregnancy* extrauterine pregnancy where the embryo develops in the uterine tube; ectopic pregnancy.

tube feeding (tyoob feeding) administration of liquid and semisolid foods through a nasogastric tube, gastrostomy tube or enterostomy tube. Tube feeds are administered to patients who are unable to take foods by mouth.

Tubegauz® (ˈtyoobˌgawz) a proprietary brand of woven circular bandage available in various sizes and applied with a special applicator.

tubercle (ˈtyoobəkəl) 1. a small nodule or a rounded prominence on a bone. 2. the specific lesion (a small nodule) produced by the tubercle bacillus.

tubercular (tyəˈbərkyələ) pertaining to tubercles.

tuberculin (tyəˈbərkyələn) the filtrate from a fluid medium in which *Mycobacterium tuberculosis* has been grown and which contains its toxins. *Old t.* is prepared from the human bacillus. It is used in skin tests in diagnosing tuberculosis. *See* MANTOUX TEST.

tuberculosis (TB) (tyəˌbərkyəˈlohsəs (tee bee)) chronic, recurrent notifiable infection, most commonly occurring in the lungs, caused by *Mycobacterium tuberculosis*; transmission is usually by inhalation of bacilli in airborne droplets. *Bovine t.* endemic in cattle and some other animals and transmissible to humans by ingestion of meat or unpasteurised milk; causes extrapulmonary (non-respiratory) TB of the tonsils, abdominal organs, joints and bones and lymph nodes (also lymphadenitis in immunosuppressed patients). *Miliary t.* severe form occurring when tubercle bacilli are spread acutely throughout the bloodstream causing extrapulmonary TB. *Open t.* any type of tuberculosis in which infectious patients are excreting bacilli from the body most often in the sputum. *Pulmonary t.* the most common form of TB, affecting the lungs. Also termed phthisis. *T. of the spine see* POTT'S DISEASE.

tuberosity (ˌtyoobəˈrosətee) an elevation or protuberance on a bone to which tendons are attached.

tuberous (ˈtyoobə·rəs) covered with tubers. *T. sclerosis* a familial disease with tumours on the surfaces of the lateral ventricles of the brain and sclerotic patches on its surface, and marked by mental deterioration and epileptic attacks.

tubule (ˈtyoobyool) a small tube. *Renal* or *uriniferous t.* the essential secreting tube of the kidney.

tularaemia (ˌtyooləˈreemi·ə) a plague-like disease of rodents, caused by *Francisella* (*Pasteurella*) *tularensis*, which is transmissible to humans. The illness can be contracted by handling diseased animals or their hides, eating infected wild game or being bitten by insects that have fed on infected animals. It causes fever and headache; the lymph glands enlarge and may suppurate.

tumefaction (ˌtyoomәˈfakshәn) a swelling or the process of becoming swollen. Tumescence.

tumescence (ˌtyooˈmesәns) 1. a swelling or enlarging of a part. 2. a swollen condition. 3. a penile erection.

tumour (ˈtyoomә) an abnormal swelling. The term is usually applied to a morbid growth of tissue which can be benign or malignant; a neoplasm. *Benign* or *innocent t.* one that does not infiltrate or cause metastases, and is unlikely to recur if removed. *Malignant t.* one that invades and destroys tissue and may spread to neighbouring tissues, and to more distant sites via the blood and the lymphatic systems.

tunica (ˈtyoonikә) a coat, a covering or the lining of a vessel. *T. adventitia*, *t. media*, *t. intima* the outer, middle and inner coats of an artery, respectively. *T. vaginalis* the membrane covering the front and sides of the testis.

tuning fork (ˈtyooning fawk) a metal instrument used for testing hearing by means of the sounds produced by its vibration. *See* RINNE'S TEST and WEBER TEST.

tunnel (ˈtunәl) in anatomy, a canal through a structure. *Carpal t.* the osteofibrous channel in the wrist between the carpal bones and tissue covering the flexor tendons. *C. t. syndrome* pain and tingling in the hand and fingers caused by compression of the median nerve in the carpal tunnel. *See also* CARPAL. *T. vision* vision that is restricted to the central field. Occurs in chronic GLAUCOMA and in RETINITIS PIGMENTOSA.

turbinate (ˈtәrbәnәt, -ˌnayt) scroll shaped. *T. bone* one of the three thin long plates that form the walls of the nasal cavity.

turgid (ˈtәrjid) swollen or distended.

turgor (ˈtәrgә) the expected resiliency of the skin caused by outward pressure of the cells and interstitial fluid. Dehydration results in decreased skin turgor, manifested by lax skin that, when grasped and raised between two fingers, slowly returns to a position level with the adjacent tissue. Oedema and ascites results in increased turgor, manifested by smooth, taut, shiny skin that cannot be grasped and raised. Loss of skin elasticity is a normal part of ageing. Evaluation of skin turgor is an important part of physical assessment.

Turner's syndrome (ˈtәrnәz ˈsinˌdrohm) *Henry Turner, American physician, 1892–1970.* A chromosomal defect in females causing short stature. Classically, an absence of one X chromosome. Affects 1 in 3000 live female births. The majority have streak ovaries, leading to an absence of puberty and infertility. Other features may include webbing of the neck, CUBITUS VALGUS, nail abnormalities and coarctation of the aorta. Intelligence is usually normal.

twilight state (ˈtwieˌliet stayt) partial disturbance of consciousness, a state that may follow an epileptic fit and may be associated with alcoholism and some confusional states. The person can still carry out some routine activities but has no awareness or memory of doing so.

twin (twin) one of a pair of individuals who have developed in the uterus together. *Binovular* (dizygotic) *t.* each twin has developed from a separate ovum; fraternal, or non-identical, twins. *Uniovular* (monozygotic) *t.* both twins have developed from the same cell; identical twins.

tympanectomy (ˌtimpəˈnektəmee) excision of the tympanic membrane.

tympanic membrane (ˌtimˈpanik ˈmembrayn) a thin semitransparent membrane in the middle ear that transmits sound vibrations to the internal ear by means of the auditory ossicles. Also called eardrum.

tympanites (ˌtimpəˈnieteez) distension of the abdomen by accumulation of gas in the intestine or the peritoneal cavity.

tympanitis (ˌtimpəˈnietəs) inflammation of the middle ear; otitis media.

tympanoplasty (ˈtimpənəˌplastee) an operation to reconstruct the eardrum and restore conductivity to the middle ear. MYRINGOPLASTY.

tympanosclerosis (ˌtimpənohskləˈrohsəs) fibrosis and the formation of calcified deposits in the middle ear which may lead to deafness.

tympanum (ˈtimpənəm) 1. the middle ear. 2. the eardrum or tympanic membrane.

type (tiep) the general or prevailing character of any particular case of disease, person, substance, etc. *Blood t.s see* BLOOD GROUPS. *Phage t.* a subgroup of a bacterial species susceptible to a particular bacteriophage and demonstrated by PHAGE TYPING. Also called lysotype and phagotype. *Pyknic t.* a type of physical constitution marked by rounded body, large chest, thick shoulders, broad head and short neck.

type A behaviour (ˌtiep ˈay beeˈhayvyə, bə-) a behaviour pattern associated with the development of coronary heart disease, characterised by excessive competitiveness and aggression, and a fast-paced lifestyle. Research has shown that this type of behaviour is associated with coronary artery disease and MYOCARDIAL INFARCTION. The opposite type of behaviour, exhibited by individuals who are relaxed, unhurried and less aggressive, is called type B and is associated with a lower risk of heart disease.

type 1 diabetes mellitus (ˌtiep wun ˌdieəˈbeeteez məlietəs) *see* DIABETES.

type 2 diabetes mellitus (ˌtiep too ˌdieəˈbeeteez məlietəs) *see* DIABETES.

type I error (ˌtiep wun ˈerə) the rejection of a null hypothesis that is actually true.

type I respiratory failure (ˌtiep wun rəˈspirətree faylyə) occurs because of lung damage. This lung damage prevents adequate oxygenation of the blood (hypoxaemia); however, the remaining normal lung is still sufficient to excrete the carbon dioxide being produced by tissue metabolism. This is possible because less functioning lung tissue is required for carbon dioxide excretion than is needed for oxygenation of the blood. Type I respiratory failure is associated with acute diseases of the lung such as cardiogenic or noncardiogenic pulmonary oedema, pneumonia and pulmonary haemorrhage. Also called hypoxaemic respiratory failure (type I).

type II error (ˌtiep too ˈerə) the acceptance of a null hypothesis that is actually false.

type II respiratory failure (ˌtiep too rəˈspirətree faylyə) occurs when alveolar ventilation is insufficient to excrete the carbon dioxide being produced. Inadequate ventilation is due to reduced ventilation effort, or inability to overcome increased resistance to ventilation—it affects the lung as a whole, and thus carbon dioxide accumulates ($PaCO_2$ higher than 50 mmHg). Underlying causes include drug overdose, neuromuscular disease, chest wall abnormalities and severe airway disorders such as chronic asthma and chronic obstructive pulmonary disease (COPD). Also called hypercapnic respiratory failure (type II).

typhoid fever (ˈtiefoyd ˈfeevə) enteric fever; a notifiable infectious disease caused by *Salmonella typhi*, which is transmitted by water, milk or other foods, especially shellfish, that have been contaminated. There is high fever, a red rash, delirium and, sometimes, intestinal haemorrhage. Recovery usually begins during the fourth week of the disease. A person who has had typhoid fever gains immunity from it but may become a carrier. Although perfectly well, the person harbours the bacteria and passes them out in the faeces. The typhoid bacillus often lodges in the gallbladder of carriers.

typhus (ˈtiefəs) an acute, notifiable, infectious disease caused by species of the parasitic microorganism *Rickettsia*. There is high fever, a widespread red rash and severe headache. Typhus is likely to occur where there is overcrowding, lack of personal cleanliness and bad hygienic conditions, because the infection is spread by bites of infected lice or by rat fleas. *Scrub t.* a form spread by mites and widespread in the Far East. *See* TSUTSUGAMUSHI DISEASE.

tyramine (ˈtierəˌmeen, ˈti-) an enzyme present in cheese, game, broad bean pods, yeast extracts, wine and strong beer, which has a similar effect in the body to that of adrenaline. Foodstuffs containing tyramine should be avoided by people taking monoamine oxidase inhibitors.

tyrosine (ˈtierəˌseen, ˈti-) an essential amino acid that is the product of phenylalanine metabolism. In some diseases, especially of the liver, it is present as a deposit in the urine. It is a precursor of catecholamines, melanin and thyroid hormones.

tyrosinosis (ˌtierohsəˈnohsəs, ˌti-) a congenital condition in which there is an error of metabolism and phenylalanine cannot be reduced to tyrosine. Hepatic failure may occur.

Uu

ulcer (ˈulsə) an erosion or loss of continuity of the skin or of a mucous membrane, often accompanied by suppuration. *Arterial u.* caused by arterial insufficiency, usually with a deep punched out appearance and is painful at rest with the legs elevated. *Decubitus u.* a pressure ulcer caused by lying immobile for long periods of time on a bony area. *Duodenal u.* a peptic ulcer in the duodenum. *Gastric u.* one in the lining of the stomach. *Gravitational u.* a varicose ulcer of the leg which heals with difficulty because of its dependent position and the poor venous return. *Gummatous u.* one arising in late non-infective syphilis; it is slow to heal. *Indolent u.* one that is painless and heals slowly. *Peptic u.* one that occurs on the mucous membrane of either the stomach or the duodenum. *Perforating u.* one that erodes through the thickness of the wall of an organ. *Rodent u.* a slow-growing EPITHELIOMA of the face which may cause local destruction and ulceration but does not give rise to metastases. *See* BASAL CELL CARCINOMA. *Trophic u.* one due to a failure of nutrition of a part. *Venous u.* gravitational ulcer. A shallow ulcer, usually on the lower leg between the knee and the ankle that is linked with varicose veins resulting in a poor circulation to and from the area. Initially, there is often an area of eczematous skin and the ulcer forms with large amounts of exudate and oozing.

ulcerative (ˈulsəˌrətiv) characterised by ulceration (the formation of ulcers). *U. colitis* inflammation and ulceration of the colon and rectum thought to be an autoimmune condition.

ulna (ˈulnə) the medial and larger bone of the forearm.

ultrasonic (ˌultrəˈsonik) relating to sound waves having a frequency range beyond the upper limit perceived by the human ear. These waves are widely used instead of X-rays, particularly in the examination of structures not opaque to X-rays.

ultrasonogram (ˌultrəˈsonəˌgram) an echo picture obtained from using ultrasound.

ultrasonography (ˌultrəsəˈnogrəfee) a radiological technique in which deep structures of the body are visualised by recording the reflections (echoes) of ultrasonic waves directed into the tissues.

ultrasound (ˈultraˌsownd) ultrasonic waves used to examine the interior organs of the body. These waves can also be used in the treatment of soft tissue pain, and to break up renal calculi or the crystalline lens when cataract is present. *U. screening* a method of body imaging based on the reflectivity of sound. Ultrasound scanning is non-invasive and is widely used in obstetrics to detect the site of the placenta, the presence of fetal abnormalities and the sex of the fetus; it will reveal a multiple pregnancy at an early stage. It is also used by other medical disciplines.

ultraviolet rays (ˌultrəˈvielət ˌrayz) short-wavelength electromagnetic rays. They are present in sunlight, and cause tanning and sunburn. *U. light* is used to promote vitamin D formation and for treatment of certain skin conditions.

umbilical cord (umˈbələkəl ˌkawd) arises from the placenta and enters the fetus at the site of the future navel, providing the nutritional, hormonal and immunological link between mother and fetus during pregnancy. *U. hernia* common in newborn infants where a part of the bowel or a section of fatty tissue protrudes through the abdominal wall near the navel.

umbilicus (umˈbiləkəs, ˌumbiˈliekəs) the navel; the circular depressed scar in the centre of the abdomen where the umbilical cord of the fetus was attached.

unconditioned response (ˈunkənˌdishən'd rəˈspons) an unlearned response, i.e. one that occurs naturally.

unconscious (unˈkonshəs) 1. insensible; incapable of responding to sensory stimuli and of having subjective experiences. 2. that part of mental activity which includes primitive or repressed wishes, concealed from consciousness by the psychological censor. *Collective u.* in Jungian psychology, the portion of the unconscious which is theoretically common to all human beings.

unconsciousness (unˈkonshəsnəs) the state of being unconscious. This may vary in depth from deep unconsciousness, when no response can be obtained, through to lesser degrees of unconsciousness, when the person can be roused by painful stimuli, to a level when the person can be roused by speech or non-painful stimuli. Deep prolonged unconsciousness is known as coma. *See* COMA.

undine (ˈundeen) a glass flask with a spout used for irrigation of the eye.

undulant (ˈundyələnt) rising and falling like a wave. *U. fever see* BRUCELLOSIS.

unguent (ungˈgwent) [L.] unguentum; an ointment or salve.

uni- (ˈyooni) a prefix meaning 'one'.

uniform resource locator (URL) (ˈyoonifawm ˈreeˌsaws ˈlohˌkaytə) in a computer, a web browser that is used in the location of specific websites. Commonly informally referred to as a web address.

unilateral (ˌyooneeˈlatə·rəl) on one side only.

union (ˈyoonyən) 1. a joining together. 2. the repair of tissue after separation by incision or fracture. *See* CALLUS and HEALING. *Immediate u.* healing by first intention.

uniovular (ˌyooneeˈohvyələ, -ˈov-) from one ovum. *U. twins* identical twins, developed from one ovum. Aso known as monozygotic twins.

unipara (ˌyooneeˈparə) a woman who has given birth to one child.

unit (ˈyoonət) 1. a single thing. 2. a standard of measurement. *Intensive care u.* a hospital department reserved for those with severe medical or surgical disorders. *International insulin u.* a measurement of the pure crystalline insulin arrived at by biological assay. *SI u.* one of the various units of measurement making up the Système International d'Unités (International System of Units).

universal precautions (UP) (ˈyooni-vərs'l prəˈcawshənz) a concept developed by nurses during the mid-1980s (largely as a response to human immunodeficiency virus, or HIV, epidemics) that assumes all patients are potentially infected with BLOOD-BORNE VIRUSES; consequently, universal blood and body fluid infection control precautions are used for all patients, all the time. This concept has been further developed and is known as STANDARD PRECAUTIONS. *See also* INFECTION CONTROL and Appendix 10.

UP *see* UNIVERSAL PRECAUTIONS.

urachal (ˌyooˈraykəl) referring to the urachus. *U. cyst* a congenital abnormality in which a small cyst persists along the course of the urachus. *U. fistula* one that forms when the urachus fails to close. Urine may leak from the umbilicus.

urachus (ˌyooˈraykəs) a tubular canal existing in the fetus, connecting the bladder with the umbilicus. In the adult, it persists in the form of a solid fibrous cord.

uraemia (yəˈreemi·ə) 1. an excess in the blood of urea, creatinine and other nitrogenous end-products of protein and amino acid metabolism; sometimes referred to as azotaemia. 2. in current usage, the entire complex of signs and symptoms of chronic renal failure. Depending on the cause, it may or may not be reversible. Uraemia leads to vomiting and nausea, headache, weakness, metabolic disturbances, convulsions and coma. *See* RENAL FAILURE.

urate (ˈyoo·rayt) a salt of uric acid. *Sodium u.* a compound generally found in concentration around joints in cases of gout.

urea (yəˈreeə, ˈyoo·ri·ə) carbamide. A white crystalline substance which is an end-product of protein metabolism and the chief nitrogenous constituent of urine. It is a diuretic. The normal daily output is about 33 g. *Blood u.* that which is present in the blood. Normal value is 3.1–8.1 mmoL/L.

ureter (yəˈreetə, ˈyoo·rətə) one of the two long narrow tubes that convey the urine from the kidney to the bladder.

ureterectomy (yəˌreetəˈrektəmee) the surgical removal of a ureter.

ureteric (yəˈreetərik) relating to the ureter. *U. catheter* a fine catheter for insertion via the ureter into the pelvis of the kidney, either for drainage or for retrograde urography. *U. transplantation* an operation which changes the way the ureter connects to the bladder by creating a new tunnel into the bladder. Congenital defects may make this necessary.

ureterocele (yəˈreetə·rəˌseel) a cystic enlargement of the wall of the ureter at its entry into the bladder.

ureterolith (yəˈreetə·rəˌlith) a calculus in a ureter.

ureterolithotomy (yəˌreetə·rohliˈ-thotəmee) removal of a calculus from the ureter.

ureterostomy (yəˌreetəˈrostəmee) the surgical creation of a permanent opening through which the ureter discharges urine.

ureterovaginal (yəˌreetə·rohvəˈ-jienəl, -ˈvajinəl) relating to the ureter and vagina. *U. fistula* an opening into the ureter by which urine escapes via the vagina.

urethra (yəˈreethrə) the canal through which the urine is discharged from the bladder. The male urethra is about 18 cm long and the female about 3.5 cm.

urethritis (ˌyoo·rəˈthrietəs) inflammation of the urethra with resulting frequency, urgency and scalding when passing urine. The condition is frequently a symptom of gonorrhoea but may be caused by other infectious organisms. *Non-specific u.* a sexually transmitted inflammation of the urethra caused by a variety of organisms other than gonococci, e.g. *Chlamydia trachomatis*, which causes 40% of cases. Also called non-gonococcal urethritis (NGU).

urethrocele (yəˈreethrohˌseel) a prolapse of the female urethral wall through the urinary meatus which may result from damage to the pelvic floor during childbirth.

urethrography (ˌyoo·rəˈthrogrəfee) radiographic examination of the urethra. A radio-opaque contrast medium is inserted by catheter.

urethroscope (yəˈreethrəˌskohp) an instrument for examining the interior of the urethra.

-uria (-yooreeə) a word termination (suffix) denoting a characteristic or constituent of the urine indicated by the stem to which it is affixed, as in oliguria and proteinuria.

uric acid (ˈyoo·rik ˈasəd) lithic acid, the end-product of nucleic acid metabolism, a normal constituent of urine. Its accumulation in the blood produces uricacidaemia. Renal calculi are frequently formed of it.

urinalysis (ˌyoo·rəˈnaləsəs) the bacteriological or chemical examination of the urine.

urinary (ˈyoorənree) relating to urine. *U. tract* the system that conducts urine from the kidneys to the exterior, including the ureters, bladder and urethra.

urination (ˌyoo·rəˈnayshən) micturition. The act of passing urine.

urine (ˈyoo·rən) the clear fluid of a varying straw colour secreted by the kidneys and excreted through the bladder and urethra. It is composed of 96% water and 4% solid constituents the most important being urea and uric acid. Specific gravity (random specimen) = 1.003–1.030; slightly acidic. *Residual u.* that which remains in the bladder after micturition. *U. retention* the inability to urinate voluntarily or to empty a full bladder.

urinometer (ˌyooriˈnomətə) an instrument used for measuring the specific gravity of urine.

URL *see* UNIFORM RESOURCE LOCATOR.

urobilin (ˌyoo·rohˈbielən) the main pigment of urine, also found in faeces, derived from urobilinogen.

urobilinogen (ˌyoo·rohbieˈlinəjən) a pigment derived from BILIRUBIN which, on oxidation, forms urobilin.

urochrome (ˈyoo·rohˌkrohm) the yellow pigment that colours urine derived from the breakdown of haemoglobin.

urodynamics (ˌyoo·rohdieˈnamiks) the dynamics of the propulsion and flow of urine in the urinary tract.

urogenital (ˌyoo·rohˈjenət'l) relating to the urinary and genital organs. Urinogenital.

urography (yəˈrogrəfee) radiographic examination of the urinary tract after the injection of a radio-opaque, water-soluble, iodine-containing medium. Also called intravenous pyelography (IVP) or pyelography.

urokinase (ˌyoo·rohˈkienayz) an enzyme in urine which is secreted by the kidneys and causes FIBRINOLYSIS. In certain diseases it may cause bleeding from the kidneys.

urolith (ˈyoo·roh ˌlith) a calculus in the urinary tract.

urology (yəˈroləjee) the study of diseases of the urinary tract.

uropathy (yəˈropəthee) any disease condition affecting the urinary tract.

urostomy (yəˈrostəmee) an artificial urinary conduit for deflecting urine from the ureters to the abdominal wall.

urticaria (ˌərtəˈkair·ri·ə) nettle rash or hives. An acute or chronic skin condition characterised by the recurrent appearance of an eruption of wheals, causing great irritation. The cause may be certain foods, infection, drugs or emotional stress. *See* ALLERGY.

uterine (ˈyootəˌrien) relating to the uterus. *U. tubes see* FALLOPIAN TUBES.

uterosalpingography (ˌyootə·roh-ˌsalpingˈgogrəfee) radiographic examination of the uterus and the uterine tubes.

uterovesical (ˌyootə·rohˈvesikəl) referring to the uterus and bladder. *U. pouch* the fold of peritoneum between the two organs.

uterus (ˈyootə·rəs) the womb: a triangular, hollow, muscular organ situated in the pelvic cavity between the bladder and the rectum. Its function is the nourishment and protection of the fetus during pregnancy, and its expulsion at term. *Bicornuate u.* one having two horns; a congenital malformation. *Gravid u.* the pregnant uterus. *U. didelphys* a double uterus caused by the failure of union of the two müllerian ducts from which it is formed.

utilitarianism (ˌyootiləˈtairee·-ənizəm) a philosophical or ethical view which holds that utility entails the greatest happiness of the greatest number of people and therefore that an action should always produce more benefits than harm.

utricle (ˈyootrikəl) a small sac. The delicate membranous sac in the bony vestibule of the ear.

uvea (ˈyoovi·ə) uveal tract. The pigmented layer of the eye consisting of the iris, ciliary body and choroid.

uveitis (ˌyooveeˈietəs) inflammation of the uveal tract.

uvula (ˈyoovyələ) the small fleshy appendage which is the free edge of the soft palate, hanging from the roof of the mouth.

Vv

vaccination (ˌvaksəˈnayshən) the introduction of vaccine into the body to produce immunity to a specific disease.

vaccine (ˈvakseen) a suspension of killed or attenuated organisms (viruses, bacteria or rickettsiae) administered for prevention, amelioration or treatment of infectious diseases. Vaccines are usually given by injection. Some require several doses spaced weeks apart, others require only a single dose. Booster doses may also be required, the interval depending upon the origin vaccine given. *Attenuated v.* one prepared from living organisms which, through long cultivation, have lost their virulence. *Bacille Calmette-Guérin v.* an attenuated bovine bacillus vaccine giving immunity from tuberculosis. *Sabin v.* an attenuated poliovirus vaccine that may be administered by mouth, in a syrup or on sugar. *Salk v.* one prepared from an inactivated strain of poliomyelitis virus. *Triple v.* one that protects against diphtheria, tetanus and whooping cough.

vaccinia (vakˈsini·ə) cowpox; a virus infection of cows, which may be transmitted to humans by contact with the lesions. A local pustular eruption is produced.

vacuum (ˈvakyoom) a space from which air or gas has been extracted. *V. extractor* an instrument known as a ventouse is used to assist delivery of the fetus. A suction cup is attached to the head and a vacuum created slowly. Gentle traction is applied which is synchronised with the uterine contractions. *V. wound drainage system* a closed suction drainage system used following surgery for wound exudates.

vagal (ˈvaygəl) relating to the VAGUS nerve.

vagina (vəˈjienə) the canal, lined with mucous membrane, that leads from the cervix of the uterus to the vulva.

vaginismus (ˌvajəˈnizməs) a painful spasm of the muscles of the vagina occurring usually when the vulva or vagina is touched, resulting in painful sexual intercourse or dyspareunia.

vaginitis (ˌvajəˈnietəs) inflammation of the vagina caused by microorganisms. *Atrophic* or *post-menopausal v.* inflammation caused by degenerative changes in the mucous lining of the vagina and insufficient oestrogen secretion. Adhesions may occur, partially closing the vagina. *Trichomonas v.* infection caused by *T. vaginalis*, a protozoon that causes a thin, yellowish discharge, giving rise to local tenderness and PRURITUS.

vagotomy (vayˈgotəmee) surgical incision of the vagus nerve or any of its branches. A treatment for gastric or duodenal ulcer when acid production cannot be reduced by other means such as medication or dietary changes. *Highly selective v.* division of only those vagal fibres supplying the acid-secreting glands of the stomach. *Medical v.* interruption of impulses carried by the vagus nerve by administration of suitable drugs.

vagus (ˈvaygəs) the 10th cranial nerves (a pair) arising in the medulla and providing the parasympathetic nerve supply to the organs in the thorax and abdomen *V. resection see* VAGOTOMY.

valgus (ˈvalgəs) a displacement outwards, particularly of the feet. *Genu valgum* knock-knee, with the ankles set apart. *Hallux v.* twisting of the big toe towards the other toes. *Talipes v.* clubfoot with the inner edge only in contact with the ground, and the foot turned outwards.

validity (vəˈlidəˌtee) the extent to which a measure, indicator or method of data collection possesses the quality of being sound or true, as far as can be judged. *Construct v.* the extent to which an instrument is said to measure a theoretical construct or trait. *Content v. the* degree to which the content of the measure represents the universe of content, or the domain of a given behaviour. *External v.* the degree to which findings of a study can be generalised to other populations or environments. *Face v.* a type of content validity that uses an expert's opinion to judge the accuracy of an instrument. *Internal v.* the degree to which it can be inferred that the experimental treatment, rather than an uncontrolled condition, resulted in the observed effects.

valine (ˈvayleen) an essential amino acid required for nitrogen equilibrium which is formed by the digestion of dietary protein.

Valsalva's manoeuvre (valˈsalvəz mənoovə) *Antonio Valsalva, Italian anatomist, 1666–1723.* Technique for increasing the intrathoracic pressure by closing the mouth and nostrils and blowing out the cheeks, thereby forcing air back into the nasopharynx. When the breath is released, the intrathoracic pressure drops and the blood is quickly propelled through the heart, producing an increase in the heart rate (tachycardia) and the blood pressure. Immediately after this event a reflex BRADYCARDIA ensues. Valsalva's manoeuvre occurs when a person strains to defecate or urinate, uses the arm and upper trunk muscles to move up in bed, or strains during coughing, gagging or vomiting. The increased pressure, immediate tachycardia and reflex bradycardia can bring about cardiac arrest in vulnerable heart patients.

valve (valv) 1. a means of regulating the flow of liquid or gas through a pipe. 2. a fold of membrane in a passage or tube, so placed as to permit passage of fluid in one direction only. Valves are important structures in the heart, in veins and in lymph vessels. *Semilunar v.* either of two valves at the junction of the pulmonary artery and aorta, respectively, with the heart.

valvotomy (valˈvotəmee) valvulotomy. A surgical operation to open up a fibrosed valve, e.g. mitral valvotomy to relieve MITRAL STENOSIS.

valvulitis (ˌvalvyəˈlietəs) inflammation of a valve, particularly of the heart.

vaporiser (ˈvaypəˌriezə) an apparatus for producing a very fine spray of a liquid.

variable (ˈvairee·əbəl) a research term that describes any factor or circumstance that is part of the study. *Confounding v.* one that affects the conditions of the independent variables unequally. *Dependent v.* one that depends on the experimental conditions. *Independent v.* the variable conditions of an experimental situation, e.g. control or experimental. *Random v.s* background factors that may affect any conditions of the independent variables equally.

variance (ˈvairee·əns) used in statistics. The distribution range of a set of results around a mean. *See* STANDARD DEVIATION.

varicella (ˌvareeˈselə) chickenpox. An infectious disease of childhood with an incubation period of 12–20 days. There is slight fever and an eruption of transparent vesicles on the chest, on the first day of disease; these appear in successive crops all over the body. The vesicles soon dry up, sometimes leaving shallow pits in the skin. The disease is usually mild, but may be severe in neonates, adults and those who are immunocompromised. Anyone who has had chicken pox may develop shingles in later life.

varicella zoster virus (VZV) (ˈvariˌ-selə zostə vierəs) a human herpes virus that causes chickenpox during childhood and may reactivate later in life to cause shingles.

varices (ˈvarəseez) alternative name for enlarged, distorted varicose veins or lymphatic vessels.

varicose (ˈvarəˌkohs) swollen or dilated. *V. ulcer* gravitational ulcer. *See* ULCER. *V. veins* a dilated and twisted condition of the veins (usually those of the leg) caused by structural changes in the walls or valves of the vessel (*see* figure, p. 491).

varus (ˈvair·rəs) a displacement inwards. *See* GENU, HALLUX, TALIPES.

vas (vas) *pl.* vasa. A vessel or duct. *V. deferens* one of a pair of excretory ducts conveying the semen from the epididymis to the urethra. Also known as Ductus (vas) deferens. *V. efferens* one of the many small tubes that convey semen from the testis to the epididymis. *Vasa vasorum* the minute nutrient vessels that supply the walls of the arteries and veins.

vascular (ˈvaskyələ) relating to or consisting largely of blood vessels. *V. system* the cardiovascular system.

vascularisation (ˌvaskyələ·rieˈzay-shən) the development of new blood vessels within a tissue that occurs during healing.

vasculitis (ˌvaskyəˈlietəs) angiitis; inflammation of a blood vessel. *Allergic v.* a severe allergic response to drugs or to cold. Arising in small arteries or veins, with fibrosis and thrombi formation.

vasectomy (vəˈsektəmee) excision of a part of the vas deferens. If performed bilaterally, sterility results. Employed as a method of contraception.

vasoconstriction (ˌvayzohkənˈstrik-shən) decrease in the diameter of a blood vessel.

vasoconstrictor (ˌvayzohkənˈstriktə) any agent that causes contraction of a blood vessel wall and therefore results in a decrease in the blood flow and a rise in the blood pressure.

vasodilator (ˌvayzohdieˈlaytə) any agent that causes an increase in the lumen of blood vessels and therefore an increase in the blood flow and a fall in the blood pressure.

vasomotor (ˌvayzohˈmohtə) controlling the muscles of blood vessels, both dilator and constrictor. *V. centre* nerve cells in the MEDULLA OBLONGATA controlling the vasomotor nerves. *V. nerves* sympathetic nerves regulating the tension of the blood vessels.

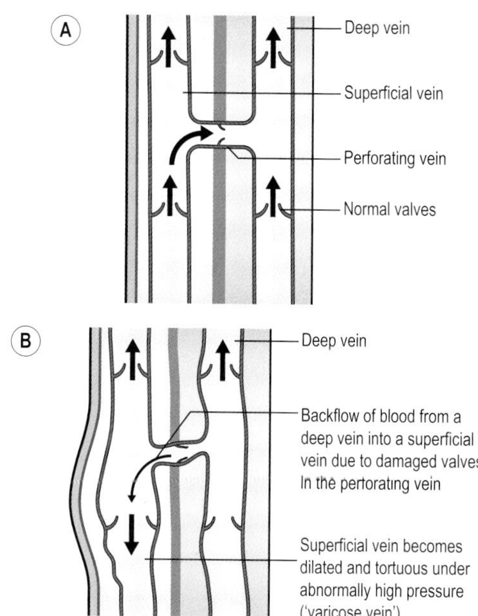

Veins of the leg and varicose vein.

vasopressin (ˌvayzohˈpresən) antidiuretic hormone (ADH). A hormone from the posterior lobe of the pituitary gland which causes constriction of plain muscle fibres and reabsorption of water in the renal tubules. Used in the treatment of DIABETES INSIPIDUS and bleeding from oesophageal varices.

vasospasm (ˈvayzohˌspazəm) constriction of a blood vessel.

vasovagal (ˌvayzohˈvaygəl) vascular and vagal. *V. attack* fainting or syncope stress, often evoked by emotional stress associated with fear and pain. There is postural hypotension.

VBI *see* VERTEBROBASILAR INSUFFICIENCY.

VDU *see* VISUAL DISPLAY UNIT.

vector (ˈvektə) 1. an animal that carries organisms or parasites from one host to another, either to a member of the same species or to one of another species, e.g. dogs, which carry rabies, and mosquitoes, which carry malaria.

2. a quantity with magnitude and direction. *Electrocardiograph v.* the method of recording the direction and magnitude of the electrical activity of the heart.

vegan (ˈveegən) a vegetarian who excludes all animal protein from the diet.

vegetarian (vejəˈtair·reeyən) a person who eats only food of vegetable origin. *V. diet* one in which no meat is eaten. *Lacto-v. diet* one that prohibits the intake of meat, poultry, fish and eggs. *Ovo-lacto-v. diet* one that allows all foods from plants plus eggs, milk and other dairy products. *Ovo-v. diet* one that allows eggs and foods of plant origin, but prohibits all animal and dairy products.

vegetation (ˌvejəˈtayshən) in pathology, a plant-like outgrowth. *Adenoid v.* overgrowth of lymphoid tissue in the nasopharynx.

vegetative (ˈvejitətəv) 1. the non-sporing stage of a bacterium. 2. profoundly lethargic and passive. *V. state* a type of deep coma that may follow severe head injuries. The person's eyes may be open with some associated random movements of the head and limbs, but there are no other signs of consciousness or response to stimuli. Only basic functions such as breathing and heartbeat are maintained.

vehicle (ˈveeəkəl) in pharmacy, a substance or medium in which a drug is administered.

vein (vayn) a vessel carrying blood from the capillaries back to the heart. It has thin walls and a lining endothelium from which the venous valves are formed.

vena cava (ˈveenə ˈkayvə) large veins returning blood to the right atrium of the heart.

venepuncture (ˈvenəˌpungkchə) the insertion of a needle into a vein for the introduction of a drug or fluid or for the withdrawal of blood.

venereal (vəˈniə·ri·əl) pertaining to, or caused by, sexual intercourse. *V. disease see* SEXUALLY TRANSMITTED INFECTION (STI).

venereology (vəˌniə·reeˈoləjee) the study and treatment of venereal diseases.

venesection (ˈvenəˌsekshən) PHLEBOTOMY. Surgical blood-letting by opening a vein or more commonly by introducing a wide-bore needle. A procedure used to collect blood from blood donors and occasionally to relieve venous congestion.

venogram (ˈveenəˌgram) 1. a graphic recording of the pulse in a vein. 2. a radiograph taken during venography.

venography (veeˈnogrəfee) radiographic examination of a vein after the instillation of a contrast medium to trace its pathway.

venom (ˈvenəm) a poison secreted by an insect, snake or other animal. *Russell's viper v.* the venom of the Russell viper (*Vipera russelli*) which acts in vitro as an intrinsic THROMBOPLASTIN and is useful in defining deficiencies of clotting factor X.

venous (ˈveenəs) pertaining to the veins. *V. sinus* one of 14 channels, similar to veins, by which blood leaves the cerebral circulation. *V. thromboembolism* abbreviated to VTE. The development of a clot. VTE is the collective name for deep vein thrombosis and pulmonary embolism. Most clots are preventable and preventative steps should be taken for patients at risk when in hospital or during periods of ill health. *V. ulcer see* ULCER.

ventilation (ˌventəˈlayshən) 1. the process or act of supplying a house or room continuously with fresh air. 2. in respiratory physiology, the process of exchange of air between the lungs and the ambient air. *Pulmonary v.* (usually measured in litres per minute) refers to the total exchange, whereas *alveolar v.* refers to the effective ventilation of the alveoli, where gas exchange with the blood takes place. 3. in psychiatry, the free discussion of one's problems or grievances.

ventilator (ˈventəˌlaytə) an apparatus designed to qualify the air that is breathed through it either intermittently or continuously. Ventilators provide an intermittent flow of air and/or oxygen under pressure and are connected to the patient by a tube inserted through the mouth, the nose or an opening in the trachea. *V.-associated pneumonia (VAP)* the most common type of nosocomial pneumonia, diagnosed in a patient breathing with a ventilator; the infection may be bacterial, viral or fungal.

Ventimask® (ˈventiˌmahsk) an oxygen mask that provides oxygen enrichment of the inspired air while eliminating the need to rebreathe the expired carbon dioxide.

ventouse (ˈvenˌtooz) *see* VACUUM EXTRACTOR.

ventricle (ˈventrikəl) a small pouch or cavity; applied especially to the lower chambers of the heart and to the four cavities of the brain.

ventricular (venˈtrikyələ) pertaining to a ventricle. *V. folds* the outer folds of mucous membrane forming the false vocal cords. *V. septal defect (VSD)* congenital abnormality in which there is communication between the two ventricles of the heart as a result of maldevelopment of the intraventricular septum. *V. fibrillation see* FIBRILLATION.

ventriculography (venˌtrikyəˈlogrəfee) 1. radiographic examination of the ventricles of the heart using a radio-opaque contrast medium. 2. radiographic examination of the ventricles of the brain after the injection of air or a contrast medium through a burr hole.

Venturi mask (venˈtyoo·ree mahsk) *Giovanni Venturi, Italian physicist, 1746–1822.* A type of disposable mask used to deliver a controlled oxygen concentration to a person. The flow of 100% oxygen through the mask draws in a controlled amount of room air (21% oxygen). Commonly available masks deliver 24%, 28%, 35%, 40% or 60% oxygen. At concentrations above 24%, humidification may be required.

Venturi nebuliser (venˈtyoo·ree ˈnebyəliezə) a type of nebuliser used in AEROSOL therapy. The pressure drop of gas flowing through the nebuliser draws liquid from a capillary tube. As the liquid enters the gas stream, it breaks up into a spray of small droplets.

venule (ˈvenyool) a minute vein which collects blood from the capillaries.

verbigeration (ˌvərbijəˈrayshən) the monotonous repetition of phrases or meaningless words.

vermicide (ˈvərməˌsied) an agent that destroys intestinal worms; an anthelmintic.

vermiform (ˈvərməˌfawm) worm-shaped. *V. appendix* the worm-shaped structure attached to the CAECUM.

vermifuge (ˈvərməˌfyooj) an agent that expels intestinal worms; an anthelmintic.

verminous (ˈvərmənəs) infested with worms or other animal parasites, such as lice.

vernix (ˈvərniks) [L.] varnish. *V. caseosa* the fatty covering on the skin of the fetus during the last months of pregnancy. It consists of cells and sebaceous material.

verruca (vəˈrookə) a wart. Condyloma. Hypertrophy of the prickle cell layer of the epidermis and thickening of the horny layer. A virus is the causative organism. *V. acuminata* a venereal wart that appears on the external genitalia. *V. plana* a small, smooth, usually skin-coloured or light-brown, slightly raised wart, sometimes occurring in great numbers; seen most often in children. Also known as flat warts. *V. plantaris* a viral epidermal tumour on the sole of the foot.

version (ˈvərshən, -zhən) the turning of a part; applied particularly to the turning of a fetus in order to facilitate delivery. *External v.* manipulation of the uterus through the abdominal wall in order to change the position of the fetus. *Internal v.* rotation of the fetus by means of manipulation with the finger of one hand in the vagina. *Podalic v.* turning of the fetus so that the head is uppermost and the feet presenting. *Spontaneous v.* one that occurs naturally without the application of force.

vertebra (ˈvərtəbrə) one of the 33 irregular bones forming the spinal column: 7 cervical, 12 thoracic, 5 lumbar, 5 sacral (sacrum) and 4 coccygeal (coccyx) vertebrae.

vertebral (ˈvərtəbrəl) pertaining to a vertebra. *V. column* the spine or backbone.

vertebrobasilar (ˌvərtəbrohˈbasələ) pertaining to the vertebral and the basilar arteries. *V. insufficiency (VBI)* a condition affecting the flow of blood through the vertebral and basilar arteries which may cause recurrent attacks of nausea, ataxia, DIPLOPIA, vertigo, dysarthria and HEMIPARESIS.

vertex (ˈvərteks) the crown of the head. *V. presentation* position of the fetus such that the crown of the head appears in the vagina first.

vertical transmission (ˈvərtik'l ˌtranzˈmishən) transmission of an infection from an infected mother to her newborn child during pregnancy, delivery or in the postpartum period through breast milk; also called perinatal or mother-to-child transmission.

vertigo (ˈvərtəˌgoh) a feeling of rotation or of going round, in either oneself or one's surroundings, particularly associated with disease of the CEREBELLUM and the vestibular nerve of the ear. It may occur in DIPLOPIA or MÉNIÈRE'S DISEASE.

vesica (ˈvesikə) a bladder; usually referring to the urinary bladder.

vesicle (ˈvesikəl) 1. in anatomy, a small bladder or blister, usually containing fluid. 2. a very small blister, usually containing serum. *Seminal v.* one of a pair of sacs which arise from the VAS DEFERENS near the bladder and contain semen.

vesicoureteric (ˌvesikoh·yoorəˈterik) relating to the urinary bladder and the ureters. *V. reflex* the passing of urine backwards up the ureter during micturition. A cause of PYELONEPHRITIS in children.

vesicovaginal (ˌvesikohvəˈjienəl) relating to the bladder and vagina. *See* FISTULA.

vesicular (vəˈsikyələ) relating to or containing vesicles. *V. breathing* the soft murmur of normal respiration, as heard on auscultation. *V. mole* hydatidiform mole.

vesiculitis (və͵sikyəˈlietəs) inflammation of a vesicle, particularly the seminal vesicles.

vessel (ˈvesəl) a tube, duct or canal for conveying fluid, usually blood or lymph.

vestibular (vəˈstibyələ) relating to a vestibule. *V. glands* those in the vestibule of the vagina, including BARTHOLIN'S GLANDS. *V. nerve* a branch of the auditory nerve supplying the semicircular canals and concerned with balance and equilibrium. *V. neuronitis* an infection of the vestibular nerve in the inner ear leading to disruption of balance. *V. schwannoma* a benign primary intracranial tumour of the myelin-forming cells of the vestibulocochlear nerve. Also known as acoustic neuroma.

vestibule (ˈvestə͵byool) a space or cavity at the entrance to another structure. *V. of the ear* the cavity at the entrance to the cochlea. *V. of the vagina* the space between the LABIA MINORA at the entrance to the vagina.

vestibulocochlear (ve͵stibyəloh-ˈkokli·ə) pertaining to the vestibule of the ear and the cochlea. *V. nerve* the eighth cranial nerve; also known as the auditory nerve.

vestigial (vəˈstijeeəl) rudimentary. Referring to the remains of an anatomical structure which, being of no further use, has atrophied.

viable (ˈvieəbəl) capable of independent life.

Vibrio (ˈvibreeoh) a genus of Gram-negative bacteria, curved and motile by means of flagellae. *V. cholerae* or *comma* that which causes cholera.

vicarious (vəˈkairi·əs) 1. obtained or undergone at second hand through sympathetic participation in another's experiences. 2. substituted for another; used when one organ functions instead of another. *V. liability* the liability of an employer for the wrongful acts of an employee committed in the course of employment.

villus (ˈviləs) a small finger-like process projecting from a surface. *Chorionic v. see* CHORIONIC. *Intestinal v.* those of the mucous membrane of the small intestine, each of which contains a blood capillary and a LACTEAL.

Vincent's angina (ˈvinsənts anˈjienə) *Henri Vincent, French physician, 1862–1950*. Infection of the gingiva or gums. Also known as acute necrotising ulcerative gingivitis (ANUG) or trench mouth.

viraemia (vieˈreemi·ə) the presence of viruses in the blood.

viral haemorrhagic fevers (ˈvieər'l ͵heməˈrajik ˈfeevəz) a group of infectious diseases prevalent in Africa that cause fever, severe malaise and headache, diarrhoea and vomiting with severe bleeding and are commonly fatal. *See* EBOLA VIRUS DISEASE, LASSA FEVER and MARBURG VIRUS DISEASE.

virilism (ˈvirə͵lizəm) masculine traits exhibited by a female owing to the production of excessive amounts of androgenic hormone either in the adrenal cortex or from an ovarian tumour.

virion (ˈviree·on) a fully developed complete infectious viral particle consisting of its nucleic acid and a surrounding coat of protein (capsid); the extracellular (cell-free) form of a virus.

virology (vie'roləjee) the scientific study of viruses, their growth and the diseases caused by them.

virulence ('virələns) the power of a microorganism to produce toxins or poisons. This depends on: (a) the number and power of the invading organisms; and (b) the power of the microorganism to overcome host resistance.

virulent ('virələnt) dangerously infectious or poisonous.

virus ('vierəs) any member of a unique class of infectious agents which were originally distinguished by their smallness and their inability to replicate outside a living host cell. Because these properties are shared by certain other microorganisms (rickettsiae, chlamydiae), viruses are now characterised by their simple organisation and their unique mode of replication. A virus consists of genetic material, which may be either DNA or RNA, and is surrounded by a protein coat and, in some viruses, by a membranous envelope. They cause many diseases, including chickenpox (varicella), herpes zoster (shingles), herpes infections, measles (rubeola), German measles (rubella), mumps, infectious mononucleosis, hepatitis A and B, yellow fever, the common cold, acquired immune deficiency syndrome (AIDS), influenza, certain types of pneumonia and croup and other respiratory infections, poliomyelitis, and several types of encephalitis. There is evidence that certain viruses might be capable of causing cancer, e.g. cancer of the liver and cervix. *See* ORTHOMYXOVIRUS.

viscera ('visə·rə) plural of viscus. The internal organs enclosed within a body cavity, including the abdominal, thoracic, pelvic and endocrine organs.

viscid ('visəd) sticky and glutinous.

viscosity (vi'skosətee) resistance to flowing. A sticky and glutinous quality.

viscus ('viskəs) any of the organs contained in the body cavities, especially in the abdomen.

vision ('vizhən) the faculty of seeing. Sight.

visual ('vizhyooəl) relating to sight. *V. acuity* sharpness of vision. It is assessed by reading test types. *V. cells* the rods and cones of the retina. *V. field* the area within which objects may be seen when looking straight ahead. *V. purple* the pigment in the outer layers of the retina. RHODOPSIN.

visual display unit (VDU) ('vizyooəl də'splay 'yoonit) the monitor screen attached to a computer.

visualisation (ˌvizyooəlie'zayshən) the technique of using the imagination and relaxation to create any desired changes in an individual's life.

vital ('viet'l) relating to life. *V. capacity* the amount of air that can be expelled from the lungs after a full inspiration. *V. signs* the signs of life; namely pulse rate, temperature, rate of respiration and usually blood pressure of a person. *V. statistics* the records kept of births and deaths among the population, including the causes of death and the factors that seem to influence their rise and fall.

vitallium (vie'tali·əm) a metal alloy used in dentistry and for prostheses in bone surgery.

vitamin ('vitəmən) any of a group of accessory food factors which are contained in foodstuffs and are essential to life, growth and reproduction.

vitiligo (ˌvitəˈliegoh) a skin disease marked by an absence of pigment, producing white patches on the face and body. LEUCODERMA.

vitrectomy (viˈtrektəmee) surgical extraction of the vitreous humour and its replacement by a physiological solution in the treatment of vitreous haemorrhage in diabetic RETINOPATHY.

vitreous (ˈvitri·əs) glassy. *V. humour* the transparent jellylike substance filling the posterior of the eye from lens to retina.

vocal (ˈvohkəl) pertaining to the voice or the organs that produce the voice. *V. cords* the two folds of tissue in the larynx, formed of fibrous tissue covered with squamous epithelium. *V. resonance* the normal sounds of speech heard through the chest wall by means of a stethoscope.

voice (voys) the acoustic sounds of speech produced by the vibrations of the vocal cords of the larynx.

void (voyd) empty or expel waste products from the body, such as urine from the bladder.

volatile (ˈvoləˌtiel) having a tendency to evaporate readily.

volition (vəˈlishən) the conscious adoption by the individual of a line of action.

Volkmann's ischaemic contracture (ˈvohlkmənz isˈkeemik kənˈtrakchə) *Richard von Volkmann, German surgeon, 1830–1889.* Contraction of the fingers and sometimes of the wrist or of analogous parts of the foot, with loss of power, after severe injury or improper use of a tourniquet or cast.

volume (ˈvolyoom) the space occupied by a substance. *Minute v.* the total volume of air breathed in or out in 1 min. *Packed cell v.* that occupied by the blood cells after centrifuging (about 45% of the blood sample). *Residual v.* the amount of air left in the lungs after breathing out fully.

voluntary (ˈvoləntree) under the control of the will. *See* INVOLUNTARY. *V. admission* a person who voluntarily agrees to enter a psychiatric unit or hospital as an inpatient. *V. muscle* a striated muscle. *See* MUSCLE. *V. organisation* a group of people who join together with a shared common purpose or cause to provide a service to others. Many of these groups are registered charities and may also have grants from state or national government. Some employ professionals and managerial staff but most remain dependent upon voluntary help. Many of these organisations provide considerable support to people, their carers and families.

volvulus (ˈvolvyələs) twisting of a loop of bowel causing obstruction. Most common in the sigmoid colon.

vomer (ˈvohmə) a thin plate of bone forming the posterior septum of the nose.

vomit (ˈvomət) 1. matter ejected from the stomach through the mouth (vomitus). 2. to eject material in this way. *Bilious v.* vomit mixed with bile. The vomit is stained yellow or green. *Coffee-ground v.* ejected matter that contains small quantities of altered blood, which has the appearance of coffee grounds. *Faecal or stercoraceous v.* vomit mixed with faeces. Occurs in intestinal obstruction when the contents of the upper intestine regurgitate back into the stomach. It is dark brown with an unpleasant odour.

vomiting (ˈvoməting) a reflex act of expulsion of the stomach contents via the oesophagus and mouth. It may be preceded by nausea and excess salivation if the cause is local irritation in the stomach. *Cyclical v.* recurrent attacks of vomiting often occurring in children and associated with acidosis. *V. of pregnancy* vomiting occurring in the months of pregnancy. MORNING SICKNESS. *Projectile v.* the forcible ejection of the gastric contents, usually without warning. Present in hypertrophic PYLORIC STENOSIS and in cerebral diseases.

von Recklinghausen's disease (von 'rekling,howzənz di'zeez) Recklinghausen's disease. *See* NEUROFIBROMATOSIS.

von Willebrand's disease (von 'vili,brants di'zeez) *Erik von Willebrand, Finnish physician, 1870–1949.* A bleeding disorder inherited as an autosomal dominant trait (rarely recessive), characterised by a deficiency of a blood protein called von Willebrand factor (vWF). vWF binds a prolonged bleeding time, deficiency of coagulation factor VIII, which is involved in the clotting process. Symptoms include EPISTAXIS and increased bleeding after trauma or surgery, MENORRHAGIA and postpartum bleeding.

voyeurism ('voyə,rizəm) sexual deviation whereby a person gains sexual satisfaction from covertly watching others who are naked or involved in sexual activity.

VSD *see* VENTRICULAR SEPTAL DEFECT.

vulnerability (,vulnə·rə'bilətee) weakness. Susceptibility to injury or infection.

vulva ('vulvə) the external female genital organs.

vulvectomy (vul'vektəmee) excision of the vulva.

vulvitis (vul'vietəs) inflammation of the vulva.

vulvovaginitis (,vulvoh,vajə'nietəs) inflammation of the vulva and vagina.

VZV *see* VARICELLA ZOSTER VIRUS.

Ww

Waldeyer's ring (ˈvaldieəz ˈring) *Wilhelm von Waldeyer-Hartz, German anatomist, 1836–1921.* The circle of lymphoid tissue in the pharynx formed by the lingual, faucial and pharyngeal tonsils.

walking belt (ˈwawking belt) a leather or nylon device with handles that is fastened around the person's waist and enables the healthcare provider to assist with the person's balance and ambulation.

Wangensteen tube (ˈwangenˌsteen tyoob) *Owen Wangensteen, American surgeon, 1898–1981.* A gastrointestinal aspiration tube with a tip that is opaque to X-rays.

wart (wawt) an elevation of the skin, often of a brownish colour, caused by hypertrophy of papillae in the dermis due to a virus infection. *See* VERRUCA and CONDYLOMA.

Wassermann test (reaction) (ˈvasəmən test (riˈakshən)) *August von Wassermann, German bacteriologist, 1866–1925.* A complement-fixation test, rarely used today, that enables the diagnosis of syphilis.

water (ˈwawtə) a clear, colourless, tasteless liquid composed of hydrogen and oxygen (H_2O). *W. balance* fluid balance. That between the fluid taken in by all routes and the fluid lost by all routes. *W.-borne* descriptive of certain diseases that are spread by contaminated water. *W. brash* the eructation of dilute acid from the stomach to the pharynx, giving a burning sensation. PYROSIS. Heartburn. *W. intoxication* a condition that results from excessive water retention in the brain, resulting in headaches, dizziness and confusion. In severe cases it may cause seizures and unconsciousness. Water intoxication can also result from the use of party drugs such as ecstasy, which may lead to excessive quantities of water being drunk. *W. seal drainage* a closed method of drainage from the pleural space allowing the escape of fluid and air but preventing air entering because the drainage tube discharges under water.

Waterhouse-Friderichsen syndrome (ˌwawtəhows ˈfreedriksən ˈsinˌdrohm) *Rupert Waterhouse, British physician, 1873–1958; Carl Friderichsen, Danish physician, 1886–1979.* An adrenal gland disease that is characterised by failure of the adrenal gland due to bleeding into the gland; marked by sudden onset fever, coma, cyanosis, haemorrhages from the skin and mucous membranes and severe shock. Also known as purpura fulminans.

Waterlow scale (ˌwawtəloh ˌskayl) *see* PRESSURE INJURY RISK ASSESSMENT SCALES.

Watson-Crick helix (ˌwotsənˈkrik ˈheeliks) *James Watson, American molecular biologist, b. 1928; Francis Crick, British molecular biologist, 1916–2004.* Double helix; a representation of the structure of DEOXYRIBONUCLEIC ACID (DNA), consisting of two coiled chains, each of which contains information completely specifying the other chain.

waxy flexibility (ˌwaksee ˌfleksə'bilətee) a psychomotor symptom associated with schizophrenia, bipolar disorder or other mental disorders in which a person's limbs are held indefinitely in any position in which they have been placed. *See* CATATONIA.

weal (weel) *see* WHEAL.

wean (ween) 1. to discontinue breast or bottle-feeding, and to substitute other feeding habits, e.g. solid foods. This should be effected gradually at about the 6th month. 2. in respiratory therapy, to gradually decrease dependence on assisted ventilation until the patient is able to breathe spontaneously.

wear and tear theory (wair ənd tair ˈthiəˌree) the concept of ageing that equates the human body with a machine, and that as parts wear out physiological functions deteriorate affecting the QUALITY OF LIFE.

web (web) a network or complex system of interconnected elements. *W. space* the soft tissue between the bases of the fingers and the toes. *W. site* in information technology, one or more pages that can be accessed through the internet to the WORLD WIDE WEB (WWW) that allows the browser to obtain specific information on the site.

webbing (ˈwebing) the state of being connected by a membrane or a fold of skin. *W. of the hands* or *feet* congenital abnormality in which the digits are not separated from each other. SYNDACTYLY. *W. of the neck* folds of skin in the neck giving it a webbed appearance. Occurs in certain congenital conditions, e.g. TURNER'S SYNDROME.

Weber test (ˈvaybə test) *Friedrich Weber Liel, German otologist, 1832–1891*. A test for hearing, in which a vibrating tuning fork is held in the centre of the forehead. Sound is normally heard equally in both ears. If the sound is heard louder in one ear, it can be indicative of conductive deafness in that ear.

Weil's disease (ˈvielz diˈzeez) *Adolf Weil, German physician, 1848–1916*. Spirochaetal jaundice. The organism *Leptospira icterohaemorrhagiae* is harboured and excreted by rats and enters through a bite or skin abrasion, or infected food or water.

Weil-Felix reaction (ˌvielˈfeeliks riˈakshən) *Edmund Weil, Austrian physician, 1880–1922*; *Arthur Felix, Czech bacteriologist, 1887–1956*. An agglutination test of blood serum used in the diagnosis of typhus.

well-baby clinic (welˈbaybee klinək) parents are encouraged to bring their infants to these clinics for assessment and monitoring of the child's health. Immunisation is available and there are opportunities for 'family' health promotion.

wellness (ˈwelnəs) the development of a personal lifestyle that promotes feelings of wellbeing, achieves the highest level of health within one's capability and minimises chances of becoming ill. It is guided by a developing sense of self-awareness and self-responsibility encompassing emotional, mental, physical, social, spiritual and environmental health.

wen (wen) a small sebaceous cyst; a STEATOMA.

Werdnig-Hoffmann disease (ˌvərdnigˈhofmən diˈzeez) *Guido Werdnig, Austrian neurologist, 1844–1919*; *Johann Hoffmann, German neurologist, 1857–1919*. A genetic condition characterised by progressive spinal muscular atrophy affecting the shoulder, neck, pelvis and, eventually, the respiratory muscles of infants. Also known as spinal muscular atrophy and autosomal recessive proximal spinal muscular atrophy.

Wernicke-Korsakoff syndrome (ˌvərnikəˈkawsəkof ˈsinˌdrohm) *Karl Wernicke, German neurologist, 1848–1905*; *Sergei Korsakoff, Russian neurologist, 1854–1900*. A disorder of the central nervous system usually associated with chronic alcoholism, nutritional deficiency and severe deficiency of vitamin B_1. It can sometimes occur with chronic illness or after weight loss (bariatric) surgery. It is characterised by a combination of motor and sensory disturbances and disordered memory function. One form is Wernicke's ENCEPHALOPATHY, a neurological condition due to vitamin B_1 deficiency. Untreated, it progresses from mental confusion and double vision to lethargy and coma.

Wertheim's operation (ˈvərt·hiemz ˌopəˈrayshən) *Ernst Wertheim, Austrian gynaecologist, 1864–1920*. *See* HYSTERECTOMY.

Wharton's jelly (ˈwawtənz ˈjelee) *Thomas Wharton, British physician, 1614–1673*. A gelatinous substance within the umbilical cord, also present in the vitreous humour of the eyeball.

wheal (weel) the dermal evidence of allergy; a raised skin lesion due to dermal swelling, often accompanied by severe itching, which has a smooth surface that characteristically evolves or disappears within minutes or up to 24 hours. Typical of URTICARIA. Called also hive, welt or weal.

wheezing (ˈweezing) breathing with a rasp or whistling sound. It results from constriction or obstruction of the throat, pharynx, trachea or bronchi. Wheezing is more common during expiration because increased intrathoracic pressure during this phase narrows the airways. Wheezing during expiration alone indicates milder obstruction than wheezing during both inspiration and expiration, which suggests more severe airway narrowing. During a most severe episode, wheezing may be absent because of the severe limitation of airflow associated with airway narrowing and respiratory muscle fatigue.

whiplash injury (ˈwipˌlash injəree) injury to the spinal cord, nerve roots, ligaments or vertebrae in the cervical region due to a sudden jerking back of the head and neck. Common in road traffic accidents where there is sudden acceleration or deceleration of the vehicle.

whiplash shake syndrome (ˈwipˌlash ˈshayk ˈsinˌdrohm) a constellation of injuries to the brain and eye that may occur when a young child is shaken vigorously with the head unsupported. This causes stretching and tearing of the cerebral vessels and brain substance, commonly leading to subdural haematomas and retinal haemorrhages. It may result in paralysis, blindness and other visual disturbances, convulsions and death. *See* SHAKEN BABY SYNDROME.

Whipple's operation (ˈwipəlz ˌopəˈrayshən) *Allen Whipple, American surgeon, 1881–1963*. Radical pancreatoduodenectomy performed for carcinoma of the head of the pancreas.

whipworm (ˈwipˌwərm) *see* TRICHURIS.

white blood cell (ˈwiet blud sel) *see* LEUCOCYTE.

white leg (ˈwiet leg) *see* PHLEGMASIA ALBA DOLENS.

whitlow (ˈwitloh) a felon; a suppurating inflammation of a finger near the nail. *Melanotic w.* a malignant tumour of the nail bed characterised by formation of melanotic tissue. Also known as subungual melanoma. *Subperiosteal w.* one in which the infection involves the bone covering. *Superficial w.* a pustule between the true skin and cuticle. *See* PARONYCHIA.

WHO *see* WORLD HEALTH ORGANIZATION. An agency of the United Nations.

whole system planning (ˈhohl ˈsistəm planing) strategic planning and commissioning across a range of services and organisational boundaries. Deals with the impact that changes in one part of the system, whether health and social care or housing, are likely to have on other parts.

whole systems approach (ˈhohl ˈsistəmz aˈprohˈch) the consideration of the interrelatedness of various elements, which come together for a common purpose and continually have an impact upon one another. The comprehension of complex systems, e.g. health care and social care; requires understanding of a diverse range of perspectives, and an appreciation that change will often be required across a number of areas to meet needs.

whooping cough (ˈhooping ˌkof) a notifiable infectious disease characterised by catarrh of the respiratory tract and paroxysms of coughing, ending in a prolonged whooping respiration; also called pertussis. The causative organism is *Bordetella pertussis.* Whooping cough is a serious disease; most cases occur in children. All babies should be immunised against whooping cough unless there is a sound medical objection.

Widal reaction (veeˈdahl riˈakshən) *Georges-Fernand Widal, French physician, 1862–1929.* A blood agglutination test for typhoid fever.

wi-fi (wie fie) the name for wireless technology used in local networks and mobile phones. A versatile system as it eliminates the need for wires, cables, switches and connectors.

Willis-Ekbom syndrome (ˈwilləs ˈekbom ˈsinˌdrohm) *Sir Thomas Willis, English physician (1621–1675); Karl-Axel Ekbom, Swedish neurologist, 1907–1977*; also known as restless leg syndrome; results in an uncontrollable urge to move the legs, possibly associated with dopamine. In some people it is temporary and in others permanent and debilitating. The temporary form is very common in pregnancy.

Wilms' tumour (vilmz ˈtyoomə) *Max Wilms, German surgeon, 1867–1918.* A highly malignant tumour of the kidney occurring in young children. A NEPHROBLASTOMA.

Wilson's disease (ˈwilsənz diˈzeez) *Samuel Wilson, British neurologist, 1878–1937.* Hepatolenticular degeneration; a genetic disorder involving the metabolism of copper leading to neurological degeneration.

wiring (ˈwieəring) the fixing together of a broken or split bone by the use of a wire. Commonly used for the jaw, the patella and the sternum.

wisdom teeth (ˈwizdəm teeth) the back molar teeth, the eruption of which is often delayed until maturity.

wish fulfilment (ˈwish ˌfuhlˈfilmənt) a desire, not always acknowledged consciously by the person, which is fulfilled through dreams or by day-dreaming.

withdrawal (withˈdrawrəl) 1. a pathological retreat from reality. 2. abstention from drugs or activities to which one is habituated or addicted; also denoting the symptoms occasioned by such withdrawal. *W. method* a contraceptive technique in coitus wherein the penis is withdrawn from the vagina before ejaculation. There is the possibility that sperm may be present in the pre-ejaculation phase and is therefore not a reliable form of contraception. Also known as coitus interruptus. *W. symptoms* symptoms brought about by abrupt withdrawal of the substance to which a person has become addicted; also called abstinence syndrome. The usual reactions to withdrawal may include anxiety, weakness, gastrointestinal symptoms, nausea and vomiting, tremor, fever, rapid heartbeat, convulsions and delirium.

Wolff-Parkinson-White syndrome (ˌwuhlf ˌpahkinsən ˈwiet ˈsin ˌdrohm) *Louis Wolff, American cardiologist, 1898–1972*; *Sir John Parkinson, British physician, 1885–1976*; *Paul White, American cardiologist, 1886–1973*. Abnormal heart rhythm caused by an accessory bundle between the atria and ventricles. A congenital disorder.

womb (woom) the uterus.

woman-centred care (ˌwomən ˌsentəd ˈkair) a collaborative and respectful partnership built on mutual trust and understanding through good communication. Each woman is treated as an individual with the aim of respecting women's ownership of their health information, rights and preferences, while protecting their dignity and empowering choice. Woman-centred practice recognises the role of family and community with respect to cultural and religious diversity.

women's health clinic (wimenz helth klinək) a health promotion clinic that offers a range of services to women including, but not limited to, screening for breast and cervical cancer, well women checks and health information, e.g. self-examination of the breasts. *See* BREAST.

Wood's light (wuhdz liet) *Robert Wood, American physicist, 1868–1955*. Ultraviolet light transmitted through a glass filter containing nickel oxide. It produces fluorescence of infected hairs when placed over a scalp affected with ringworm.

woolsorter's disease (ˈwuhl ˌsawtəz diˈzeez) pulmonary form of anthrax.

word blindness (werdˈbliendnəs) *see* DYSLEXIA.

word salad (ˈwərd ˌsaləd) speech in which the words are strung together without meaning.

World Health Organization (WHO) (wərld helth ˈawgənie ˌzayshən) the specialised agency of the United Nations that is concerned with health on an international level. WHO organises health campaigns against infectious diseases and sponsors research in medical laboratories. It also provides expert advice on all matters directly or indirectly concerned with physical or mental health to all member states.

World Wide Web (WWW) (wərld wied web) an information space where documents and other resources are stored and interlinked and accessed via the internet.

worm (wərm) any one of a number of groups of long soft-bodied invertebrates, some of which are parasitic to humans.

wound (woond) a cut or break in continuity of any tissue caused by injury or operation. It is classified according to its nature. *Abrased w.* the skin is scraped off but there is no deeper injury. *Contused w.* with bruising of the surrounding tissue. *Incised w.* usually the result of operation and produced by a knife or similar instrument. The edges of the wound can remain in apposition, and it should heal by first intention. *Lacerated w.* one with torn edges and tissues, usually the result of accident or injury. It is often septic and heals by second intention. *Open w.* a gaping wound on the body surface. *Penetrating w.* often made by gunshot, shrapnel, etc. There may be an inlet and outlet hole, and vital organs are often penetrated by the missile. *Punctured w.* made by a pointed or spiked instrument. *Septic w.* any type into which infection has been introduced, causing suppurative inflammation. It heals by second intention. *W. dressing* material applied to a surgical or medical wound to provide protection and assist healing. Dressings are made from a variety of materials with or without medication, e.g. hydrocellular or alginate dressings used in the management of cavities or exuding wounds, and low-adherent absorbent dressings used for clean wounds. The aim is that the dressing should be comfortable, permit the exchange of gases but be impermeable to bacteria, prevent adherence to the wound, and therefore reduce damage to new tissue when it is removed. *W. healing* the restoration of integrity to injured tissues by replacement of dead tissue with viable tissue. In wound healing there are four stages—haemostasis, inflammation, proliferation (or granulation) and maturation—which may take several months to complete. Wound healing may be delayed by physical stress, inadequate blood supply or by more general factors that include malnutrition, ageing, drugs such as corticosteroids, etc. The process starts immediately after an injury and may continue for months or years. *See* HEALING.

wrist (rist) the point of the carpus and bones of the forearm. *W. drop* loss of power in the muscles of the hand. It may be due to nerve or tendon injury, but can result from lack of sufficient support by splint or sling.

writer's cramp (ˌrietəz ˈkramp) a colloquial term for painful spasm of the hand and forearm, caused by excessive writing and poor posture. *See* REPETITIVE STRAIN INJURY.

wryneck (ˈrieˌnek) *see* TORTICOLLIS.

Wuchereria (ˌvookəˈriə·ri·ə) a genus of nematode worms which are the principal vector of FILARIASIS. *W. bancrofti* the most common species in tropical and subtropical areas.

WWW *see* WORLD WIDE WEB.

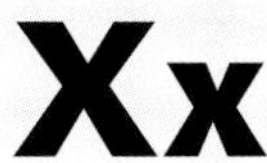

X-linked (eks lingk'd) pertaining to the genes, or the effect of these genes, situated on the X chromosome. X-linked disorders are those caused by the genes on the X chromosome.

X-rays (ˈeksˌrayz) electromagnetic waves of short length which are capable of penetrating many substances and of producing chemical changes and reactions in living matter. They are used both to aid diagnosis and to treat disease. Also called Röentgen radiation.

xanthelasma (ˌzanthəˈlazmə) a disease marked by the formation of flat or slightly raised yellow fatty deposits on or around the eyelids.

xanthine (ˈzantheen) a compound found in plant and animal tissues; a rare genetic disorder, xanthinuria, results from a lack of xanthine oxidase and an inability to convert xanthine to uric acid.

xanthochromia (ˌzanthohˈkrohmi·ə) 1. the presence of yellow patches on the skin. 2. the yellow colouring of cerebrospinal fluid seen in people who have had a subarachnoid haemorrhage.

xanthoma (zanˈthohmə) the presence in the skin of flat areas of yellowish pigmentation due to deposits of lipids. There are several varieties. *X. palpebrarum* XANTHELASMA.

xanthopsia (zanˈthopsi·ə) a disturbance of vision in which all objects appear yellow.

xanthosis (zanˈthohsəs) a yellow skin discolouration of degenerating tissue, seen in malignant neoplasms.

X chromosome (eks ˈkrohməˌsohm) the female sex chromosome, being present in all female gametes and only half the male gametes. When union takes place, two X chromosomes result in a female child (XX) but one of each results in a male child (XY). *See* Y CHROMOSOME.

xenophobia (ˌzeenəˈfohbi·ə) a fear or dislike of strangers, of foreigners or of anything that is strange or foreign.

Xenopsylla (ˌzenopˈsilə) a genus of fleas, some of which are vectors of plague. *X. cheopis* the rat flea which transmits bubonic plague and murine typhus.

xero- (ˈziə·roh-) combining form meaning dryness.

xeroderma (ˌziə·rohˈdərmə) also known as xerosis cutis. Dry skin occurring most commonly on the scalp, lower legs, arms, hands, abdomen and thighs. A very common condition, especially in winter. *X. pigmentosum* (XP) a rare disorder of DNA repair where the ability to repair damage caused by ultraviolet light is deficient. It begins in childhood and rapidly progresses. The formation of malignant neoplasms of the skin is common and is a common cause of death in people with XP.

xerophthalmia (ˌziə·rofˈthalmi·ə) a condition in which the cornea and conjunctiva become dry, thin and wrinkled. It may be caused by a deficiency of vitamin A. Also known as xeroma.

xerosis (zəˈrohsəs) a condition of dryness, especially of the eyes, mouth, vagina or skin.

xerostomia (ˌziə·rohˈstohmi·ə) dryness of the mouth due to a failure of salivary gland secretion or a change in the composition of saliva.

xiphoid process (ˈzifoyd proses) a small cartilaginous process (extension) of the lower part of the sternum which is usually ossified in the adult human. Also called xiphisternum.

xylose (ˈzielohz) a pentose sugar found in connective tissue (and sometimes in urine) which is not metabolised in the body. *X. absorption test* an investigation for malabsorption.

XXY syndrome (ˌeksˌ eksˌ ˈwie ˈsinˌdrohm) a syndrome where boys are born with an additional X chromosome. *See* KLINEFELTER'S SYNDROME.

XYY syndrome (ˌeks ˌwie ˈwie ˈsinˌdrohm) an extremely rare condition in males in which there is an extra Y chromosome, making a total of 47 chromosomes in each body cell. Also known as Jacob's syndrome.

Yy

yarn (yahn) to talk.

yarning (yahning) a form of storytelling and an Indigenous cultural form of conversation where the oral tradition dominates. Aboriginal yarning or storytelling from an Aboriginal and Torres Strait Islander perspective is both an ongoing fluid process and an exchange. Yarning encompasses elements of respect and engagement as individuals interact to preserve and pass on cultural knowledge. Yarning is emerging as a collaborative research method and has wide-ranging potential to shape conventional research. *Clinical y.* a patient-centred approach that integrates Aboriginal and Torres Strait Islander cultural communication preferences with biomedical understandings of health and disease. Clinical yarning consists of three interrelated areas: the social yarn, in which the practitioner aims to find common ground and develop the interpersonal relationship; the diagnostic yarn, in which the practitioner facilitates the patient's health story while interpreting it through a biomedical or scientific model; and the management yarn, which employs stories and metaphors as tools for patients to assist them to understand a health issue so a collaborative management approach can be employed. Clinical yarning has the potential to improve health outcomes for patients and practitioners.

yawning (ˈyawning) a reflex in which the mouth is opened wide and air is drawn in and exhaled. It may accompany tiredness or boredom.

yaws (yawz) framboesia. An infection of the skin, bones and joints common in tropical countries. Caused by *Treponema pallidum pertenue*, it is common among people (especially children) who live in poor conditions in equatorial Africa, South America and the East and West Indies. The World Health Organization (WHO) aimed to eradicate yaws by 2020.

Y chromosome (ˈwie ˌkrohmə ˌsohm) the male sex chromosome, being present in half the male gametes and none of the female. Y is the sex determining chromosome. *See* X CHROMOSOME.

yeast (yeest) any of the fungi of the genus *Saccharomyces*. They produce fermentation in malt and in sweetened fruit juices, resulting in the formation of alcoholic solutions such as beer and wine.

yellow fever (ˈyeloh ˈfeevə) an acute, notifiable, infectious disease of the tropics caused by a virus and transmitted by the bite of an infected female mosquito (*Aedes aegypti*). The virus attacks the liver and kidneys and the symptoms include rigor, headache, pain in the back and limbs, high fever and nausea. Haemorrhage from the intestinal mucous membrane may occur. There is a high mortality rate. A vaccine is available.

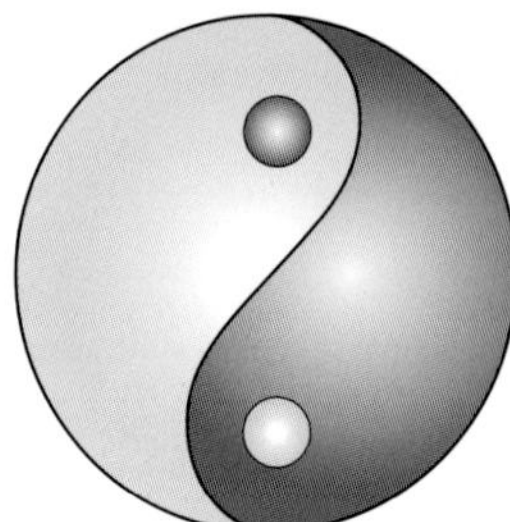

The Chinese symbol for yin–yang.

Yersinia (yər'sinyə) a genus of Gram-negative bacteria containing the pathogen *Y. pestis* responsible for the bubonic plague. *Yersinia* is also responsible for a variety of other infections, e.g. gastroenteritis in the young and septicaemia in adults.

yin and yang (yin ənd yang) describes how seemingly opposite forces may be complementary—the principles of this Chinese philosophy are incorporated into traditional Chinese medicine. Yin is the black side, dark and negative; yang is the white side, bright and positive. Together, the yin–yang interaction and balance is believed to maintain the harmony of the body and, in a healthy person, to maintain a state of dynamic balance (*see* figure).

yoga ('yohgə) a Hindu discipline which emphasises personal physical preparation using meditation, relaxation, breathing control and the attainment of defined body positions to achieve relaxation, with physical and emotional harmony and wellbeing.

yolk sac (yohk sak) a membranous sac attached to an embryo and which is important for the blood supply of the early embryo.

yttrium ('itryəm) *symbol* Y. A rare chemical element, which in its radioactive form is sometimes used in cancer therapy and the treatment of severe arthritis.

Zz

Z-plasty (ˈzed ˌplastee) a plastic surgery technique for removing and repairing deformity resulting from a contraction scar (*see* figure).

Z-track injection (ˈzed ˌtrak inˈjekshən) an intramuscular injection technique which allows a medication, e.g. an iron preparation, to be given, but which prevents the leakage and the staining of tissues surrounding the site. *See* INJECTION.

Zen (zen) Zen Buddhism is the teaching that a form of meditation consisting of the contemplation of one's essential nature to the exclusion of everything else is the way to true enlightenment.

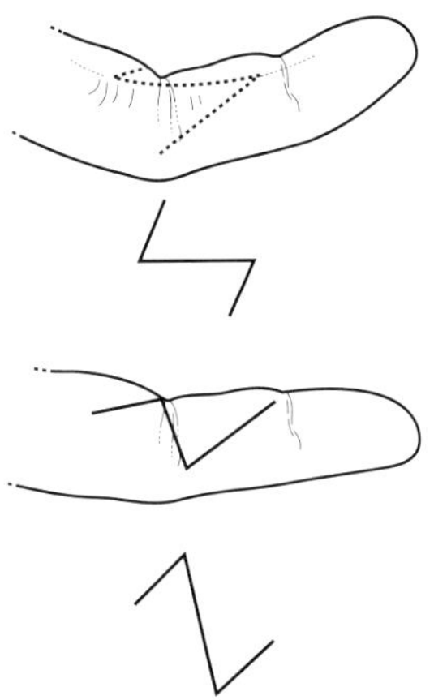

Z-plasty.

zenith (ˈzenəth) the highest point. The opposite is NADIR.

zero (ˈziəroh) nought; *symbol* 0. In the Celsius thermometer 0°C is the melting point of ice; in the Fahrenheit thermometer, 0°F is 32° below the melting point of ice. *See* CELSIUS and FAHRENHEIT.

Ziehl-Neelsen method (ˌzielˈneel-sən ˈmethuhd) *Franz Ziehl, German bacteriologist, 1857–1926*; *Friedrich Neelsen, German pathologist, 1854–1894*. A method of staining tubercle bacilli for microscopic study. Also known as the acid-fast stain.

zika virus (ˈzeeka ˈvierəs) (also known as zika fever) a viral disease mainly spread by mosquitoes which is serious for pregnant women as it is thought to cause birth defects—particularly microcephaly (small head). There is currently no vaccine.

Zimmer® (ˈzimə) the trade name of a metal, lightweight walking aid commonly applied to other products of similar design and weight. Predominantly used by older people to assist the person in walking and in rehabilitation.

zinc (zingk) *symbol* Zn. A trace element which is essential in the body for cell growth and multiplication. The recommended daily intake of zinc is 12 mg for an adult male and 8 mg for an adult female. A severe deficiency of zinc can retard growth in children, cause a low sperm count in adult males and retard wound healing.

Zn *symbol* for ZINC.

Zollinger-Ellison syndrome (ˌzolinjə ˈelisən ˈsinˌdrohm) *Robert Zollinger, American surgeon, 1903–1992; Edwin Ellison, American surgeon, 1918–1970.* A rare condition in which a pancreatic tumour causes excessive outpouring of gastric juice. PEPTIC ULCERS may occur.

zona (ˈzohnə) a zone. *Z. pellucida* the membrane surrounding the ovum.

zone therapy (ˈzohn ˌtherəpee) reflex zone therapy; the feet are palpated in order to alleviate pain and/or treat symptoms by stimulating the self-healing capacity of the body.

zonula (ˈzonyələ) a zonule. In anatomy, a small, usually circular, area. *Ciliary z.* the area surrounded by the suspensory ligaments of the eye.

zoonosis (ˌzoh·əˈnohsəs, ˌzooəˈnoh-səs) a disease of animals that is transmissible to humans, e.g. ebola, rabies, cat-scratch fever, toxoplasmosis.

zoster (ˈzostə) *see* HERPES.

zygoma (zieˈgohmə, zi-) zygomatic bone commonly referred to as the cheek bone or molar bone.

zygote (ˈziegoht, ˈzi-) a single cell formed from the union of a male and a female gamete.

zymosis (zieˈmohsəs) fermentation.

APPENDIX 1

Commonly used prefixes, suffixes and combining forms

Medical and nursing terms can often be broken down into separate components. There are five possible parts to a word: prefix, suffix, root, combining vowel and combining form. A root is the foundation of a word. The prefix comes before the root, and the suffix comes after the root. A combining vowel is used to combine words. A combining form is made up of a root plus the combining vowel.

Prefix, suffix, combining form	Meaning
a-	without, not
ab-	away from
abdomin/o-	pertaining to the abdomen
acanth/o-	thorny
acou-	pertaining to hearing
acr/o-	pertaining to the extremities
ad-	to, towards
aden/o-	pertaining to the glands
adip/o-	pertaining to fat
-aemia, -emia	pertaining to blood
aer/o-	pertaining to air, gas
-aesthesia, -esthesia	pertaining to feeling or sensation
-agog, -agogue	an agent that promotes the expulsion of a substance
alg-, algesi-	pertaining to pain
-algia	painful
allo-	reversed or differing from normal
ambi-	pertaining to both sides
andr/o-	pertaining to the male
angi/o-	pertaining to a vessel, especially a blood vessel
ant-, -anti-	against
ante-	before, in front of

Prefix, suffix, combining form	Meaning
arthr/o-	pertaining to a joint
-asthenia	depleted vitality
audi/o-	hearing
aur/i, aur/o-	pertaining to the ear
aut/o-	pertaining to the self
bar/o-	pertaining to pressure
-basia	ability to walk
bi-	two or twice, double
bili-	pertaining to bile
blephar/o-	pertaining to the eyelids or eyelash
brachy-	short
brady-	slow
bronch/o-	pertaining to the bronchus
bucc/o-	pertaining to the cheek
carcin-	pertaining to cancer
cardi/o-	pertaining to the heart
cata-	against
-cele	swelling or tumour
-centesis	to puncture or cut
cephal/o-	pertaining to the head
cerebr/o-	pertaining to the cerebrum
cervic-	pertaining to the neck
cheir/o-, chir/o-	pertaining to the hand
chemo-	chemical
-chesia	pertaining to the discharge of substances
chol/e-, chol/o-	pertaining to bile
circum-	around
-clasia	crushing or breaking up
-coele	cavity, space
col/o-	pertaining to the colon, bowel
colp/o-	pertaining to the vagina
contra-	opposed, against

Prefix, suffix, combining form	Meaning
copr/o-	pertaining to faeces
cortic-	pertaining to the cortex or bark
crani/o-	pertaining to the cranium or skull
cry/o-	cold
crypt/o-	concealed or hidden
cut-	pertaining to the skin
cyan-	blue
cyst/o-	pertaining to the bladder
cyt/o-	cell or cytoplasm
-dactyl	digit
de-	away from
derm/a-, derm/o-	pertaining to the skin
di-	twice or two
dipl/o-	double
-dipsia	thirst
dia	separation
dors/i-, dors/o-	pertaining to the dorsum or back
duoden/o-	pertaining to the duodenum of intestine
dys-	painful or disordered
ecto-	outside
-ectomy	the surgical removal of, excision
-ectopia	the displacement of a part or organ
electro-	electrical
end-, endo-, ent-, ento-, enter/o	within, inner, pertaining to the intestines
epi-	upon, on, over
eu-	good or well
eurythr/o-	red
faci/o-	pertaining to the face
-faction	the process of making
-fibroma	benign tumour consisting of fibrous tissue
ferr-	pertaining to iron

Prefix, suffix, combining form	Meaning
fiss-	split, cleft
flex-	bend
fore-	in front of, before
galact/o-	pertaining to milk
gastr/o-	pertaining to the stomach
-genesis	beginning process, origin
gen/o-	producing
glio-	pertaining to the neuroglia, or a gluey substance
gloss/o-	pertaining to the tongue
gluc/o-, glyc/o-	pertaining to glucose, or sweetness
gnath-	pertaining to the jaw
-gram, -gramme	a drawing
-gravida	pregnant woman with (specified) quantity of pregnancies
gynaec/o-, gyn/o-	pertaining to woman
haem-, hem-	pertaining to blood
hemi-	half
hepat-	pertaining to the liver
heter/o-	pertaining to another
hist/o-	pertaining to the tissues
holo-	pertaining to the whole
home/o-, hom/o-	the same
hydr/o-	pertaining to water or hydrogen
hyper-	excess or above
hypo-	beneath or deficient
hyster/o-	pertaining to the uterus
-iasis	produced by or producing disease
ile/o-	ileum of intestine
ili/o-	ilium (upper part of hip bone)
immuno-	immunity
inter-	situated between
intra-	situated within

Prefix, suffix, combining form	Meaning
ischi/o-	pertaining to the hip, or ischium
iso-	equal
jejun/o-	jejunum of intestine
kerat-	horn, skin, cornea
kin/e-, kin/o-, kinesi/o-	movement, motion
-lalia	a disorder of speech
lamin-	layer
lapar-	pertaining to the abdomen
laryng/o-	pertaining to the larynx
later/o-	pertaining to the side
leuco-, leuko-	white, pertaining to the white corpuscles
lip/o-	pertaining to fat, fatty acids
-lipoma	tumour consisting of fatty tissue
lith/o-	stone or calculus
lymph/o-	pertaining to lymph
-lysis	detachment or breaking down, dissolving
macr/o-	large or abnormal size
mal-	bad or abnormal
-malacia	softening of tissue
man-	pertaining to the hand
mast/o-	pertaining to the breast
mega-	large or great
melan-	black
mening/o-	pertaining to the meninges
meta-	change, beyond
micro-	small
mon/o-	one
morph/o-	form, structure, shape
multi-	many
myc/o-	pertaining to fungus
myel/o-	pertaining to bone marrow or spinal cord
my/o-	pertaining to muscle

Prefix, suffix, combining form	Meaning
myring/o-	pertaining to the eardrum
narc/o-	pertaining to stupor
nas/o-	pertaining to the nose
necr/o-	pertaining to death
neo-	new, recent
nephr/o-	pertaining to the kidneys
neur/o-	pertaining to the nerves
nutri-	pertaining to nourishment
ocul/o-	pertaining to the eye
-odynia	a state of pain
olig/o-	few or little
-oma	a tumour
onc/o-	pertaining to a swelling or tumour
oo-	pertaining to an egg or ovum
ophthalm/o-	pertaining to the eye(s)
orch/i-, orchi/do-, orch/o-	pertaining to the testis or testes
-orexia	pertaining to the appetite
or/o-	pertaining to the mouth
orth/o-	straight or normal
-osis	a pathological condition
oste/o-	pertaining to bone
-ostomy	to form a new opening or pertaining to a mouth-like opening
oto-	pertaining to the ear
paedia-, pedia-	pertaining to a child
-penia	deficiency of, lack of
pan-	all
para-	beside, beyond, after
path/o-	related to disease
ped-, pod-	pertaining to the foot
pell-	pertaining to the skin
-pepsia	pertaining to digestion

Prefix, suffix, combining form	Meaning
peri-	around
-pexy	surgical fixation
phag/o-	pertaining to eating
pharyng/o-	pertaining to the pharynx
-phasic	speech disorder
-phily	fondness or affinity for something
phleb/o-	pertaining to a vein
-phobe	one who fears
-phyma	a swelling or tumour
pil/o-	resembling hair
-plasty	surgical shaping or forming
-plegic	pertaining to paralysis
plex-	a stroke
pneum/o-	of or related to the lungs, air or breathing
-pnoea, -pnea	breathing or breath
-poiesis, -poesis	production of
poli/o-	pertaining to the grey matter in the central nervous system
poly-	many
post-	after or behind
-praxia	pertaining to the performance of movements
pre-	before
proct/o-	pertaining to the rectum
psor-	pertaining to itching
pseud/o-	false
psych-	pertaining to the mind
-ptosis	a prolapse of an organ
pulm/o-	pertaining to the lungs
pyel/o-	pertaining to the pelvis or the kidney
py/o-	pertaining to pus
quadr/i-	four
rachi/o-	pertaining to the spine

Prefix, suffix, combining form	Meaning
re-	backward; again
ren/o-	pertaining to the kidneys
retin/o-	pertaining to the retina
retro-	located behind
rhin/o-	pertaining to the nose
-rrhagia	to pour or burst forth
-rrhoea, -rrhea	flow or discharge
ruber-, rubor-	red, redness
sacr/o-	pertaining to the sacrum
salping/o-	pertaining to the fallopian tube or eustachian tube
sangui-	pertaining to blood
sarc/o-	pertaining to flesh or muscular substance
scler/o-	hard
scoli/o-	twisted, crooked
-scope	instrument for examining
semi-	half
sero-	serum
somat/o-	pertaining to the body
sphygm/o-	pertaining to the pulse
spondyl/o-	pertaining to the vertebra or spinal column
-stasis	a stoppage or inhibition
sten/o-	narrow
steth/o-	pertaining to the chest
-stomy	a surgical opening
-strophy	twisting
sub-	under, beneath
super-, supra-	above, superior, excess
sym-, syn-	together, with
tachy-	fast or rapid
tend/o-, ten/o-, tenont/o, tendin/o-	pertaining to tendon(s)
-thelioma	a tumour in cellular tissue

Prefix, suffix, combining form	Meaning
therm/o-	pertaining to heat
thorac/o-	pertaining to the chest or thorax
thromb/o-	pertaining to a clot, or thrombus
-tomy	a surgical incision
-tony	pertaining to motor control
trache/o-	pertaining to the trachea
trans-	across or through
-tresia	a perforation
tri-	three
-trophy	a condition of growth
uni-	one
ure-	pertaining to urine or the urinary tract
-uria	the presence of a substance in the urine
uter-	uterus
vas/o-	pertaining to a vessel
ven/e-, ven/i, ven/o-	pertaining to vein(s)
ventr/i-, ventr/o-	pertaining to the front of the body or belly
vesic/o-	pertaining to the bladder or a blister
xen/o-	strange
xer/o-	dry

APPENDIX 2

Commonly used nursing abbreviations

Abbreviations in use can vary widely from place to place. Each institution's list of acceptable abbreviations is the best authority for its records.

See page 527 for abbreviations used in prescriptions.

Abbreviation	Meaning
AAA	abdominal aortic aneurysm
ABG	arterial blood gases
ABO	the three basic blood groups
ACE	angiotensin-converting enzyme
ACS	acute coronary syndrome
ACTH	adrenocorticotrophic hormone
ADH	antidiuretic hormone
ADHD	attention deficit hyperactivity disorder
ADL	activities of daily living
AED	automated external defibrillator
AF	atrial fibrillation
AFB	acid-fast bacillus
AIDS	acquired immunodeficiency syndrome
AIN	assistant in nursing
AK	above the knee
ALS	advanced life support; amyotrophic lateral sclerosis
am	morning
AMI	acute myocardial infarction
AML	acute myeloblastic/myeloid leukaemia
ANOVA	analysis of variance
ANS	autonomic nervous system
APKD	acute polycystic kidney disease
ARDS	adult respiratory distress syndrome
ARM	artificial rupture of membranes

Abbreviation	Meaning
BGL	blood glucose level
BiPAP	bi-directional positive airway pressure
BK	below the knee
BLS	basic life support
BMD	bone mineral density
BMI	body mass index
BMR	basal metabolic rate
BP	blood pressure
BPH	benign prostatic hypertrophy
bpm	beats per minute
BSE	breast self-examination
Bx	biopsy
·/c	with
C	Celsius/Centigrade
Ca	carcinoma
CABG	coronary artery bypass graft
CAPD	continuous ambulatory peritoneal dialysis
CAT	computerised (axial) tomography
CAUTI	catheter-associated urinary tract infection
CCF	congestive cardiac failure
CCU	coronary care unit; critical care unit
CF	cystic fibrosis
CHF	congestive heart failure
CHO	carbohydrate
CI	cardiac index; cardiac insufficiency; cerebral infarction
CINAHL	Cumulative Index to Nursing and Allied Health Literature
CJD	Creutzfeldt-Jakob disease
CMV	cytomegalovirus
CNC / CMC	clinical nurse/midwife consultant
CNE / CME	clinical nurse/midwife educator
CNS / CMS	clinical nurse/midwife specialist
CNS	central nervous system; clinical nurse specialist
c/o	complains of/complaints of

Abbreviation	Meaning
COLD	chronic obstructive lung disease
COPD	chronic obstructive pulmonary disease
CPAP	continuous positive airway pressure
CPD	continuing professional development
CPR	cardiopulmonary resuscitation
CSSD	Central Sterile Supplies and Disinfection Unit
CSF	cerebrospinal fluid
CT	computed tomography
CVA	cerebrovascular accident
CVP	central venous pressure
CVS	chorionic villi sampling; cardiovascular system
CXR	chest X-ray
D&C	dilation (dilatation) and curettage
DB&C	deep breathing and coughing
DEXA	dual energy X-ray absorptiometry
DIC	disseminated intravascular coagulopathy/coagulation
DKA	diabetic ketoacidosis
DNA	deoxyribonucleic acid
DOA	dead on arrival
DOB	date of birth
DOE	dyspnoea on exertion
DON	director of nursing
DRG	diagnostic-related groups
DT	delirium tremens
DVT	deep venous thrombosis
EBP	evidence-based practice; epidural blood patch
ECG	electrocardiogram; electrocardiograph
ECHO	echocardiography
ED	emergency department
EEG	electroencephalogram; electroencephalograph
EEN	endorsed enrolled nurse
EMLA	eutectic mixture of local anaesthetics
EN	enrolled nurse

Abbreviation	Meaning
ENT	ears, nose and throat
EPS	electrophysiology study
ESR	erythrocyte sedimentation rate
ESRD	end-stage renal disease
F	Fahrenheit
FBC	fluid balance chart; full blood count
FEV	forced expiratory volume
FH, Fhx	family history
FSE	fetal scalp electrode
FSH	follicle-stimulating hormone
GFR	glomerular filtration rate
GI	gastrointestinal; glycaemic index
GORD	gastro-oesophageal reflux disease
GP	general practitioner
GTT	glucose tolerance test
GU	genitourinary
GVHD	graft versus host disease
HAI	healthcare associated infection
Hb, Hgb	haemoglobin
HbA_{1c}	glycosylated haemoglobin
HCT	haematocrit
HDL	high-density lipoprotein
HDU	high dependency unit
HIV	human immunodeficiency (AIDS) virus
Hx, hx	history
IBS	irritable bowel syndrome
ICP	intracranial pressure
ICU	intensive care unit
IDC	indwelling catheter
Ig	immunoglobulin
IM	intramuscular
IOP	intraocular pressure
IPPB	intermittent positive pressure breathing

Abbreviation	Meaning
IPPV	intermittent positive pressure ventilation
ISBAR	Introduction, situation, background, assessment, recommendations
IV	intravenous
IVF	in vitro fertilisation
IVP	intravenous pyelogram
KPI	key performance indicator
Lab	laboratory
LDL	low density lipoprotein
LFT	liver function tests
LMP	last menstrual period
LOC	level of consciousness; loss of consciousness
LP	lumbar puncture
MAOI	monoamine oxidase inhibitor
MAU	medical assessment unit
MDT	multidisciplinary team
MI	myocardial infarction
MND	motor neuron disease
MRI	magnetic resonance imaging
MS	multiple sclerosis
MSU	midstream specimen of urine
MVA/MVC	motor vehicle accident/collision
N/A	not applicable; not available
NAD	no abnormalities detected; non-adherent dressing
NBM	nil by mouth
NG, ng	nasogastric
NICU	neonatal intensive care unit
NM	nurse manager
NOF	neck of femur
NP	nurse practitioner
NRT	nicotine replacement therapy
NS, N/S	normal saline
NSAID	non-steroidal anti-inflammatory drug

Abbreviation	Meaning
NST	newborn screening test (Guthrie)
NSTEMI	non ST-segment elevation myocardial infarction
NUM / MUM	nursing / midwifery unit manager
O/A	on admission
OCD	obsessive compulsive disorder
O/E	on examination
OTC	over-the-counter
Pap test	Papanicolaou smear
PBS	Pharmaceutical Benefits Scheme
PCA	patient-controlled analgesia
PCI	percutaneous coronary intervention
PCOS	polycystic ovary syndrome
PET	positron emission tomography
pH	hydrogen ion concentration (alkalinity and acidity in urine and blood analysis)
PID	pelvic inflammatory disease
PKU	phenylketonuria
pm	afternoon/evening
PMT	premenstrual tension
PR	per rectum; pulse rate
PRN, prn	as required (*pro re nata*)
PTSD	post-traumatic stress disorder
PUO	pyrexia of unknown origin
PVC	premature ventricular contraction
RBC	red blood cell; red blood count
RCT	randomised controlled trial
RDI	recommended daily intake
Rh	Rh factor
RN / RM	registered nurse/midwife
ROM	range of motion
rpm	revolutions per minute; respirations per minute
SD	standard deviation
s/s, S&S	signs and symptoms

Abbreviation	Meaning
SG, sp.gr.	specific gravity
SGOT	serum glutamic oxaloacetic transaminase
SIDS	sudden infant death syndrome
SLE	systemic lupus erythematosus
SMART	specific, measurable, achievable, realistic, time-bound
SOB	shortness of breath
SOBOE	shortness of breath on exertion
SR	sedimentation rate
SROM/PROM	spontaneous or premature rupture of membranes
staph	*Staphylococcus*
Stat	immediately (statim)
STEMI	ST-segment elevation myocardial infarction
STI	sexually transmitted infection
strep	*Streptococcus*
subcut	subcutaneous
SVT	supraventricular tachycardia
T1D or T1DM	type 1 diabetes mellitus
T2D or T2DM	type 2 diabetes mellitus
TB	tuberculosis; tubercle bacillus
TED/S	thromboembolism deterrent stockings
TENS	transcutaneous electrical nerve stimulation
TIA	transient ischaemic attack
TPN	total parenteral nutrition
TPR	temperature, pulse and respiration
TSH	thyroid-stimulating hormone
Tx, Rx	treatment
UA	urinalysis
URTI	upper respiratory tract infection
UTI	urinary tract infection
VAC	vacuum assisted closure
VF	ventricular fibrillation
VSD	ventricular septal defect
WBC, wbc	white blood cell; white blood count

Abbreviation	Meaning
WCC	white cell count
WHO	World Health Organization
wt	weight
WWW	World Wide Web
X-ray	roentgen ray

Abbreviations used in prescriptions

English is the preferred language for the writing of prescriptions, rather than the traditional Latin. The use of abbreviations in prescriptions in both English or Latin is potentially dangerous and should be discouraged. Hospitals usually have a list of abbreviations approved for use in that institution. Nurses might still encounter the following Latin abbreviations.

Abbreviation	Latin	English
a.c.	ante cibum	before food
b.d. or b.i.d.	bis in die	twice a day
gtt	guttae	drops (of liquid)
mane	omni mane	every morning
nocte	omni nocte	every night
p.c.	post cibum	after food
PO or p.o.	per orem	by mouth
p.r.n.	pro re nate	whenever necessary
q.d.s.	quaque die sumendum	four times daily
q.i.d.	quater in die	four times a day
q.q.h.	quater quaque hora	every four hours
stat.	statim	at once
t.d.s.	ter die sumendum	three times daily
t.i.d.	ter in die	three times a day

APPENDIX 3
Units of measurement

SI units (Système Internationale d'Unités)

Base units

Physical quantity	Name of unit	Symbol
Mass	kilogram	kg
Length	metre	m
Time	second	s
Electric current	ampere	A
Temperature	kelvin	K
Luminous intensity	candela	cd
Amount of substance	mole	mol
Volume	litre	L

Derived units

Derived units to measure other quantities are obtained by multiplying or dividing any two or more of the eight base units. Some of these have their own names and symbols. For example:

Physical quantity	Name of unit	Symbol	Base or derived units
Force	newton	N	$kg{\cdot}m{\cdot}s^{-2}$
Pressure	pascal	Pa	$N{\cdot}m^{-2}$
Energy, work, heat	Joule	J	$N{\cdot}m$
Power	Watt	W	$J{\cdot}s^{-1}$

Prefixes used for multiples

Factor	Prefix	Symbol
10^{-15}	femto	f
10^{-12}	pico	p
10^{-9}	nano	n
10^{-6}	micro	μ
10^{-3}	milli	m
10^{-2}	centi	c
10^{-1}	deci	d
10	deca	da
10^{2}	hecto	h
10^{3}	kilo	k
10^{6}	mega	M
10^{9}	giga	G
10^{12}	tera	T

Capacity

The SI unit of volume is the cubic metre (m^3), but the litre (L) is more commonly used and accepted.

1000 microlitres (microL)	= 1 millilitre (mL)
1000 millilitres	= 1 litre (L)
1 cubic centimetre (cm^3)	= 1 millilitre
1 teaspoon	= 5 mL
1 dessertspoon	= 10 mL
1 tablespoon	= 15 mL
1 cup	= 250 mL
1 tumbler	= 285 mL

Weight

1000 micrograms (microg)	= 1 milligram (mg)
1000 milligrams	= 1 gram (g)
1000 grams	= 1 kilogram (kg)
1000 kilograms	= 1 metric tonne

Energy

The body needs energy for growth, metabolism and activity. Energy is provided by carbohydrates, fat, proteins and alcohol. It is measured in either kilocalories (usually called 'Calories' with a capital 'C') or kilojoules (kJ). A dietetic Calorie is the amount of heat required to raise the temperature of 1 litre of water by 1°C and is equal to 4.184 kilojoules.

- 1 Calorie (1 kilocalorie) = 4.184 kilojoules
- 1 g of carbohydrate (sugar and starches) yields 4 Calories = 17 kilojoules
- 1 g of fat yields 9 Calories = 38 kilojoules
- 1 g of protein yields 4 Calories = 17 kilojoules
- 1 g of alcohol yields 7 Calories = 29 kilojoules.

Comparative temperatures

Celsius (°C)	Fahrenheit (°F)	Celsius (°C)	Fahrenheit (°F)
100.0 (boiling point)	212	38.5	101.3
95	203	38	100.4
90	194	37.5	99.5
85	185	37	98.6
80	176	36.5	97.7
75	167	36	96.8
70	158	35.5	96
65	149	35	95
60	140	34	93.2
55	131	33	91.4
50	122	32	89.6
45	113	31	87.8
44	112.2	30	86
43	109.4	25	77
42	107.6	20	68
41	105.8	15	59
40	104	10	50
39.5	103.1	5	41
39	102.2	0 (freezing point)	32

To convert readings on the Fahrenheit scale to Celsius, subtract 32, multiply by 5 and divide by 9. $T_{(°C)} = (T_{(°F)} - 32) \times 5 \div 9$ where T means temperature.

For example, convert 98 degrees Fahrenheit to degrees Celsius:

$$98 - 32 = 66 \times 5 = 330 \div 9 = 36.6°C.$$

To convert readings on the Celsius scale to Fahrenheit, multiply by 9, divide by 5, and add 32. $T_{(°F)} = T_{(°C)} \times 9 \div 5 + 32$.

For example, convert 36.6 degrees Celsius to degrees Fahrenheit:

$$36.6 \times 9 = 330 \div 5 = 66 + 32 = 98°F.$$

The term 'Celsius' (after the Swedish astronomer who invented the scale in 1742) is now used internationally instead of 'centigrade', a term used in some countries to denote fractions of an angle.

APPENDIX 4
Table of normal values

Normal values for adults based on those obtained from major teaching hospitals. These reference ranges can vary, depending on age, gender, pregnancy and the assay used in particular laboratories.

Haematology	
Haemoglobin	M: 130–180 g/L F: 115–165 g/L
Haematocrit	M: 0.38–0.52 F: 0.32–0.46
Mean corpuscular volume (MCV)	80–100 fL
Platelet count	150–400 × 10^9/L
Reticulocytes	10–100 × 10^9/L
White cell count (WCC)	4.0–11.0 × 10^9/L
WCC differential	
Neutrophils	2.0–8.0 × 10^9/L
Lymphocytes	1.0–4.0 × 10^9/L
Monocytes	0.2–1.0 × 10^9/L
Eosinophils	0–0.5 × 10^9/L
Basophils	0–0.1 × 10^9/L
Erythrocyte sedimentation rate (ESR)	0–15 mm/hr
Coagulation	
Fibrinogen	2.0–4.0 g/L
Partial thromboplastin time activated (aPTT)	24–35 seconds
Prothrombin time (PT)	11–16 seconds
Thrombin time	15–19 seconds
Blood gases	
Arterial pCO_2	M: 35–45 mmHg F: 32–45 mmHg
Arterial pO_2	75–105 mmHg

Haematology	
Arterial O_2 saturation	95–100%
Arterial bicarb	22–28 mmol/L
Arterial pH	7.35–7.45
Biochemistry	
Alanine aminotransferase (ALT)	< 55 U/L
Albumin	35–52 g/L
Alkaline phosphatise (ALP)	30–110 U/L
Ammonia	11–55 micromol/L
Aspartate aminotransferase (AST)	12–36 U/L
Bicarbonate	22–32 mmol/L
Bilirubin	3–20 micromol/L
Calcium	2.1–2.6 mmol/L
Chloride	95–110 mmol/L
Creatinine	M: 60–110 micromol/L F: 45–90 micromol/L
Creatinine kinase (CK)	M: 30–200 U/L F: 29–168 U/L
Ferritin	M: 30–300 microgram/L F: 30–200 microgram/L
Gamma glutamyl transferase (GGT)	M: 12–64 U/L F: 9–36 U/L
Glucose, fasting	3.5–5.5 mmol/L
Iron	M: 11–30 micromol/L F: 8–30 micromol/L
Lactate	0.5–2.3 mmol/L
Lactate dehydrogenase (LD)	120–250 U/L
Lipase	8–78 U/L
Magnesium	0.7–1.1 mmol/L
Osmolality	274–296 mmol/kg (water)
Phosphate	0.75–1.5 mmol/L
Potassium	3.5–5.2 mmol/L
Protein	60–80 g/L

Haematology	
Sodium	135–145 mmol/L
Transferrin	M: 1.74–3.64 g/L
	F: 1.80–3.82 g/L
Troponin 1	M: < 26 ng/L
	F: < 16 ng/L
Urate	M: 0.24–0.48 mmol/L
	F: 0.16–0.43 mmol/L
Urea	3.1–8.1 mmol/L
Lipids and lipoproteins	
Cholesterol	< 5.5 mmol/L
Triglyceride	< 2.0 mmol/L
High-density lipoprotein (HDL) cholesterol	> 1.0 mmol/L
Non HDL-cholesterol	< 2.5 mmol/L
Endocrinology	
Adrenocorticotrophic hormone (ACTH)	7.2–63.3 ng/L
Calcitonin	0–20 ng/L
Cortisol	AM: 100–535 nmol/L
	PM: 80–480 nmol/L
Urinary free cortisol	< 300 nmol/24 hrs
C peptide	260–1730 pmol/L
Glycosylated haemoglobin (HbA_{1c})	4.0–6.0%
Parathyroid hormone (PTH)	15–68 ng/L
Prolactin	M: 73–410 mIU/L
	F: 110–560 mIU/L
Sex hormone binding globulin (SHBG)	M: 11–78 nmol/L
	F: 12–140 nmol/L
Free triiodothyronine (free T3)	2.6–6.0 pmol/L
Free thyroxine (free T4)	9.0–19.0 pmol/L
Testosterone	M > 16 years: 8–30 nmol/L
	F > 16 years: 0.4–2.0 nmol/L
Thyroid-stimulating hormone (TSH)	0.4–3.5 mIU/L

Haematology	
Vitamin D (1-25-dihydroxy)	60–210 pmol/L
Vitamin D (25OH)	50–130 nmol/L
Cerebrospinal fluid	
CSF glucose	2.5–5.6 mmol/L
CSF protein	0.15–0.45 g/L
Urine	
Albumin	< 30 mg/L
Albumin excretion rate (AER)	< 20 microgram/min
Albumin/creatinine ratio	M: < 2.5 mg/mmol
	F: < 3.5 mg/mmol
Calcium	1.25–7.50 mmol/24 hours
Calcium/creatinine ratio	Adult: < 0.61 mmol/mmol creatinine
Magnesium	2.5–8.0 mmol/24 hours
Phosphate	13–42 mmol/24 hours
Protein	< 0.15 g/24 hours
Urea	430–710 mmol/24 hours

M = males F = females
For further information please see LabInfoTest Directory at www.palms.com.au/php/labinfo/index.php

APPENDIX 5

Medication calculations and administration

Medications are drugs or other forms of medicines used to diagnose, prevent or treat medical conditions or diseases. As a result they are one of the most commonly used management strategies in healthcare. Nurses and midwives working in direct patient care in healthcare settings or in the community spend a significant amount of time preparing and administering medications to patients. Medication calculations, preparation and administration are all associated with a high incidence of errors and adverse events that can occur at any point in the medication administration process. The outcome related to errors or adverse events may lead to a longer hospital stay, increased hospital costs or has life or death consequences for the patient. As nurses and midwives consistently administer medications they are ideally placed to take a more proactive and risk reduction approach, not only to medication administration but also to prevention of medication errors. To implement the principles of safe medication administration nurses and midwives need to be aware of their professional responsibilities and demonstrate proficiency in dosage calculation skills, including those involving prescriptions and medication labels.

Professional responsibilities

To ensure a safe environment for preparation and administration of medications, nurses and midwives must be familiar with and adhere to relevant legislation and regulations, comply with guidelines and codes of conduct published by their national board, be aware of the National Medication Standard (Standard 4) and be familiar with local policies and procedures related to the administration of medications.

1 Legislation and regulations

Nurses and midwives have a particular responsibility and accountability in relation to medications under legislation. Although Acts and Regulations may vary in each state and territory, three relevant ones are:

- *Poisons and Therapeutic Goods Act 1966 and related Poisons and Therapeutic Goods Regulation 2008.*

This Act and associated Regulation deals with drug schedules and the storage and accountability related to medications.

- *Misuse and Trafficking Act 1985 and the Misuse and Trafficking Regulation 2011.*

This Act and associated Regulation highlights that it is a criminal offence to possess and supply certain drugs of addiction.

- *Nurses & Midwives Act 1991.*

This Act provides authorisation for nurse practitioners or midwife practitioners to possess, use, supply or prescribe any such substance dealt with under the *Poisons and Therapeutic Goods Act 1966.*

2 National Safety and Quality Health Service (NSQHS) Standards

The Medication Safety Standard (Standard 4) requires that health services have strategies and systems in place that are designed to minimise the causes of medication errors. The intention of this standard is that all health facilities will have clear policies and procedures in place to ensure healthcare professionals safely prescribe, dispense and administer appropriate medicines, and monitor medicine use and errors associated with the administration of medications. In response to this standard, healthcare facilities develop local policies, procedures and protocols around medication management. It is the responsibility of nurses and midwives to access, read and adhere to these within the particular healthcare facility where they work.

See Appendix 11 for information related to NSQHS Standards.

3 Professional standards

The Nursing and Midwifery Board of Australia (NMBA) regulates the practice of nursing and midwifery in Australia, and one of its key roles is to protect the public. The NMBA does this by developing standards, codes and guidelines that together establish the requirements for the professional and safe practice of nurses and midwives in Australia. It is the responsibility of each nurse and midwife to be familiar with the codes of conduct, standards for practice and codes of ethics and any obligations concerning medication management, including safety requirements. See Appendix 8 for a synopsis of these documents.

To ensure medications are prepared and administered safely, it is the professional responsibility of each nurse and midwife to be familiar not only with relevant legislation, regulations and standards, but also to know how to access relevant resources. Some useful web resources are included at the end of this Appendix.

Dosage calculation skills including prescriptions and medication labels

A comprehensive understanding of mathematics (fractions and ratios) is essential for the skill of safe medication administration in the healthcare setting. The main system in use for medication administration is the metric system (multiples of 10), which is based on SI Units (Systéme International d'Unités). For example:

1 kilogram (kg) = 1000 grams (g)
1 gram (g) = 1000 milligrams (mg)
1 milligram (mg) = 1000 micrograms*
1 litre (L) = 1000 millilitres (mL)
0.5 litre = 500 millilitres (mL)

* *Note:* Always write micrograms in full. The use of the 'micro' symbol ('μ') has been phased out due to potential confusion with 'm' (used for 'milli').

Patient safety depends on the ability of the nurse or midwife to calculate medication dosages accurately and in a timely manner. When in doubt about the answer to a calculation, verifying the correct dosage with another responsible registered nurse/midwife or medical officer is to be encouraged.

Pharmacists also have a wealth of information about medications and can be another resource, if available, to check your calculation.

Medications may be administered via several routes, including oral (tablets or liquids) or parenteral (injections or intravenous).

The following dosage calculations are examples of the types of problems that may be encountered by nurses or midwives in daily practice.

1. Calculation for oral medications (tablets, capsules)

$$\text{Formula: number required (NR)} = \frac{\text{dose required (DR)}}{\text{stock strength (SS)}}$$

Number required refers to the number of tablets, capsules etc.

The formula can be shortened to: $NR = \frac{DR}{SS}$

Example 1

A patient has been ordered ranitidine 300 mg. The stock strength of the drug is 150 mg per tablet. How many tablets would you administer?

$$NR = \frac{DR}{SS}$$

$$NR = \frac{300 \text{ mg}}{150 \text{ mg}}$$

$$NR = \frac{300}{150}$$

$$NR = \frac{2}{1} \text{ tablet}$$

$$= 2 \text{ tablets}$$

Example 2

A patient is ordered 0.25 mg of digoxin orally. The digoxin is available in tablets containing 125 micrograms. How many tablets would you administer?

Step 1. Change both strengths to the same units: 0.25 mg = 250 micrograms.

Step 2. Then apply the above formula: $NR = \frac{DR}{SS}$

$$NR = \frac{250 \text{ micrograms}}{125 \text{ micrograms}}$$

$$NR = \frac{250}{125}$$

$$NR = \frac{2}{1} \text{ tablets}$$

$$= 2 \text{ tablets}$$

Example 3

Administering an oral medication (tablets) using a prescription and medication label.

A patient is to be given their next mane (morning) dose of ramipril. Using the prescription below, how many Tritace tables should be given?

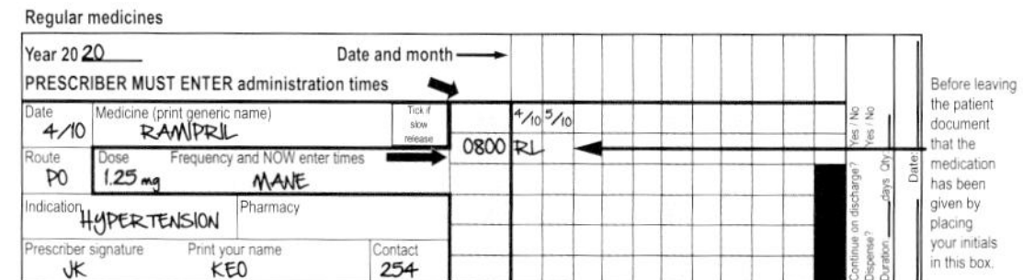

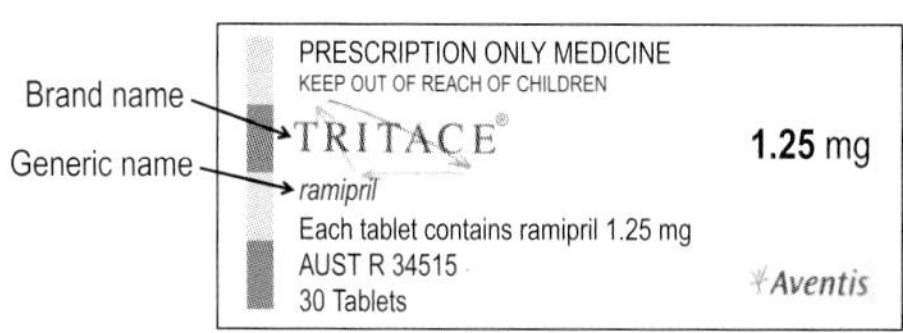

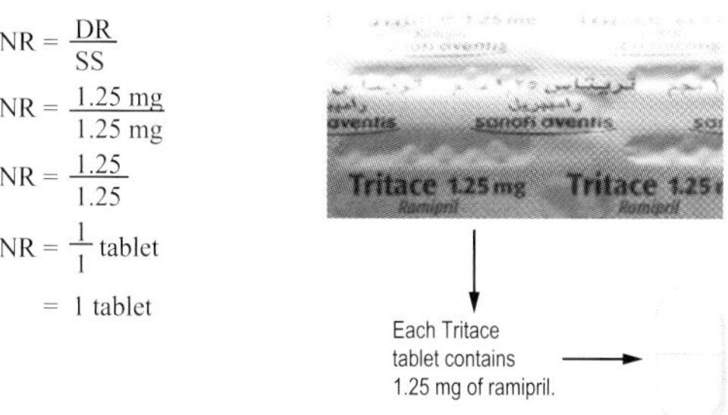

$$NR = \frac{DR}{SS}$$

$$NR = \frac{1.25 \text{ mg}}{1.25 \text{ mg}}$$

$$NR = \frac{1.25}{1.25}$$

$$NR = \frac{1}{1} \text{ tablet}$$

$$= 1 \text{ tablet}$$

2. Calculation for oral medications (liquids)

Oral medications are also available in liquid form and come in a variety of forms, such as syrups, elixirs, solutions or suspensions.

Formula:

$$\text{volume required (VR)} = \frac{\text{dose required (DR)}}{\text{stock strength (SS)}} \times \text{volume of stock solution (VS)}$$

$$VR = \frac{DR}{SS} \times \frac{VS}{1}$$

Example 1

A patient is ordered 750 mg of erythromycin orally. The stock suspension contains 250 mg/5 mL. Calculate the volume to be administered.

$$VR = \frac{DR}{SS} \times \frac{VS}{1}$$

$$VR = \frac{750\ \text{mg}}{250\ \text{mg}} \times \frac{5\ \text{mL}}{1}$$

$$VR = \frac{750}{250} \times \frac{5\ \text{mL}}{1}$$

$$VR = \frac{3}{1} \times \frac{5\ \text{mL}}{1}$$

$$= 15\ \text{mL}$$

Recommended administration time for morning (mane) medications is 0800.

Important note. Liquids can separate on standing (e.g. suspensions) and must be thoroughly rotated to remix before measuring the required volume.

Example 2

Administering an oral medication (liquid) using a prescription and medication label.

A patient is to be given their 2000 dose of chlorpromazine. How many mL of Largactil syrup should be given for the prescription below?

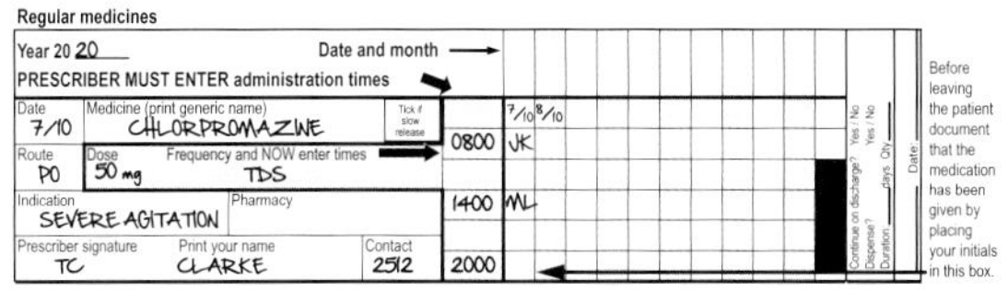
Regular medicines
Year 20 20
Date and month
PRESCRIBER MUST ENTER administration times
Date: 7/10
Medicine (print generic name): CHLORPROMAZINE
Tick if slow release
Route: PO
Dose: 50 mg
Frequency and NOW enter times: TDS
Indication: SEVERE AGITATION
Pharmacy
Prescriber signature: TC
Print your name: CLARKE
Contact: 2512

Time	7/10	8/10
0800	JK	
1400	ML	
2000		

Continue on discharge? Yes / No
Dispense? Yes / No
Duration ___ Days Qty ___
Date:
Before leaving the patient document that the medication has been given by placing your initials in this box.

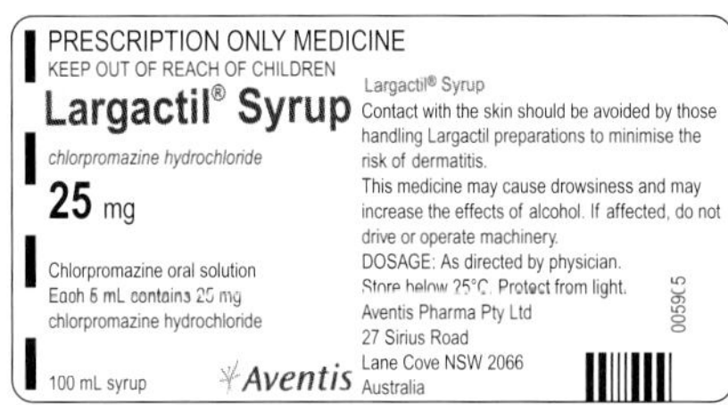

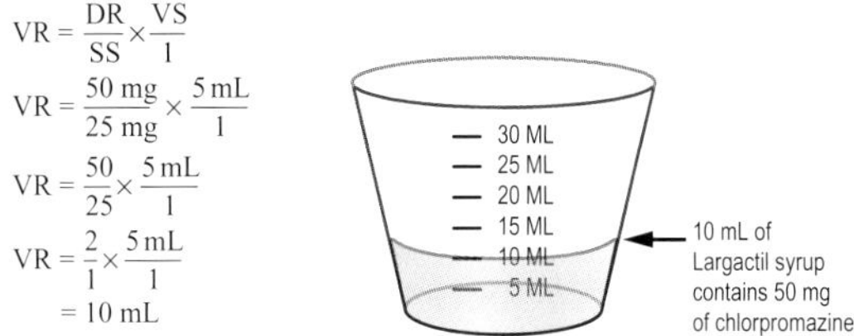

$$VR = \frac{DR}{SS} \times \frac{VS}{1}$$

$$VR = \frac{50 \text{ mg}}{25 \text{ mg}} \times \frac{5 \text{ mL}}{1}$$

$$VR = \frac{50}{25} \times \frac{5 \text{ mL}}{1}$$

$$VR = \frac{2}{1} \times \frac{5 \text{ mL}}{1}$$

$$= 10 \text{ mL}$$

Recommended administration times for three times per day (TDS) medications are 0800, 1400 and 2000.

3. Calculation for parenteral administration (injections)

Formula:

$$\text{volume required (VR)} = \frac{\text{dose required (DR)}}{\text{stock strength (SS)}} \times \text{volume of stock solution (VS)}$$

$$\text{VR} = \frac{\text{DR}}{\text{SS}} \times \frac{\text{VS}}{1}$$

Example 1

A patient is ordered 75 mg of pethidine for pain. The ampoule contains 100 mg in 2 mL. What volume would you administer?

$$\text{VR} = \frac{\text{DR}}{\text{SS}} \times \frac{\text{VS}}{1}$$

$$\text{VR} = \frac{75 \text{ mg}}{100 \text{ mg}} \times \frac{2 \text{ mL}}{1}$$

$$\text{VR} = \frac{75}{100} \times \frac{2 \text{ mL}}{1}$$

$$\text{VR} = \frac{3}{4} \times \frac{2 \text{ mL}}{1}$$

$$\text{VR} = \frac{6}{4}$$

$$= 1.5 \text{ mL}$$

Example 2

Administering a parenteral medication (injection) using a prescription and medication label.

A patient is commenced on frusemide. What time would frusemide be given and how many mL of Lasix would be drawn up and given?

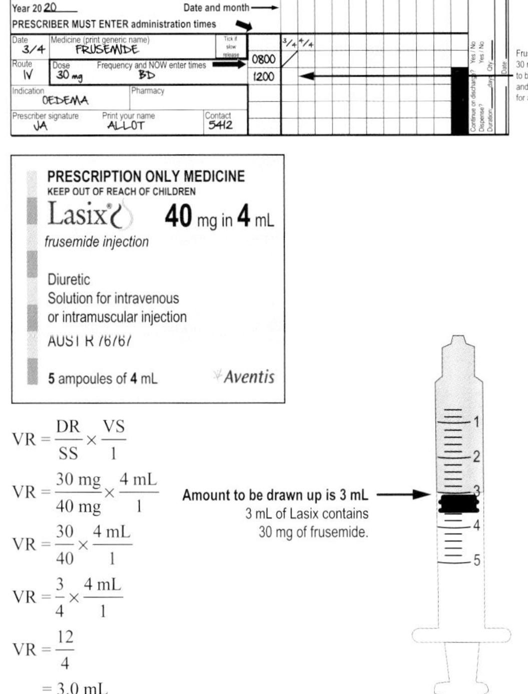

$$VR = \frac{DR}{SS} \times \frac{VS}{1}$$

$$VR = \frac{30\text{ mg}}{40\text{ mg}} \times \frac{4\text{ mL}}{1}$$

$$VR = \frac{30}{40} \times \frac{4\text{ mL}}{1}$$

$$VR = \frac{3}{4} \times \frac{4\text{ mL}}{1}$$

$$VR = \frac{12}{4}$$

$$= 3.0\text{ mL}$$

Recommended administration times for twice per day (BD) medications are 0800 and 2000. One exception is frusemide (Lasix), which is given at 0800 and 1200.

4. Calculation for parenteral administration (intravenous fluids)

When administering intravenous fluids, infusion rates (mL/hour) and drop factors (macrodrop = 20 drops per minute and microdrop = 60 drops per minute) need to be considered.

Infusion rates

To determine intravenous infusion rates (mL/hr)

Formula:

$$\text{rate (mL / hr)} = \frac{\text{total volume to be given (mL)}}{\text{time (hr)}}$$

Example

A patient is to receive 1000 mL of normal saline over 8 hours. How many millilitres per hour should the pump be set at?

$$\text{rate (mL/hr)} = \frac{\text{total volume to be given (mL)}}{\text{time (hr)}}$$

$$\text{Rate} = \frac{1000 \text{ mL}}{8 \text{ hrs}}$$

$$= \frac{1000}{8} \text{ mL/hr}$$

$$= 125 \text{ mL/hour}$$

Drops per minute

To calculate the drops per minute

When the time is given in minutes use:

Formula:

$$\text{drops per minute} = \frac{\text{total volume to be given (mL)} \times \text{drop factor (drops / mL)}}{\text{time (minutes)}}$$

When the time is given in hours use:

Formula:

$$\text{drops per minute} = \frac{\text{total volume to be given (mL)} \times \text{drop factor (drops / mL)}}{\text{time (hours)} \times 60}$$

Example 1

A patient is to receive 500 mL of normal saline over 6 hours (360 minutes). An IV set that delivers 20 drops per mL (i.e. a drop factor of 20 drops/mL) will be used. Calculate the required drops per minute.

$$\text{drops / minute} = \frac{\text{total volume to be given (mL)} \times \text{drop factor (drops / mL)}}{\text{time (hours)} \times 60}$$

$$\text{drops / minute} = \frac{500\ (\text{mL}) \times 20\ \text{drops / mL}}{6\ \text{hrs} \times 60}$$

$$\text{Since } \frac{20}{60} = \frac{1}{3}$$

$$\text{drops / minute} = \frac{500}{6} \times \frac{1}{3}$$

$$\text{drops / minute} = \frac{500}{18}$$

$$= 27.7^{*} \text{ rounded to nearest whole number } = 28 \text{ drops / minute}$$

* If the outcome of the equation results in a number which is not a whole number, round up/down to the nearest whole number.

Example 2

An infant is ordered 150 mL of normal saline to run over 10 hours (600 minutes). The microdrip delivers 60 drops per mL (i.e. a drop factor of 60 drops/mL). Calculate the required drops per minute.

$$\text{drops / minutes} = \frac{\text{total volume to be given (mL)} \times \text{drop factor (drops / mL)}}{\text{time (hours)} \times 60}$$

$$\text{drops / minutes} = \frac{150\ (\text{mL}) \times 60\ (\text{drops / mL})}{10\ \text{hrs} \times 60}$$

$$\text{Since } \frac{60}{60} = \frac{1}{1}$$

$$\text{drops / minute} = \frac{150}{10} \times \frac{1}{1}$$

$$\text{drops / minute} = \frac{150}{10}$$

$$= 15 \text{ drops / min}$$

Important note: Before commencing the calculation, make sure that you know the drop factor of the drip chamber of the giving set being used. For example, a drip chamber that delivers 60 drops per mL has a drop factor of 60 drops/mL (microdrop) while another giving set may deliver 20 drops per mL and therefore has a drop factor of 20 drops/mL (macrodrop).

Useful resources

Nurses and Midwives Act 1991, https://legislation.nsw.gov.au/#/view/act/1991/9/historical 2007-04-02/full

National Inpatient Medication Chart – Adult versions, www.safetyandquality.gov.au/our-work/medication-safety/medication-charts/national-standard-medication-charts/national-inpatient-medication-chart-adult-versions

Nursing and Midwifery Board - Professional Standards, www.nursingmidwiferyboard.gov.au/Codes-Guidelines-Statements/Professional-standards.aspx

National Safety and Quality Health Service (NSQHS) Standards, www.safetyandquality.gov.au/standards/nsqhs-standards

Source

Sections of the National Inpatient Medication Chart (NIMC) – Acute copied with permission from Australian Commission on Safety and Quality in Health Care.

APPENDIX 6

Resuscitation

This Appendix concentrates on basic life support (BLS) and is based on guidelines published in 2016 by the Australian and New Zealand Committee on Resuscitation (ANZCOR). The ANZCOR guidelines replace earlier Australian Resuscitation Council (ARC) and New Zealand Resuscitation Council (NZRC) guidelines and are endorsed by both councils. The guidelines are regularly revised to reflect new evidence on best practice in resuscitation. Further information on current guidelines can be obtained by visiting the Australian Resuscitation Council website at https://resus.org.au/

The central focus of resuscitation is the protection of the brain and heart from ischaemia, and the steps involved in resuscitation are systematic and implemented in order of priority. The principles of basic life support include: (a) establishing and maintaining an airway; (b) breathing; and (c) circulation—the objective being to provide the brain and heart with an oxygenated blood supply. Effective BLS techniques rely on rapid assessment of the situation and initiating procedures that facilitate and maintain an adequate supply of oxygenated blood to the brain before irreversible damage occurs. Advanced life support (ALS) techniques include a range of therapeutic and technological interventions carried out by trained health personnel. These are not discussed here.

Basic life support

If a person collapses, the rescuer must: assess the situation quickly; ensure the safety of the rescuer, person in need and bystanders; send for help (call an ambulance); and commence appropriate treatment following the BLS guidelines. When there is more than one person requiring assistance, priority of care should be given to those who are unconscious.[1] A popular way to remember the sequence of steps in basic life support is DRS ABCD (see flow chart[2]):

D = Danger

R = Response

S = Send for help

A = Airway

B = Breathing

C = CPR

D = Defibrillation

Danger

Prior to commencing BLS, consider the safety or risks involved. Assess the area for danger. Check for and remove any hazards prior to approaching the person who has collapsed.

Response

The level of consciousness is determined by the use of verbal and tactile stimuli. Check for response of a collapsed person by giving a loud simple command close to the person's ear, such as 'open your eyes; squeeze my hand'. Then firmly grasp and squeeze the person's shoulders to elicit a response.[3] These stimuli should never reach a level that causes or aggravates injury, and infants and small children should never be shaken. If conscious, the person will respond. Allow the person to adopt a comfortable position, and observe them closely for any changes in condition.[3]

If there is no response to the stimuli, the person is unconscious. If only a minor response is displayed, such as groaning without opening of the eyes, the person should be treated as though they are unconscious. Anyone who fails to respond to touch or the spoken word is considered to be unconscious and more vigorous efforts to obtain a response (such as painful stimuli) are not warranted.[3]

Send for help

If the person is unconscious, send for help. Call an ambulance (000; 111 in NZ).

Airway

The key to successful resuscitation is a clear airway. In an unconscious victim, care of the airway takes precedence over any injury, including the possibility of spinal injury.[4] Current recommendations are to leave the person in the position found unless the airway is obstructed by fluid or vomit.[4] If it is necessary, move the head gently to obtain a clear airway. Where possible, an assistant should support the head when an injured victim is being moved. The mouth should be open and turned slightly downwards to allow any foreign material to be expelled. Should regurgitation or vomiting occur during resuscitation, the person should be turned on their side and the airway manually cleared.[4] All unconscious victims should be handled gently and care should always be taken to avoid twisting or forward movement of the head and spine.

Airway management

Airway assessment and management can take place with the person lying on their side or back. In some instances, lying on the side is preferable for the reasons stated above. If the person is breathing spontaneously, they can be left lying on their side. If they are not breathing normally, they should be rolled onto their back so that resuscitation can be started.

The steps involved in airway management include the following.

- *Clear the airway.* Remove loose-fitting dentures and any visible foreign material from the mouth. Allow fluids or vomitus to drain by turning the face slightly downwards.
- *Open the airway.* Use the head tilt-chin lift manoeuvre, i.e. tilt the head backwards and support the jaw. The head (NOT the neck) is tilted

backwards by placing one hand on the forehead and supporting the jaw at the point of the chin in such a way that there is no pressure on the soft tissues of the neck. This brings the jaw and tongue forwards and opens the airway.[4]

Children should be managed in the same manner as adults. Infants (those less than 1 year of age) can have their upper airway easily obstructed because of narrow airways. The trachea is easily distorted if the head is tilted excessively, so the head should be kept in a neutral position. The lower jaw should be supported at the chin and the mouth maintained in an open position. The head can be tilted backwards very slightly only if a clear airway is not obtained with the head in a neutral position.[4]

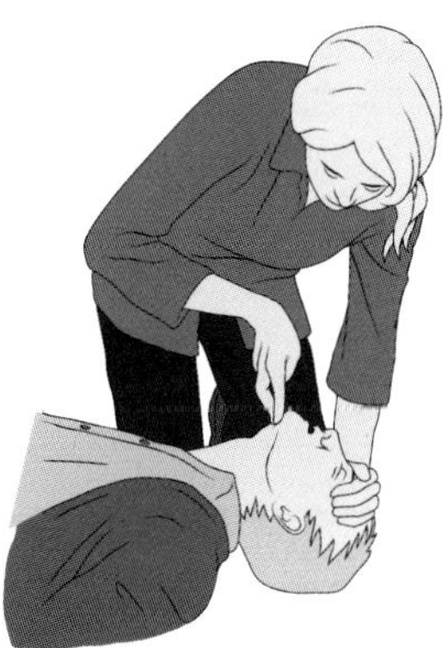

Head tilt and chin lift.
Source: Perkins, G.D., Handley, A.J., Koster, R.W., et al, on behalf of the Adult Basic Life Support and Automated External Defibrillation Section Collaborators. European Resuscitation Council Guidelines for Resuscitation 2015. Resuscitation 2015;95:81–99, Fig. 2.4. Copyright European Resuscitation Council.

Recognition of airway obstruction

If the airway is partially or completely occluded, attempts to breathe result in:

- noisy and laboured respiratory efforts if the airway is partially obstructed, and no movement of air if completely obstructed
- flaring of the nostrils
- use of accessory muscles, evidenced by sucking in of the soft tissues of the neck and upper chest, in-drawing of the chest and out-pushing of the abdomen.

Note: There might be no attempt to breathe at all and airway obstruction might not be apparent in the non-breathing unconscious person until rescue breathing is attempted.

Management of foreign body airway obstruction

A foreign body airway obstruction is a life-threatening emergency. In conscious adults and children over 1 year of age, chest thrusts or back blows may be effective in dislodging the foreign body. Abdominal thrusts may be effective in clearing the airway, but have also been associated with complications, so are not routinely recommended. If the person is unconscious, a finger sweep can be used to remove solid, visible material from the airway before commencing cardiopulmonary resuscitation (CPR).[4]

Breathing

Once the airway is open, the unconscious person's breathing should be checked. With an ear placed over the person's nose and mouth, the rescuer should:

- *look* AND *feel* for movement of the chest or upper abdomen
- *listen* for the passage of air into and out of the mouth and nose.

If breathing is *present*, leave the person on their side, ensuring that the airway remains open, and observe closely for any changes in condition.

If, after the airway has been cleared, breathing is *absent* or the person is not breathing normally, the rescuer must immediately commence chest compressions and then rescue breathing. Give 30 compressions and then two breaths (over approximately one second each).[5] If the rescuer is unwilling to perform ventilation, they may proceed with compression-only CPR.

If the chest does not rise, assess for possible causes, including:

- airway obstruction or ineffective opening of the airway
- insufficient air being delivered with each breath
- a poor seal around the mouth and/or nose causing air to leak.

Note: Distension of the stomach with air occurs if the breaths delivered are too hard or are delivered when the airway is partially obstructed. This can precipitate regurgitation and vomiting, and can further compromise the airway.

Methods of expired air resuscitation (EAR) include mouth-to-mouth respiration, mouth-to-nose respiration, mouth-to-stoma respiration and mouth-to-mask respiration.[5]

Cardiopulmonary resuscitation (CPR)

Unresponsiveness and absence of normal breathing indicates the need for resuscitation. Palpation of a pulse is not reliable and does not need to be performed to confirm the need for resuscitation. Even if the person is taking occasional gasps, CPR should be commenced, beginning with chest

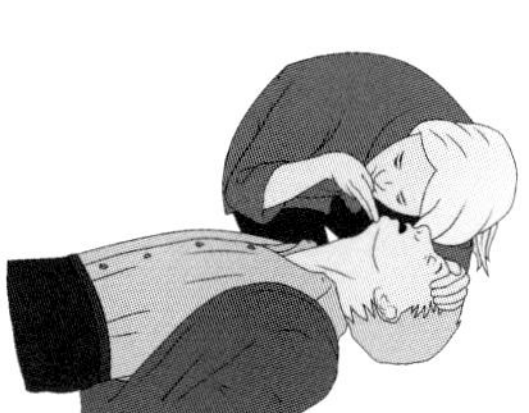

Blow steadily into the mouth while watching the chest rise.

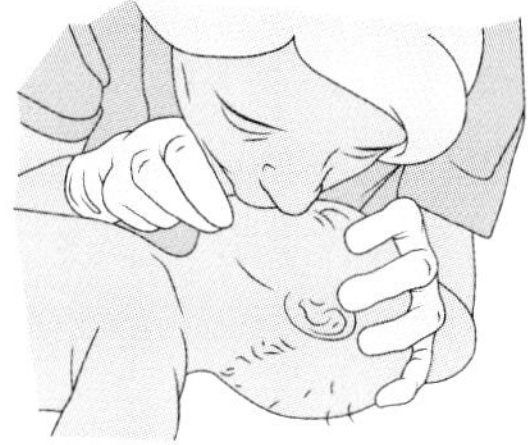

Mouth-to-mouth and nose ventilation: infant.

Source: Perkins, G.D., Handley, A.J., Koster, R.W., et al, on behalf of the Adult Basic Life Support and Automated External Defibrillation Section Collaborators. European Resuscitation Council Guidelines for Resuscitation 2015. Resuscitation 2015;95:81–99, Fig. 2.4. Copyright European Resuscitation Council.

compressions. People requiring chest compressions should be placed on a firm, flat surface in a supine position before compressions are commenced. The heel of the hand should be placed in the centre of the chest with the other hand on top. Steps should be taken to avoid compressions below the lower limit of the sternum as this may lead to organ damage or an increased chance of regurgitation. Placement on the upper half of the sternum may result in ineffective compressions.[6] Compressions should be rhythmic and the same amount of time used for compression and relaxation. Interruptions to chest compressions must be minimised as interruption to compressions is associated with lower survival rates.

Methods of compression differ for infants and children. For infants, the two-finger technique should be used. For children, a one- or two-hand technique can be used, depending on the child's size.[6]

Depth and rate of compression

The lower half of the sternum should be compressed approximately one-third of the depth of the chest with each compression. This equates to more than 5 cm in adults, approximately 5 cm in children and 4 cm in infants. Allow the chest to return to its normal position between compressions. The rate of compression is 100 to 120 times per minute, for both children and adults. This equates with almost two compressions per second.[6] During external cardiac compression (ECC), the heel of the hand remains on the sternum. To maintain the quality of compressions, rescuers should be changed every 2 minutes, if possible. This should be done to minimise interruptions to compressions. There is no need to interrupt compressions to check for response or breathing.

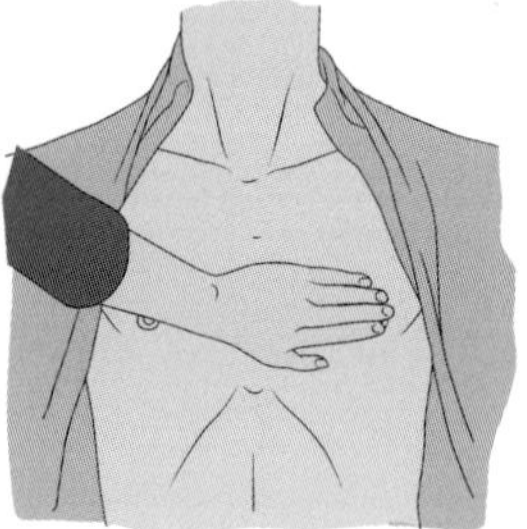

Place the heel of one hand in the centre of the victim's chest.

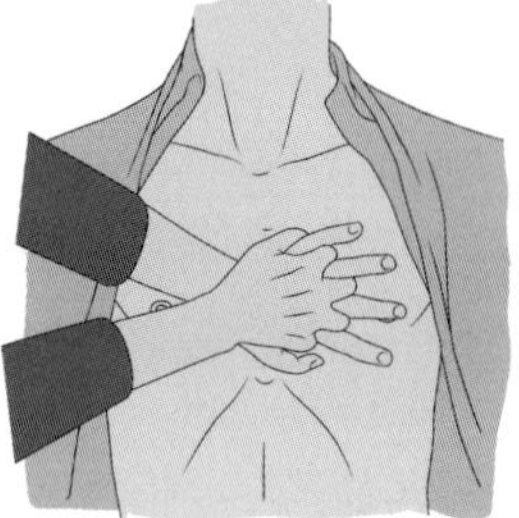

Place the heel of your other hand on top of the first hand.

Source: Perkins, G.D., Handley, A.J., Koster, R.W., et al, on behalf of the Adult Basic Life Support and Automated External Defibrillation Section Collaborators. European Resuscitation Council Guidelines for Resuscitation 2015. Resuscitation 2015;95:81–99, Fig. 2.4. Copyright European Resuscitation Council.

Rate of compressions to inflations

For all ages, the ratio is 30 compressions (at 100 to 120 compressions per minute) to two breaths for both one- and two-person CPR. This should result in the delivery of five cycles in approximately 2 minutes. If rescuers are unwilling or unable to perform rescue breathing, they should provide chest compressions at a rate of 100 to 120/min.[7]

CPR is continued until the person recovers, or until a health professional arrives and takes over or directs that the CPR should be ceased. In some cases the rescuer may be too exhausted to continue CPR. Multiple rescuers have the advantage of being able to assist with providing compressions, ensuring help is summoned and obtaining additional equipment, such as an automatic external defibrillator (AED). Correctly performed, CPR can re-establish cardiac function, or at least maintain an artificial circulation sufficient to preserve neurological function until personnel trained in ALS arrive at the scene.

Automated external defibrillation

The first priority for the unconscious, non-breathing patient is the commencement of cardiac compressions. The importance of defibrillation is well established and time to defibrillation is a key factor that influences survival. Automated external defibrillators (AEDs) mean that defibrillation can now be incorporated into BLS and their use is not restricted to trained personnel.[8]

CPR must be continued until the AED is turned on and defibrillator pads attached. The rescuer should then follow the AED prompts. Defibrillation pads are placed on the exposed chest in an anterior-lateral position. Diagrams for appropriate placement are provided on the pads to assist rescuers to achieve correct placement. Contact of the pad with the skin is important and may

Basic Life Support

D	**Dangers?**
R	**Responsive?**
S	**Send** for help
A	Open **Airway**
B	Normal **Breathing?**
C	Start **CPR** **30 compressions : 2 breaths**
D	Attach **Defibrillator (AED)** **as soon as available, follow prompts**

Continue CPR until responsiveness or normal breathing return

January 2016

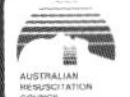

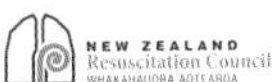

Basic Life Support Flowchart

Source: ANZCOR. Basic Life Support Flowchart. 2016 Available from: https://resus.org.au/guidelines/flowcharts-3/

require removal of moisture or excessive hair. If a person has an implantable device, such as a pacemaker, the pad should be placed at least 8 cm away from the device. Medication patches should likewise be avoided and can be removed before attaching the electrode pad. Any residual medication should be wiped away before pad placement.[8]

For children over the age of 8 years, a standard adult AED and pads can be used. For children between the ages of 1 and 8 years, paediatric pads and an AED with paediatric capability should be used. Pad placement is the same as for adults. If the AED does not have a paediatric mode or if paediatric pads are not available, a standard adult AED can be used, provided the pads do not touch each other.[8]

Safety for the rescuer is important and care should be taken to avoid touching the person during shock delivery.

References

1. Australian and New Zealand Committee on Resuscitation (ANZCOR). Guideline 2: Managing an emergency. 2016. Online 24 July 2019. Available: https://resus.org.au/guidelines/.
2. ANZCOR. Basic Life Support Flowchart. 2016. Online 24 July 2019. Available: https://resus.org.au/guidelines/flowcharts-3/.
3. ANZCOR. Guideline 3: Recognition and first aid management of the unconscious person. 2016. Online 24 July 2019. Available: https://resus.org.au/guidelines/.
4. ANZCOR. Guideline 4: Airway. 2016. Online 24 July 2019. Available: https://resus.org.au/guidelines/.
5. ANZCOR. Guideline 5: Breathing. 2016. Online 24 July 2019. Available: https://resus.org.au/guidelines/.
6. ANZCOR. Guideline 6: Compressions. 2016. Online 24 July 2019. Available: http://resus.org.au/guidelines/.
7. ANZCOR. Guideline 8: Cardiopulmonary resuscitation. 2016. Online 24 July 2019. Available: https://resus.org.au/guidelines
8. ANZCOR. Guideline 7: External automated defibrillation in basic life support. 2016. Online 24 July 2019. Available: https://resus.org.au/guidelines.

APPENDIX 7
Immunisation

The Australian Immunisation Handbook

The Australian Immunisation Handbook (2018 updated 2019) provides clinical guidelines for healthcare professionals and others about using vaccines safely and effectively. These guidelines were developed by the Australian Technical Advisory Group on Immunisation (ATAGI) and approved by the National Health and Medical Research Council (NHMRC).

National Immunisation Program (NIP)

The National Immunisation Program (NIP) was set up by the Commonwealth and state and territory governments in 1997. It aims to increase national immunisation coverage to reduce the number of cases of diseases that are preventable by vaccination in Australia. The NIP provides free vaccines to eligible people to help reduce diseases that can be prevented by vaccination. Eligible people include babies, young children, teenagers and older Australians. The program also targets people of all ages who are at greater risk of serious harm from certain diseases.

The National Immunisation Program (NIP) Schedule

The document on the following pages outlines a series of immunisations given at specific times ranging from birth through to adulthood. The current Schedule was updated in April 2019. The NIP Schedule is continuously updated and any person using this Schedule should refer to the latest information for advice, as new vaccines are added and others may be taken off the NIP Schedule.

If you have any questions about the National Immunisation Program (NIP) Schedule, talk to your medical doctor or healthcare provider.

Useful resources

https://beta.health.gov.au/health-topics/immunisation

https://immunisationhandbook.health.gov.au/

https://beta.health.gov.au/initiatives-and-programs/national-immunisation-program

https://beta.health.gov.au/sites/default/files/nip-childhood-immunisation-schedule-portrait.pdf

Copied with permission from the *Australian Immunisation Handbook*, (2018 and updated April 2019). Full document available online at: https://immunisationhandbook.health.gov.au/

National Immunisation Program Schedule
From 1 April 2019

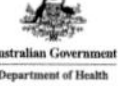

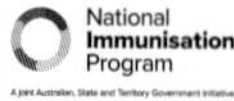

Age	Disease	Vaccine Brand
Childhood vaccination (also see influenza vaccine)		
Birth	• Hepatitis B (usually offered in hospital)[a]	H-B-Vax® II Paediatric or Engerix B® Paediatric
2 months Can be given from 6 weeks of age	• Diphtheria, tetanus, pertussis (whooping cough), hepatitis B, polio, *Haemophilus influenzae* type b (Hib) • Pneumococcal • Rotavirus[b]	Infanrix® hexa Prevenar 13® Rotarix®
4 months	• Diphtheria, tetanus, pertussis (whooping cough), hepatitis B, polio, *Haemophilus influenzae* type b (Hib) • Pneumococcal • Rotavirus[b]	Infanrix® hexa Prevenar 13® Rotarix®
6 months	• Diphtheria, tetanus, pertussis (whooping cough), hepatitis B, polio, *Haemophilus influenzae* type b (Hib)	Infanrix® hexa
Additional vaccines for Aboriginal and Torres Strait Islander children (QLD, NT, WA and SA) and medically at-risk children[c]	• Pneumococcal	Prevenar 13®
12 months	• Meningococcal ACWY • Measles, mumps, rubella • Pneumococcal	Nimenrix® M-M-R® II or Priorix® Prevenar 13®
Additional vaccines for Aboriginal and Torres Strait Islander children (QLD, NT, WA and SA)	• Hepatitis A	Vaqta® Paediatric
18 months	• *Haemophilus influenzae* type b (Hib) • Measles, mumps, rubella, varicella (chickenpox) • Diphtheria, tetanus, pertussis (whooping cough)	ActHIB® Priorix-Tetra® or ProQuad® Infanrix® or Tripacel®
Additional vaccines for Aboriginal and Torres Strait Islander children (QLD, NT, WA and SA)	• Hepatitis A	Vaqta® Paediatric
4 years	• Diphtheria, tetanus, pertussis (whooping cough), polio	Infanrix® IPV or Quadracel®
Additional vaccines for medically at-risk children[c]	• Pneumococcal	Pneumovax 23®

National Immunisation Program Schedule
From 1 April 2019

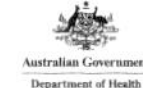

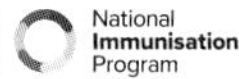

Age	Disease	Vaccine brand
Adolescent vaccination (also see influenza vaccine)		
12–<13 years (School programs[d])	• Human papillomavirus (HPV)[e] • Diphtheria, tetanus, pertussis (whooping cough)	Gardasil®9 Boostrix®
14–<16 years (School programs[d])	• Meningococcal ACWY	Nimenrix®
Adult vaccination (also see influenza vaccine)		
15–49 years Aboriginal and Torres Strait Islander people with medical risk factors[c]	• Pneumococcal	Pneumovax 23®
50 years and over Aboriginal and Torres Strait Islander people	• Pneumococcal	Pneumovax 23®
65 years and over	• Pneumococcal	Pneumovax 23®
70–79 years[f]	• Shingles (herpes zoster)	Zostavax®
Pregnant women	• Pertussis (whooping cough)[g] • Influenza[h]	Boostrix® or Adacel®

Funded annual influenza vaccination[h]

- **6 months and over with certain medical risk factors[c]**
- **All Aboriginal and Torres Strait Islander people 6 months and over**
- **65 years and over**
- **Pregnant women**

[a] Hepatitis B vaccine: Should be given to all infants as soon as practicable after birth. The greatest benefit is if given within 24 hours, and must be given within 7 days.
[b] Rotavirus vaccine: First dose must be given by 14 weeks of age, the second dose by 24 weeks of age.
[c] Refer to the current edition of *The Australian Immunisation Handbook* for all medical risk factors.
[d] Contact your state or territory health service for school grades eligible for vaccination.
[e] Observe Gardasil®9 dosing schedules by age and at-risk conditions. 2 doses: 9 to <15 years—6 months mininimum interval. 3 doses: ≥15 years and/or have certain medical conditions—0, 2 and 6 month schedule. Only 2 doses funded on the NIP unless 12-13 year old has certain medical risk factors.
[f] All people aged 70 years old, with a five year catch-up program for people aged 71–79 years old until 31 October 2021.
[g] Single dose recommended each pregnancy, ideally between 20–32 weeks, but may be given up until delivery.
[h] Refer to annual influenza information for recommended vaccine brand for age.

- Contact your State and Territory Health Department for further information on any additional immunisation programs specific to your State or Territory.
- All people aged less than 20 years are eligible for free catch up vaccines.
- Adult refugees and humanitarian entrants are eligible for free catch up vaccines.

For more information

health.gov.au/immunisation

State/Territory	Contact Number
Australian Capital Territory	(02) 6205 2300
New South Wales	1300 066 055
Northern Territory	(08) 8922 8044
Queensland	13 HEALTH (13 4325 84)
South Australia	1300 232 272
Tasmania	1800 671 738
Victoria	1300 882 008
Western Australia	(08) 9321 1312

APPENDIX 8

Code of conduct and Code of ethics for nurses and Code of conduct and Code of ethics for midwives

Part A: Code of conduct for nurses and Code of conduct for midwives

Preamble

In 1993, under the auspices of the then Australian Nursing and Midwifery Council, a Code of professional conduct and a Code of ethics were developed for nurses in Australia. These codes were revised in 2002 and 2003, respectively. These earlier codes were intended to cover both nurses and midwives; however, in 2008 new codes were developed and published to acknowledge the many and varied differences between these two professions.

With the introduction of the National Scheme in 2010, the Nursing and Midwifery Board of Australia (NMBA) undertakes functions as set out by the Health Practitioner Regulation National Law (the National Law). One of these functions is to regulate the practice of nursing and midwifery in Australia; this is achieved by further developing registration standards, professional codes, guidelines and standards for practice, which, along with other documents, establish the requirements for the professional and safe practice of nurses and midwives in Australia.

Following a systematic review of the literature, comparisons with current and other codes, and extensive consultation with the profession, public and professional organisations, the NMBA developed a contemporary Code of conduct for nurses and a Code of conduct for midwives, which comply with the National Law and cover all contexts where nursing and midwifery are practised. Incorporated in the codes is also content related to professional boundaries (previously known as Professional boundaries for nurses and Professional boundaries for midwives). This inclusion means that all aspects of expected conduct and behaviour can be accessed in one document.

In addition, the codes provide guidance on cultural safety and respectful practice. These areas identify many factors, such as social, historical and structural factors that can have an impact on the health and health outcomes of Aboriginal and/or Torres Islander peoples. Culturally safe and respectful practice requires nurses and midwives to challenge biases and beliefs based on assumption. Such assumptions according to the codes are based on gender, disability, race, ethnicity, religion, sexuality, age or political beliefs.

Further, the codes acknowledge that bullying and harassment are generally workplace and performance issues; however, the evidence from the reviews undertaken by the NMBA indicated that a separate section needed to be included in the codes specifying that 'bullying and harassment is not acceptable and should not be tolerated'.

The codes consist of seven principles of conduct, grouped into four domains, each with an explanatory value statement. The following are abridged versions of the codes. For the complete versions of the Code of conduct for nurses and the Code of conduct for midwives, go to the NMBA website: www.nursingmidwiferyboard.gov.au (see the professional codes and guidelines section).

Code of conduct for nurses

The code applies to all nurses.

The principles of the code apply to all types of nursing practice in all contexts. This includes any work where a nurse uses nursing skills and knowledge, whether paid or unpaid, clinical or non-clinical. This includes work in the areas of clinical care, clinical leadership, clinical governance responsibilities, education, research, administration, management, advisory roles, regulation or policy development. The code also applies to all settings where a nurse may engage in these activities, including face-to-face, publications or via online or electronic means.

Code of conduct for nurses: domains, principles and values

These domains, principles and values set out legal requirements, professional behaviour and conduct expectations for all nurses. The principles apply to all areas of practice, with an understanding that nurses will exercise professional judgement in applying them, with the goal of delivering the best possible outcomes.

(*Note:* Person or people is used to refer to those individuals who have entered into a therapeutic and/or professional relationship with a nurse.)

Domain: Practise legally

Principle 1: Legal compliance—Nurses respect and adhere to their professional obligations under the National Law, and abide by relevant laws.

Value: Nurses respect and adhere to professional obligations under the National Law, and abide by relevant laws.[1]

[1]The code does not address in detail the full range of legal and ethical obligations that apply to nurses. Examples of legal obligations include, but are not limited to, obligations arising in Acts and Regulations relating to privacy, the aged and disabled, child protection, bullying, anti-discrimination and workplace health and safety issues. Nurses should ensure they know all of their legal obligations relating to professional practice, and abide by them.

Domain: Practise safely, effectively and collaboratively

Principle 2: Person-centred practice

Value: Nurses provide safe, person-centred, evidence-based practice for the health and wellbeing of people and, in partnership with the person, promote shared decision-making and care delivery between the person, nominated partners, family, friends and health professionals.

Principle 3: Cultural practice and respectful relationships

Value: Nurses engage with people as individuals in a culturally safe and respectful way, foster open, honest and compassionate professional relationships and adhere to their obligations about privacy and confidentiality.

Domain: Act with professional integrity

Principle 4: Professional behaviour

Value: Nurses embody integrity, honesty, respect and compassion.

Principle 5: Teaching, supervising and assessing

Value: Nurses commit to teaching, supervising and assessing students and other nurses in order to develop the nursing workforce across all contexts of practice.

Principle 6: Research in health

Value: Nurses recognise the vital role of research to inform quality healthcare and policy development, conduct research ethically and support the decision-making of people who participate in research.

Domain: Promote health and wellbeing

Principle 7: Health and wellbeing

Value: Nurses promote health and wellbeing for people and their families, colleagues, the broader community and themselves in a way that addresses health inequality.

Code of conduct for midwives

This code applies to all midwives

The principles of the code apply to all types of midwifery practice in all contexts. This includes any work where a midwife uses midwifery skills and knowledge, whether paid or unpaid, clinical or non-clinical. This includes work in the areas of clinical care, clinical leadership, clinical governance responsibilities, education, research, administration, management, advisory roles, regulation or policy development. The code also applies to all settings where a midwife may engage in these activities, including face-to-face, publications or via online or electronic means.

Code of conduct for midwives: domains, principles and values

These domains, principles and values set out legal requirements, professional behaviour and conduct expectations for all midwives. The principles apply to all areas of practice, with an understanding that midwives will exercise professional judgement in applying them with the goal of delivering the best possible outcomes.

(*Note:* Woman or women is used to refer to those individuals who have entered into a therapeutic and/or professional relationship with a midwife.)

Domain: Practise legally

Principle 1: Legal compliance

Value: Midwives respect and adhere to professional obligations under the National Law, and abide by relevant laws.[2]

Domain: Practise safely, effectively and collaboratively

Principle 2: Woman-centred practice

Value: Midwives provide safe, woman-centred, evidence-based practice for the health and wellbeing of women and, in collaboration with the woman, promote shared decision-making and care delivery between the woman and baby, nominated partners, family, friends and health professionals.

Principle 3: Cultural practice and respectful relationships

Value: Midwives engage with women as individuals in a culturally safe and respectful way, foster open, honest and compassionate professional relationships and adhere to their obligations about privacy and confidentiality.

Domain: Act with professional integrity

Principle 4: Professional behaviour

Value: Midwives embody integrity, honesty, respect and compassion.

Principle 5: Teaching, supervising and assessing

Value: Midwives commit to teaching, supervising and assessing students and other midwives in order to develop the midwifery workforce across all contexts of practice.

Principle 6: Research in health

Value: Midwives recognise the vital role of research to inform quality healthcare and policy development, conduct research ethically and support the decision-making of women who participate in research.

Domain: Promote health and wellbeing

Principle 7: Health and wellbeing

Value: Midwives promote health and wellbeing for women and their families, colleagues, the broader community and themselves and in a way that addresses health inequality.

Part B: Code of ethics for nurses and Code of ethics for midwives

Preamble

The Nursing and Midwifery Board of Australia (NMBA) and other relevant nursing and midwifery organisations jointly agreed to adopt the International Council of Nurses Code of ethics for nurses (ICN Ethics)* and the International

[2]The code does not address in detail the full range of legal and ethical obligations that apply to midwives. Examples of legal obligations include, but are not limited to, obligations arising in Acts and Regulations relating to privacy, the aged and disabled, child protection, bullying, anti-discrimination and workplace health and safety issues. Midwives should ensure they know all of their legal obligations relating to professional practice, and abide by them.

Confederation of Midwives Code of ethics for midwives (ICM ethics) as the guiding documents for ethical decision-making for nurses and midwives in Australia. These documents replace the previous NMBA Code of ethics for nurses in Australia (2006) and Code of ethics for midwives in Australia (2006).

The ICN Code of ethics for nurses and the ICM Code of ethics for midwives was adopted for all nurses and midwives in Australia on 1 March 2018.

The ICN Code of ethics for nurses and the ICM Code of ethics for midwives are dynamic and evolving documents, and nurses and midwives need to be familiar with and reflect on the code's standards and apply them to everyday nursing and midwifery healthcare amid a changing society. Nurses and midwives also need to be aware that the new codes are admissible as evidence in any Nursing and Midwifery Board regulatory or disciplinary proceedings as to what constitutes acceptable professional standards from March 2018.

International Council of Nurses Code of ethics for nurses

The ICN's Code of ethics for nurses contains elements that define standards of ethical conduct for nurses, such as respecting human rights, including cultural rights, demonstrating compassion and integrity, advocating for equity in access to healthcare, maintaining standards of personal conduct that uphold the profession's values, implementing standards of clinical practice and fostering collaborative and respectful relationships with colleagues. Within each principle element of the code is a guide for practitioners and managers, educators and researchers and national nursing associations.

In summary, the code addresses:

- nurses and people
- nurses and practice
- nurses and the profession
- nurses and co-workers.

International Confederation of Midwives Code of ethics for midwives

The code encourages midwives to acknowledge the rights of women and families, ensure equity in access to healthcare, provide culturally appropriate and respectful care and base relationships on mutual respect, trust and the dignity of all members of society. The code also provides relevant supporting statements and a guide for the education, practice and research of the midwife.

In summary, the code addresses:

- midwifery relationships
- practice of midwifery
- the professional responsibilities of midwives
- advancement of midwifery knowledge and practice.

Sources

Part A: Code of conduct for nurses, and Code of conduct for midwives (2017) at www.nursingmidwiferyboard.gov.au/codes-guidelines-statements/codes-guidelines.aspx

Part B: International Council of Nurses (ICN) Code of ethics for nurses at www.icn.ch/sites/default/files/inline-files/2012_ICN_Codeofethicsfornurses_%20eng.pdf; and the International Confederation of Midwives Code of ethics for midwives at www.internationalmidwives.org/assets/files/general-files/2019/10/eng-international-code-of-ethics-for-midwives.pdf

Note: This information is continuously updated and any person requiring details about the Codes of ethics and Codes of conduct for nurses and midwives in Australia should refer to the Nursing and Midwifery Board of Australia website at www.nursingmidwiferyboard.gov.au. Copyright NMBA, reproduced with permission.

APPENDIX 9

Aspects of nursing and the law

Nursing practice is governed and regulated in various ways. The most important of these for nurses and midwives are:

- professional regulation
- codes, guidelines and standards
- parliamentary or statute law
- civil law
- employment contracts.

The Australian Health Practitioner Regulation Agency (AHPRA) is the organisation responsible for the implementation of the National Registration and Accreditation Scheme across Australia. AHPRA's operations are governed by the *Health Practitioner Regulation National Law Act 2009*, which came into effect on 1 July 2010. AHPRA supports the Nursing and Midwifery Board of Australia (NMBA). The functions of the board include:

- registering nursing and midwifery practitioners and students
- developing standards, codes and guidelines for the nursing and midwifery profession
- handling notifications, complaints, investigations and disciplinary hearings
- assessing overseas trained practitioners who wish to practise in Australia
- approving accreditation standards and accredited courses of study.

The National Board has established state and territory boards to support the work of the National Board. The National Board sets policy and professional standards and the state and territory boards make individual notification and registration decisions affecting individual nurses and midwives. The national standards are supported by the Code of ethics, the Code of conduct and National Competency Standards. The Code of conduct does not replace any Act or Regulation. The criminal law and relevant legislation still apply to nurses and midwives and where there is any conflict between the Code of conduct and provisions of any Act or Regulation, the latter apply.

The practice of nursing and midwifery is limited by Acts of Parliament, commonly referred to as legislation. Acts of Parliament often have a separate document, known as Regulations, which give directions that must be followed in order to comply with the intent of the Act. Where there is no legislation, the courts will interpret the law in civil law courts.

Employment contracts give rise to the rights and obligations between the employer and employee; therefore, it is important that nurses and midwives have a good understanding of employment conditions within the healthcare sector. There are several state, territory and federal Acts, which control areas such as equal opportunity, workers' compensation, occupational health and safety, complaints and industrial awards.

Examples of some Australian law statutes
Aged Care Act 1997 (Cwlth)
Aged Care Quality and Safety Commission Act 2018 (Cwlth)
Anti-Discrimination Act 1991 (Qld)
Children and Young Persons (Care and Protection) Act 1998 (NSW)
Child Protection Act 1993 (SA)
Crimes Act 1900 (NSW)
Disability Services Act 1986 (Cwlth)
Freedom of Information Act 1982 (Cwlth)
Good Samaritan laws
• *Most Australian states and territories have some form of good Samaritan protection, e.g. Civil Liability Act 2002 No. 22 (NSW) Part 8*
Guardianship Act 1987 (NSW)
Health Care Act 2008 (SA)
Health Care Liability Act 2001 (NSW)
Health Complaints Act 1995 (Tas)
Health Practitioners Act 2015 (NT)
Health Practitioner Regulation National Law Act 2009 (Qld)
Health Records Act 2001 (Vic)
Health Records and Information Privacy Act 2002 (NSW)
Health Services Act 1988 (Vic)
Hospital and Health Services Act 1927 (WA)
Human Tissue Act 1982 (Vic)
Coroners and Human Tissue Acts (Amendment) Act 2006 (Vic)
Medicines, Poisons and Therapeutic Goods Act 2008 (ACT)
Mental Health Act 2007 (NSW)
National Health Act 1953 (Cwlth)
Narcotic Drug Act 1967 (Cwlth)
Poisons Act 1964 (WA)
Private Health Facilities Act 1999 (Qld)
Privacy Act 1988 (Cwlth)
Public Health Act 1997 (Tas)
Therapeutic Goods Act 1989 (Cwlth)
Work Health and Safety Act 2011 (NSW)

Four aspects of law affecting nursing practice are professional negligence, consent, confidentiality and documentation.

Professional negligence

Negligence is a tort, or civil wrong, that regulates the rights and responsibilities of one individual towards another. To succeed in a claim of negligence, the patient (plaintiff) must be able to establish, on the balance of probability, all the following elements:

- The patient was owed a duty of care by the health professional (defendant). In the nursing and midwifery contexts, it is well established that such a duty is owed to patients and fellow employees. Inherent in the concept of a duty of care is the existence of an appropriate standard of care.
- There was a breach of that duty in that the health professional's conduct fell below the required standard of care.
- This conduct caused the damages suffered by the patient. No compensation will be awarded if no harm was suffered or if the harm did not arise as a direct consequence of the negligent act.
- The loss or damage suffered was reasonably foreseeable.

If a healthcare professional negligently injures a patient in the course and scope of his or her employment, the professional's employer might be held liable. This is the doctrine of vicarious liability.

Consent

The law requires consent to be obtained before providing treatment. Failure to do this could result in an action for assault. Additionally, the common law places a duty on healthcare providers to adequately inform a patient of the significant risks involved in a particular treatment and the available alternatives.

The onus for ensuring that a patient is properly informed and that consent has been obtained for a procedure, operation or treatment rests with the professional who will be providing the treatment. Health services and hospitals may also have legal responsibilities in this area. The requirements for obtaining a valid consent are as follows:

- The person must have the capacity to give consent and be capable of understanding the implications of having treatment.
- The consent must be given freely and voluntarily.
- The consent must be specific and is valid only in relation to the treatment or procedure for which the patient has been informed and has agreed to.
- The person must be informed in broad terms of the procedure which is intended, in a way they can understand.

Consent can be 'expressed' either orally or in writing, or it can be 'implied' from a person's conduct; e.g. a patient may hold out their arm to receive an injection.

No consent is required where the person is unconscious or seriously ill and immediate intervention is required to save his or her life. In such an emergency, the overriding duty of care negates the need for consent based on the principle of necessity.

The law relating to consent for children and in emergency situations can vary in different states and territories.

Mental health legislation in each state and territory gives limited power to detain, admit and treat patients against their will. Other legislation, such as the Commonwealth *Quarantine Act 1908* and child protection legislation, also provides statutory power to detain and treat people.

Confidentiality

Nurses are required to collect highly sensitive information from patients and must observe a duty of confidentiality and respect for patient privacy. This is spelt out in the Code of conduct, Code of ethics and privacy laws. Nurses may also owe a common law duty of confidentiality to their patients. A breach of confidentiality can lead to substantial penalties including prosecution, removal from the register and dismissal for breach of contract.

There are a number of exceptions, including:

- where the patient consents to disclosure
- where the information is required to continue the patient's care
- where the law requires disclosure, e.g. assisting police in investigating a criminal offence, reporting of notifiable diseases
- where public interest is deemed of greater importance than confidentiality, e.g. child abuse, drug-related offences.

Documentation

The purpose of maintaining a health record is to facilitate optimal patient care and outcomes. Documentation should be accurate, objective and a contemporaneous description of care. Nurses and midwives should ensure their documentation is clear, concise and based on fact, not subjective or emotive. Health records are a method of communication. They may be used for educational or research purposes and could be used as evidence in legal proceedings.

For more information regarding all areas of law relating to nursing practice, see Forrester K, Griffiths D. Essentials of law for health professionals. 4th ed. Sydney: Mosby, 2015.

APPENDIX 10

Infection prevention and control guidelines

Healthcare-associated infections (HAIs) are infections acquired as a direct or indirect result of healthcare. They are a major concern in Australian healthcare facilities because HAIs are strongly associated with poor outcomes for patients. One of the main strategies for effective prevention of the transmission of HAIs from person to person within the Australian healthcare setting is the development and implementation of best practice infection control guidelines and policies. To establish a nationally accepted approach to infection prevention and control and to assist healthcare organisations with implementing best practice, the Australian Commission on Safety and Quality in Health Care and the National Health and Medical Research Council released the *Australian guidelines for the prevention and control of infection in healthcare* in 2010. The guidelines were updated in May 2019 and are focused on the following core principles:

- an understanding of the modes of transmission of infectious agents and of risk management
- effective work practices that minimise the risk of transmission of infectious agents
- governance structures that support the implementation, monitoring and reporting of infection prevention and control work practices
- compliance with legislation, regulations and standards relevant to infection control.

The guidelines contained in this document are intended as a resource that outlines a two-tiered approach encompassing 'standard precautions' and 'transmission-based precautions' as strategies to integrate a risk management approach into daily work practices that involve infection control.

This approach is intended to provide high-level protection to patients, healthcare professionals and other people in healthcare settings.

- *Standard precautions* are work practices that constitute the first-line approach to infection prevention and control in the healthcare environment. They apply to everyone and are required to achieve a basic level of infection control in healthcare settings; they are recommended for the management and care of all patients. Implementing standard precautions has the potential to reduce the risk of transmission of infectious agents from person to person, even in high-risk situations.

- *Transmission-based precautions* are additional work practices for specific situations where a particular infectious agent and its mode of transmission might not be contained by standard precautions alone.

Standard precautions

Standard precautions minimise the risk of transmission of HAIs; therefore, it is essential that standard precautions are applied at all times. This is because:

- people may be placed at risk of infection from others who carry infectious agents
- people may be infectious before signs or symptoms of disease are recognised or detected, or before laboratory tests are confirmed in time to contribute to care
- people may be at risk from infectious agents present in the surrounding environment, including environmental surfaces or from equipment
- there may be an increased risk of transmission associated with specific procedures and practices.

Standard precautions consist of:

- hand hygiene, as consistent with the 5 moments for hand hygiene (see section below)
- the use of appropriate personal protective equipment (PPE) (see section below)
- the safe use and disposal of sharps
- routine environmental cleaning
- reprocessing of reusable medical equipment and instruments
- respiratory hygiene and cough etiquette
- aseptic technique
- waste management
- appropriate handling of linen.

Standard precautions should be used in the handling of: blood (including dried blood); all other body substances, secretions and excretions (excluding sweat), regardless of whether they contain visible blood; non-intact skin; and mucous membranes.

Transmission-based precautions

Transmission-based precautions are recommended as extra work practices in situations where standard precautions alone may be insufficient to prevent transmission. Transmission-based precautions are also used in the event of an outbreak (e.g. gastroenteritis), to assist in containing the outbreak and preventing further infection. Therefore:

- transmission-based precautions are applied in addition to standard precautions
- the aim of instituting early transmission-based precautions is to reduce further transmission opportunities that may arise due to the specific route of transmission of a particular pathogen
- while it is not possible to prospectively identify all patients needing transmission-based precautions, in certain settings, recognising an increased risk warrants their use while confirmatory tests are pending.

Transmission-based precautions consist of:

- continued implementation of standard precautions
- appropriate use of PPE (see section below)
- patient-dedicated equipment
- allocation of single rooms or cohorting of patients
- appropriate air handling requirements
- enhanced cleaning and disinfecting of the patient environment
- restricted transfer of patients within and between facilities.

Hand hygiene: five moments for hand hygiene

There are many times when hand hygiene is essential in the clinical area as a means of reducing the risk of healthcare-associated infections in the work environment. Hand Hygiene Australia has identified five critical times when hand hygiene should be performed. These are:

1. before touching a patient
2. before a procedure
3. after a procedure or body substance exposure risk
4. after touching a patient
5. after touching a patient's surroundings.

Hand hygiene is also performed before putting on gloves and after the removal of gloves.

Personal protective equipment (PPE)

Personal protective equipment (PPE) refers to a variety of barriers, used alone or in combination, to protect mucous membranes, airways, skin and clothing from contact with infectious agents. Selection of protective equipment must be based on assessment of the risk of transmission of infectious agents to the patient or carer, and the risk of contamination of the clothing or skin of

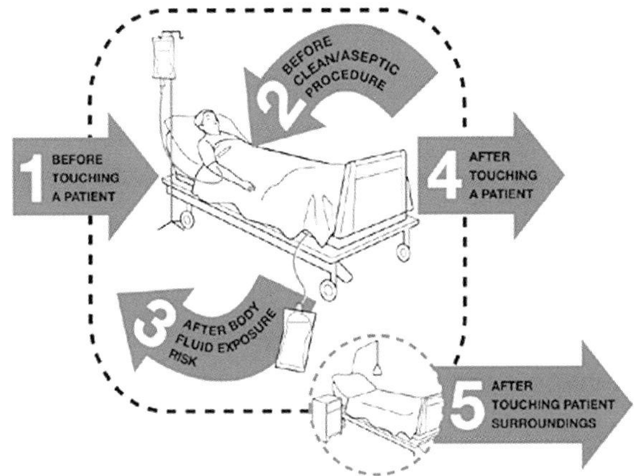

Five moments for hand hygiene

Source: World Health Organization. www.who.int/infection-prevention/campaigns/clean-hands/5moments/en/

For further information on hand hygiene go to: www.who.int/gpsc/5may/background/5moments/en/.

healthcare workers or other staff by patients' blood, body substances, secretions or excretions.

Local policies and current health and safety legislation should also be taken into account.

Factors to be considered are:

- probability of exposure to blood and body substances
- type of body substance involved
- probable type and probable route of transmission of infectious agents.

PPE used as part of standard precautions includes aprons, gowns, gloves, surgical masks, protective eyewear and face shields.

Checklist of standard precautions for procedures

The table on pages 572–573 outlines the use of standard precautions for a range of procedures. It is assumed that there is no known or suspected infection. Decision-making about the level of protection required involves a risk assessment of the procedure to be performed, e.g. usual wound irrigation is unlikely to require surgical mask and eye protection in primary care, but may be required more often in the healthcare setting.

Checklist of standard precautions for procedures

Procedure	Hand hygiene	Gloves	Sterile gloves	Surgical mask	Eye protection	Gown
Activities of daily living (washing, toileting etc.)	✓	—*	—	—	—	—
Routine observations (e.g. blood pressure measurement)	✓	—	—	—	—	—
General medical examination	✓	✓ For contact with broken skin/rash/ mucous membrane	—	✓ If splash risk likely	✓ If splash risk likely	✓ If splash risk likely
Wound examination/ dressing	✓	✓ For contact with body substances	✓ For direct contact with wound	✓ For wound irrigation if splash likely	✓ For wound irrigation if splash likely	✓ For grossly infected wounds
Blood glucose and haemoglobin monitoring	✓	✓	—	—	—	—
Vaginal delivery	✓	—	✓	—	✓	✓
Intravenous cannula insertion	✓	✓	—	—	✓ If splash risk likely	—
Intravascular access device insertion	✓	—	✓	✓	✓	✓ (Where max. barrier precautions are used)
Intravascular access device care	✓	—	✓	—	—	—

Continued

Checklist of standard precautions for procedures—cont'd

Procedure	Hand hygiene	Gloves	Sterile gloves	Surgical mask	Eye protection	Gown
Surgical aseptic technique procedure (e.g. lumbar puncture)	✓	—	✓	✓	✓	✓
Insertion of urinary catheter	✓	—	✓	✓ If exposure risk likely	✓ If exposure risk likely	✓ If exposure risk likely
Urinary catheter care	✓	✓	—	—	✓ When emptying drainage bag	✓ If exposure risk likely
Suctioning: endotracheal tube, tracheostomy	✓	—	✓ Dominant hand (open suction system)	✓	✓	✓ If exposure risk likely
Major dental procedures**	✓		✓	✓	✓	✓
Routine intra-oral dental procedures	✓	✓	—	✓	✓	✓ If exposure risk likely

*In general, most activities of daily living (ADLs) will not require gloves; however, ADL is an extremely broad term and some activities will require gloves, therefore a risk assessment must be undertaken for each person requiring assistance. Examples where gloves should be worn are when skin is not intact, rashes are evident, performing oral hygiene or washing the genital area. Another example would be when toileting a person.

**Including most dental implants, surgical removal or exposure of completely impacted teeth or tooth fragments, vital endodontics, surgical periodontics, maxillo-facial surgery.

Source: National Health and Medical Research Council. Australian Guidelines for the Prevention and Control of Infection in Healthcare. Australian Government. Online. Available: www.nhmrc.gov.au/about-us/publications/australian-guidelines-prevention-and-control-infection-healthcare-2019; 2019. For all enquires regarding the guidelines, contact: nhmrc.publications@nhmrc.gov.au

APPENDIX 11

National Safety and Quality Health Service (NSQHS) Standards

Background

The Australian Commission on Safety and Quality in Health Care

As part of the Australian Government's endeavour to improve the quality and safety of Australia's healthcare, the Australian Commission on Safety and Quality in Health Care (the Commission) was established in January 2006 as a government-funded organisation to lead and coordinate national improvements in safety and quality within healthcare across Australia.

The Commission released the first edition of the NSQHS Standards in 2011 with implementation commencing in 2013. Using the NSQHS Standards, health service organisations have put in place safety and quality systems that have improved patient safety. For example, the rates of healthcare-associated infections have decreased, in-hospital cardiac arrests have decreased, adverse drug reactions and medication histories are better documented and fewer antibiotics are prescribed due to improvements in antibiotic stewardship.

Under the auspices of the Commission, and in collaboration with the Australian Government, states and territories, the private sector, clinical experts, patients and carers the second edition of the NSQHS Standards was released in 2017, with health service organisations being assessed against these standards from January 2019.

National Safety and Quality Health Service (NSQHS) Standards

The second edition of the NSQHS Standards addresses gaps identified in the first edition, including mental health, cognitive impairment, health literacy, end-of-life care and Aboriginal and Torres Strait Islander health. It also updates the evidence for actions, consolidates and streamlines standards and actions to make them clearer and easier to implement and reduces duplication.

The primary aims of the NSQHS Standards are to:

- protect the public from harm, and
- improve the quality of health care provision.

The second edition of the NSQHS Standards comprises eight standards and provides a nationally consistent statement about the standard of care consumers can expect from their health service organisations. They also describe the level of care that should be provided by health service organisations and the systems that are needed to deliver such care. The eight NSQHS Standards are:

1. **Clinical Governance**, which aims to ensure that there are systems in place within health service organisations to maintain and improve the reliability, safety and quality of health care.

2. **Partnering with Consumers**, which aims to ensure that consumers are partners in the design, delivery and evaluation of healthcare systems and services and that patients are given the opportunity to be partners in their own care.
3. **Preventing and Controlling Healthcare-Associated Infection**, which aims to reduce the risk of patients getting preventable healthcare-associated infections, manage infections effectively if they occur and limit the development of antimicrobial resistance through the appropriate prescribing and use of antimicrobials.
4. **Medication Safety**, which aims to ensure that clinicians safely prescribe, dispense and administer appropriate medicines and monitor medicine use. It also aims to ensure that consumers are informed about medicines and understand their own medicine needs and risks.
5. **Comprehensive Care**, which aims to ensure that patients receive comprehensive health care that meets their individual needs, and that considers the impact of their health issues on their life and wellbeing. It also aims to ensure that risks to patients during health care are prevented and managed through targeted strategies.
6. **Communicating for Safety**, which aims to ensure that there is effective communication between patients, carers and families, multidisciplinary teams and clinicians and across the health service organisation, to support continuous, coordinated and safe care for patients.
7. **Blood Management**, which aims to ensure that patients' own blood is safely and appropriately managed, and that any blood and blood products that patients receive are safe and appropriate.
8. **Recognising and Responding to Acute Deterioration**, which aims to ensure that acute deterioration in a patient's physical, mental or cognitive condition is recognised promptly and appropriate action is taken.

Each standard contains:

- a description of the standard
- a statement of intent
- a list of criteria that describe the key areas covered by the standard
- explanatory notes on the content of the standard
- item headings for groups of actions in each criterion
- actions that describe what is required to meet the standard.

Implementing the NSQHS Standards

A range of supporting resources to assist health service organisations to implement the NSQHS Standards are available on the Commission's website. The Advice Centre provides support for health service organisations, surveyors and accrediting agencies on NSQHS Standards implementation.

Contact details

Email: accreditation@ safetyandquality.gov.au
Phone: 1800 304 056

Further information

A full explanation of the NSQHS Standards (second edition) is available on the Commission's website at www.safetyandquality.gov.au.

Source

Copied with permission from the Australian Commission on Safety and Quality in Health Care. National Safety and Quality Health Service Standards. 2nd edn. Sydney: ACSQHC, 2017.

APPENDIX 12

Useful addresses

Australian Nursing and Midwifery Accreditation Council
Level 1, 15 Lancaster Place
Majura Park
Canberra Airport ACT 2609
Postal address:
PO Box 400
Canberra City ACT 2601
Ph: (02) 6257 7960
Email: anmac@anmac.org.au
Web: www.anmac.org.au

Australian Nursing and Midwifery Federation
Head office
Unit 3, 28 Eyre Street
Kingston ACT 2604
Ph: (02) 6232 6533
Fax, (02) 6232 6610
Email: anmfcanberra@anmf.org.au
Web: www.anmf.org.au

Branches

Australian Capital Territory
2/53 Dundas Court,
Phillip ACT 2606
Postal address:
PO Box 4
Woden ACT 2606
Ph: (02) 6282 9455
Fax: (02) 6282 8447
Email: anmfact@anmfact.org.au
Web: www.actanf.org.au

New South Wales
Sydney—NSW Nurses and Midwives' Association
50 O'Dea Avenue
Waterloo NSW 2017
Ph: (02) 8595 1234 (metro)
Regional: 1300 367 962
Fax: (02) 9662 1414
Email: gensec@nswnma.asn.au
Web: www.nswnma.asn.au

Northern Territory
16 Caryota Court
Coconut Grove NT 0810
Postal address:
PO Box 42533
Casuarina NT 0811
Ph: (08) 8920 0700
Fax: (08) 8985 5930
Email: info@anmfnt.org.au
Website: www.anmfnt.org.au

Queensland
Queensland Nurses & Midwives Union
Main Office
106 Victoria St
West End, QLD 4101
Postal address:
GPO Box 1289
Brisbane QLD 4001
Ph: (07) 3840 1444
Toll free: 1800 177 273
Fax: (07) 3844 9387
Email: qnmu@qnmu.org.au
Web: www.qnmu.org.au

South Australia
191 Torrens Rd
Ridleyton, SA 5008
Postal address:
Reply Paid 861
PO Box 861
Regency Park BC SA 5942
Ph: (08) 8334 1900
Toll free: 1800 809 642
Fax: (08) 8334 1901
Email: enquiry@anmfsa.org.au
Web: www.anmfsa.org.au

Tasmania
Hobart office:
182 Macquarie Street
Hobart TAS 7000
Ph: (03) 6223 6777
Toll free: 1800 001 241
Fax: (03) 6224 0229
Launceston office:
Fax: (03) 6334 3928
Email: enquiries@anmftas.org.au
Web: www.anmftas.org

Victoria
Head office:
535 Elizabeth Street
Melbourne VIC 3000
Postal address:
PO Box 12600
A'Beckett Street
Melbourne VIC 3000
Ph: (03) 9275 9333
Toll free: 1800 133 353
Fax: (03) 9275 9344
Email: records@anmfvic.asn.au
Web: www.anmfvic.asn.au

Western Australia
260 Pier Street
Perth WA 6000
Postal address:
PO Box 8240
Perth Business Centre WA 6849
Ph: (08) 6218 9444
Fax: (08) 9218 9455
Toll free: 1800 199 145
Email: anf@anfwa.asn.au
Web: www.anfiuwp.org.au

International Council of Nurses

3, Place Jean Marteau
1201—Geneva
Switzerland
Ph: +41 22 908 0100
Fax: +41 22 908 0101
Email: icn@icn.ch
Web: www.icn.ch

Australian Nursing and Midwifery Registering Authority

Nursing and Midwifery Board of Australia
GPO Box 9958
Melbourne VIC 3001
Web: www.nursingmidwiferyboard.gov.au

Australian Health Practitioner Regulation Agency (AHPRA)
Ph: (03) 9275 9009 (Metro)
Regional: 1300 419 495
Web: www.ahpra.gov.au

Australian Capital Territory
RSM Bird Cameron Building
Ground Floor
50 Blackall Street
Barton
ACT 2600
Postal address:
GPO Box 9958
Canberra ACT 2601

New South Wales
Level 51, 680 George Street
Sydney NSW 2000
Postal address:
GPO Box 9958
Sydney NSW 2001

Northern Territory
Level 5, 22 Harry Chan Ave
Darwin NT 0800
Postal address:
GPO Box 9958
Darwin NT 0801

Queensland
Level 4, 192 Ann Street
Brisbane QLD 4000
Postal address:
GPO Box 9958
Brisbane QLD 4001

South Australia
Level 11, 80 Grenfell Street
Adelaide SA 5000
Postal address:
GPO Box 9958
Adelaide SA 5001

Tasmania
Level 5, 99 Bathurst Street
Hobart TAS 7000
Postal address:
GPO Box 9958
Hobart TAS 7001

Victoria
Level 8, 111 Bourke Street
Melbourne VIC 3000
Postal address:
GPO Box 9958
Melbourne VIC 3001

Western Australia
Level 1, 541 Hay Street
Subiaco WA 6008
Postal address:
GPO Box 9958
Perth WA 6001

New Zealand Nursing Registering Authority

Nursing Council of New Zealand
Postal address:
PO Box 9644
Wellington 6141
New Zealand
Ph: +64 4 385 9589
Fax: +64 4 801 8502
Email: reception@nursingcouncil.org.nz
Web: www.nursingcouncil.org.nz

Coalition of National Nursing Organisations (CoNNO)

The CoNNO is an alliance of various organisations that represent the nursing profession. The website contains a directory and links to members of the CoNNO.
Web: www.conno.org.au

Australian College of Nursing

Sydney office
Level 6
9 Wentworth Street
Parramatta NSW 2150
Postal address:
PO Box 650
Parramatta NSW 2124
Ph: (02) 9745 7500
Toll free: 1800 265 534
Web: www.acn.edu.au

Canberra office
1 Napier Close
Deakin West ACT 2600
PO Box 219
Deakin West ACT 2600
Ph: (02) 6283 3400
Toll free: 1800 061 660
Fax: (02) 6282 3565
Email: acn@acn.edu.au

New Zealand Nurses Organisation

National Office
Level 3, Willbank Court
57 Willis Street
Wellington
Postal address:
PO Box 2128
Wellington 6140
New Zealand
Ph: +64 4 499 9533
Toll free: +64 800 28 38 48
Fax: +64 4 382 9993
Email: nurses@nzno.org.nz
Web: www.nzno.org.nz

Congress of Aboriginal and Torres Strait Islander Nurses and Midwives (CATSINaM)

Level 1, 15 Lancaster Place
Majura Park ACT 2609
Ph: (02) 6262 5761
Web: www.catsinam.org.au

Physiotherapy

Australian Physiotherapy Association
National
Level 1, 1175 Toorak Road
Camberwell VIC 3124
Ph: (03) 9092 0888
Fax: (03) 9092 0899
Email: info@australian.physio
Web: www.physiotherapy.asn.au

Chiropractic

Australian Chiropractors Association
National
Level 1 / 75 George Street
Parramatta, NSW 2150
Postal address:
PO Box 255, Parramatta NSW 2124
Toll Free 1800 075 003
Ph: (02) 8844 0400
Fax (02) 8844 0499
Web: www.chiropractors.asn.au

Pharmacy

Society of Hospital Pharmacists of Australia
National
Suite 3, 65 Oxford Street
Collingwood VIC 3066
PO Box 1774
Collingwood VIC 3066
Ph: (03) 9486 0177
Fax: (03) 9486 0311
Email: shpa@shpa.org.au
Web: www.shpa.org.au

Occupational therapy

Occupational Therapy Australia
National
OT Australia National Office
6/340 Gore St
Fitzroy VIC 3065
Toll free: 1300 682 878
Email: info@otaus.com.au
Web: www.otaus.com.au

Speech pathology

Speech Pathology Australia
National
Level 1 / 114 William Street
Melbourne VIC 3000
Ph: (03) 9642 4899
Fax: (03) 9642 4922
Web: www.speechpathologyaustralia.org.au

Departments of Health

Australian government
Department of Health
Central Office postal address:
GPO Box 9848
Canberra ACT 2601
Australia
Ph: (02) 6289 1555
Toll free: 1800 020 103
Email: enquiries@health.gov.au
Web: www.health.gov.au

State/territory governments

ACT
ACT Health
GPO Box 825
Canberra City,
ACT 2601
Ph: 13 2281
Email: HealthACT@act.gov.au
Web: www.health.act.gov.au

New South Wales
NSW Ministry of Health
Locked Mail Bag 961
North Sydney NSW 2059
Ph: (02) 9391 9000
Fax: (02) 9391 9101
Web: www.health.nsw.gov.au

Northern Territory
Department of Health
PO Box 40596
Casuarina NT 0811
Ph: (08) 8999 2400
Fax: (08) 8999 2700
Web: www.health.nt.gov.au

Queensland
Queensland Health
GPO Box 48
Brisbane QLD 4001
Ph: (07) 3022 0001
Web: www.health.qld.gov.au

South Australia
SA Health
PO Box 287
Rundle Mall
Adelaide SA 5000
Ph: (08) 8226 6000
Fax: (08) 8226 6899
Email: communications@health.sa.gov.au
Web: www.sahealth.sa.gov.au

Tasmania
Department of Health and Human Services
GPO Box 125
Hobart TAS 7001
Ph: (03) 6233 3185 (Metro)
Regional: 1300 135 513
Web: www.dhhs.tas.gov.au

Victoria
Department of Health & Human Services
50 Lonsdale Street
Melbourne VIC 3000
Ph: 1300 650 172
Web: www.health.vic.gov.au

Western Australia
Department of Health
PO Box 8172
Perth Business Centre
Perth WA 6849
Ph: (08) 9222 4222
Fax: (08) 9222 4046
Web: www.health.wa.gov.au

CREDITS

Body Atlas 1 and 2: Harris P, Nagy S, Vardaxis N. Mosby's dictionary of medicine, nursing and health professions. 3rd Australian and New Zealand ed. Sydney: Elsevier; 2014, p. A-2. Body Atlas 3: Harris P, Nagy S, Vardaxis N. Mosby's dictionary of medicine, nursing and health professions. 3rd Australian and New Zealand ed. Sydney: Elsevier; 2014, pp. 234, A-7. Body Atlas 4 and 5: Harris P, Nagy S, Vardaxis N. Mosby's dictionary of medicine, nursing and health professions. 3rd Australian and New Zealand ed. Sydney: Elsevier; 2014, pp. A-8 and A-9. Body Atlas 7: Dorland WAN. Dorland's illustrated medical dictionary. 32nd ed. Philadelphia: Elsevier Saunders; 2012, Plate 32. Body Atlas 8 and 9: Harris P, Nagy S, Vardaxis N. Mosby's dictionary of medicine, nursing and health professions. 3rd Australian and New Zealand ed. Sydney: Elsevier; 2014, pp. A-12, A-13. Body Atlas 11: Harris P, Nagy S, Vardaxis N. Mosby's dictionary of medicine, nursing and health professions. 3rd Australian and New Zealand ed. Sydney: Elsevier; 2014, p. A-16. Body Atlas 10 (top): Dorland WAN. Dorland's illustrated medical dictionary. 32nd ed. Philadelphia: Elsevier Saunders; 2012, p. 826. Body Atlas 10 (bottom): Harris P, Nagy S, Vardaxis N. Mosby's dictionary of medicine, nursing and health professions. 3rd Australian and New Zealand ed. Sydney: Elsevier; 2014, p. 415. Body Atlas 12: Harris P, Nagy S, Vardaxis N. Mosby's dictionary of medicine, nursing and health professions. 3rd Australian and New Zealand ed. Sydney: Elsevier; 2014, p. A-19. Body Atlas 13: Harris P, Nagy S, Vardaxis N. Mosby's dictionary of medicine, nursing and health professions. 3rd Australian and New Zealand ed. Sydney: Elsevier; 2014, p. A-21. Body Atlas 14 and 15: Harris P, Nagy S, Vardaxis N. Mosby's dictionary of medicine, nursing and health professions. 3rd Australian and New Zealand ed. Sydney: Elsevier; 2014, pp. A-24, A-25, A-26. Body Atlas 14: Harris P, Nagy S, Vardaxis N. Mosby's dictionary of medicine, nursing and health professions. 3rd Australian and New Zealand ed. Sydney: Elsevier; 2014, p. A-27 (top picture only). Body Atlas 18 and 19: Harris P, Nagy S, Vardaxis N. Mosby's dictionary of medicine, nursing and health professions. 3rd Australian and New Zealand ed. Sydney: Elsevier; 2014, pp. A-28, A-29. Body Atlas 20 and 21: Harris P, Nagy S, Vardaxis N. Mosby's dictionary of medicine, nursing and health professions. 3rd Australian and New Zealand ed. Sydney: Elsevier; 2014, p. A-31. Body Atlas 22 (top): Harris P, Nagy S, Vardaxis N. Mosby's dictionary of medicine, nursing and health professions. 3rd Australian and New Zealand ed. Sydney: Elsevier; 2014, p. A-33 (top 2 figures only). Body Atlas 22: Harris P, Nagy S, Vardaxis N. Mosby's dictionary of medicine, nursing and health professions. 3rd Australian and New Zealand ed. Sydney: Elsevier; 2014, pp. A-34 to A-42.

p. 1: Waugh A, Grant A. Ross and Wilson: Anatomy and physiology in health and illness. 9th ed. London: Churchill Livingstone; 2001, Figure 3.37. p. 6: Weller B. Baillière's nurses' dictionary. 26th ed. Edinburgh: Baillière Tindall Elsevier; 2014, p. 5. p. 18: Weller B. Baillière's nurses' dictionary. 26th ed. Edinburgh: Baillière Tindall Elsevier; 2014, p. 15. p. 23: Weller B. Baillière's nurses' dictionary. 26th ed. Edinburgh: Baillière Tindall Elsevier; 2014, p. 20. p. 24: Symonds EM, Symonds IM. Essential obstetrics and gynaecology. 3rd ed. Edinburgh: Churchill Livingstone; 1997, Figure 6.15. p. 28: Weller B. Baillière's nurses' dictionary. 26th ed. Edinburgh: Baillière Tindall Elsevier; 2014, p. 24. p. 35: Winson NV, McDonald S. Illustrated dictionary of midwifery. Edinburgh: Elsevier Butterworth–Heinemann; 2005, p. 28. p. 50: Wilson J. Infection control in clinical practice. 2nd ed. Edinburgh: Baillière Tindall; 2001, Figure 1.2. p. 57: Weller B. Baillière's nurses' dictionary. 26th ed. Edinburgh: Baillière Tindall Elsevier; 2014, p. 48. p. 65: Weller B. Baillière's nurses' dictionary. 26th ed. Edinburgh: Baillière Tindall Elsevier; 2014, p. 55. p. 68: Waugh A, Grant A. Ross and Wilson: Anatomy and physiology in health and illness. 9th ed. London: Churchill Livingstone; 2001, Figure 16.3. p. 71: Weller B. Baillière's nurses' dictionary. 26th ed. Edinburgh: Baillière Tindall Elsevier; 2014, p. 60. p. 72: Source: UNICEF Australia, Baby Friendly Health Initiative. http://www.unicef.org.au/Discover/Australia-s-children/Baby-Friendly-Hospital-Initiative.aspx. p. 88: Waugh A, Grant A. Ross and Wilson: Anatomy and physiology in health and illness. 9th ed. London: Churchill Livingstone; 2001, Figure 3.1. p. 90: Waugh A, Grant A. Ross and Wilson: Anatomy and physiology in health and illness. 9th ed. London: Churchill Livingstone; 2001, Figure 7.16. p. 98: Jennett S. Dictionary of sport and exercise science and medicine. Edinburgh: Churchill Livingstone; 2008, pp. 95, 316. p. 99: Porter S. Dictionary of physiotherapy. Elsevier Butterworth–Heinemann; 2005, pp. 67, 166. p. 132: Weller B. Baillière's nurses' dictionary. 26th ed. Edinburgh: Baillière Tindall Elsevier; 2014, p. 117. p. 155: King J, Hawley R. Australian nurses' dictionary. 5th ed. Baillière Tindall; 2012, p. 152. p. 160: Waugh A, Grant A. Ross and Wilson: Anatomy and physiology in health and illness. 9th ed. London: Churchill Livingstone; 2001, Figure 19.10. p. 167: Weller B. Baillière's nurses' dictionary. 26th ed. Edinburgh: Baillière Tindall Elsevier; 2014, p. 145. p. 185: Waugh A, Grant A. Ross and Wilson: Anatomy and physiology in health and illness. 9th ed. London: Churchill Livingstone; 2001, Figure 16.15. p. 188: Weller B. Baillière's nurses' dictionary. 26th ed. Edinburgh: Baillière Tindall Elsevier; 2014, p. 164. p. 200: Weller B. Baillière's nurses' dictionary. 26th ed. Edinburgh: Baillière Tindall Elsevier; 2014, p. 174. p. 212: Nicol M, Bavin C, Cronin P, et al. Essential nursing skills. 4th ed. Edinburgh: Mosby; 2012. Adapted from National Patient Safety Agency Clean Your Hands Campaign © 2011 NHS England. Adapted from WHO http://whqlibdoc.who.int/publications/2009/9789241597906_eng.pdf. p. 214: World Health Organization (WHO). p. 218: Weller B. Baillière's nurses' dictionary. 26th ed. Edinburgh: Baillière Tindall Elsevier; 2014, p. 191. p. 220: Weller B. Baillière's nurses' dictionary. 26th ed. Edinburgh: Baillière Tindall Elsevier; 2014, p. 193. p. 245: King J, Hawley R. Australian nurses' dictionary. 5th ed. Baillière Tindall; 2012, p. 251. p. 248: Weller B. Baillière's nurses' dictionary. 26th ed. Edinburgh: Baillière Tindall Elsevier; 2014, p. 218. p. 270: Weller B. Baillière's nurses' dictionary. 26th ed. Edinburgh: Baillière Tindall Elsevier; 2014, p. 236. p. 277: Weller B. Baillière's nurses' dictionary. 26th ed. Edinburgh: Baillière Tindall Elsevier; 2014, p. 242. p. 278: Waugh A, Grant A. Ross and Wilson: Anatomy and physiology in health and illness. 9th ed. London:

Churchill Livingstone; 2001, Figures 4.6 and 4.9. p. 286: Adapted from Waugh A, Grant A. Ross and Wilson: Anatomy and physiology in health and illness. 11th ed. Edinburgh: Elsevier; 2010. p. 287: Adapted from Wong DL, Hockenberry MJ, Wilson D, et al. Wong's nursing care of infants and children. 7th ed. St Louis: Mosby; 2003. p. 295: Weller B. Baillière's nurses' dictionary. 26th ed. Edinburgh: Baillière Tindall Elsevier; 2014, p. 256. p. 297: Monahan FD, Sands JK, Neighbors M, et al. Phipps' medical-surgical nursing. 8th ed. St Louis: Mosby; 2007, Figure 2.15A and B. p. 344: Waugh A, Grant A. Ross and Wilson: Anatomy and physiology in health and illness. 9th ed. London: Churchill Livingstone; 2001, Figure 8.13. p. 351: Beare PG, Myers JL. Adult health nursing. 3rd ed. St Louis: Mosby; 1998. p. 353: Nicol M, Bavin C, Cronin P, et al. Essential nursing skills. 4th ed. Edinburgh: Mosby; 2012, Figure 2.15A and B. p. 355: Waugh A, Grant A. Ross and Wilson: Anatomy and physiology in health and illness. 9th ed. London: Churchill Livingstone; 2001, Figure 12.36. p. 374: Jennett S. Dictionary of sport and exercise science and medicine. Edinburgh: Churchill Livingstone; 2008, pp. 95, 316. p. 385: Weller B. Baillière's nurses' dictionary. 26th ed. Edinburgh: Baillière Tindall Elsevier; 2014, p. 332. p. 387: Weller B. Baillière's nurses' dictionary. 26th ed. Edinburgh: Baillière Tindall Elsevier; 2014, p. 333. p. 399: Weller B. Baillière's nurses' dictionary. 26th ed. Edinburgh: Baillière Tindall Elsevier; 2014, p. 345. p. 409: Waugh A, Grant A. Ross and Wilson: Anatomy and physiology in health and illness. 9th ed. London: Churchill Livingstone; 2001, Figure 7.27. p. 427: Weller B. Baillière's nurses' dictionary. 26th ed. Edinburgh: Baillière Tindall Elsevier; 2014, p. 369. p. 439: Lewis SM, Heitkemper MM, Dirksen SR. Medical-surgical nursing: assessment and management of clinical problems. 8th ed. St Louis: Mosby, 2011. p. 455: Weller B. Baillière's nurses' dictionary. 26th ed. Edinburgh: Baillière Tindall Elsevier; 2014, p. 392. p. 460: Weller B. Baillière's nurses' dictionary. 26th ed. Edinburgh: Baillière Tindall Elsevier; 2014, p. 397. p. 491: Bale S, Jones V. Wound care nursing: a patient-centred approach. London: Baillière Tindall; 1997. p. 508: Weller B. Baillière's nurses' dictionary. 26th ed. Edinburgh: Baillière Tindall Elsevier; 2014, p. 437. p. 509: Weller B. Baillière's nurses' dictionary. 26th ed. Edinburgh: Baillière Tindall Elsevier; 2014, p. 438.